Handbuch der experimentellen Pharmakologie

Handbook of Experimental Pharmacology

Heffter-Heubner New Series

Herausgegeben von/Edited by

O. Eichler
Heidelberg

A. Farah
Rensselaer, N Y

H. Herken
Berlin

A. D. Welch
New Brunswick, N J

Vol. XVI/2

Springer-Verlag Berlin · Heidelberg · New York 1969

Erzeugung von Krankheitszuständen durch das Experiment

Teil 2

Atemwege

Bearbeitet von

J. E. Alberty · O. Eichler · H. Friebel · K. Karzel

J. Lulling · J. Prignot

Herausgeber

Oskar Eichler

Mit 59 Abbildungen

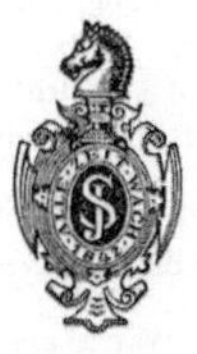

Springer-Verlag Berlin · Heidelberg · New York 1969

ISBN-13: 978-3-642-48083-6 e-ISBN-13: 978-3-642-48082-9
DOI: 10.1007/978-3-642-48082-9

Titel-Nr. 5711

Inhalt

Mitarbeiterverzeichnis

Professor Dr. J. E. Alberty, Kajavatie 1, Helsinki 20, Finnland

Professor Dr. O. Eichler, Pharmakologisches Institut der Universität, 6900 Heidelberg, Hauptstr. 47—51

Professor Dr. med. H. Friebel, World Heath Organisation. CH-1211 Genf, Avenue Appia

Dozent Dr. K. Karzel, Pharmakologisches Institut der Universität, 5300 Bonn, Reuterstr. 2b

Dr. J. Lulling, Pharmacological Department of the Research and Development Direction, UCB-DIPHA, Brüssel, Belgien

Professor Dr. J. Prignot, Clinique pneumologique de l'Université de Louvain, Mont, Godinne, Belgien

Experimental Chronic Aspecific Respiratory Affections

J. Prignot and J. Lulling

With 4 Figures

A. Introduction

From the close relationship between chronic bronchitis and emphysema on both pathological and clinical fields results the necessity of a combined study of the experimental methods which have been used until now for their production and investigation in animals.

These numerous techniques have been inspired, specially, by the diverse conceptions concerning the aetiopathogeny of bronchitis and emphysema.

Those who consider them to be the result of *bronchiolar obstruction* have used methods aimed at reproducing this mechanism, by acting on the animal through the *airways*.

Thus, in many publications, attempts have been made to induce inflammation in the lower respiratory tract by introducing — by instillation, aerolisation or simple inhalation —, toxic gases, dusts, cigarette smoke, car exhaust fumes, enzymes, bacteria or mycoplasma, in other words, a number of irritants, either simultaneously or successively.

Several authors used mechanical means to provoke broncho-pulmonary hyperdistension and inflammation. They have also studied the combined effects of both hyperdistension and inflammation.

Exposure of the animal to hypoxia and hypercapnia, results in hyperventilation which can also produce the same type of morphological changes.

A few tentative experiments were stimulated by the *thoracogenic concept* of emphysema, regarding the distension of the thoracic cage as the causal factor of the disease.

Those who attribute a primary rôle to *vascular factors* in the pathogenesis of emphysema have tried to produce obstruction of the pulmonary arteries by means of dyes, or of the bronchial arteries by highly irritant substances like chlorpromazine, in the hope of thus obtaining atrophy of the alveolar walls and the development of the histopathological picture of emphysema.

It is probably by the same mechanism that some have obtained lesions resembling those of bronchial emphysema after external irradiation of the lung (Devilliers, 1964).

More recently, certain authors consider that bronchial emphysema could be attributed to *auto-immune phenomena*. Various experiments based on the subcutaneous injection of homologous pulmonary tissue have tried to confirm this hypothesis.

Finally, the pathological interpretation of the phenomena observed in the living animal can be facilitated by certain studies carried out mainly *in vitro*.

We shall mention those which deal with ciliary activity, with the study of the surface properties of the lung, and with the effect of toxic substances on the activity of pulmonary cells in tissue cultures.

B. Experimental Methods Acting Via the Respiratory Tract

I. Methods Aiming to Produce Broncho-Pulmonary Inflammation

1. Use of Toxic Gases

These consist mainly of SO_2, NO_2, $COCl_2$ (phosgene), and O_3 (ozone). They have long been used in animal experiments. However the motivation of the authors has undergone a considerable evolution over the course of the years. At first, it consisted of the pathological study of the changes resulting from the sudden and brief inhalation of a large quantity of toxic substances, such as in industrial accidents or, after the use of war gases in 1914—18 (Coman *et al.*, 1947).

While some authors attribute a rôle in the genesis of bronchial emphysema to these single, accidental inhalations, it is obvious that work employing repeated exposures to relatively small doses of the toxic agent are more likely to furnish useful information for our purpose.

Many authors have devoted themselves to this, either in the study of the consequences (pulmonary and general) of atmospheric pollution or by interesting themselves in the threshold levels of various toxic agents in work places (Wagner *et al.*, 1965; Freeman *et al.*, 1966; Steadman *et al.*, 1966).

But the most interesting research aimed at reproducing in animals the usual stigmata of bronchial emphysema in man.

In 1957, Stokinger *et al.* observed a thickening of the bronchiolar walls in animals which had been chronically exposed to low concentrations of *ozone*.

In 1960, Ball *et al.* studied the survival of rats which had been chronically exposed to *sulfur dioxide*.

However, one of the leading investigations in this field remains that of Reid (1963), who exposed young rats to an atmosphere containing about 300 to 400 parts per million (ppm) of SO_2, for 5 hours a day, five days a week during six successive weeks, and then studied mainly the histopathological broncho-pulmonary changes arising in these animals.

These rats, whose tracheo-bronchial tree in its normal state bears numerous secreting cells, developed from the 4rth week of exposure a considerable mucus hypersecretion, with mucus impaction in the bronchioles and the alveoli. The number of goblet cells in the bronchi increased considerably. They were even seen to appear in the peripheral bronchioles, where they are normally absent. The bronchiolar changes were of irregular distribution, some normal bronchioles vicining others rich in goblet cells. Reid's data also suggest that hypersecretion favours infection, a raised percentage of positive cultures having been obtained from animals in which mucus hypersecretion was macroscopically seen. Finally, the same work suggests that after cessation of exposure to toxic agents, the goblet cell increase does not continue or even shows a tendency to reversal. As the period of observation of the rats did not extend beyond three months, no definitive conclusions can be drawn in this respect.

Quevauviller and Huyen (1966), carried out a similar experiment and observed the bronchi and their contents with the binocular magnifying glass. In this manner, they noted that repeated exposures to SO_2 led the hypersecretion which was responsible for obstructive phenomena both in the main and more peripheral bronchi.

Superinfections were frequent. The same method was used by Huyen *et al.* (1966) for studying the effects of a mucolytic, S-carboxymethylcysteine which markedly reduced after oral administration the frequency of mucopurulent intrabronchial obstruction.

The interpretation of the observations in rats must take account of the high frequency of idiopathic bronchopneumopathies, which were already recognized by Cruikshank (1948), and which according to Mosinger and Luccioni (1967) affect 80—83% of rats more than 2 years old. It is necessary therefore to use, as was done by Reid, young rats which are only slightly affected, or to include control groups.

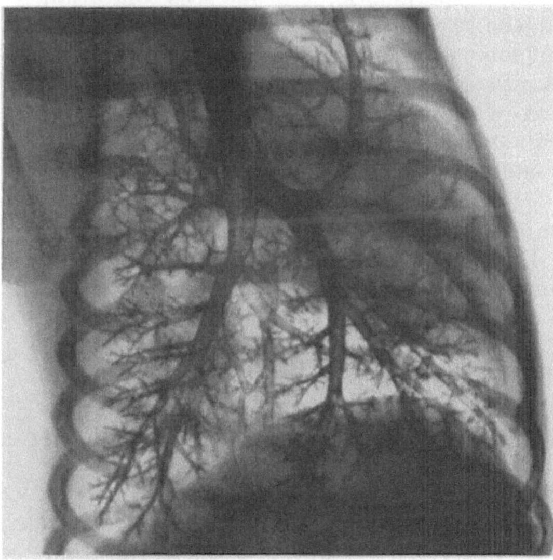

a

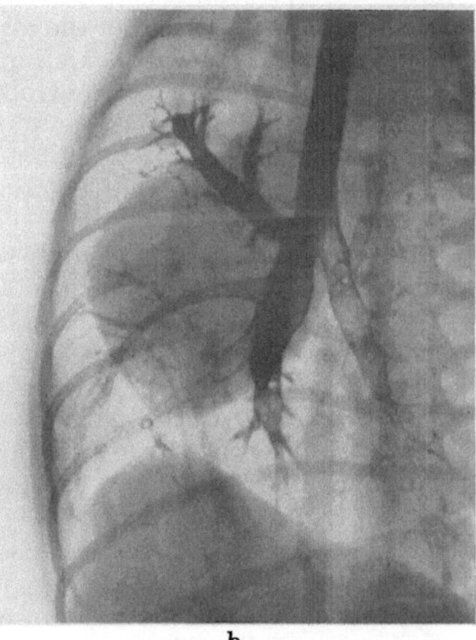

b

Fig. 1. Examples of bronchograms. Left: Normal dog. Position right anterior oblique. Right: Exposed dog (10 hours in 12 months). Position left anterior oblique. Dilatation of the right main bronchi, and irregular bronchiolar-filling

Elmes and Bell (1963) found almost no difference between control rats and those which had been exposed to chlorine gas from the 20th week of life onwards, whilst in the younger exposed animals they noted glandular hyperplasia, centrilobular emphysema and a peripheral pulmonary arteriolitis much more frequently than in the control group.

In a later investigation the same authors (Bell and Elmes, 1965) used specific pathogen free rats whose epithelium is poor in goblet cells and in·lymphoid reactions. These rats can tolerate chlorine gas in much higher doses than the sick rats. Furthermore, the histological lesions produced by the toxic agent were much less severe and much less like those of chronic human bronchitis than in rats "spontaneously" sick and exposed to gas.

It is likely that the "spontaneous" disease is due to a mycoplasma (Klieneberger-Nobel, 1962), which is a saprophyte of the upper respiratory tract of the rat (Ventura and Goucher, 1966).

Nitrogen dioxide was used by Kleinerman and Wright (1962) at different concentrations, intermittently and during periods of up to 21.5 months.

These authors noted in 50% of guinea pigs exposed for 15 to 18 months to 20—25 ppm for 2 hours a day, 4 days a week, a marked dilatation of the proximal respiratory bronchioles, whereas proximal respiratory bronchioles and alveolar canals appeared normal. There was almost no inflammatory reaction.

Whereas these authors did not observe such lesions in the rabbit or in the rat, Freeman and Haydon (1964) and, later Haydon *et al.* (1965) obtained hypertrophy and bronchial glandular hyperplasia as well as emphysema in rats exposed to NO_2. Afterwards, Haydon *et al.* (1967) also used NO_2 in rabbits which they exposed continually to concentrations of 8 to 12 ppm during 3 months. The histopathological changes are of the same order as those obtained in the rat: the bronchiolar epithelium is hypertrophic and hyperplastic, and one sees dilatation of the alveolar canals and of the alveoli. The proliferative bronchiolitis disappears 3 months after cessation of exposure, but some peripheral hyperdistension persists.

Here also, the need for controlled studied arises from the existence of a high frequency of "spontaneous" emphysema in these animals either in a generalized form (present in 50% of old rabbits) or in a form localised to the lobular margins, or even in the shape of vesiculation sometimes associated with a chronic interstitial pneumonia (Strawbridge, 1960a).

The small laboratory animals which are suitable for epidemiological survival studies or for the histopathological investigation of large series exposed to different conditions, pose, on the other hand, complex problems when it comes to the study of the clinical, radiological, and above all the functional symptomatology of the experimental disease.

Following the work of Rossing (1962), who had developed a technique for the study of ventilatory mechanics in the dog, Lulling *et al.* (1968) produced a bronchopneumopathy by exposing adult Colley dogs to an atmosphere containing 500 ppm SO_2 in a gas chamber of 1 m^3 during 1 to 4 hours a day (depending on tolerance) from thrice to once a week, then at progressively longer intervals as the symptoms disappeared. These animals were examined clinically, radiographically, bronchographically and bronchoscopically. The evolution of the respiratory function was followed up regularly by arteriopuncture (with measure of blood gases and of the acid-base balance) and, above all, by the study of the ventilatory mechanics. The latter was carried out in the conscious animal, lying down, by measurements of the oesophageal pressure with the balloon technique and that of volumes, flow and pressures of the respiratory tract, intubated by means of a rigid cannula attached to a pneumotachograph, and to differential manometers. The lungs of a few dead dogs were subjected to a detailed histophatological study after insufflation with an aqueous formol solution.

It was possible to observe the development of a clinical syndrome very close to human bronchitis, including cough, the expectoration of muco-purulent or purulent sputum, often expiratory dyspnoea, with recession and working of the accessory muscles of respiration. Auscultation often revealed rhonchi and sibilants. X-rays were generally normal, but sometimes showed bronchopneumonic foci at the bases, which regressed after antibiotic therapy. Bronchography often showed dilatation of the main bronchi, and irregular bronchiolar filling (Fig. 1). Bronchoscopy revealed a congested, oedematous mucosa, which was fragile and, exceptionally, had a granular or polypoid appearance.

A single exposure to SO_2 lead to a marked rise in the pulmonary resistance (LR) and less marked in the elastance (LE), maximal after 48 hours, and followed by a progressive decrease during several days. Repeated exposures to SO_2 lead to an obstructive syndrome which became more and more marked, and more and more persistent in spite of spacing out the exposures. On average, the pulmonary resistance is 10 times and the pulmonary elastance $1^1/_2$ to $3^1/_2$ times above the normal values. The pressure-volume and the pressure-flow curves take on an abnormal appearance (Fig. 2). In those dogs in which the pulmonary resistance is highest, the respiratory rate is lower than in normal dogs. Furthermore, a lowering of the oxygen saturation and an increase in the Pa CO_2 were observed in the arterial blood compared to the values observed in normal dogs.

Bacteriological examination of the sputum showed that Gram negative organisms dominate the picture. The flora is rich, and similar in all dogs.

Macroscopical examination shows bullows emphysema (Fig. 3). Histopathological examination of two dogs that died respectively after 13 and 9 months of exposure to the toxic agents, showed the following elements: an intense desquamation of the tracheobronchial epithelium appeared in the exposed

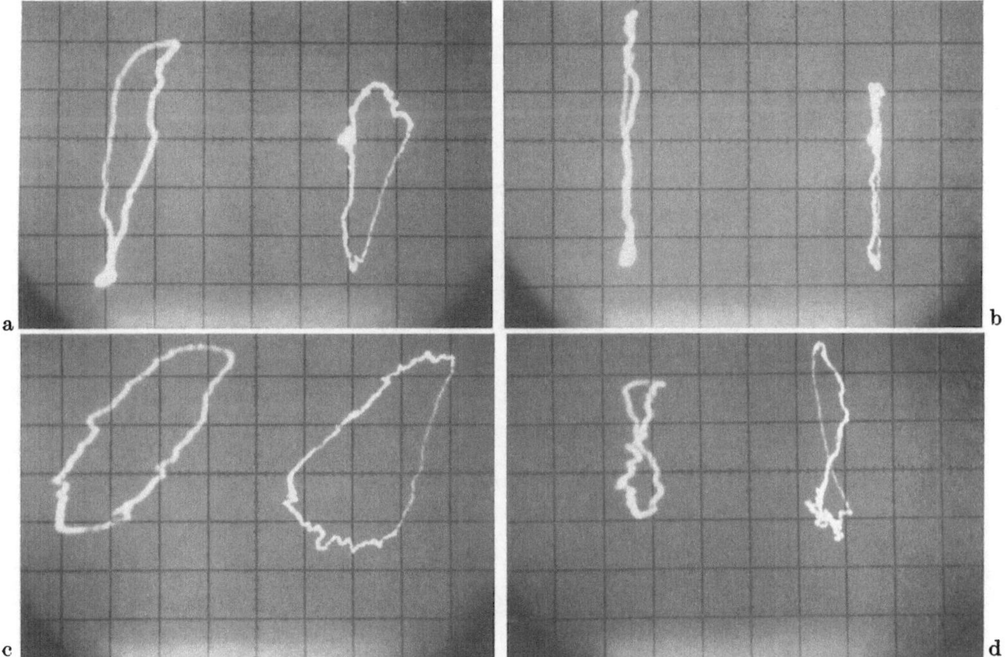

Fig. 2 a—d. Examples of pressure-volume and pressure-flow diagrams. The vector loops: transpulmonary pressure (abscissae) volume (ordinates) on the left of Figs. a, b, c and d and the loops: transpulmonary pressure (abscissae) air flow (ordinates), on the right of Figs. a, b, c and d are represented simultaneously on an oscilloscope Hewlett-Packard, 140 A and photographed with a scope camera Hewlett-Packard 197 A. Figs. a and b concern normal dogs; Figs. c and d bronchitic dogs. Figs. a and c refer to uncorrected loops; Figs. b and d to loops corrected as follows: One subtracts electrically from the transpulmonary pressure signal ($P(t)$) two linear terms $R\dot{v}$ and Kv, where v represents the volume displacement, R the viscous resistance, and K the elastance. The subtraction of $R\dot{v}$ transforms the pressure-volume loop to a sloping straight line, while that of Kv brings that straight line to the vertical (Fig. b, left). On the pressure-flow diagram, the subtraction of Kv, annuling $P(t)$ at the point of zero flow, converts the loop to a sloping straight line, while that of $R\dot{v}$ brings that line back to the vertical (Fig. b, right). The operation achieves the complete annulment of the transpulmonary pressure signal, provided that the linear model $P(t) = R\dot{v} + Kv$ is adequate. For a satisfactory approximation, this is only true in the case of a healthy animal (Fig. b). On the other hand, in an animal suffering from an obstructive syndrome, the initial loops are wider (Fig. c) and the anulmennt of $P(t)$ is only possible at one point in the cycle, as shown by the eight-shaped appearance of the corrected loops in Fig. d. This reflects the intervention of non linear terms linked to resistance changes occuring during one single respiratory cycle animal 5 days before death. In both animals, there was a discrete hypertrophy of the bronchial glands, some inflammatory polyps in the lumen of the large bronchi, a bronchiolitis and a peripheral peribronchiolitis with areas of centrilobular emphysema, sometimes independent of the bronchiolitis (Fig. 4). The pulmonary parenchyma, normal in places, showed atelectasis and extensive areas of broncho pneumonia in the lower lobes. Intrabronchial and intraalveolar fibromata of an unusual appearance were also observed.

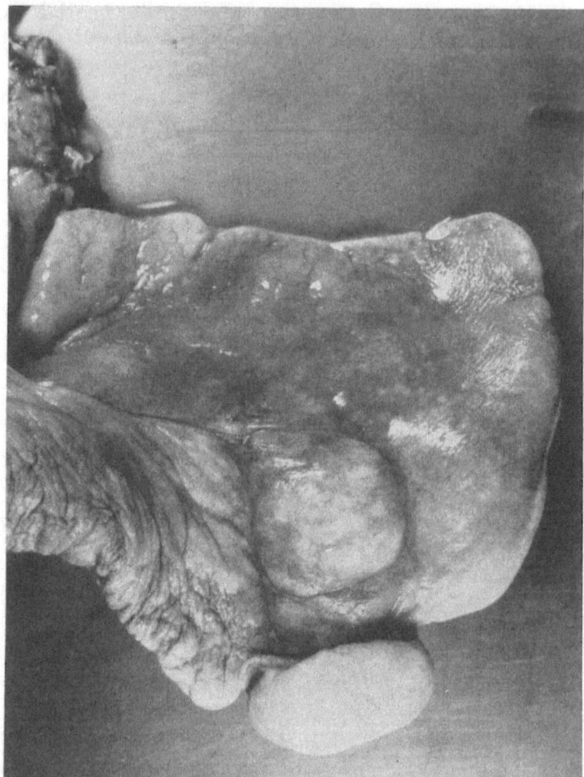

Fig. 3. Macroscopic aspect of the lung of an exposed dog: Bullous emphysema

This experimental model was used for the pharmacological study of various bronchodilators, which brought about a fairly marked regression of the broncho-obstructive phenomena. Similarly, some mucolytics administered as aerosols appreciably altered the ratio of dry weight of the sediment to the dry weight of the supernatant, evidence of an action on the mucopurulent secretions of this experimental bronchitis.

Thus, in adapting the duration of exposure to the individual susceptibility of the animals and of their bronchi, it was possible to reproduce a persistent, experimental bronchopneumopathy, closely resembling that found in man, and involving profound alterations, partially reversible, of the ventilatory mechanics. As the increase in the pulmonary resistance is reversible, it cannot be entirely attributed to irreversible anatomical abnormalities such as obliterative bronchitis. The rise in the pulmonary elastance which, to a great extent, is also corrected by the bronchodilators, can be related to the bronchial obstruction, which results in ventilatory inequalities and asynchronism.

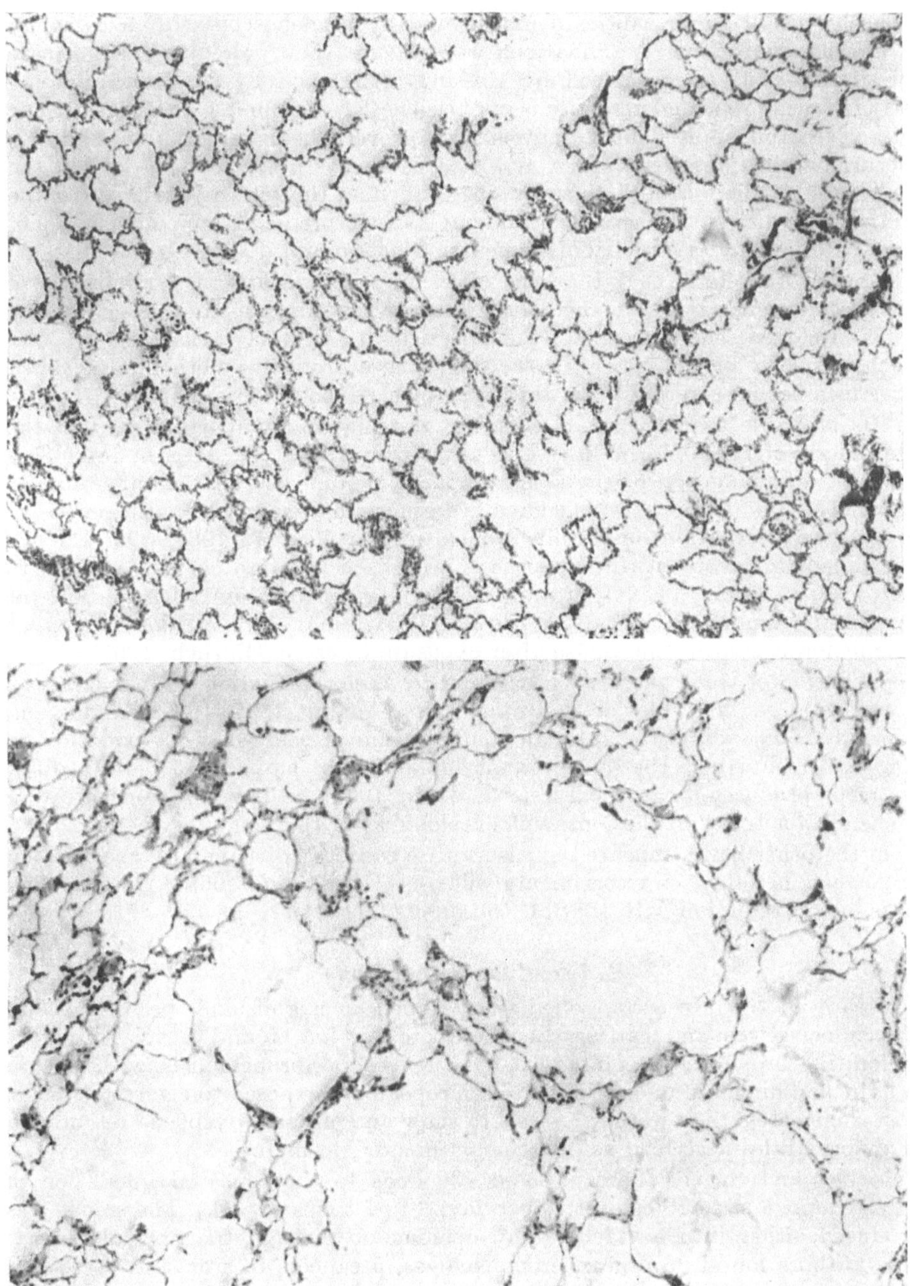

Fig. 4. Microscopic aspect (Stain Hemalun-Eosine-Saffron; magnification 80 ×). Above: Normal dog. Normal calibre of alveolar canals and alveoli. Below: Exposed dog. Advanced centri-acinar emphysema

A syndrome of alveolar hypoventilation was also found in the dog, and was not obtained by Davidson *et al.* (1967) after the continuous exposure of rabbits to 8 to 12 ppm NO_2.

The bronchial abnormalities demonstrated by bronchoscopy, bronchography and morbid anatomical examinations were severe. The pulmonary lesions are very similar to those described by Rossing (1964) and by Clay and Rossing (1964), following repeated inhalations of phosgene (24—40 ppm). One finds a chronic obliterative bronchiolitis and emphysema. However, the hypertrophy of secreting structures, so characteristic of rat and man, is always much less marked in the dog. Therefore, there is nothing surprising in the fact that chemical analysis of the secretions sampled in the bronchitic animal shows a predominance of elements of plasmatic origin and a paucity of elements of local origin.

It seems, therefore, that the type of lesion observed after the inhalation of toxic gases depends more on the constitution of the mucosae concerned than on the gas employed. The mucosae of the rat, rich in secretory structures, respond by a hyperplasia of the latter. In the dog, whose bronchial epithelium is much poorer in mucous-secreting cells, this hyperplasia is much less marked.

It is probable that bronchial infection also plays an important part in the pathogenesis of the abnormalities encountered: perhaps the SO_2, in producing an abrupt desquamation of the respiratory epithelium, acts in a manner similar to that of viral infections, which have been incriminated in the pathogenesis of some acute exacerbations in chronic bronchitics (Carilli *et al.*, 1964). One can see an argument in favour of this hypothesis in the sensitization of mice exposed to small doses (3.5 ppm) of NO_2, towards experimental infection with aerosols of Klebsiella pneumoniae (Purvis and Ehrlich, 1961, 1963; Ehrlich, 1966). A similar phenomenon is seen in the mouse after exposure to ozone (Ehrlich, 1963).

The action of toxic gases is potentiated by their association with inhalations of aerosols of sodium chloride and other salts (Amdur, 1957, 1959; Amdur and Underhill, 1968), doubtless through solubilization of the SO_2 and oxidation to form H_2SO_4. Further, the concomitant inhalation of gas and of certain dusts like carbon produces larger focal lesions (Boren, 1964), probably by concentrating the chemical activity in the most vulnerable areas of the lung.

On the other hand, repeated exposure to NO_2 does not have any accelerating or collagenizing effect on experimental silicosis (Gross *et al.*, 1968). This observation is in contradiction with that of Robson *et al.* (1934).

2. Use of Cigarette Smoke

Already in 1958, in a controlled study aimed at establishing the relationship between cigarettes and cancer, Leuchtenberger *et al.*, found a very frequent proliferative bronchitis accompanied by a severe peribronchiolitis with pus in the bronchial lumen in mice that had been repeatedly exposed to cigarette smoke.

In some cases, they were even able to show an epithelial dysplasia resembling the abnormalities described as "carcinoma in situ" in man.

Rockey and Speer (1966) exposed 130 dogs to the repeated inhalation of cigarette smoke (1 to 10 cigarettes per day, 3 to 7 times a week). The smoke was introduced either into a tracheotomy opening or through the normal airway. These authors found 26 precancerous changes, 5 cancers in situ, and 7 cases of emphysema.

Auerbach *et al.* (1967) obtained fibrosis and emphysema in 5 dogs submitted to repeated inhalation of cigarette smoke through a tracheotomy.

The controlled trials of Hernandez *et al.* (1966) who exposed 15 greyhounds during 2 to 20 months to inhalations of cigarette smoke for 30 to 45 minutes per day, 5 days a week, allow them to demonstrate areas of dilatation and parenchymal destruction which, when examined microscopically, were closely related to an inflammatory component, and closely resembled the lesions of emphysema encountered in man.

According to Guillerm *et al.* (1967) 3 puffs of cigarette smoke applied to guinea pigs with sectioned spinal cords, and artificially ventilated, sufficed to produce a marked elevation of the dynamic expiratory resistance and a much less well marked decrease in the compliance at moments of zero flow. These observations join and complete these of Loomis who, since 1956, has stated that the inhalation of cigarette smoke led to an increase in the global transpulmonary pressure.

3. Use of Car Exhaust Gases

Accroding to Murphy *et al.* (1963), exposure, even of short duration (2 to 6 hours) of rats, mice and guinea pigs to car exhaust gases leads to a temporary increase of the resistance of the respiratory tract, particularly if the pollutants had been previously exposed to U.V. irradiation in the spectrum of sun light.

4. Enzyme Action

One can speculate that some enzymes, by altering the pulmonary framework, favour the development of emphysema. It was only recently that Gross *et al.* (1965) succeeded in provoking the development of enphysematous lesions in the rat six hours after the intratracheal injection of papain: the lesions (centri-lobular, then planlobular and sometimes destructive) are correspondingly more severe as the dose is higher, or the survival of the animal prolonged. Animals that had been rendered artificially silicotic are less sensitive to the action of papain than non-silicotic animals. In any case, the pneumoconiotic foci are not involved in the localisation of the emphysema, whether experimental or spontaneous (Gross *et al.*, 1968).

According to Goldring *et al.* (1968), the inhalation of aerosols of a 3% solution of papain, during a single 4 hour session, leads, in the course of the next few hours, to an acute respiratory distress syndrome linked with pulmonary oedema with hypercongestion and petechiae. After an interval of several weeks a panlobular emphysema develops, without any sign of mucus hypersecretion.

5. Action of Microorganisms

The acute experimental bronchitis of mice infected with influenza virus or with the swine virus is characterized in the large bronchi by a phase of epithelial degeneration with nuclear pycnosis, followed by a phase of regeneration of normal epithelium (Straub, 1937; Straub, 1940).

Of greater interest are the observations concerning Mycoplasma pneumoniae.

Ventura and Goucher (1966) insisted on the major role played by this agent in the proliferation of mucus-secreting elements at different levels of the respiratory tree of the animal.

This Mycoplasma, saprophyte of the upper respiratory tract of the normal rat, can invade the lower respiratory tract, for example, at the time of surgical trauma.

The sequence described by Reid (hypersecretion followed by infection) is contested by these authors, according to whom the hypersecretion could be the result of latent infections by viruses or Mycoplasma pneumoniae.

Blake (1962) inoculated pullets with the virus of infectious bronchitis, and with a PPLO[1]. The former produced an acute symptomatology, while the latter led to a more chronic and also less frequent symptomatology.

[1] Pleuro-pneumonia-like-organism.

Laurenzi *et al.* (1965) showed the great resistance of normal mice to the aerosolisation of the staphylococcus aureus, due to a very effective bacterial clearance in the lungs. Alcohol and cigarette smoke interfered considerably with this bacterial clearance, which was studied by culturing the homogenate of the lungs of mice sacrificed at various intervals after the inhalation of the organisms.

II. Methods Aimed at Obtaining Mechanical Hyperdistension of the Lung

These techniques which were extensively used in the past, have been reviewed by Strawbridge (1960b).

The simplest of these consisted in producing an atelectasis or in resecting a part of the lung, in order to obtain a compensatory emphysema in the remaining areas (Nissen, 1927). It is well known, however, that such compensatory emphysema is anatomically and functionally different from obstructive emphysema.

The creation of an artificial partial tracheal stenosis by means of encercling the organ with a lead wire kept in place for several weeks, enabled Kohler (1877) to obtain an alveolar hyperdistension in the rabbit, but not a true emphysema.

Similar results were obtained by Rasmussen and Adams (1942) by submitting their experimental animals to positive pressure insufflations over a period of several months. Tura (1960) arrived at lesions of the same kind by making rats swim to exhaustion, i.e. for 15 to 20 minutes a day for 90 consecutive days: the "emphysema" was assessed by measuring the percentage of light transmission after scanning chest X-rays, and by histological studies. The difference in density ranged from 15 to 24% according to the level, between the rats who had been subjected to forced excercise and the controls. In the histological examinations, the "emphysema" (characterized by a breakdown of the alveolar walls and the formation of lacunae) was generally slight, although it was very marked in some cases. The rats also had a mild polycythemia, associated with adrenal hypertrophy.

Other authors have attempted to induce pulmonary hyperdistension by introducing valves into the trachea (Harris and Chillingworth, 1919). The pulmonary distension observed was hardly greater than that obtained by means of a simple endotracheal tube without valve.

The various later attempts having recourse to similar techniques also failed to induce a true emphysema (Hinshaw, 1938; Paine, 1940).

A tracheal obstruction can also be achieved by means of the simple implantation of an endotracheal tube which is narrowed at one end. This produces an expiratory turbulence (and hence an increased resistance to flow), which is greatly above that observed at inspiration (Eiseman *et al.*, 1959). However, the physiological pressures attained in this way are not sufficient to cause the rupture of normal alveolar walls.

In consideration of these failures, Krahl (1959) attempted to produce a more peripheral bronchial stenosis in the lobar or segmental bronchi. He used a valve system in polyethylene, which he introduced into the right inferior lobar bronchus of the rat, and which he left in place for from 2 to 12 weeks. The corresponding area on the left served as control. On macroscopic examination, the right lower lobe generally collapsed less well than the others. Histological examination showed an increase in the calibre of the peripheral airways, degeneration of the interalveolar septa, and the development of abnormally large air spaces.

After special staining, he noted severe changes in the number and disposition of the elastic fibres (rupture, retraction and rearrangement of the bronchiolar fibres, retraction of the interalveolar septa, and even, in places, the disappearance, of the latter). One must bear in mind that the lesions observed by Krahl could be the result of both the obstruction and the inflammation due to the presence of the valve. But these lesions, although less severe than those seen in man, nevertheless bear of a great similarity to them.

Aczuy *et al.* (1961) succeeded in producing a barrel shaped thorax in the dog by means of a valve producing mechanical pulmonary hyperdistension.

Anderson *et al.* (1963, 1964) stated that, after introducing a venturi valve into the trachea of greyhounds, they obtained very little more emphysema than in untreated animals, this in spite of a considerable increase of the expiratory resistance. On the other hand, the instillation of a 1% nitric acid solution characteristically increased the frequency of emphysema in the animals with an implanted valve. It would appear, therefore, that an NO_2 alveolitis is necessary to diminish the alveolar resistance to mechanical factors of hyperdistension, and thus to allow the development of a true experimental emphysema.

Palecek *et al.* (1967) also succeeded in inducing various stigmata of emphysema in young rats of 5 weeks by means of repeated injections of dilute papain into the trachea, and by producing a tracheal constriction with the help of a loop positioned around it surgically. These authors found, in animals treated in this manner, that there was an increase in the resistance and a lowering of the compliance (measured with a body plethysmograph), an increase in the $PaCO_2$ and finally, in the histological sections a hyperdistension of the airways compared to the control groups.

Finally, Rainer *et al.* (1967), produced histopathological signs of emphysema in rabbits challenged with repeated inhalation of 75 to 125 ppm NO_2, after tracheal insertion of a stenosing tube.

Among the methods acting via the respiratory tract one can also class those which try to achieve hyperventilation by placing the animal in an abnormal atmosphere.

Campbell (1927) and Prinzmetal (1933, 1934) obtained only a pulmonary hyperdistension without true emphysema in subjecting their animals to hypoxia.

Glauser (1966, 1968), exposed young rats and young piglets to an atmosphere poor in O_2 and enriched in CO_2. The hyperventilation which resulted produced in the rat areas of atelectasis, and other areas of hyperdistension, with some fibrotic lesions. In the new-born piglet, there were even morphological abnormalities of the emphysematous type. In any case, the addition of CO_2 had a potentiating effect on the hypoxic hyperventilation.

C. Parietal Methods

Some authors, referring to the hypothesis of Freund, according to whom emphysema has a parietal cause, tried to enlarge the thoracic cage, by placing a metal bar between the sternum and the ribs of the dogs (Nissen, 1927).

Others (Paine, 1940) worked by suturing reefs in the diaphragm and thus lowering the diaphragmatic dome. All these techniques achieved no much more than a simple pulmonary hyperdistension without true emphysema.

D. Experimental Methods Acting through Vascular Routes

The importance of the destruction of the pulmonary capillary bed in emphysema in man is a generally admitted phenomenon. The question which remains open is whether these vascular lesions are a causal pathogenic factor, acting early into the genesis of emphysema, or whether they are a late consequence of its development, and thus a terminal phenomenon. If emphysema results from an ischaemic atrophy, it ought to be possible to induce it by disturbing the circulation through the lungs, even in the absence of parenchymatous hyperdistension.

Various authors have investigated the pulmonary consequences of experimental vascular lesions of the pulmonary and bronchial arteries.

I. Pulmonary Arteries

Obviously, complete occlusions of the pulmonary arteries are inadequate, because they produce pulmonary infarcts and not emphysema.

Strawbridge (1960b) worked with the repeated intravenous injection of an amorphous dye, Caledon blue RC, in a particulate state (average size between 10 and 20 μ), insoluble in water and in organic solvents. He was able to show that, by blocking the peripheral pulmonary vessels in rabbits, a pulmonary ischaemia was produced, and as a result, an increased occurence of interstitial pneumonia and a greater prevalence of emphysema than in the control animals. He observed no pulmonary infarcts, nor fibrosis or granulomatous reactions. The incidence of generalized emphysema increased with the repetition of the Caledon blue injections.

II. Bronchial Arteries

Complete interruption of the bronchial arterial flow by simple ligature seems impossible because of the numerous anastomoses with the oesophageal, mediastinal and intercostal arteries.

Under these conditions, it is preferable to have recourse to occlusion of the artery over a considerable length, by injection of a fairly inert plastic substance, such as vinyl acetate, which solidifies on exposure to moisture. The injection is made during thoracotomy, after cannulation of the intercostal artery, which gives rise to the right posterior bronchial artery (Ellis *et al.*, 1951).

In this manner, these authors produced an infarction and ulceration of the central bronchi of the operated side, with bilateral pneumonia. The bronchi lying distant from the hilum remained normal, except for a slight sub-mucosal congestion: this could be explained by the double circulation — pulmonary and bronchial — which exists at this level. By this method, therefore, one cannot produce either bronchiolitis or emphysema.

It would however, be incorrect to transpose the results obtained in the dog to the horse or to man, since the distribution of the bronchial artery differs according to the species: its perfusion areas are far more peripheral in the horse and in man than in the dog. This is the reason why McLaughlin *et al.* (1965) tried to obtain experimental emphysema in the horse by injecting chlorpromazine during thoracotomy into a proximal branch of a bronchial artery. This highly irritant product produces an endarteritis obliterans.

The early lesions observed in the parenchyma consist of severe necrosis with oedema, interstitial haemorrhage and inflammatory reaction. Twelve weeks later, the lesions assume an atrophic appearance, and closely resemble that of pulmonary emphysema observed in man. When the injection is made into the distal portion of the bronchial artery, the same endarteritis obliterans is accompanied by dense parenchymatous scarring, but never by emphysema. These last investigations suggest that a vascular element, particularly at the level of the bronchial artery, could play a part in the pathogenesis of emphysema.

E. Injcetion of Homologous Pulmonary Tissue

Some authors have put forward a hypothesis of the pathogenic role played by auto-immunisation in emphysema: the inhalation of some toxic agents (cigarette smoke, gas), might transform the pulmonary proteins into foreign substances able to induce an antigen-antibody reaction.

Crowle (1959) injected 3 guinea pigs subcutaneously with Freund's adjuvant and with an homogenate of lung taken from a guinea-pig killed with nitrogen oxide. He found an allergic pneumonitis with, in places, areas of blebs formed by hyperdistended lung.

In the same way, Balchum *et al.* (1964) succeeded in the guinea pig in setting up an intense interstitial pneumonia with oedema and thickening of the walls and round cells, and less often polynuclear infiltrations, by injecting it intradermically with extracts from normal guinea pig lungs, or from guinea pigs which had been exposed to toxic gases (NO_2, NO, NO—NO_2 mixture). They did not observe any lesions resembling human emphysema. It is possible that this interstitial pneumonia could be the result of an antigen-antibody reaction.

Boren *et al.* (1965) recently repeated Crowle's experiments, by using 86 guinea pigs, males and females, and injecting them with extracts of normal lungs, or of lungs that had been exposed to sublethal and lethal concentrations of NO_2, sometimes with adjuvants, and including control animals in their series. The lesions obtained were of the lymphoid hyperplastic, or rather round cell hyperplastic type, but after 4 to 6 months observation there was still no emphysema.

These various investigations therefore, do not allow to conclude up to now that auto-immune phenomena play a rôle in the genesis of bronchial emphysema.

F. Investigations Aimed at Pathogenic Interpretation of the Phenomena Observed in vivo

I. Studies on the "Flow" of Tracheo-Bronchial Mucus and on Ciliary Activity

The bronchial mucus lining propelled by ciliary activity causes clearing or removal of impinged foreign material from the trachea and the bronchi. The ciliary activity can be studied by direct observation, or indirectly by measuring the speed of displacement of solid particles of small size, on the mucous lining. The latter method is less precise, because the particular displacement depends not only on the activity of the cilia, but also on the volume and rheological characteristics of the mucus.

Battigelli *et al.* (1966) recently summarized in a general review the numerous earlier observations on the subject.

The effect of exhaust gas provokes in the dissected trachea of the rat a slowing of the clearance, which can often be demonstrated at low concentrations, still inactive on the airway resistance of man. The clearance is rapidly reestablished after interruption of exposure.

According to Dalhamn and Rhodin (1966) who examined rats exposed to 10 ppm of SO_2 for 6 hours a day, during 10 weeks, the flow of mucus is slowed although the ciliary kinetics are not affected. This could be explained by a thickening of the mucus layer and perhaps by an increase in its viscosity.

According to Guillerm *et al.* (1961), cigarette smoke inhibits ciliary activity.

The transport of mucus is also slowed, according to Dalhamn (1966) by cigarette smoke. But this depressor effect is greatly weakened if the cigarette smoke is filtered before being projected unto the mucosa. Kensler and Battista had already arrived at similar conclusions in 1963.

Kaminski *et al.* (1968) further demonstrate, in vivo, that the ciliary depressant effect of cigarette smoke was weakened if it was used after passing through a chamber containing moist surfaces (as is the case in the buccal cavity), no doubt as a result of the solution of some of its components.

Finally, Falk *et al.* (1963) studied the effects of various atmospheric pollutants and of cigarette smoke on the displacement of mucus in the oesophagus of the frog, which is covered by an epithelium equivalent to that of the respiratory tree. They noted a distinct slowing of the displacement of carbon particles observed by stereomicroscopy. These effects can be prevented by prior administration of acetylcholine, eserine or arecoline: the participation of the parasympathetic system in this reflex mechanism should be admitted.

II. Studies of the Properties of the Lung Surfaces

The alveolar surfactant is one of the important factors of alveolar stability, opposing collapse. It is conceivable that an increase in the secretion of surfactant, by reducing the surface element among the forces tending to retract the lungs, should favor alveolar distension, and thence prepare for emphysema. Many experiments have attempted to define the effect of toxic gases on the surface tension of the lungs.

Kahana and Aronovitch (1966) carried out such experiments on the isolated lungs of male albino rats subjected to mechanical respiratory measures during fluid and air filling after single or repeated exposures to fairly strong concentrations of SO_2. An acute exposure leads to reduction in surface forces, while repeated exposures give results which are more difficult to interprete but suggest a similar effect.

The same type of finding was observed with ozone, cigarette smoke, and particles of aluminium oxide. This might have been caused by an increased secretion at the alveolar surface producing a greater concentration of surfactant in the alveolar lining film.

The surface properties of the alveolar fluid can also be studied in vitro. The surface pressure of the products obtained by washing the lungs of white mice increases when they are exposed to the action of ozone (Mendenhall and Stokinger, 1962).

The surface pressure of lung extracts also increases after exposure to cigarette smoke (Miller and Bondurant, 1962). These different phenomena could play a rôle in the pathogenesis of emphysema.

III. Studies of the Inhibiting Properties of Mucus with Regard to Viruses

According to Falk *et al.* (1963), the mucus of the common garden snail looses a significant fraction of its inhibitory capacity with regard to the virus P-R_8, following contact with ozone.

IV. Studies on Cell Cultures

The alveolar macrophage contribute considerably to pulmonary clearing, with regard to dusts and microbial contaminants: this phagocytic activity constitutes one of the most important of the anti-infectious mechanisms present in the lung.

This mechanism is disturbed under the influence of cigarette smoke. Green and Carolin (1967), demonstrated on cultures of alveolar macrophages from the lungs of rabbits that their phagocytic activity towards the Staphylococcus albus and their capacity to digest this organism was depressed in proportion to the quantity of cigarette smoke with which they had been in contact, and that this depression was a function of the type of cigarette used and of the filter employed. The toxic agent was present in the gaseous filtrable phase of the smoke.

Cultures of pulmonary cells from guinea pigs which had been exposed to SO_2 were much more frequently superinfected with Pseudomonas than those coming from control animals, even though bacteriological investigations of the living animals did not show this organism (Richters *et al.*, 1966).

Finally, cell cultures show very little resistance to the action of NO_2; concentrations of 10 ppm lead to the death of the greater part of the cells after a few days. The tolerance of different cell lines in tissue culture is greatly increased by the presence of serum in the medium (Pace *et al.*, 1961).

It is evident, therefore, that different irritant agents, used to produce experimental bronchitis, induce major disturbances in the cells, and that these disturbances can be elegantly studied by the methods of tissue culture.

G. Conclusions

The investigations carried out up to now on experimental bronchitis and emphysema are particularly numerous and varied. So many different methods and such different criteria of assessment were used that comparison of the results is particularly difficult.

It is however, possible to conclude that purely mechanical methods, and those consisting of the injection of pulmonary homogenates have been especially disappointing, while those trying to obtain broncho-pulmonary ischemia, or inflammation, with or without mechanical distension, have produced lesions which much more closely resemble those observed in man. It is therefore probable that these latter mechanisms acting simultaneously or successively play a rôle in the pathogenesis of the illness.

In the future, very special attention should be paid to the choice of the experimental animals. The frequency of spontaneous broncho-pulmonary pathology, the greater or lesser quantity of mucous secreting structures, and the distribution of bronchial and pulmonary arterial branches vary considerably from one species to another.

In the experiments making use of toxic gases, special care must be brought to the methods of dilution, or distribution, and of measurement of the agents used, as was done by Hinners *et al.* (1966).

Finally, assessment of the results obtained should be based on precise anatomical and functional methods.

Histological examinations must include the large bronchi, but should also permit the distinction between simple pulmonary hyperdistension and the destructive alveolar wall phenomena characteristic of true emphysema: use of special staining techniques of the elastic tissue facilitate interpretation in this respect (Eiseman *et al.*, 1959).

Measurements of respiratory mechanics (making use either of oesophageal balloons or of plethsmography for the smallest animals) must be completed by studies of blood gases and the acid-base balance.

Under these rigorous conditions, one may, thanks to experimental methods, hope to achieve a better understanding of the pathogenesis of human bronchitis and emphysema, and, through this, to develop preventive measures regarding the tabacco habits, pollution, vaccinations etc....

On the other hand, one can apply the experimental model to pharmacological studies: this was only still exceptionnally realised by few authors in the past. The results of Huyen *et al.* (1966) and of Lulling *et al.* (1968), prove that bronchodilators and mucolytics can be experimented on provoked bronchitis in the animal. They suggest that such methods should be more extensively applied to investigation of drugs intended for the treatment of aspecific respiratory affections.

References

Amdur, M. O.: The physiological responses of guinea pigs to atmospheric pollutants. Int. J. Air Pollut. **1**, 170—183 (1959).

— The influence of aerosols upon the respiratory response of guinea pigs to sulfur dioxide. Amer. industr. Hyg. Ass. Quart. **18**, 149—155 (1957).

—, and D. Underhill: The effect of various aerosols on the response of guinea pigs to sulphur dioxide. Arch. environm. Hlth **16**, 460—468 (1968).

Anderson, A. E., Jr., A. Azcuy, T. Batchelder, and A. G. Foraker: Morphogenesis of pulmonary emphysema. Dis. Chest. **43**, 350—357 (1963).

— — — — Experimental analysis in dogs of the relationship between pulmonary emphysema, alveolitis and hyperinflation. Thorax **19**, 420—432 (1964).

Auerbach, O., E. G. Hammond, D. Kirman, and L. Garfinkel: Emphysema produced in dogs by cigarette smoking. J. Amer. med. Ass. **199**, 241—246 (1967).

Azcuy, A., A. E. Anderson, T. Batchelder, and A. G. Foraker: Experimentally induced barrel deformity of the chest in dogs. Amer. Rev. resp. Dis. **84**, 680—683 (1961).

Balchum, O. J., R. Buckley, S. Levey, J. Bertolino, H. Swann, and T. Hall: Studies in experimental emphysema. Arch. environm. Hlth **8**, 132—138 (1964).

Ball, C. O. T., R. M. Heyssel, O. J. Balchum, G. O. Elliott, and G. R. Meneely: Survial of rats chronically exposed to sulfur dioxide. Physiologist **3**, 15 (1960).

Battigelli, M. C., F. Hengstenberg, R. J. Mannella, and A. P. Thomas: Mucociliary activity. Arch. environm. Hlth **12**, 460—466 (1966).

Bell, D. P., and P. C. Elmes: The effects of chlorine gas in the lungs of rats without spontaneous pulmonary disease. J. Path. Bact. **89**, 307—317 (1965).

Blake, J. T.: Effects of experimental chronic respiratory disease and infectious bronchitis on pullets. Amer. J. vet. Res. **23**, 847—854 (1962).

Boren, H. G.: Carbon as a carrier mechanism for irritant gas. Arch. environm. Hlth **8**, 119—124 (1964).

— A. B. Delahaut, and W. Steenken Jr.: Reaction of guinea pig lungs to injected lung homogenates. Med. Thorac. **22**, 355—364 (1965).

Campbell, J. A.: Note on some pathological changes in tissues during attempted acclimatization to alterations of oxygen pressure in air. Brit. J. exp. Path. **3**, 347—351 (1927).

Carilli, A. D., R. S. Gold, and W. Gordon: A virologic study of chronic bronchitis. New Engl. J. Med. **270**, 123—126 (1964).

Clay, J. R., and R. G. Rossing: Histopathology of exposure to phosgene. An attempt to produce pulmonary emphysema experimentally. Arch. Path. **78**, 544—551 (1964).

Coman, D. R., H. D. Bruner, R. C. Horn, M. Friedman, R. D. Boche, M. D. McCarthy, M. H. Gibbon, and J. Schultz: Studies on experimental phosgene poisoning — 1. The pathologic anatomy of phosgene poisoning with special reference to the early and late phases. Amer. J. Path. **23**, 1037—1074 (1947).

Crowle, A. J.: An attempt to produce emphysema in the guinea pig. Amer. Rev. resp. Dis. **80**, 153—154 (1959).

Cruickshank, A. H.: Bronchiectasis in laboratory rats. J. Path. Bact. **60**, 520—521 (1948).

Dalhamn, T.: Effects of cigarette smoke on ciliary activity. Amer. Rev. resp. Dis. **93**, 108—114 (1966).

—, and J. Rhodin: Mucous flow and ciliary activity in the trachea of rats exposed to pulmonary irritant gas. Brit. J. industr. Med. **13**, 110—113 (1956).

Davidson, J. T., G. A. Lillington, G. B. Haydon, and K. Wasserman: Physiologic changes in the lungs of rabbits continuously exposed to nitrogen dioxide. Amer. Rev. resp. Dis. **95**, 790—796 (1967).

De Villiers, A. J.: Morphologic changes induced in lungs of hamsters and rats by external radiation (X-rays). A study of experimental carcinogenesis. Thesis Univ. of Pittsburg, 1964.

Ehrlich, R.: Effects of air pollutants on respiratory infection. Arch. environm. Hlth **6**, 638—642 (1963).

— Effect of nitrogen dioxide on resistance to respiratory infection. Bact. Rev. **30**, 604–614 (1966).

Eiseman, B., T. Petty, and W. Silen: Experimental emphysema. Amer. Rev. resp. Dis. **80**, 147—152 (1959).

Ellis, F. H., Jr., J. H. Grindkay, and J. E. Edwards: The bronchial arteries — I. Experimental occlusion in dogs. Surgery **30**, 810—826 (1951).

Elmes, P. C., and D. Bell: The effects of chlorine gas on the lungs of rats with spontaneous pulmonary disease. J. Path. Bact. **86**, 317—326 (1963).

Falk, H. L., P. Kotin, and W. Rowlette: The response of mucus secreting epithelium and mucus to irritants. Ann. N.Y. Acad. Sci. **106**, 583—608 (1963).

Freeman, G., J. Furiosi, and G. B. Haydon: Effects of continuous exposure of 0.8 ppm NO_2 on respiration of rats. Arch. environm. Hlth **13**, 454—456 (1966).

—, and G. B. Haydon: Emphysema after low level exposure to NO_2. Arch. environm. Hlth 8, 125—128 (1964).

Glauser, E. M.: Experimental production of acute pulmonary emphysema in newborn piglets. Amer. Rev. resp. Dis. (to be published).

Goldring, I. P., L. Greenburg and I. M. Ratner: On the production of emphysema in Syrian hamsters by aerosol inhalation of papain. Arch. environm. Hlth **16**, 59—60 (1968).

Green, G. M., and D. Carolin: The depressant effect of cigarette smoke on the in vitro antibacterial activity of alveolar macrophages. New Engl. J. Med. **276**, 421—427 (1967).

Gross, P., R. T. P. de Treville, M. A. Babyak, M. Kaschak, and E. B. Tolker: Experimental emphysema. Effect of chronic nitrogen dioxide exposure and papain on normal and pneumoconiotic lungs. Arch.environm. Hlth **16**, 51—58 (1968).

— E. A. Pfitzer, E. B. Tolker, M. A. Babyak, and M. Kaschak: Experimental emphysema. Its production with papain in normal and silicotic rats. Arch. environm. Hlth **11**, 50–58 (1965).

Guillerm, R., R. Badri et B. Vignon: Inhibition de la ciliomotricité par la fumée de cigarettes. Bull. Acad. nat. Méd. (Paris) **145**, 416—423 (1961).

— A. Saindelle, P. Faltot et J. Hee: Action de la fumée de cigarettes et de quelques uns de ses constituants sur les résistances ventilatoires chez le cobaye. Arch. int. Pharmacodyn. **167**, 101—114 (1967).

Harris, W. H., and F. P. Chillingworth: The experimental production in dogs of emphysema with associated asthmatic syndrome by means of an intratracheal ball valve. J. exp. Med. **30**, 75—85 (1919).

Haydon, G. B., J. J. Davidson, G. A. Lillington, and K. Wasserman: Nitrogen dioxide induced emphysema in rabbits. Amer. Rev. resp. Dis. **95**, 797—805 (1967).

— G. Freeman, and N. J. Furiosi: Covert pathogenesis of NO_2-induced emphysema in rat. Arch. environm. Hlth **11**, 776—783 (1965).

Hernandez, J. A., A. E. Anderson Jr., W. L. Holmes, and A. G. Foraker: Pulmonary parenchymal defects in dogs following prolonged cigarette smoke exposure. Amer. Rev. resp. Dis. **93**, 78—83 (1966).

Hinners, R. G., J. K. Burkart, and G. L. Contuer: Animal exposure chambers in air pollution studies. Arch. environm. Hlth **13**, 609—615 (1966).

Hinshaw, H. C.: Experimental production of chronic obstructive pulmonary emphysema in animals. Proc. Mayo Clin. **13**, 599—600 (1938).

Huyen, V. N., S. Garcet et L. Lakah: Hypersécrétion expérimentale du mucus bronchique chez le rat. II. Application à l'étude d'un agent dit mucolytique: la S carboxyméthyl cystéine. C.R. Soc. Biol. (Paris) **160**, 1849—1851 (1966).

Kahana, L. M., and M. Aronovitch: Effects of sulfur dioxide on surface properties of the lung. Amer. Rev. resp. Dis. **94**, 201—207 (1966).

Kaminski, E. J., O. E. Fancher, and J. C. Calandra: In vivo studies of the ciliastatic components of tobacco smoke. Absorption of ciliastatic components by wet surfaces. Arch. environm. Hlth **16**, 188—193 (1968).

Kensler, C. J., and S. P. Battista: Components of cigarette smoke with ciliary depressant activity. Their selective removal by filters containing activated charcoal granules. New Engl. J. Med. **269**, 1161—1166 (1963).

Kleinerman, J., and G. W. Wright: Experimental production of a lesion ressembling human microbullous emphysema. Fed. Prod. **21**, 439 (1962).

Klieneberger-Nobel, E.: Pleuropneumonia-like organisms (PPLO). — Mycoplasmataceae. London: Acad. Press 1962 (157 pp.)

Kohler, H.: Ueber die Compensation mechanischer Respirationsstörungen und die physiologische Bedeutung der Dyspnoe. Naunyn-Schmiedebergs Arch. exp. Path. Pharmak. **7**, 1 (1877).

Krahl, V. E.: The experimental production of pulmonary emphysema. A preliminary report. Amer. Rev. resp. Dis. **80** (Suppl.) 158—168 (1959).

Laurenzi, G. A., J. J. Guarneri, and R. B. Endriga: Important determinants in pulmonary resistance to bacterial infection. Med. Thor. **22**, 48—59 (1965).

Leuchtenberger, C., R. Leuchtenberger, and P. F. Doolin: A correlated histological, cytological, and cytochemical study of the tracheabronchial tree and lungs of mice exposed to cigarette smoke. I. Bronchitis with atypical epithelial changes in mice exposed to cigarette smoke. Cancer (N.Y.) **11**, 490—506 (1958).

Loomis, T. A.: Bronchoconstrictor factor in cigarette smoke. Proc. Soc. exp. Biol. (N.Y.) **92**, 337—340 (1956).

Lulling, J., J. Prignot, and P. Lievens: Experimental bronchopneumopathy due to SO_2 in the dog. Naunyn-Schmiedebergs Arch. exp. Path. Pharmak. **261**, 1—25 (1968).

McLaughlin, R. F., Jr., W. S. Tyler, D. W. Edwards, G. L. Creushaw, R. O. Canada, M. A. Fowler, E. A. Parker, and G. H. Reifenstein: Chlorpromazine induced emphysema. Amer. Rev. resp. Dis. **92**, 597—608 (1965).

Mendenhall, R. M., and H. E. Stokinger: Films from lung washings as a mechanism model for lung injury by ozone. J. appl. Physiol. **17**, 28—32 (1962).

Miller, D., and S. Bondurant: Effects of cigarette smoke on surface characteristics of lung extracts. Amer. Rev. resp. Dis. **85**, 692—696 (1962).

Mosinger, M., et R. Luccioni: Recherches épidémiologiques sur la bronchopneumopathie chronique des rangeurs en comparaison avec la bronchite chronique de l'homme. Symposium Bronchite-Emphysème, CECA Luxembourg, 1967, p. 248—251.

Murphy, S. D., J. K. Leng, C. E. Ulrich, and H. V. Davis: Effects on animals of exposure to auto-exhaust. Arch. environm. Hlth **7**, 60—70 (1963).

Nissen, R.: Experimentelle Untersuchungen zur Theorie der Entstehung des Lungen-Emphysems. Dtsch. Z. Chir. **200**, 177—205 (1927).

Pace, D. M., J. R. Thompson, B. Th. Aftonomos, and H. G. O. Holck: The effects of NO_2 and salts of NO_2 upon established cell lines. Canad. J. Biochem. **39**, 1247—1255 (1961).

Paine, J. R.: Studies in experimental production of emphysema. J. thorac. Surg. **10**, 150—175 (1940).

Paleck, F., M. Palecekova, and D. M. Aviado: Emphysema in immature rats: condition produced by tracheal constriction and papain. Arch. environm. Hlth **15**, 332—342 (1967).

Prinzmetal, M.: The relation of inspiratory distension of the lungs to emphysema. J. Allergy **5**, 493 (1933—1934).

Purvis, M. R., and R. Ehrlich: Effects of atmospheric pollutants on susceptibility to respiratory infection. II. Effect of nitrogen dioxide. J. infect. Dis. **113**, 72—76 (1963).

— S. Millers, and R. Ehrlich: Effects of atmospheric pollutants on susceptibility to respiratory infection. I. Effect of ozone. J. infect. Dis. **109**, 238—242 (1961).

Quevauviller, A., et V. N. Huyen: Hypersécrétion expérimentale du mucus bronchique chez le rat. I. Méthode d'appréciation anatomo-pathologique. C.R. Soc. Biol. (Paris) **160**, 1845—1848 (1966).

Rainer, W. G., D. L. Kelble, J. P. Newby, and M. Sanchez: Experimental emphysema. Ann. thorac. Surg. **3**, 539—546 (1967).

Rasmussen, R. A., and W. E. Adams: Experimental production of emphysema. Arch. intern. Med. **70**, 379—395 (1942).

Reid, L.: An experimental study of hypersecretion of mucus in the bronchial tree. Brit. J. exp. Path. **44**, 437—445 (1963).

Richters, V., R. P. Sherwin, R. Buckley, O. Balchum, and D. Ivler: Pseudomonas: delayed occurrence in lung tissue cultures from guinea pigs exposed to nitrogen dioxide. Amer. Rev. resp. Dis. **94**, 569—573 (1966).

Rockey, E. E., and F. D. Speer: The ill effects of cigarette smoking in dogs. Int. Surg. **46**, 520—530 (1966).

Rossing, R. G.: Airflow resistance in lower airways of the dog. J. appl. Physiol. **17**, 877–884 (1962).

— Physiologic effects of chronic exposure to phosgene in dogs. Amer. J. Physiol. **207**, 265—272 (1964).

Steadman, B. L., R. A. Jones, D. E. Rector, and J. Siegel: Effects on experimental animals of long term continuous inhalation of nitrogen dioxide. Toxicol. appl. Pharmacol. **9**, 160—170 (1966).

Stokinger, H. E., W. D. Wagner, and O. J. Dobrogorski: Ozone toxicity studies. III. Chronic injury to lungs of animals following exposures at a low level. Arch. industr. Hlth **16**, 514—522 (1957).

Straub, M.: Microscopal changes in lungs of mice infected with influenza virus. J. Path. Bact. **45**, 75—78 (1937).

— Histology of catarrhal influenzal bronchitis and collapse of lung in mice infected with influenza virus. J. Path. Bact. **50**, 31—36 (1940).

Strawbridge, H. T. G.: Chronic pulmonary emphysema (an experimental study). II. Spontaneous pulmonary emphysema in rabbits. Amer. J. Path. **37**, 309—331 (1960a).

— Chronic pulmonary emphysema (an experimental study). III. Experimental pulmonary emphysema. Amer. J. Path. **37**, 391—407 (1960b).

Tura, S.: Pulmonary emphysema and polycythemia induced in rats by forced swimming. Proc. Soc. exp. Biol. (N.Y.) **103**, 713—715 (1960).

Ventura, J., and S. Goncher: Bronchial epithelial mucus in rats infected with mycoplasma pulmonis. Arch. environm. Hlth **13**, 593—596 (1966).

Wagner, W. D., B. R. Duncan, P. G. Wright, and H. E. Stokinger: Experimental study of threshold limit of NO_2. Arch. environm. Hlth **10**, 455—466 (1965).

Experimenteller Husten*

H. Friebel

Mit 16 Abbildungen

Niesen und Husten wird durch chemische, mechanische oder thermische Reize, im Experiment auch durch elektrische Stimulation ausgelöst. Beide Vorgänge kommen reflektorisch zustande. Sie sind durch kurzfristige Änderung der Atemmotorik charakterisiert.

A. Niesreflex

Niesen tritt vorwiegend nach Reizung sensibler Trigeminusfasern der Nasenschleimhaut auf. Der afferente Teil der Reflexbahn verläuft für die vorderen und oberen Bezirke der Nase, ihre Scheidewand, die Nebenhöhlen und vorderen Siebbeinzellen in den N. ethmoidales, für den Nasenboden in den N. nasales post. und inf. aus dem Ganglion pterygopalatinum. Starke Geruchsreize können über den N. olfactorius den Niesreflex auslösen.

Die Niesreaktion verläuft in den zentrifugalen Hirnnervenfasern, die sich im N. hypoglossus, N. accessorius, N. glossopharyngicus und N. facialis finden, ferner im N. vagus. An ihr ist die Gesamtheit der Atemmuskulatur beteiligt. Die Reizantwort kann je nach dem Grad der Reizung in verschiedener Intensität und Ausbreitung auf diesen Bahnen erfolgen. Als geringster Reflexerfolg kommt es in der Nase zur Vasoconstriction oder Vasodilatation, bei stärkerer Reaktion zum reflektorischen Mundverschluß und Atemausstoß durch die Nase nach maximaler Einatmung mit geöffnetem Mund. Als Hemmung wirken der Wille, Gegenreize sensibler Art und Schockwirkung. Die Reflexzeit, d.h. das Intervall zwischen dem Augenblick des Reizes und der reflektorischen Beantwortung ist in Abhängigkeit von der Reizstärke variabel, auch unterschwellige Reize können bei entsprechend langer Wirkdauer zum Erfolg führen. Niesen verläuft stets unwillkürlich (Rein-Schneider; Grosse-Brockhoff).

Die physiologische Zweckbestimmung des Niesreflexes ist Warnung bzw. Reinigung der oberen Luftwege von reizenden Stimuli. Als selbständiges Krankheitssymptom hat der Niesreflex keine Bedeutung. Unterdrücken des Niesreflexes ist kein Objekt der Arzneimittelforschung geworden.

Niesen wird an dieser Stelle erwähnt, weil es bei der experimentellen Provokation von Husten als Nebenreaktion auftreten kann und seine Abgrenzung vom Husten nicht immer leicht ist.

B. Hustenreflex

I. Morphologie der Hustenreflexbahn

a) Afferente Elemente

Die peripheren sensiblen Elemente der Hustenreflexbahn findet man im Parenchym des Larynx, der Trachea, den tieferen Atemwegen und der Pleura. Es sind Endorgane markhaltiger Nerven und sensorische Anteile von Vagus und

* Mit einem Abschnitt von O. Eichler (C. III. n).

Sympathicus. Man hat mehrere Formen afferenter Nervenendigungen kennengelernt (Elftman). Im Bronchialepithel der Kaninchen fanden Larsell und Burget zwei Typen: Solche mit knopfförmiger Endigung und andere mit abgeflachtem Endorgan. Von den ersteren nehmen sie an, daß sie taktile Reize übermitteln, denn es gelang ihnen, durch Stimulation derartiger afferenter Endigungen in den Hauptbronchien reflektorischen Husten auszulösen. Die abgeflachten Endorgane halten Larsell und Dow für Chemoreceptoren. Einige dieser Endigungen scheinen Kapseln zu haben, andere sind offenbar nackt. Widdicombe (1954), der die sensiblen Receptoren in der Trachea und in den Bronchien der Katze untersuchte, fand, daß drei Typen von Mechanoreceptoren im Epithel des Tracheo-Bronchialbaumes nachweisbar sind: Solche bei denen eine Adaption an Dehnung und Entlastung der Atemwege langsam erfolgt, solche, deren Reizung sehr kurze Entladungen hervorruft — die er als verantwortlich für den mechanisch ausgelösten Husten ansieht — und weiterhin solche, die ebenfalls Änderungen des Bronchiallumens mit kurzen Entladungen beantworten, die zugleich aber auch durch reizende Gase erregt werden. Letztere werden als Hustenreceptoren für die chemische und mechanische Stimulation angesehen. Offen bleibt, ob und wieweit diese an einzelnen Tierarten erhaltenen Resultate verallgemeinert werden können.

Nervenspindeln sind auch in der Bronchialmuskulatur nachgewiesen worden; sie werden vermutlich durch Längsänderungen der Muskelfasern erregt, stellen also Dehnungsreceptoren dar. Afferente Nervenendigungen kommen auch in der Adventitia der Lungenarterien und im Perichondrium der Bronchialknorpelplatten vor (Larsell; Larsell und Dow). Im Hilusgebiet ist die Anwesenheit sensibler Nervenendigungen noch nicht sicher bewiesen. Die Verteilung der sensiblen Endorgane entlang der Atemwege wechselt offenbar von Tierart zu Tierart.

Fasern, in denen afferente Impulse fortgeleitet werden, verlaufen im wesentlichen mit dem Vagus, beim Hund zum Teil auch mit sympathischen Fasern (Craigie) und durch das Ganglion stellatum (Cromer, Young und Ivy). Die von pulmonalen Dehnungsreceptoren kommenden Fasern werden beim Kaninchen im Vagus gefunden (Weidmann, Berde und Bucher). Am Menschen haben Morton u. Mitarb. nachgewiesen, daß nach Vagusdurchtrennung dicht unterhalb der Einmündung des Recurrens elektrisch induzierter Husten und Bronchialschmerz erlöschen.

b) Zentraler Teil

Die zentralen Anteile der Reflexbahn, in denen afferente Impulse zum explosiven Exspirationsstoß umgeformt werden, liegen nach Borison in der dorsolateralen Region des Myencephalon, einschließlich der Strukturen, die dem absteigenden Tract. vestibularis und zugehörigen Nucleus, dem Tract. solitarius nebst Kern sowie den Wurzeln des Vagus und Glossopharyngeus entsprechen. Dieser von ihm als Koordinationszentrum angesehene Bereich läßt sich nach seinen an Katzen durchgeführten Versuchen vom eigentlichen Atemzentrum anatomisch und funktionell abgrenzen. Chakravarty u. Mitarb. ergänzten diese Befunde dahingehend, daß das medulläre hustenregulierende System als supraregulatorisches System aufzufassen sei, das den basalen vom Atemzentrum ausgehenden Rhythmus zu Hustenstößen aktiviert. Nach Befunden von Dubi ist in höheren Abschnitten des Zentralnervensystems, in der cranialen Hälfte der Pons ein Substrat gelegen, bei dessen Ausfall der Husten nur noch schwach auftritt. Dieses Substrat scheint mit den bekannten vagalexspiratorischen Substraten im Pons nicht identisch zu sein. Ihm kommt eher eine hustenverstärkende als husteninduzierende Funktion zu.

Die Feinstruktur des medullären Koordinationszentrums wurde kürzlich von Engelhorn und Weller (1965) untersucht. Sie beobachteten im exspiratorischen Gebiet der Medulla von Katzen 2 Typen von Neuronen. Sie nennen sie E_α- und E_β-Neurone. E_α-Neurone waren während der normalen Ausatmung aktiv, E_β-Neurone stumm. E_β-Neurone wurden erst durch die mechanische und chemische Erregung der Receptoren in der Trachealschleimhaut oder die elektrische Reizung ihrer afferenten Bahnen angestoßen. Die Autoren fanden noch weitere stumme Neurone im gleichen Gebiet, deren Verhalten von dem der E_β-Neurone abwich. Die Zahl der durch elektrische Reizung des N. laryngeus superior aktivierbaren Neurone war etwa gleich groß wie die der phasensynchron entladenden E_α-Neurone. E_α- und E_β-Neurone wurden histologisch im oder am caudalen Ende des Nucleus ambiguus lokalisiert. Wieweit sie mit den von Porter (1962, 1963) in demselben Bereich gefundenen Elementen verwandt sind, konnte nicht entschieden werden. Eine genaue Zuordnung zu einer bestimmten Zellstruktur war wegen der durch Elektrocoagulation gesetzten Läsionen nicht möglich.

Die Existenz von Verbindungen zwischen der zentralen Repräsentation hustenwirksamer Afferenzen zu anderen Arten nervöser Elemente kann aus funktionellen Befunden abgeleitet werden. Engelhorn und Weller (1965) beschreiben die Miterregung von E_α-Neuronen bei Hustensalven; die Ausbreitung der Erregung des „Hustenzentrums" auf das Brechzentrum ist bekannt; willkürliche Kontrolle, bzw. Unterdrückung des Hustens ist möglich (Kuhn und Friebel, 1960; Engelhorn und Weller, 1961; Friebel und Hahn, 1966; Hahn und Friebel, 1966).

c) Efferenter Teil

Die efferenten Bahnen verlaufen im N. recurrens, im N. phrenicus und in den zur Thoraxmuskulatur ziehenden Nerven des Rückenmarks. Efferente bronchoconstrictorische Nervenfasern haben Job und Schaumann im Halsvagus und Widdicombe im Lungenvagus nachgewiesen. Nervenendigungen, die in der Bronchialmuskulatur gefunden wurden, stammen wahrscheinlich aus Nerven pulmonaler Ganglien. Andere, für den Hustenreflex wohl weniger wichtige Fasern endigen in den Schleimdrüsen, in der glatten Muskulatur der pulmonalen Bronchialarterien oder umziehen netzförmig die Lungencapillaren und endigen in deren Wandung (Larsell und Dow).

II. Mechanismus des Hustens

a) Funktion der Bronchien

Der Hustenstoß wurde ursprünglich einer beschleunigten energischen Ausatmung gleichgesetzt. Tierexperimentelle Untersuchungen haben aber gezeigt, daß doch wesentliche Unterschiede gegenüber der forcierten Exspiration bestehen. Sie wurden von Bucher und seinen Mitarbeitern untersucht und diskutiert (Bucher, 1958, 1965). Nach Di Rienzo ist der Husten ein dynamischer Akt, bei dem Luft und Sekret durch schnelle peristaltische Wellenbewegungen der Bronchialschleimhaut nach außen gefördert werden. Er beobachtete am Röntgenschirm, daß der Hustenakt mit einer Streckung der Bronchialäste beginnt, worauf in den feinen Bronchialverzweigungen eine schnelle peristaltische Welle entsteht und in der Stimmritze ihren Abschluß findet. Doch fand weder Widdicombe (1954) Peristaltik, — er spricht lediglich von aktiver Bronchoconstriction —, noch gelang es Ross, Gramiak und Rahn derartige Vorgänge röntgenkinematographisch zu erfassen. Diese fanden auch keinen Anhalt für aktive bronchoconstrictorische Durchmesserveränderungen. Sie halten den Hustenstoß vielmehr für ein Produkt von erheblicher intrapleuraler Druckerhöhung und passiver Verkleinerung des Bronchiallumens. Die Lumenverengung tritt bei hohem intrapleuralem Druck während der Glottisöffnung auf. Sie resultiert aus der Druckdifferenz zwischen Innen- und Außenseite von Trachea und Bronchien, da beim Öffnen der Glottis die Druckentlastung primär in den Bronchien und in der Trachea eintritt. Sie betonen, daß diese Lumenverengung den Hustenstoß von einer kräftigen exspiratorischen Bewegung unterscheidet. Wenn diese Anschauung richtig ist, muß dem initialen Glottisverschluß eine maßgebliche Teilfunktion beim Hustenstoß zukommen.

b) Funktion der Glottis

Floersheim, der die Glottisfunktion an der narkotisierten Katze untersuchte, fand, daß die Glottis beim Exspirationsstoß des Hustens folgenden Bewegungsablauf erkennen läßt: Zunächst kommt es — noch bei Normalatmung — zur Verengung, dann — nach Anstieg des intrapleuralen Druckes — zur Erweiterung und anschließend wieder zur Verengung. Die Bewegungen treten unabhängig davon auf, ob Luft durch die Glottis geht oder nicht. Es handelt sich um aktive Bewegungen, von denen die initiale Verengung wahrscheinlich primär vom Zentralnervensystem gesteuert wird, während die folgenden Bewegungen möglicherweise einen peripher induzierten Reflexvorgang darstellen. Interessant ist nun, daß in Floersheims Versuchen aus dieser Bewegungsfolge eine im ganzen nur geringe intrapleurale Druckzunahme resultiert. Wenn er den Hustenstoß unterhalb der Glottis nach außen leitete, war der maximale intrapleurale Druck nur um 20% niedriger, als wenn durch die Glottis gehustet wurde. So hält er die Bedeutung der Glottis für die Druckbildung beim Exspirationsstoß für gering. Ob diese an narkotisierten Katzen gewonnenen Ergebnisse allgemeinere Bedeutung haben, bedarf der Nachprüfung, denn Hahn und Friebel fanden, daß bei hexobarbitalbehandelten Meerschweinchen mit zunehmender Somnolenz und Narkose nicht nur eine Erhöhung der Hustenreizschwelle, sondern auch ein Übergang des Hustens in geräuscharme Exspirationen nachweisbar war. Die Windgeschwindigkeiten, die in den Atemwegen des wachen Menschen beim Husten auftreten, sind nach Rohrer im Glottisbereich wesentlich höher als in den sonstigen Teilen der Lunge.

c) Funktion der Dehnungsreceptoren

Auf zwei weitere Merkmale des Hustenvorgangs wurde von Bucher und seinen Mitarbeitern (Bucher, 1958, 1965) hingewiesen. 1. Sie fanden bei narkotisierten Katzen eine Vergrößerung des Atemvolumens infolge einer Verschiebung der inspiratorischen Endlage (Kroepfli). 2. Sie konnten bei narkotisierten Katzen nur nach vorausgegangener Inspiration Hustenstöße auslösen, wobei weniger die inspiratorische Aktivität des Atemzentrums, als vielmehr der inspiratorische Bewegungserfolg am peripheren Atmungsorgan wichtig war. Verhinderung der inspiratorischen Vergrößerung der Lunge unterdrückte den Hustenstoß, während bei Inspirationsstellung des Thorax der Hustenanfall selbst unter Trachealverschluß weiterging. Graduell war eine Hustenhemmung, die durch Trachealverschluß bewirkt wurde, um so schwächer, je weiter die Lunge über die exspiratorische Ruhestellung entfaltet war. Infolgedessen wird der Erregung der Dehnungsreceptoren eine wesentliche Rolle beim Zustandekommen des Hustenstoßes zugeschrieben (Weisser).

Demgegenüber fanden Sell u. Mitarb., daß nach Vagusdurchschneidung, peripher der Einmündungsstelle des Nervus laryngicus cranialis, keine wesentliche

Verminderung der Hustenreizbarkeit über diesen Nerv eintritt, obwohl die Durchschneidung den Einfluß der Dehnungsreceptoren ausschaltet. Widdicombe (1954) sowie Trendelenburg vertreten die Ansicht, daß dem Husten nicht in jedem Fall eine Inspiration bzw. keine tiefe Inspiration vorausgehen muß. Kuhn und Friebel (1960) registrierten bei nicht narkotisierten Meerschweinchen eine weitgehende Unabhängigkeit des Hustenstoßes von der Lungenentfaltung. Engelhorn und Weller (1961) haben nachgewiesen, daß die durch Hustenstöße ausgelösten Reaktionen exspiratorischer Neurone des Rhombencephalon ohne vorausgegangene tiefe Inspiration bzw. ohne Verlängerung inspiratorischer Spikeserien vorkommen. In späteren Versuchen (1965) wurde von ihnen der Zeitpunkt der maximalen Erregbarkeit der hustenspezifischen E_{β}-Neurone bestimmt. Dazu wurden zunächst nacheinander und in gleichen Abständen bei der narkotisierten Katze drei Einzelreize von submaximaler Stärke am N. laryngicus superior gesetzt. Der erste fiel in die Inspiration, der zweite zusammen mit der inspiratorischen Endlage und der dritte an den Anfang der Exspiration. Mit jedem Reiz nahm die Zahl der im Zentrum auftretenden Spikes zu, d.h. die E_{β}-Neurone waren in Inspiration schwerer erregbar als in Exspiration, aber sie waren in jeder Atemphase erregbar. In Versuchen von Friebel und Hahn (1966) traten bei nicht narkotisierten Meerschweinchen in 85% der Fälle die explosiven Exspirationen während der Inspirationsphase, in 12% während der Exspirationsphase und in 3% bei vollständiger Exspirationsstellung auf. Nach Behandlung mit Hexobarbital kam es zu Abweichungen von der Norm; den Hustenstößen ging dann ausnahmslos eine Inspiration voraus. Andere Pharmaka verschoben die Einordnung des Hustenstoßes in den Atemrhythmus zur exspiratorischen Seite (Hahn und Friebel). Offenbar reicht bei nicht narkotisierten Meerschweinchen der durch die Reserveluft gegebene Füllungszustand aus, um jederzeit während des Atemcyclus einen Hustenstoß von normaler Stärke zu ermöglichen. Der Hustenreflex scheint aufgrund dieser Befunde wenigstens partiell, wenn nicht ganz unabhängig von der Tätigkeit pulmonaler Dehnungsreceptoren zu sein (Friebel und Kuhn, 1962; Kuhn und Friebel, 1960). Für diese Ansicht finden sich auch im klinischen Schrifttum Belege (Staehelin).

d) Funktion des zentralen Teils der Reflexbahn

Über die Arbeitsweise des hustensteuernden Systems wissen wir wenig. Man darf vermuten, daß es sowohl der „Summation" als auch der Verarbeitung hustenstimulierender Afferenzen dient (Stefko und Benson; Bucher, 1958), und weiterhin der Koordination der am Hustenstoß beteiligten Muskulatur. Man möchte vermuten, daß die beiden ersten Funktionen im atmungssteuernden System nicht vertreten sind (Friebel und Kuhn, 1962). Hinsichtlich der letztgenannten dürften Beziehungen bestehen.

Die Fähigkeit der Hustenreflexbahn, unterschwellige Reize zu speichern und bis zur Schwellenüberschreitung zu „summieren", wurde von Friebel und Hahn an nicht narkotisierten Meerschweinchen nachgewiesen. Bei Reizung ihrer trachealen Mucosa mit elektrischen Stimuli recht unterschiedlicher Art und Stärke reagierten sie durchschnittlich 2,8 sec nach Reizungsbeginn mit einer explosiven Exspiration. Wenn aber sehr schwach, knapp oberhalb des Schwellenwertes gereizt wurde, trat eine Verlängerung der Latenzzeit bis zu 16 sec auf. Stimulationen, die innerhalb von 16 sec nicht zum Erfolg führten, blieben vollkommen unproduktiv. Die Fähigkeit zum „Summieren" oder zum „Bahnen" — charakterisiert durch die Latenzzeit zwischen hustenerzeugender Reizung und explosiver Exspiration — ist demnach limitiert. So erhöht diese Fähigkeit einerseits den protektiven Wert des Hustenreflexapparates, und schützt ihn andererseits auch vor unproduktiver Tätigkeit.

Die Variabilität der Latenz war die einzige spezifische Modifikation der Charakteristika des einzelnen Hustenstoßes, die durch Abwandlung von Intensität, Dauer und Frequenz der Reizströme bewirkt werden konnte. Der zentrale Teil des Reflexbogens kann offenbar Afferenzen, durch recht variable Reizqualitäten ausgelöst, dahingehend verarbeiten, daß die efferenten Reaktionen weitgehend normiert ablaufen; die einzelne Hustenreaktion verläuft, wenn sie einmal in Gang gesetzt ist, beurteilt nach Stärke und Charakteristik recht uniform (Friebel und Hahn).

Die efferenten Impulse des Hustenreflexmechanismus aktivieren Muskulatur, die normalerweise die Atmungsbewegungen ausführt, wobei der Ablauf des normalen Atemcyclus unterbrochen oder zeitlich nachgeordnet wird. Nur selten ist bei hustenerzeugender Reizung eine zunehmende Acceleration und Akzentuierung der Atemzüge bis zur typischen Hustenreaktion hin beobachtet worden (Kuhn und Friebel, 1960). Immerhin weist diese gelegentliche synchrone Einordnung des Hustens in die Atemrhythmik auf funktionelle Beziehungen zwischen Neuronen, die efferente Impulse im Rahmen des Hustenreflexes und des Atemzuges steuern, hin (Kuhn und Friebel, 1960; Friebel und Hahn). Engelhorn und Weller (1965) registrierten bei Stimulierung hustenreizsensibler Elemente eine Hemmung der Aktivität exspiratorischer Neurone zugunsten von hustenspezifischen Neuronen. War der sensible Einstrom aus der Peripherie aber groß genug, so kam es zu einer allgemeinen Erregung des ganzen Systems und zu einer Rekrutierung weiterer — sonst stummer — exspiratorischer Einheiten.

Soweit neuere Befunde Rückschlüsse auf die Organisation und Funktion des Hustenreflexmechanismus zulassen, stützen sie die Vorstellungen von

a) der prinzipiellen Selbständigkeit des Hustenreflexmechanismus,

b) seiner Fähigkeit, afferente hustenauslösende Impulse zu „summieren",

c) dem Vorrang überschwelliger Impulse vor der Atmungsrhythmik bei der Inanspruchnahme des pneumotaktischen Apparates.

Die Funktionen des Hustenreflexes als Warn- und Schutzmechanismus sind:

a) Warnung vor schädigender Reizung der Atemwege durch inhalierte Chemikalien und Fremdkörper,

b) Reinigung der Atemwege durch Eliminierung der Irritantien.

III. Husten als Krankheitssymptom

Husten tritt bei einer großen Zahl und Vielfalt von Krankheitszuständen als Symptom auf. Entzündung des Atemtraktes kann von erhöhter Empfindlichkeit der sensiblen Receptoren und Nervenfasern begleitet sein. Intrapulmonale Tumoren können durch Druck auf Receptoren und Fasern Husten verursachen. Bekannt ist Husten, der über den auriculären Zweig des Vagus durch Entzündungen oder andere Ursachen im äußeren Gehörgang hervorgerufen wird. Husten kann Ausdruck einer allergischen Reaktion sein, er kann beim Versagen des Kreislaufs oder psychiatrisch bedingt auftreten. Üblicherweise wird er durch Reizung der im Atemtrakt gelegenen Receptoren durch Infektionen oder mechanische Irritation (Bickerman, 1960b) oder durch Inhalation von verunreinigter Luft oder Tabakrauch (Herzog; Phillips u. Mitarb.) hervorgerufen. Vom klinischen Gesichtspunkt her ist Husten möglicherweise der bedeutendste unter den Mechanismen, die für die Reinigung der Atemwege sorgen (Bickerman, 1960a).

Wenn Husten längere Zeit anhält, kann „Gewöhnung" in der Weise eintreten, daß der Patient seinen chronischen Husten nicht mehr wahrnimmt. Andererseits können empfindsame Individuen die Tendenz zeigen, Intensität und Schwere ihrer Hustenattacken zu steigern. Wenn der Husten in der Regel auch reflektorisch abläuft, so kann er doch auch willkürlich in Gang gesetzt und bis zu einem gewissen Grade auch willkürlich unterdrückt werden (Bickerman, 1960a, b).

Husten, der seine Warnfunktion erfüllt oder die Reizursache aus den Atemwegen entfernt hat, aber dennoch persistiert (unproduktiver, nutzloser Husten), wird zum behandlungsbedürftigen Krankheitssymptom. Wenn der Husten untauglich oder unwirksam ist, den hustenprovozierenden Stimulus zu entfernen, resultiert tussive Insuffizienz. Auch sie ist behandlungsbedürftig. Bei vielen eitrigen Lungenerkrankungen kann die dicke, zähe, mucopurulente Sekretion, die ständig als Infektionsfolge gebildet wird, durch Husten nicht entfernt werden. Der trockene, irritierende Husten, der bei akuten Infektionen wie Laryngitis, Tracheitis, Bronchitis und Pertussis auftritt, kann durch sich selbst zu einem Faktor werden, der die Wiederherstellung verzögert, weil er den Schlaf raubt, appetitlos macht, Schwindel und Erbrechen verursacht. Bei obstruktiven Erkrankungen des Tracheobronchialbaumes, wie Tumoren, Fremdkörpern und chronischem Asthma kann der Hustenreflex zu einem sich selbst unterhaltenden Mechanismus werden. Die resultierenden schweren Paroxysmen können eine erhebliche Entkräftung der chronisch kranken Patienten verursachen (Bickerman, 1960b; Banyai und Joannides, 1956). Andere Folgen von schwerem protrahierten Husten sind pulmonales Emphysem, Frakturen von Rippen und gelegentlich auch von Wirbelkörpern, Bewußtlosigkeit, Harninkontinenz, postoperativer Narbenbruch, Spontanpneumothorax. Die Notwendigkeit der antitussiven Therapie ist daher in vielen Fällen von pathologischem Husten unbestritten (Friebel, 1963).

Die Arzneibehandlung des Hustens nimmt in der ärztlichen Praxis einen breiten Raum ein, zumal der Prozentsatz der „chronischen Huster" in der Bevölkerung nicht gering ist. So wird in den USA, in denen 13% der Bevölkerung älter als 65 Jahre sind, der Anteil der „chronischen Huster" in diesem Personenkreis auf 6% oder 1,3 Mill. geschätzt (Bickerman, 1960a). Im britischen Health Service betrafen 1958 11% aller Verschreibungen Hustenmittel. Wertmäßig waren es 4—5% der gesamten Arzneikosten. Es ist verständlich, daß diesem Therapiebereich in den letzten Jahren viel Beachtung geschenkt worden ist.

Zur Bereicherung des Arzneimittelschatzes dürfte die Entwicklung tierexperimenteller Methoden zur Hustenprovokation erheblich beigetragen haben.

C. Tierexperimentelle Provokation von Husten

I. Allgemeines

Für die experimentelle Provokation von Husten ergeben sich folgende Möglichkeiten: Husten kann

1. über die Stimulation von Mechano-Receptoren,
2. durch Reizung von Chemo-Receptoren,
3. durch elektrische Stimulation von afferenten Fasern,
4. durch Stimulation des Hustenzentrums selbst ausgelöst werden.

Chemische und mechanische Reizungen sind sowohl bei Menschen als auch bei Tieren vorgenommen worden. Für die experimentelle Reizung der afferenten Bahnen und des Hustenzentrums selbst kommt nur das Versuchstier in Frage. Nach Schroeder soll eine tierexperimentelle Methode nach Möglichkeit 3 Forderungen erfüllen:

1. die Untersuchung soll am wachen Tier erfolgen,
2. die Hustenreize sollen genau dosierbar sein und
3. das Tier soll durch die Untersuchung nicht geschädigt werden.

Tabelle 1

	Reizmittel	Reizort	Narkose-mittel	Tierart	Autor
Mechanische Reizung	Nylonbürste	intra-tracheal	—	Hund	Kasé, (1952, 1954)
	Kamelhaar-bürste	intra-tracheal	Urethan	Kaninchen	Larsell u. Burget
	Polyäthylen-katheter	intra-tracheal	Pento-barbital-Na	Katze	May u. Widdicombe
	bewegliche Eisenröhrchen	intra-tracheal	—	Hund	Tedeschi u. Mitarb.
	digital	extra-tracheal	—	Meer-schweinchen	Kuhn u. Friebel (1960)
Chemische Reizung	Ammoniak-, Äther-, Essigsäure-dampf	intra-pulmonal	Urethan	Kaninchen	Larsell u. Burget
	SO_2-Gas-Luft-gemisch	intra-pulmonal	—	Meer-schweinchen	Friebel u. Mitarb., (1955, 1960, 1962)
	SO_2-Gas-Luft-gemisch	intra-pulmonal	—	Ratte	Reichle u. Friebel
	H_2SO_4-Aerosol	intra-pulmonal	—	Hund	Winter u. Flataker
	H_2SO_4-Aerosol	intra-pulmonal	Urethan	Hund	de Vleesch-houwer
	Ammoniak-Aerosol	intra-pulmonal	—	Meer-schweinchen	Winter u. Flataker
	Ammoniak-Gas-Luft-gemisch	intra-pulmonal	—	Hund	Rosiere und Mitarb.
	Ammoniak-Gas-Luft-gemisch	intra-pulmonal	Narkoticum nicht genannt	Katze	Stefko und Denzel
	Acroleindampf	intra-pulmonal	—	Meer-schweinchen	Silvestrini und Maffii
	Citronensäure-Spray	intra-pulmonal	—	Meer-schweinchen	Gösswald
	Waschpulver	intra-pulmonal	Apro-barbital	Katze	Kroepfli
Elektrische Reizung	spitze Spannungs-stöße, 2 V, 20—30 Hz,	Vagus-schlinge	—	Hund	Schroeder
	ca. 100 mV, 30—100 Hz, 1 sec	Submucosa der Trachea	—	Hund	Stefko u. Benson
	0,15—3,0 V, 5 Hz, 5—15 sec	N. Laryng. sup.	Apro-barbital	Katze	Domenjoz
	0,15—3,0 V, 5 Hz, 5—15 sec	N. Laryng. sup.	Pento-barbital-Na	Katze	Toner u. Macko

Tabelle 1 (Fortsetzung)

	Reizmittel	Reizort	Narkose-mittel	Tierart	Autor
	wellenförmige Stromstöße, 1—5 V, 6—10 Hz, 3,5—10 sec	zentrales Ende des durch-trennten N. Laryng. sup.	Pento-barbital-Na	Katze	Green u. Ward
	rechteckige Impulse, 0,3—0,6 mA, 60 Hz, 5—10 sec	beide N. Laryng. sup.	Pernocton	Katze	Sell u. Mitarb.
	rechteckige Impulse, 5—15 mA, 10 Hz, 10 sec	Tracheal-schleimhaut	Urethan	Meer-schwein-chen	Krause
	rechteckige Impulse, 0,5—5 V, 10—20 Hz, 10—15 sec	Medulla obl.	decerebr.	Katze	Chakravarty u. Mitarb.
	rechteckige Impulse, 1—10 mA, 15—80 Hz, 2—8 msec, max. 10 sec	Tracheal-schleim-haut	—	Meer-schweinchen	Kuhn u. Friebel (1960), Friebel u. Hahn

Aus dem Folgenden ist ersichtlich, daß zahlreiche Methoden weniger vollkommen sind und dennoch im Rahmen ihrer Zweckbestimmung brauchbar; neben das Bestreben, den Husten des Kranken im Tierversuch nachzuahmen und seinen Mechanismus zu studieren, trat der Wunsch, einfache Verfahren zu besitzen, die das Auffinden neuartiger Antitussiva erleichtern. So kann man heute zwischen recht verschiedenartigen Methoden wählen, von denen die bekannteren in der Tabelle 1 zusammengestellt sind.

Historisch gesehen wurde der Husten im Tierexperiment zuerst 1819 von Krimer provoziert. Er reizte die Kehlkopfschleimhaut mechanisch und chemisch. Die elektrische Reizung von afferenten Nerven der Hustenreflexbahn gelang erstmals Nothnagel sowie Kohts. Mayer, Magne und Plantefol sowie Craigie bemühten sich im wesentlichen um die Aufklärung der hustenempfindlichen Areale der Trachealschleimhaut, des sensorischen und zentralen Teiles der Hustenreflexbahn.

Die erste zum systematischen Studium der antitussiven Wirkung von Pharmaka brauchbare Methode wurde 1938 von Ernst publiziert. Er erzeugte bei Katzen durch die Injektion von Lugolscher Lösung in den Pleuraspalt eine chronische Pleuritis und erreichte damit eine so weitgehende Herabsetzung der Schwelle für artifizielle Hustenreizung, daß durch Beklopfen oder schwaches Kneifen Husten ausgelöst werden konnte. Die gesteigerte Reizempfindlichkeit wird durch Antitussiva gedämpft. Mit dieser Methode hat Schaumann (1953) die antitussive Wirkung von Pethidin nachgewiesen.

Etwa zur gleichen Zeit entwickelten auch Eichler und Smiatek eine zur Arzneimittelprüfung geeignete Methode. Bei Meerschweinchen wurde durch

Inhalation reizender Gase und Nebel Husten hervorgerufen. Sie erprobten eine große Zahl verschiedenartiger Reizmittel und fanden, daß sich mehrere für diesen Zweck eignen, z.B. Ammoniak, Schwefeldioxyd, Schwefelsäure, Amylacetat u.a. Reizhusten, der mit Schwefelsäure erzeugt wurde, bewährte sich bei der vergleichenden Prüfung von antitussiv wirkenden Pharmaka (Morphin, Dihydrocodein) am besten. Die Methode ist darüber hinaus für künftige Entwicklungen wertvoll; man kann mit ihr neben akutem Reizhusten auch chronische Katarrhe im Atemtrakt hervorrufen, d.h. man kann im Experiment Krankheitsbilder erzeugen, die der chronischen Bronchitis des Menschen ähnlicher sind als die akute im Tierexperiment übliche Stimulierung des Hustenreflexmechanismus [detaillierte Beschreibung der Herstellung von reizenden Nebeln bei Eichler (1961)].

Kasé veröffentlichte 1952 eine Methode zur mechanischen Stimulation der reizsensiblen Receptoren durch die operativ eröffnete Trachea.

Schroeder führte 1951 die elektrische Reizung der Hustenreflexbahn ein.

Die in der Folgezeit publizierten Methoden sind im wesentlichen Modifikationen dieser grundlegenden Verfahren.

II. Mechanische Stimulation

a) Methode von Kasé (1952, 1954, 1955)

Vorbereitende Operation: Hunde, im Gewicht von 6 kg oder mehr, werden mit Äther oder Morphium und Urethan narkotisiert und in Rückenlage fixiert. Nach Rasur und Desinfektion der Haut des Halses, Hautschnitt in der Mittellinie und Freilegen der Trachea. 1 cm unterhalb des C. cricoides wird ein Teil der vorderen Trachealwand entfernt, um eine Öffnung für die Einführung einer Trachealkanüle zu schaffen. Blutungen aus der Wand der Trachea werden durch Kauterisation oder lokale Anwendung von Adrenalin verhütet; Vorsorge vor Aspiration von Blut- und Fremdmaterial ist notwendig. Drei Tage nach der Operation sind die Tiere für die Prüfung von Antitussiva verwendbar.

Durchführung des Versuchs: Die Tiere werden ohne Anaesthesie und ohne Zwang in Seitenlage fixiert und die Trachealfistel desinfiziert. Eine Y-förmige sterilisierte Glaskanüle wird mit dem nicht gegabelten Ende in die Trachea eingeführt und mit einer Bandage am Hals befestigt. Von den freien Enden wird das eine mit einer Mareyschen Kapsel verbunden, deren Bewegungen auf ein Kymographion übertragen werden, das andere wird zur Einführung eines mechanischen Stimulators verwendet. Dieser besteht aus etwa 5 cm langen gekrümmten Schweine- oder Nylonborsten, die an einem Draht von ungefähr 30—40 cm Länge befestigt und verschieblich in einem Nélaton-Katheter (Nr. 5 oder 6) untergebracht sind. Der Katheter ist markiert, damit er stets gleich tief in die Trachea eingeführt werden kann. Das aus ihm herausragende freie Ende des Bürstendrahtes ist ebenfalls markiert, damit das Herausstoßen der Bürste aus dem Katheter und die Reizung der Trachealwand in gleichbleibender Weise vorgenommen werden kann. Die Borsten sollen bis zur Teilungsstelle der Trachea herabgeführt werden, weil dieser Teil der Luftröhre beim Hund am empfindlichsten ist.

Zur Provokation von Hustenattacken wird die Bürste mit einer Hand wiederholt aus dem Katheter herausgestoßen und wieder eingezogen, während die andere Hand die Lage des Katheters in der Kanüle fixiert. Die Hustenattacken sistieren sofort nach Beendigung der mechanischen Reizung. Eine einmalige Stimulation dauert 20—40 sec, sie kann in Intervallen von etwa 2 min wiederholt werden. Nach Beendigung eines Experimentes wird die Trachealkanüle entfernt, Haut und Trachealfistel werden mit 2%iger Mercurochrom-Lösung desinfiziert. Tägliche

Wiederholungen des Experimentes sind möglich, so daß nicht nur die akute antitussive Wirkung eines Pharmakons, sondern auch Gewöhnung an Hustensedativa nachgewiesen werden kann. Es ist günstig, ruhige Tiere zu verwenden. Das Winseln und Bellen nervöser Hunde läßt sich auf der Kurve schlecht von Hustenreaktionen unterscheiden.

b) Methode von Larsell und Burget

Kaninchen erhalten mit der Magensonde Urethan und zusätzlich Ätherinhalationen oder ausschließlich Äther, bis die operativen Vorbereitungen beendet sind. Hautschnitt in der Mittellinie, Freilegen der Trachea, Einbinden einer Y-förmigen Trachealkanüle, von der ein Seitenarm mit einer Mareyschen Kapsel verbunden wird. Durch den anderen kann die Trachealschleimhaut mit einer feinen Kamelhaarbürste, die am Ende eines dünnen Messingdrahtes befestigt ist, bestrichen werden. Die Reizempfindlichkeit der Trachea ist an der Teilungsstelle der Trachea am stärksten, tiefere Anteile des Tracheo-Bronchialbaums liefern weniger kräftige Reizantworten; auch sind diese Teile leichter verletzbar (Hämorrhagie). Nach der mechanischen Reizung verliert das betroffene Areal für 2—5 min seine Empfindlichkeit. Bei der Durchführung von Versuchen werden die Tiere unter leichter Äthernarkose gehalten. Infektionen der Atemwege verändern die Empfindlichkeit, vielleicht wegen der Bedeckung der Schleimhaut mit Sekreten.

c) Methode von May und Widdicombe

Einer Katze wird in Pentobarbital-Na-Narkose (32 ml/kg Nembutal i.p.) eine Trachealkanüle eingebunden. Das Tier wird dann in den Körper-Plethysmographen von Dawes, Mott und Widdicombe eingeschlossen und mit einem Polyäthylenkatheter durch kurzes Betupfen der Trachealschleimhaut in der Gegend der Bifurkation gereizt. Der Husten wird kymographisch über eine schwimmende Kapsel registriert; zusätzliche Registrierung von Atemvolumen und Reserveluft, von intratrachealem und intraoesophagalem Druck sowie von arteriellem Blutdruck.

Husten wird als Quotient aus:

$$\frac{\text{Volumen des initialen exspiratorischen Hustenstoßes}}{\text{durchschnittliches Volumen von 10 vorausgehenden Exspirationen}}$$

ausgedrückt.

Durchführung des Versuchs: Arzneimittel werden im 5 min- (Morphin und Pentobarbital) oder 10 min-Intervall (Codein und Pholcodin) intravenös verabfolgt. Sie werden in steigender Dosis gegeben, so daß die Einzeldosen summiert werden. Der Gesamtversuch dauert nicht länger als 1 Std. Nach jeder Injektion wird mehrere Minuten gewartet, ehe die Prüfung der Reflexerregbarkeit erfolgt. Im unmittelbaren Anschluß daran wird die nächste Prüfstoffinjektion gegeben.

Die Wirkung von Antitussiva wird aus Änderungen des o. a. Quotienten abgelesen und in Prozent des Ausgangswertes angegeben.

d) Methode von Tedeschi u. Mitarb.

Vorbereitende Operation: Bastardhunde mit einem Gewicht von 12—25 kg werden mit Pentobarbital-Na (30 mg/kg i.v.) narkotisiert. Hautschnitt in der Mittellinie des Halses, Freilegen der Trachea, 2 schmale Querincisionen in die Trachea zwischen 2 Knorpelringen (1,5 cm unterhalb des C. cricoides und 6 cm unterhalb des ersten Einschnittes). Durch die Incision wird eine Gummischlaufe mit einem aufgefädelten Eisenröhrchen eingeführt. Es ist ein mit schneckenförmiger Außenwindung und Innenbohrung versehener Eisenzylinder von 4 mm Durchmesser und 15 mm Länge. Die Gummischlaufe wird intratracheal mit Hilfe eines dünnen Drahtes an zwei metallischen Haltern aufgehängt, die in das Lumen der Trachea hineinragen. Sicherung der Metallarme in der Trachealwand durch Nähte von rostfreiem Stahldraht. Einfache Nähte — an die Enden der Einschnitte in die Trachea gelegt — beschränken die Möglichkeit zur Emphysembildung. Sorgfältiges Vernähen der Muskelfascie und Haut. Zur Unterstützung der postoperativen Pflege werden 10 mg Chlorpromazin i.m. und 300000—1000000 IE Penicillin i.m. verabfolgt. Nach der Operation wird eine Ruhepause von 1 bis 3 Wochen eingelegt.

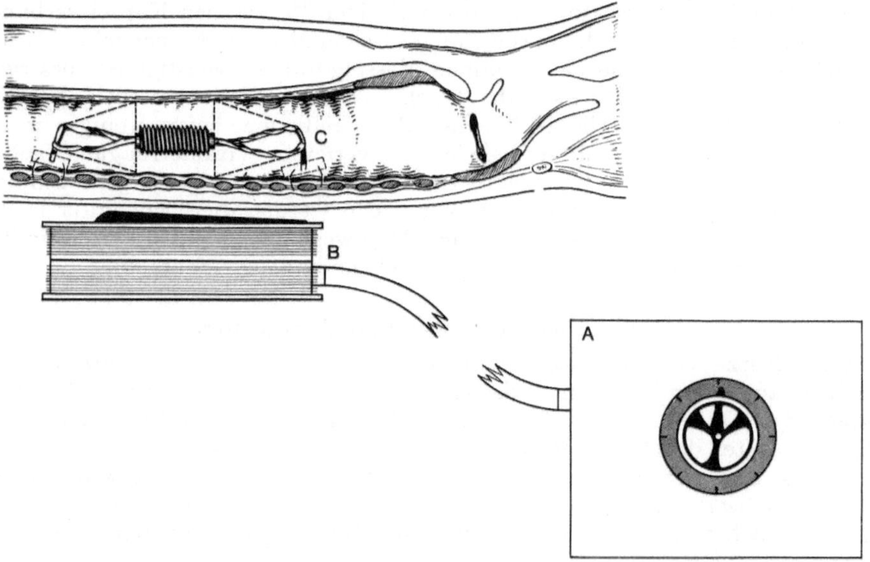

Abb. 1. Position des Eisenröhrchens in der Trachea in Ruhe und unter Magneteinwirkung. *A* Wchselstrom-Rheostat, *B* Elektromagnet, *C* Eisenröhrchen, in der Trachea aufgehängt. [Aus: Tedeschi et al.: J. Pharmacol. exp. Ther. **126**, 338 (1959)]

Husten wird durch vibrierende Schläge des Röhrchens gegen die Trachealwand erzeugt. Die Vibration wird durch einen Druck-Zugmagneten hervorgerufen (Modell Nr. K 200-MP I, National Acme Company, Cleveland 8, Ohio; in zweckdienlich modifizierter Form). Ein Transformator (Superior Electric Comp., Bristol, Connectic., Eingang: 120 V, Frequenz 50/60, Ausgang: 0—140 V, max. 45 A, 6,3 kVA) ermöglicht eine graduelle Steigerung der magnetischen Energie. Bei der „kritischen elektromagnetischen Kraft" werden die Mechanoreceptoren in der Trachea durch das Vibrieren des Eisenröhrchens gerade erregt. Bei der Prüfung von Pharmaka am hustenden Tier wird der Ausgang des Transformators um 20% über diesen Schwellenwert erhöht.

Durchführung des Versuchs: Der energiedurchflossene Elektromagnet wird 3 sec lang in Höhe des Eisenröhrchens an den Hals des Hundes gehalten. Dann folgt eine Ruhepause von 30 sec. Während dieses 33 sec-Intervalls werden die Hustenstöße in Form von Thoraxbewegungen mit einem Sphygmomanometer kymographisch registriert; gewöhnlich sind es 3—5. Diese Prozedur wird bei jedem Versuch 5mal wiederholt. Bei Arzneimittelprüfungen wird ein Leerversuch ausgeführt, dann wird der Prüfstoff s.c. oder oral (in Kapseln) verabreicht;

1—2 Std später wird erneut stimuliert. Gewöhnlich werden 3 Dosierungen von jedem Prüfstoff untersucht, jede Dosis an mindestens 5 Tieren. Abschließend wird die Dosis, die die Zahl der Hustenstöße um 50% reduziert, (ED_{50}), aus der Regressionsgeraden abgelesen. Dosisberechnung mit Grenzen für 95% Wahrscheinlichkeit nach Finney.

III. Chemische Stimulation

a) Methode von Larsell und Burget

Kaninchen in Äther- bzw. Urethan-Äthernarkose (s. S. 29). Freilegen der Trachea und Einbinden einer Y-förmigen Trachealkanüle. Ein Arm der Kanüle wird für die Registrierung von Hustenstößen mit einer Mareyschen Kapsel verbunden, durch den anderen wird aus einer Gummiblase Ammoniakdampf, Ätherdampf, Essigsäuredampf, Tabakrauch oder Formaldehyd eingeblasen. Im Augenblick der Reizgaszuführung atmet das Tier Frischluft mit starker Beimischung der irritierenden Stoffe ein. (Genauere Angaben über das Mischungsverhältnis von Reizgas und Luft sind nicht angegeben.) Vorsorglich wird verhütet, daß die reizenden Dämpfe die Nasenschleimhäute erreichen. Es gelingt, nahezu gleichmäßige Stimulationsperioden von 4—5 min Dauer zu erzeugen. Ammoniak-, Äther- oder Essigsäuredampf verursachen eine kräftige exspiratorische Reizantwort, die sich mehrere Male wiederholt. Anschließend kommt es, wenn Ammoniak in stärkerer Konzentration verwendet wird, zu einer 5—6 sec dauernden Apnoe, schließlich zur Polypnoe. Bei mehrfacher aufeinanderfolgender Reizung müssen Ruheperioden von 2—5 min zwischen Einzelreizungen eingelegt werden.

b) Methode von Friebel, Reichle und v. Graevenitz

Modifiziert von Friebel und Kuhn (1962), Kuhn und Friebel (1960)

Meerschweinchen werden einem Gemisch von SO_2 und Luft ausgesetzt. SO_2 wird einer handelsüblichen Gasflasche entnommen. Reduktion des Gasdruckes in 2 Stufen auf etwa 1 atü und dann mit einem Feinventil auf etwas mehr als 20 mm Hg. Der Betriebsdruck von genau 20 mm Hg wird mit einem Überlaufventil eingestellt und konstant erhalten, indem die überschießende Gasmenge über den offenen Schenkel eines in 10%ige Kochsalzlösung eintauchenden T-Stückes abgeleitet wird. Das mit 20 mm Hg Druck vor einer Glascapillare angestaute Gas fließt durch die Capillare dem Versuchsraum zu (10,6, 11 bzw. 13,4 ml SO_2/min), wird aber, bevor es den Versuchsraum erreicht, mit 15 l/min Preßluft gemischt. Das SO_2-Luftgemisch erfüllt den Versuchsraum und strömt aus ihm über eine Rohrleitung ins Freie ab. Ein Dreiwegehahn — zwischen die Capillare und den Zusammenfluß von Preßluft und SO_2 geschaltet — der gleichzeitig auch einen unmittelbaren Anschluß an die ins Freie führende Rohrleitung hat, gibt die Möglichkeit, das kontinuierlich der Flasche entströmende SO_2-Gas während der Pause zwischen 2 Versuchen unter Umgehung des Versuchsraumes direkt ins Freie zu leiten. Der Versuchsraum besteht aus einem Glastrog zur Aufnahme der Versuchstiere. In diesen Glastrog wird das Gas-Luftgemisch von unten her eingeleitet. Durch einen anderen Ansatzstutzen strömt es wieder nach unten ab. Ein dritter Ansatzstutzen dient zur Aufnahme von Harn und Kot. Über den Glastrog wird ein Glaszylinder gestülpt, der oben durch eine Cellophanmembran verschlossen ist. Auf den oberen Rand dieses Zylinders und über die Cellophanmembran wird ein mit Filz abgedichteter Deckel aus Holz gesetzt, der in einer flachen Höhlung zwei Mikrophone enthält, welche die im Zylinder entstehenden Geräusche aufnehmen. Ein Mikrophon ist über einen Verstärker mit einem Lautsprecher verbunden. Das andere Mikrophon ist an einen direktschreibenden Elektrokardiographen angeschlossen.

Durchführung der Versuche: Ein Meerschweinchen wird aufrecht in den Glastrog des Versuchsraumes gesetzt; dann wird der Glaszylinder über den Glastrog gestülpt. Anschließend wird mit dem Dreiwegehahn der SO_2-Strom — nach Durchmischung mit Preßluft — in den Versuchsraum eingeleitet. Nach 30—40 sec ist der Versuchsraum mit dem Gas-Luftgemisch gefüllt. Bei dieser Hahneinstellung werden die Tiere 2 min lang im Versuchsraum belassen und beobachtet. Zeitkontrolle mit der Stoppuhr. Husten sie während dieser Zeit, so wird die Zahl der Hustenstöße gezählt und notiert. 2 min nach Versuchsbeginn wird durch Drehen des Dreiwegehahns der SO_2-Strom unter Umgehung des Versuchsraumes in die Außenluft abgeführt, während die weiterhin hindurchströmende Preßluft den Versuchsraum in 10 sec von Gasresten freispült. Anschließend wird der Glaszylinder abgehoben und das Meerschweinchen herausgenommen. Unmittelbar

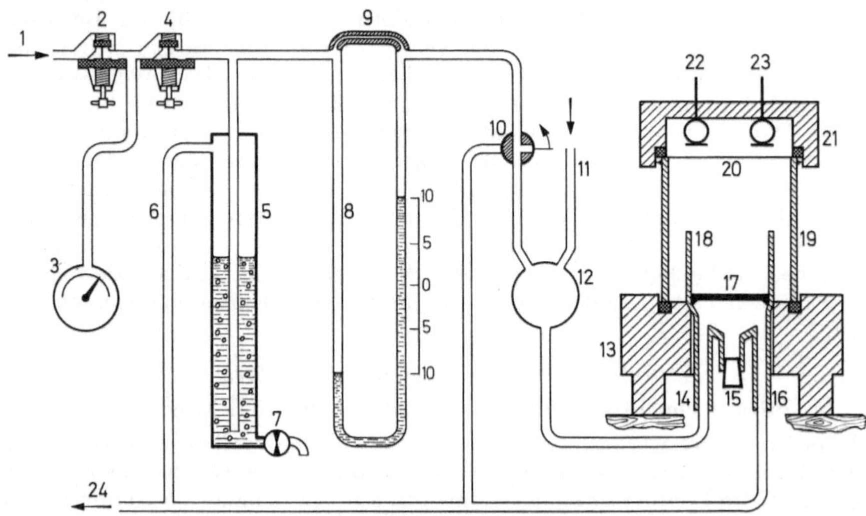

Abb. 2. Schema des Gerätes. *1* SO_2-Eingang, *2* Druckminderer, 1. Stufe, *3* Manometer, *4* Druckminderer, 2. Stufe, *5* T-förmiges Glasrohr und Überlaufgefäß zum Abführen der überschießenden Gasmenge, *6* Ableitung für überschüssiges Gas, *7* Füllstutzen, *8* Manometer, *9* Capillare. *10* Dreiwegehahn, *11* Preßluft-Eingang, *12* Mischkugel, *13* Fußteil des Versuchsraumes, *14* Ansatzstutzen für die Gas-Luftzuführung, *15* Ansatzstutzen für Harn- und Kotentleerung, *16* Ansatzstutzen für die Gas-Luftableitung, *17* Bodenplatte, *18* Glastrog zur Aufnahme des Versuchstieres, *19* Glaszylinder, *20* Cellophanmembran, *21* Holzdeckel, *22* u. *23* Mikrophon, *24* Abführung des SO_2-Luftgemisches ins Freie

anschließend kann das nächste Tier in den Glastrog gesetzt und in derselben Weise behandelt werden. Auf diese Weise wird alle 3 min ein Testergebnis erhalten.

Die Reizbarkeit der Tiere und die Zahl der von den einzelnen Tieren gelieferten Hustenstöße schwankt von Versuch zu Versuch, soweit sie an verschiedenen Tagen durchgeführt werden. Werden die Tiere aber zweimal innerhalb 1 Std dem SO_2-Gemisch ausgesetzt, so husten sie mit großer Regelmäßigkeit zum zweiten Male (96,2% der Tiere). Es werden daher die jeweils reizempfindlichsten Tiere unmittelbar vor dem Versuch aus einem größeren Tierkollektiv ausgewählt. Wenn zwischen 2 Versuchstagen einwöchige Ruhepausen eingeschaltet werden, können die Tiere mehrmals zu Versuchen herangezogen werden. In den Wintermonaten haben Meerschweinchen vielfach eine erhöhte Reizbarkeit, die berücksichtigt werden muß.

Bei der Arzneimittelprüfung werden jeweils 20 mit derselben Arzneimitteldosis vorbehandelte Meerschweinchen hintereinander in den Versuchsraum gebracht. Die arzneibedingte Herabsetzung der Reizempfindlichkeit wird in der Regel 30 min nach der Injektion eines Medikamentes geprüft. Die hustenverhütende Wirkung einer Prüfsubstanz wird im Einzelfall als bewiesen angesehen, wenn 30 min nach der s.c. Arzneimittelinjektion kein einziger Hustenstoß mehr registriert wird. Prüfung jeder Arzneimitteldosis an 20 Meerschweinchen, mathematische Behandlung der Versuchsergebnisse nach Litchfield und Wilcoxon. Im Laufe eines Arbeitstages können, einschließlich der Auswahl reizempfindlicher Meerschweinchen, an 40 Tieren Arzneimittelprüfungen durchgeführt werden.

c) Methode von Kelentey u. Mitarb. (1957)

Bei Meerschweinchen und Mäusen wird ein 1%iges SO_2-Luftgemisch zur Auslösung von Husten verwendet. Die Reduktion der Hustenfrequenz durch Pharmaka gibt ein Maß für die antitussive Wirkung.

d) Methode von Reichle und Friebel

Bei der Verwendung von Ratten kann bis auf geringfügige Änderungen mit der von Friebel, Reichle und v. Graevenitz (S. 31) beschriebenen Methode gearbeitet werden. Die Konzentration von SO_2 im SO_2-Luftgemisch muß auf 18,2 cm^2/min erhöht und der Versuchsraum abgeändert werden. Zu- und Ableitung des Gas-Luftgemisches in einem Glaskäfig ($23 \times 13 \times 13$) mit Metallrahmen, dessen Deckplatte das Mikrophon trägt. Öffnen des Versuchsraumes durch Abnehmen einer Seitenwand. Als Versuchstiere werden weibliche Albinoratten im Gewicht von 120—200 g verwandt. Die Arbeitsweise entspricht sonst völlig den früheren Angaben. Die Tiere verhalten sich im gasdurchströmten Versuchsraum ähnlich wie Meerschweinchen, sie niesen aber häufiger und die Hustenstöße sind weniger kräftig und daher schwerer zu hören. Husten und Niesen lassen sich aber bei ständigem Beobachten sicher unterscheiden. Wie Meerschweinchen zeigen auch die Ratten jahreszeitlich bedingte Veränderungen der Hustenbereitschaft und Arzneiempfindlichkeit, wenn auch in geringerem Maße. Darüber hinaus beeinflussen Alter und Gewicht die Testergebnisse, junge Tiere sind reizempfindlicher. Auswechseln der Versuchstiere nach 3monatiger Verwendung.

e) Methode von Winter und Flataker (1952)

Ein Hund wird in einen aus Holz und Glas hergestellten Käfig von ungefähr 56 cm Breite und Länge und 42 cm Höhe gesetzt. Durch 2 Öffnungen wird aus preßluftbetriebenen (400 mm Hg) Vaponephrin-Verneblern ein feines N/2 H_2SO_4-Aerosol eingeleitet. Expositionszeit 5 min. Übertragung des Hustengeräusches von einem Kehlkopfmikrophon am Hund zum Kopfhörer des Beobachters.

Durchführung der Versuche: Vor der Anwendung von Pharmaka werden 2 Leerversuche durchgeführt. Zuführung von Pharmaka in Form von Gelatinekapseln oder in wäßriger Lösung mit der Magensonde nach 18stündigem Fasten oder durch s.c. Injektion. Nachfolgend stündlich erneute Hustenprovokation bis zum Abklingen der Wirkung. Bewertet wird die Abnahme der Hustenfrequenz. Zwischen 2 Expositionen wird eine Ruhepause von einer Woche eingelegt. Toleranz, wachsende Empfindlichkeit oder Erkrankungen der Luftwege treten unter dieser Arbeitsweise nicht auf.

f) Methode von de Vleeschhouwer

Sie ist eine Modifikation der Methode von Winter und Flataker (S. 33). Den Hunden wird 2 Std vor Versuchsbeginn 0,25 g/kg Urethan i.m. verabfolgt, um die allgemeine Erregbarkeit herabzusetzen. Das H_2SO_4-Aerosol wird mit einem Druck von 175 bzw. 380 mm Hg (= 0,5—0,7 kg/cm³) entwickelt. Der Käfig ist etwas größer als der von Winter und Flataker (70 × 40 × 40), er kann mit Luft durchströmt werden.

g) Methode von Winter und Flataker (1954)

Meerschweinchen werden in zylindrische Glasröhrchen von 23 cm Länge und 10,5 cm Durchmesser gesetzt. Die Enden der horizontal liegenden Rohre werden

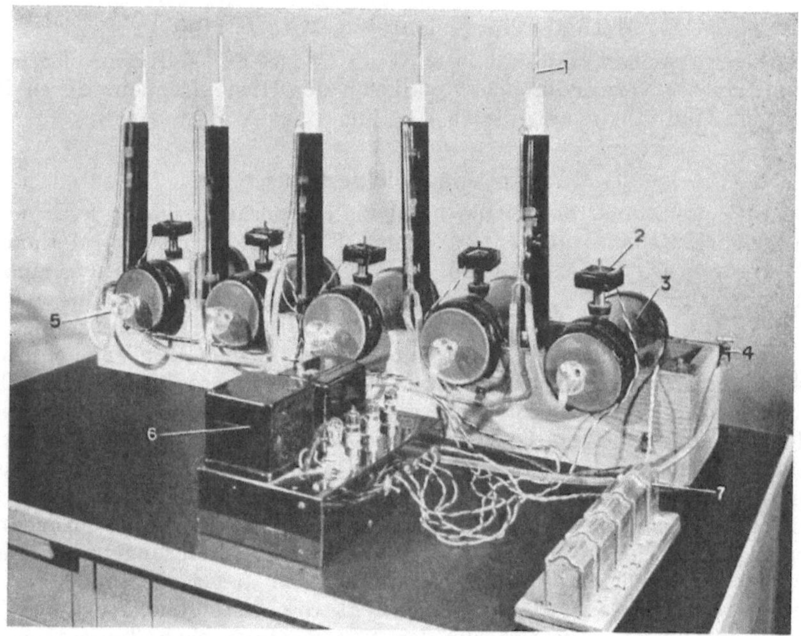

Abb. 3. Gerät zur Registrierung von Husten bei Meerschweinchen (rückwärtige Ansicht). *1* Quecksilber-Manometer, *2* Detektor, *3* Tierkammer, beachte die steife Drahtgaze, die das Tier hindert, den Luftzu- und -abfluß zu blockieren, *4* Druckluftventil, *5* Vernebler, *6* elektronische Schalteinrichtung, *7* Zählwerke. [Aus: Winter u. Flataker: J. Pharmacol. exp. Ther. **112**, 99 (1954)]

mit Gummistopfen verschlossen. Durch einen Stopfen wird das Mundstück eines Vaponephrin-Verneblers geleitet, durch den gegenüberliegenden Stopfen wird das Aerosol abgesaugt. Der Vernebler wird mit 2 ml einer 28%igen Ammoniaklösung gefüllt und 3 min lang mit Preßluft (100 mm/Hg) betrieben. Fünf derartige Kammern können gleichzeitig betätigt werden. Nach jedem Einzelversuch muß der im Vernebler bleibende Ammoniakrest entfernt werden.

Nachweis von Husten mit einem Detektor, einer kleinen Bakelitkapsel, die mit Hilfe eines Gummistopfens in das Glasrohr eingefügt ist. Er enthält eine auf eine Gummimembrane aufgeklebte Metallplatte, die bei Druckschwankungen (Husten) gegen eine Metallschraube geschleudert wird. Die Empfindlichkeit des Detektors kann durch Verstellen der Schraube geändert werden, so daß Hustenstöße ohne oder mit begleitenden Atmungsbewegungen registriert werden.

Summierung der Impulse und automatische Einschaltung von Registrierperioden über ein elektrisches Relais. Für Arzneimittelprüfungen werden Tiere ausgewählt, die bei 3 min dauernder Ammoniakeinwirkung 10—40 Hustenstöße liefern. Die Empfindlichkeit einzelner Tiere kann von Tag zu Tag wechseln, aber bei Versuchen, die an demselben Tag im 1 Std-Intervall vorgenommen werden, bleibt sie gleich.

Durchführung der Versuche: Zunächst wird ein Leerversuch vorgenommen, dann das Arzneimittel injiziert und eine Std später erneut getestet. Kontrolltiere werden mit physiologischer Kochsalzlösung behandelt. Aus der Reduktion der Hustenfrequenz wird auf antitussive Wirkung geschlossen.

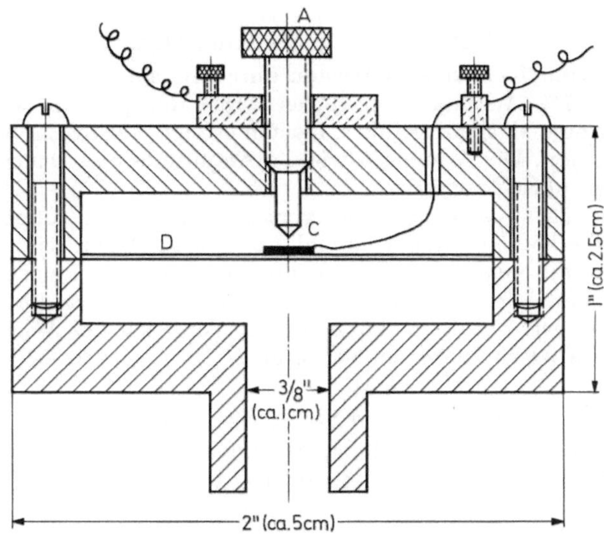

Abb. 4. Aufriß des Detektors (Teil 2 der Abb. 3). *A* verstellbare Schraube, *C* Metallplatte, befestigt auf *D* Gummimembran. [Aus: Winter u. Flataker: J. Pharmacol. exp. Ther. **112**, 99 (1954)]

h) Methode von Rosiere, Winder und Wax

Vorbereitende Operation: Hunde werden in kurzdauernder Barbiturat-anaesthesie unter septischen Bedingungen operiert. Hautincision seitwärts der Mittellinie, Eröffnung der Trachea. Etwa 3 cm unterhalb des Larynx wird eine Polyäthylenkanüle (Durchmesser 3,7 mm innen, 4,8 mm außen) in die Trachea eingelegt, über die 2 Halbzylinder als Flansch geschoben sind. Der eine Halbzylinder wird mit einem Kanülende in die Trachea eingebracht, der andere so über die Trachea gelegt, daß die Öffnung von beiden Seiten bedeckt wird. Mit vier feinen Nähten aus rostfreiem Stahldraht werden sie miteinander verbunden. Das Ende der Kanüle ragt ungefähr 2,5 cm über die Haut hinaus. Hautverschluß mit Wundklammern, Schlußdesinfektion des Operationsgebietes, 300000 bis 1000000 IE Procain-Penicillin. Trockene Bandage.

Durchführung der Versuche: Ungefähr eine Woche nach der Operation werden die Hunde für den Versuch trainiert. Nach 24stündigem Hunger und ohne die Möglichkeit, die experimentellen Manipulationen beobachten zu können, werden die Tiere über die Trachealkanüle mit Ammoniakgas gereizt. Zunächst wird durch die Kanüle ein konstanter vorgewärmter und in Wasserdampf gesättigter Luftstrom von 0,7 l/min geleitet. Diesem wird bei Bedarf 0,9—2,1 ml reines wasserfreies Ammoniakgas, unter atmosphärischem Druck in einer Spritze aufgezogen, beigemischt. Die Empfindlichkeit der Tiere bleibt bei wiederholten Versuchen in der Regel gleich, nur gelegentlich, z. B. bei freudiger Erregung tritt spontanes Husten auf. Zum Erbrechen kommt es erst bei beträchtlicher Erhöhung der Ammoniakkonzentration. Der Husten ist gut hörbar. Verwechslungen mit Niesen oder anderen Atmungsreflexen kamen nicht vor. Der Husten wird durch eine Kombination von Pneumogramm, Beobachten der Tiere und akustischer Wahrnehmung des Hustens registriert, wobei der Ton das wesentlichste Kriterium ist. Mit der Überlebenszeit operierter Tiere von durchschnittlich mehr als 157 Tagen kann gerechnet werden.

i) Methode von Stefko und Denzel

Bei narkotisierten Katzen wird Husten durch Inhalation von Frischluft und Beimischung von 7% Ammoniak produziert. Das Reizgas wird am Ende einer Exspiration über eine Maske zugeführt. Husten erfolgt regelmäßig bei der darauffolgenden Inspiration. Die Atmung sowie die Amplitude und Dauer des Hustens werden pneumographisch registriert.

Durchführung der Versuche: Die vorausgehende Kontrollperiode dauert 12 min; das Tier erhält alle 3 min einmal Ammoniak. Dann wird der Prüfstoff oral oder parenteral zugeführt. Die Veränderungen der Reizempfindlichkeit werden anschließend alle 5 min aufgezeichnet, bis die Ausgangsempfindlichkeit wieder eingetreten ist. Die Tiere können zum Vergleich der Wirksamkeit verschiedener Stoffe wiederholt verwendet werden.

k) Methode von Silvestrini und Maffii

Meerschweinchen werden durch Acroleindampf zum Husten gereizt. Die hustenhemmende Wirkung wird anhand der Reduktion der Hustenfrequenz bewertet.

l) Methode von Gösswald

Meerschweinchen inhalieren 2 min lang 20%igen Citronensäurespray. Der Prozentsatz der Tiere, bei denen Antitussiva den Husten vollständig unterdrücken, wird bestimmt.

m) Methode von Kroepfli

Katzen werden mit 60—70 mg/kg Aprobarbital i.p. und 20 γ/kg Atropin sulf. s.c. narkotisiert. Freilegung und Querdurchschneidung der Trachea. Eine Spezialkanüle mit zwei Seitenästen wird in die Trachea gelegt, durch die die Atemluft ihren natürlichen Weg nehmen kann. Husten wird durch Einblasen von Seifenpulverpartikelchen, die ca. 30 μ Durchmesser haben und unregelmäßig gezackt sind, erzeugt. Das Einblasen erfolgt über den einen Seitenast der Kanüle.

Durchführung der Versuche: In einer Delle des zum Einblasen bestimmten Seitenastes werden 8 mg Seifenpulver deponiert. Dann wird seine Verbindung zur Trachea abgeklemmt und in ihm mit Hilfe eines Druckreservoirs von ca. 40 ml ein Überdruck von ca. 0,1 atü erzeugt. Schließlich wird das Pulver durch Öffnen einer Klemme mit genau 4 ml Luft gegen die Bifurcatio geblasen. Das Einblasen wird zu Beginn einer Inspiration vorgenommen. Die eingeblasene Luftquantität muß bei der Ermittlung der Atemlage in Rechnung gestellt werden. Der ausgelöste Hustenanfall besteht aus 5—15 einzelnen Hustenstößen. Das Charakteristische des Hustens wird darin gesehen, daß während der Exspiration der Trachealseitendruck abrupt und über die Norm hinaus ansteigt. Er wird über den zweiten Seitenast der Trachealkanüle gemessen. Die erreichte Druckhöhe gibt ein gewisses Maß für die Luftströmungsgeschwindigkeit und die Stärke des

Hustens. Beim einzelnen Hustenanfall werden die Hustenstöße bis zum 5. Hustenstoß zunehmend stärker. Reizungen werden in viertelstündigem Intervall vorgenommen, wobei die Hustenanfälle im ganzen allmählich schwächer werden, die einzelnen Hustenstöße innerhalb eines Anfalls aber stärker. Zuführung von Arzneimitteln i.v., Steigerung der Dosis bis zur Feststellung der sicher hustenmindernden Grenzdosis. Filmbildung auf der Trachealschleimhaut und hiervon ausgehende Änderungen der Ansprechbarkeit müssen beachtet werden (Pellmont und Bächtold).

n) Methode von Eichler und Smiatek[1] (1940)

Als Reizstoff werden Nebel von H_2SO_4 verwendet. Diese werden aber auf eine besondere Art hergestellt. Die Anordnung (nach Eichler, 1961) sei auf Abb. 5 wiedergegeben, weil sie wichtig zu sein scheint.

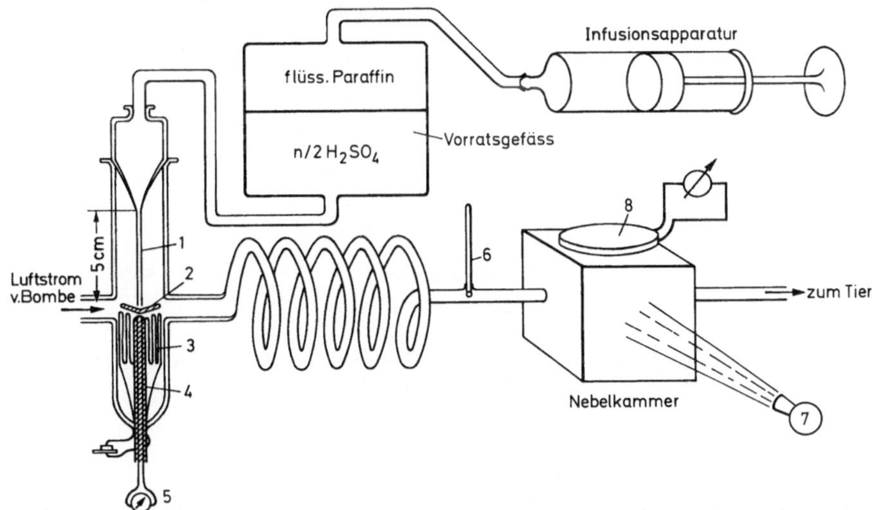

Abb. 5. Arch. int. Pharmacodyn. **133**, 11 (1961). *1* Quarzcapillare, durch die die n/2 H_2SO_4 durchgedrückt wird (0,001—0,01 ml/min). *2* Quarztrichter zum Verdampfen. *3* Heizkörper aus Platindraht. *4* Röhre mit Thermosäule aus Pt-Platin Iridium zur Kontrolle der Temperatur. *5* Galvanometer zur Messung des Thermostroms. *6* Thermometer zur Kontrolle der Lufttemperatur (< 25°). *7* Bogenlampe zur Erzeugung des Tyndallichtes, das durch Photozelle *8* gemessen wird

Die Temperatur auf dem Quarztrichter muß auf 800—900° gesteigert werden, um einen dann aber für viele Stunden absolut gleichmäßigen Nebel zu liefern. Der Heizkörper aus Platindraht selbst hergestellt, kam zur Glut. Vielleicht spendet er zugleich auf diese Weise die Kondensationskeime.

Die verdampfte Schwefelsäure wurde mit getrockneter Luft (ca. 1 l/min) fortgeführt. Die dann eingeatmeten Nebelteilchen erreichten so eine Konzentration von 60—70% H_2SO_4.

Wie auf Abb. 6 wiedergegeben, kann die Konzentration durch Zusatz von Luft verdünnt werden, wodurch die Schwefelsäurekonzentration natürlich weitersteigt. Wichtig ist, daß der so erzeugte Nebel nicht einem Gefäß zugeführt wird, in dem sich das Tier befindet. Durch den Wasserdampf der Ausatmungsluft wird die Säurekonzentration der Nebelteilchen herabgesetzt und sie verlieren ihre

1 Von O. Eichler.

Wirksamkeit. Der Nebel muß den Tieren in stetem Strom durch eine Maske zugeführt werden. Das kann man gleich dazu benutzen, um die Hustenstöße mit einer Mareykapsel zu registrieren. Durch die Einrichtung der Ventile und einer Drosselung kann es gelingen, daß man vorwiegend die Hustenstöße bei ganz kleiner Atmung registriert. Sicher gibt es teurere Vorrichtungen, die diese Aufgabe besser erfüllen, wie auf verschiedenen Seiten dieses Buches dargestellt wird (s. Methode Friebel S. 45 und Methode S. 35).

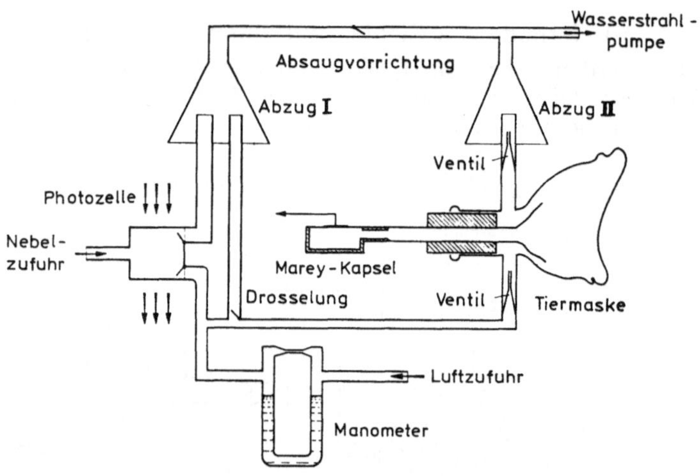

Abb. 6. Naunyn-Schmiedebergs Arch. exp. Path. Pharmakol. **194**, 622, Abb. 1 (1940) nach Eichler und Smiatek

Die Aerosole erwiesen sich aus drei Gründen als brauchbar.

1. Sie sind bei der Einatmung fein dispers und können so leicht an den oberen Atemwegen vorbeigeführt werden. Der Dispersitätsgrad wurde nicht gemessen, sondern nur aus der etwas bläulichen Farbe erschlossen.

2. Die Teilchen gewinnen durch Aufnahme von Wasserdampf an Durchmesser, so daß weniger ausgeatmet werden. Die Zunahme des Volumens der neuen Partikel ließ sich durch größere Dichtigkeit des Nebels mit der Photozelle nachweisen.

3. Die Säurekonzentration ist so groß, daß die Bronchialwände geschädigt werden. Verdampft man $n/4$ H_2SO_4, so geht die Wirksamkeit zurück. Es entsteht ein Husten, der viele Wochen anhält, und durch den Hustenmittel nachgewiesen werden können. Die Registrierung erfolgt mit der obigen Vorrichtung, aber ohne Nebelzufuhr.

In der betreffenden Arbeit werden die Mengen des eingeatmeten Nebels durch das Produkt Konzentration × Zeit angegeben, wie es Flury bei der Beurteilung von Kampfstoffen definiert hat. Konzentration in mg im l, Zeit in min der Einatmung. Uns erwiesen sich $c \cdot t$-Produkte von 2000—3000 als geeignet. Gezählt wurde die Zahl der Hustenstöße. Geprüft wurde Morphin und Dicodid, Gabe von Cardiazol führte nicht zur Reduktion der Wirksamkeit von Dicodid. In einer späteren Arbeit (O. Eichler und Scholtze, 1940) wurde noch ein Präparat aus Lactuca virosa schwach wirksam gefunden.

o) Methode von Sanzari et al.

Man hat schon früher beim Menschen beobachtet, daß durch intravenöse Injektion von Lobelin ein Hustenanfall erfolgte, dem eine langdauernde Tachypnoe folgte. Das wurde auch zur Testung von hustendämpfenden Mitteln am Menschen benutzt (s. S. 65). Der Erfolg war nicht gut, weil im Lobelin eine Wirkung zur zentralen Erzeugung von Husten einherging mit einer lähmenden Wirkung über die Ganglien. Außerdem zeigte sich eine Tachyphylaxie. Diese Symptome lassen sich nach Sanzari *et al.* (1968) vermeiden, wenn man eine andere Substanz anwendet, die auch ganglienblockierend wirkt, nämlich 1,1-Dimethyl-4-phenylpiperaziniumjodid (DMPP).

Die Zufuhr muß intravenös und rasch erfolgen. Als Versuchstiere dienten gesunde erwachsene Katzen, die mit 80 mg/kg i.p. Chloralose narkotisiert wurden. Das Narkoticum unterdrückte keine Reflexe. Die Dosierung hat in dem Bereich von 5—100 μg/kg zu erfolgen, denn hier steigt die Zahl der Hustenstöße mit der Dosis. In höheren Gaben können sich spastische Hustenanfälle und schließlich eine Ganglienblockade bemerkbar machen. Bei Dosen von mehr als 10 μg/kg findet sich vorher eine kurze Hypotonie, anschließend eine Apnoe, auch eine Blutdrucksteigerung und Bradykardie. Alle Symptome sind in 5 min abgeklungen, so daß eine neue Testung vorgenommen werden kann. Es gibt weder Kumulation noch Tachyphylaxie.

Bei der Testung kann man auf zwei Wegen vorgehen. Entweder werden im Abstand von 5 min 5, 10, 15, 20, 25, 50 und 100 μg/kg verabfolgt, nachdem 10 min vorher die zu testende Substanz gegeben wurde. Oder man verwendet eine einzelne fixierte Dosis DMPP, läßt die zu testende Substanz folgen und schließlich gibt man wieder die vorherige Dosis. Gerechnet wird nach der Zahl der Hustenstöße. Beide Methoden geben dieselben relativen Werte. Eine große Zahl von Substanzen wird mit d-Metorphon verglichen.

Substanzen, die ganglioplegisch wirken, dürfen nicht verwendet werden, weil sie den DMPP-Husten unterdrücken können.

IV. Elektrische Stimulation

a) Methode von Schroeder

Der Vagus von Hunden wird an einer Halsseite operativ in einen Hautschlauch verlagert und am wachen Tier durch einen in Form und Stärke genau dosierbaren elektrischen Reiz erregt. Die Operation entspricht im Prinzip derjenigen der Carotisschlinge. Sie muß streng aseptisch vorgenommen werden, um eine entzündliche Reizung des Vagus zu vermeiden. Hautschnitt in der Mittellinie, 7 cm lang, am unteren Rande des Cricoid beginnend. Ein zweiter Hautschnitt wird im Abstand von 3—3,5 cm vom ersten entfernt angelegt, er verläuft über 5 cm parallel und endet cranial und caudal bogenförmig, wie in der Abb. 7 angegeben. Die beiden Zwickel, die so entstehen, werden später unter der gebildeten Schlinge eingeschlagen. Dann wird die Hautbrücke zwischen den beiden parallelen Schnitten einschließlich der Zwickel von der Subcutis gelöst und durch einen breiten, mit physiologischer Kochsalzlösung angefeuchteten Gazestreifen lateralwärts gezogen. Nach Durchtrennung der oberflächlichen Muskeln und Fascien des Halses präpariert man zwischen dem M. sternocleidomastoideus und M. sternohyoideus stumpf in die Tiefe, bis die Gefäßnervenscheide mit der A. carotis und dem N. vagus in einem Bereich von 10 cm freiliegt. Nun wird der Nerv in dem ganzen Bereich von 10 cm bis an die Teilungsstelle für den Abgang der A. thyreoidea sup. aus der Scheide herausgelöst und zur Hautbrücke in den Gazestreifen hineingenommen. Der Nerv muß über eine ausreichende Strecke freipräpariert werden, damit er bei der folgenden Verlagerung nicht zu stark gezerrt wird. Der anschließende Wundverschluß erfolgt schichtweise und mit solcher Sorgfalt, daß Nachblutungen und damit Druckschädigungen durch Hämatome vermieden werden. Zunächst wird der Muskelspalt durch fünf versenkte Catgutnähte wieder verschlossen. Dabei ist besonders darauf zu achten, daß die Stelle des Nervendurchtrittes nicht zu eng und nicht zu weit wird. Die letzte Muskelnaht soll etwa 1 cm vom Nerven entfernt sein. Diese Nahtstelle muß besonders gut versenkt werden, um eine Druckschädigung des Nerven durch das Nahtmaterial zu vermeiden. Bevor der Muskelspalt verschlossen wird, ist es zweckmäßig, einen etwa 1 cm breiten Streifen des medialen Randes des M. sternocleidomastoideus zu entfernen. Hierzu klemmt man ein entsprechendes Stück des mittleren Muskelrandes in zwei

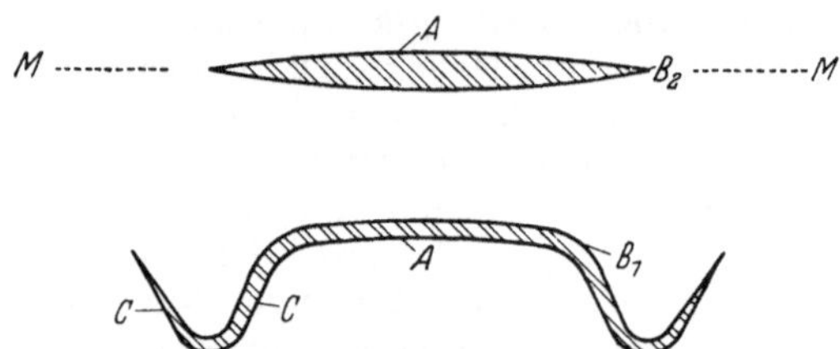

Abb. 7. Schnittführung bei der Vagusschlingenoperation. Die Subcutis, welche infolge des Auseinanderklaffens der Wundränder sichtbar wird, ist gestrichelt gezeichnet. $M \ldots M$ Mittellinie des Halses. A wird an A, B_1 unter der hochgehobenen Hautbrücke an B_2 und C an C angenäht. [Aus: Schroeder: Naunyn-Schmiedebergs Arch. exp. Path. Pharmak. **212**, 433 (1951)]

scharfe Klemmen, schneidet dazwischen durch und reißt die in die Klemmen eingefaßten Muskelfasern nach cranial und caudal möglichst weit bis zum Muskelansatz ab. Erst dann werden die Muskelstümpfe mit dem Messer abgetrennt. Jetzt wird die Haut über dem verschlossenen Muskelspalt durch kräftige subcutane Catgutfäden (von A nach A der Abb. 7) zusammengezogen und danach die Subcutis der Hautbrücke um den Nerven durch feine Catgutfäden zu einer Schlinge zusammengefügt. Man beginnt in der Mitte der Hautbrücke und setzt die Nähte möglichst weit vom Nerven entfernt so weit ein, daß die Hautränder gut adaptiert werden. In den Ecken müssen die Zwickel in der Weise eingeschlagen werden, daß die Zwickelspitzen in die Mittellinie zu liegen kommen. Der Punkt B_1 wird unter der Hautbrücke an den Punkt B_2 herangebracht und durch feine (subcutane) Catgutfäden angenäht. Durch die Zwickel wird erreicht, daß alle Nähte in den „Ecken" nervenfern liegen und der Nerv weder durch Nahtdruck noch durch eine lokale Infektion beim Aufgehen einer Nahtstelle unmittelbar geschädigt werden kann. Wenn alle Catgutnähte gelegt sind, kann die Schlinge durch feine Seidenknopfnähte (im Abstand von 1 cm) endgültig verschlossen werden. Für die Nähte zwischen A—A und C—C (das ist der Hautbereich, aus dem der Zwickel stammt), sollen kräftige Seidenfäden verwendet werden. Bei einigen Hunden, die eine sehr straffe Haut besitzen, müssen die seitlichen Hautpartien in einem Bereich von 3—4 cm von ihrer Unterhaut gelöst werden, um zu vermeiden, daß die Hautnähte unter eine zu große Spannung geraten. Bei der ganzen Operation ist auf eine sorgfältige Blutstillung zu achten, damit der Nerv nicht durch den Druck eines Hämatoms geschädigt wird.

Nach der Operation wäscht man die Schlinge mit steriler Kochsalzlösung, jodiert die Nähte und füllt den Raum unter der Schlinge *reichlich* mit 1%iger sterilisierter Silbernitratsalbe aus. Auf das gesamte Operationsgebiet kommt eine ebenfalls dick mit Silbernitratsalbe bestrichene Mullage, die locker mit sterilen

Papierbinden (keine Mullbinden, welche die Schlinge strangulieren) befestigt wird. Die Salbe wirkt als Schmiermittel, in dem die Schlinge bei Bewegungen des Halses gleiten kann. Beim trocknenen Wundverband pflegt die Schlinge mit der Umgebung zu verkleben, wodurch die Nähte bei Bewegungen des Halses leicht aufgerissen werden können. Nun folgt eine doppelte Wattelage, wieder Papierbinden und schließlich ein Gipsverband, der an den Ohren beginnt und den ganzen Thorax einschließt. Der Gipsverband muß auf der Rückseite durch zwei Aluminiumschienen verstärkt werden.

Der erste Verbandwechsel erfolgt am 5. Tage nach der Operation. Hierzu wird der Gipsverband auf beiden Seiten des Halses durchtrennt und die untere U-

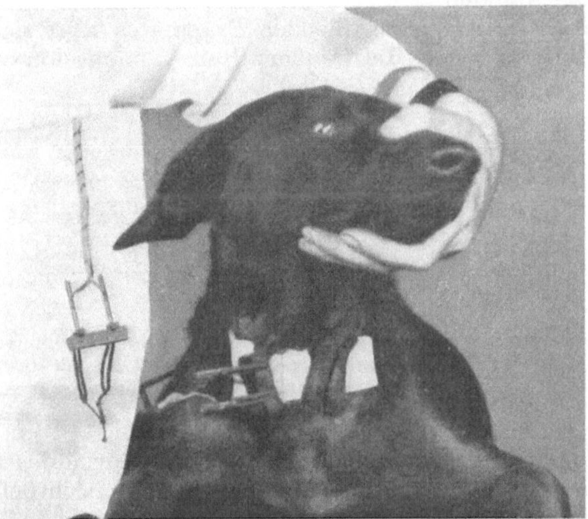

Abb. 8. Originalphoto eines Hundes mit 2 Vagusschlingen und 1 Carotisschlinge (in der Mitte). An der rechten Vagusschlinge ist eine Reizelektrode angelegt, deren Konstruktion aus der hängenden Elektrode (auf der linken Bildseite) ersichtlich ist. [Aus: Schroeder: Naunyn-Schmiedebergs Arch. exp. Path. Pharmak. **212**, 433 (1951)]

förmige Schale abgenommen. Dann wird die Watte mit der Mullage entfernt und das Wundgebiet mit einem sterilen, trockenen Tupfer vorsichtig gesäubert. Anschließend deckt man die Wunde durch eine sterile, mit Silbernitratsalbe dick bestrichene Mullage ab und wickelt die mit Watte frisch gepolsterte Gipsschale mit einer Gipsbinde wieder an. Am 8. Tag nach der Operation entfernt man den ganzen Verband und zieht die vorher jodierten Fäden. Nochmaliger Salbenverband, der nach Wattepolsterung mit 1—2 Gipsbinden am Hals fixiert werden muß, damit der Hund durch Kratzen den Verband nicht entfernen kann. Im Abstand von 2—3 Tagen müssen die Verbände bis zur vollständigen Abheilung wiederholt werden, wobei jedesmal das ganze Wundgebiet mit Wundbenzin gereinigt wird. Wichtig ist, daß der Hund nach dem Abheilen etwa 4 Wochen lang eine breite Ledermanschette um den Hals trägt, um ein Kratzen an der Schlinge zu verhindern. Nach dieser Zeit sind die Haare an der Schlingenhaut wieder gewachsen und stellen einen natürlichen Schutz derselben dar, so daß sich die Ledermanschette nach dieser Zeit erübrigt. Vier Wochen nach der Operation kann das Tier bereits zu Versuchen benutzt werden.

Für die elektrische Reizung der Vagusschlinge benötigt man ein Gerät, mit dem man die Reizfrequenz von 0,1—100 Hz regeln kann. Das von Wagner und Wetterer angegebene Gerät wird empfohlen. Reizung mit den von dem Gerät gelieferten „sehr kurzen spitzen" Spannungsstößen. Als Elektroden dienen 2—3 cm dicke, mit physiologischer Kochsalzlösung angefeuchtete Wollfäden, welche die Schlinge in einem Abstand von 2,5 cm umfassen. Die Wollfäden besitzen an ihrem Ende je ein dünnes Gummiband, das mit einer Öse an die Metallstifte der Stromzuführung angehängt wird (s. Abb. 8). Die Spannung der Gummibänder darf nur geradeso groß sein, daß sich die Wollfäden gut anlegen. Ein zu starker Druck auf den Vagus macht sich bald durch eine Erhöhung der Herzfrequenz bemerkbar. Um eine gleichmäßige Durchfeuchtung der Wollfäden über 2—3 Std zu garantieren, empfiehlt es sich, jeden Metallstift der Elektroden mit einem wattegefüllten Metallröhrchen zu umgeben und jeweils einen kleinen Wattezipfel an einen Wollfaden anzubinden.

Die Wirksamkeit eines hustenstillenden Präparates zeigt sich an einer charakteristischen Änderung der Reizfrequenz-Reizspannungskurve. Es ist daher

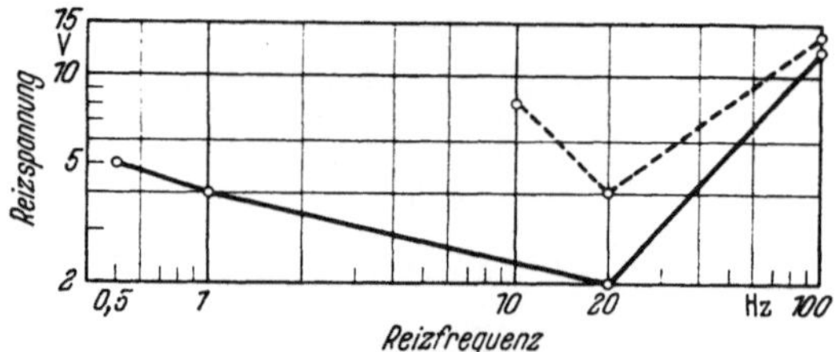

Abb. 9. Reizfrequenz-Reizspannungskurve. Ausgezogene Linie: normales Tier, gestrichelte Linie: 10 min nach der i.v. Injektion von 0,25 mg/kg 1-Polamidon. *Hz* Reizfrequenz in Hertz, *V* Reizspannung in Volt. [Aus: Schroeder: Naunyn-Schmiedebergs Arch. exp. Path. Pharmak. **212**, 433 (1951)]

notwendig, zunächst die Reizfrequenz-Reizspannungskurve des normalen Tieres zu ermitteln. Ihr typischer Verlauf ist aus der Abb. 9 ersichtlich.

Die Werte der „normalen" Kurve sind jedoch beim gleichen Tier nicht immer konstant, sondern zeigen sowohl für die Reizfrequenz als auch für die Reizspannung von Tag zu Tag geringe Differenzen. Die unterschiedliche Reizspannung dürfte im wesentlichen von der immer etwas verschiedenen Lage der Elektroden abhängen, wodurch der elektrische Widerstand der Schlinge (zwischen 4000—5000 Ω) wechselt. Die Frequenzschwelle, d.h. die langsamste, gerade noch wirksame Reizfrequenz (0,15—0,7 Hz) ist bei jedem Hunde verschieden, sie schwankt beim gleichen Tier von Tag zu Tag um 0,1—0,2 Hz. Diese Änderung ist von der „vegetativ-nervösen Ausgangslage" abhängig. Die Frequenzschwelle ist aber in jeder Ausgangslage scharf ausgeprägt und experimentell genau bestimmbar. Bei höheren Reizfrequenzen nimmt die benötigte Reizspannung etwas ab und durchläuft bei Frequenzen zwischen 20—30 Hz ein flaches Minimum. Bei Reizfrequenzen über 50 Hz muß die Reizspannung auf das 2—3fache erhöht werden, um den gleichen Reizerfolg zu erhalten. Als Reizerfolg wird ein dreimaliger Hustenstoß angesehen. Für den Nachweis der Wirksamkeit eines Präparates genügt die Untersuchung weniger Punkte der Reizfrequenz-Reizspannungskurve. Kritik der Methodik bei Schlez.

b) Methode von Stefko und Benson

Der Hustenreiz wird bei wachen Hunden ausgelöst, in deren Trachealschleimhaut Elektroden operativ eingebettet sind. Die Operation wird unter aseptischen Bedingungen in Narkose durchgeführt. Incision in der Mittellinie in der Höhe des Cricoidknorpels. Abwärts gerichtete Schnittführung, wobei Haut, subcutanes Gewebe und Platysma auf eine Distanz von 6 cm durchschnitten werden. Das oberflächliche Gewebe wird von der vorderen Halsfascie abgestreift. Die Fascie wird entlang der Mittellinie eingeschnitten und die Trachea freigelegt. Unter einem der Trachealringe hindurch werden 2 Kanäle gebohrt, die die Submucosa durchstoßen. Zwei Elektroden aus Platin, Silber, Kupfer oder Stahl werden durch die Kanäle gefädelt und am Knorpel befestigt.

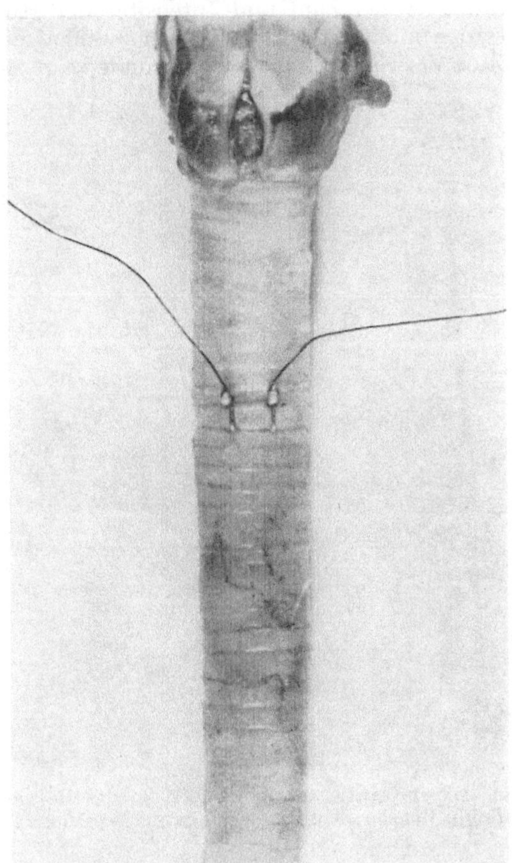

Abb. 10. Position und Sicherung der Elektroden an einem Trachealring. [Aus: Stefko u. Benson: J. Pharmacol. exp. Ther. **108**, 217 (1953)]

Von jeder wird ein isolierter Draht durch die Muskulatur, das Subcutangewebe und die Haut nach außen geführt. Ein schützendes Halsband wird angelegt, um Schädigungen des Operationsfeldes zu vermeiden.

Nach Wiederherstellung des Tieres wird die Leitung mit einem Stimulator verbunden, der 1—250 mV liefert und dessen Frequenz von 1—100 Hz abgestuft werden kann. Jedes Tier wird daraufhin getestet, welche Stromstärke und -frequenz notwendig ist, um eindeutigen Husten zu erhalten. Gewöhnlich sind es 100 mV und 100 Hz. Es wird mit geringer Voltzahl und Frequenz begonnen, bis der Husten in reproduzierbarer Weise eintritt. Die Hustenreaktion wird graduiert in

+ = seufzende oder gesteigerte Exspiration bis zu schwachem Husten,
++ = mäßig starken Husten,
+++ = bemerkenswert starken Husten.

Die ++-Stärke wird gewöhnlich als Standardhusten gewählt.

Durchführung der Versuche: Das Tier wird in Intervallen von 5 sec für die Dauer von 1 sec 10mal hintereinander gereizt. Dieser Kontrolltest wird dreimal ausgeführt. Wenn eine ausreichende Reaktion erhalten wird, werden die Testdrogen s.c. verabreicht. Die Hustenreaktion wird nach 15, 30, 60 und 120 min erneut gemessen. Hustenhemmende Wirkung wird an der Abschwächung der Normalreaktion erkannt, wobei Zahl und Intensität der Hustenstöße als Maß dienen. Die Tiere werden nicht öfter als ein- oder zweimal pro Woche herangezogen. Bei wiederholter Verwendung derselben Hunde zeigt sich bei einigen eine

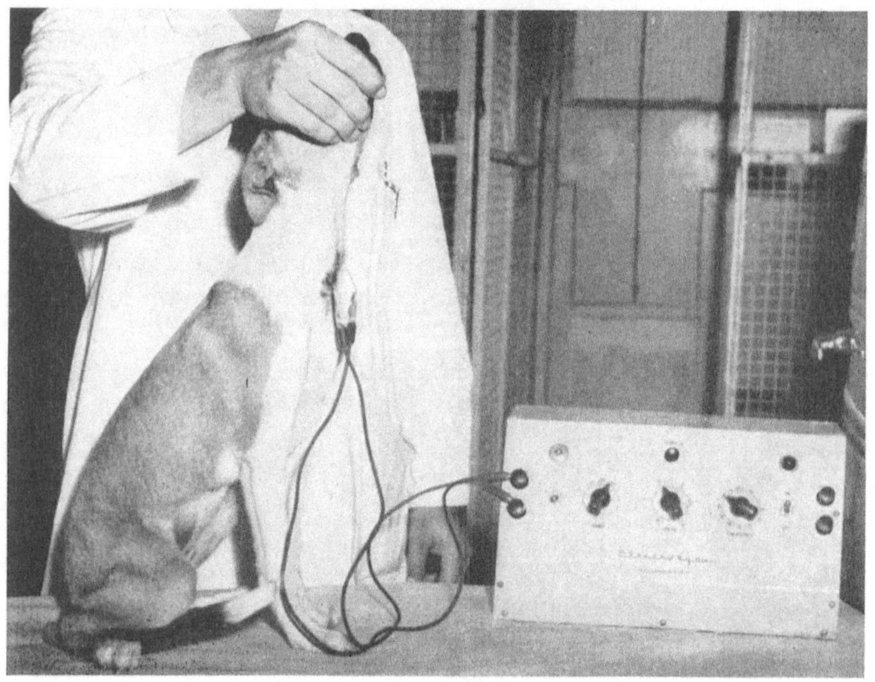

Abb. 11. Versuchstier mit implantierten Elektroden an das Reizgerät angeschlossen. [Aus: Stefko u. Benson: J. Pharmacol. exp. Ther. **108**, 217 (1953)]

Tendenz zur Erhöhung der Reizschwelle, in anderen Fällen bleibt die Empfindlichkeit über 3—6 Wochen lang gleich. Die Autoren glauben, daß die gelegentliche Erhöhung der Reizschwelle durch die Entwicklung von fibrotischen Belägen auf den Elektroden bedingt ist.

c) Methode von Krause

Modifikation der Methode von Stefko und Benson (S. 42). Der Hustenreiz wird bei Meerschweinchen in Urethannarkose (1,2 g/kg s.c.) durch elektrische Reizung der Trachealschleimhaut mit Hilfe einer in die Luftröhre eingeführten Platinelektrode ausgelöst. Mit dem Reizgerät „Megatest" werden rechteckige Stromstöße (Impulsdauer 5 m/sec, Intensität 5—15 mA, Frequenz 10 Hz) 10 sec lang verabfolgt. Registrierung der Hustenstöße über einen an der Bauchdecke befestigten Stirnschreiber. Antitussive Wirkung wird dann als positiv bewertet, wenn die Reizantwort vollständig ausbleibt. Berechnung der ED_{50} nach Litchfield und Wilcoxon.

d) Methode von Kuhn und Friebel (1960), Friebel und Hahn, Hahn und Friebel

Modifikation der Methode von Krause (S. 44). Männlichen Meerschweinchen, 250—400 g schwer, werden Trachealelektroden implantiert, Kabel aus vier 30 cm langen lackierten Kupferdrähten (0,05 mm Cu mit 0,005 mm Polyurethanlack) oder nylonisierten Silberdrähten (0,025 mm Ag mit 0,015 Nylon), bei denen in der Mitte (auf einer Strecke von 1 mm) und an den Enden die Isolationsschicht entfernt wird. Implantation in Hexobarbitalnarkose unter aseptischen Bedingungen. Nach Freilegen der Trachea wird in der Höhe des oberen Sternumrandes eine Elektrode unter einer Trachealspange hindurchgezogen, eine weitere unter einer 3 Knorpelringe höher liegenden Spange. Jede wird dicht neben dem Knorpeln ein- und ausgeführt, um die im Zwischenknorpelraum verlaufenden Gefäße nicht zu verletzen, und so gelagert, daß ihr nicht isolierter Anteil der Mucosa aufliegt. Zur Fixierung werden die Schenkel jedes Kabels über der Spange zu einem Strang gedreht. Jede Elektrode wird in weiten Schlingen — die caudale rechts, die craniale links — 2 cm seitlich der medianen Schnittlinie nach außen geführt und dann unter ebenfalls schlingenförmigem Verlauf in einem Halsverband fixiert.

Eine locker ansitzende, um Hals, Schultern, Brust und Rücken reichende „Weste“ ermöglicht über Steckkontakte die Verbindung der Elektrodenkabel mit den Leitungen vom Reizgerät. Die Tiere werden aufrecht in einen zylindrischen Plexiglasbehälter mit verstellbarer Sitzplatte gesetzt. Verschluß des Behälters durch einen Deckel mit zentraler Öffnung für Kopf und Hals des Tieres. Abdichtung zwischen Deckel und Hals mit konisch geschnittenen Schaumgummimanschetten. Der Innenraum des Behälters steht mit einer Mareyschen Kapsel in Verbindung, die die Volumenänderungen des Tierkörpers auf ein Kymographion überträgt. Über dem Kopf der Tiere hängt ein Kristallmikrophon, das Hustengeräusche über einen regulierbaren Hochfrequenzverstärker auf einen Lautsprecher und parallel dazu auf den Endverstärker eines Elektrographen (System Schwarzer) überträgt. Letzterer zeichnet mit einem Registriersystem die geräuschbedingten Impulse auf eine Kymographionschleife. Auf der Schleife werden außerdem die Reizdauer und Zeitsignale markiert. Reizimpulse liefert ein Reizgerät, Typ Medeor (Fa. Netheler & Hinz, Hamburg), mit variablen Frequenz-, Impulsdauer- und Stromstärkebereichen. Zur Ausschaltung von Schwankungen der Reizstromstärke bei Veränderungen des Übergangswiderstandes zwischen Elektroden und Gewebe liegt parallel zum Ausgang des Reizgerätes ein 100 kΩ Widerstand.

Hustenprovokation durch manuelle Betätigung eines Stromschalters im Elektrodenstromkreis. Reizdauer bis zum Auftreten eines Hustenstoßes; bei Ausbleiben einer Reizantwort aber in der Regel nicht länger als 10 sec. Zwischen zwei aufeinanderfolgenden Hustenprovokationen wird eine Pause von 2 min eingehalten. Jedes Tier wird im Durchschnitt 35—45mal aufeinanderfolgend stimuliert. Die Tiere werden erstmals 24 Std nach der Operation und nur während der ersten 3 Tage nach der Elektrodenimplantation verwendet, da die Reizempfindlichkeit danach schnell abnimmt. Die Erhöhung der Reizschwelle war in den Versuchen von Friebel und Hahn offenbar nicht durch Widerstandserhöhung zwischen den Elektroden bedingt, denn ein Ansteigen des normalen Widerstandes von 1,4—6 kΩ, gemessen mit der Universalmeßbrücke Philoskop II, wurde nicht beobachtet. Versuche, bei denen sich die anfängliche Reizempfindlichkeit ändert, werden abgebrochen.

Im Versuch werden die Tiere mit Serien rechteckiger Impulse verschiedener Dauer, Stärke und Frequenz zum Husten gereizt. Bei jedem Versuch wird einer dieser drei Faktoren konstant gehalten, die beiden anderen systematisch verändert und so kombiniert, daß abwechselnd leicht überschwellige und gering unterschwellige Reizungen zustande kommen. Die Ergebnisse der Einzelreizungen werden, den Größen der variierten Faktoren zugeordnet, in ein doppelt logarithmisches System eingezeichnet. Zwischen den Markierungen für über- und unterschwellige Reizungen wird die individuelle Reizschwellenkurve gefunden. Aus individuellen Kurven von mehreren Tieren, die gleichartig gereizt werden, werden Mittelwertskurven gebildet.

Bei der Untersuchung von hustenhemmenden Pharmaka werden je fünf Meerschweinchen unter gleichbleibenden Bedingungen mit derselben Versuchssubstanz behandelt. Der Husten wird mit einem Reizstrom von 60 Hz, 6 msec Impulsdauer und leicht überschwelliger Stromstärke ausgelöst unter Wechsel der Stromflußrichtungen von Reizung zu Reizung. Bezugspunkt für prüfstoffbedingte Veränderungen der Hustenreizschwelle ist der im unbehandelten Zustand ermittelte Schwellenwert der Stromstärke.

Nach der Ermittlung der Ausgangsempfindlichkeit und Sicherung dieses Befundes durch viermalige Kontrolle im Abstand von 2 min wird der Prüfstoff unter die Bauchhaut injiziert. Prüfstoffbedingte Veränderungen der Hustenreizschwelle werden fortlaufend durch Anpassung der Reizstromstärke in Stufen von 1 mA gerade so weit ausgeglichen, daß auch unter dem Einfluß von Prüfstoffen Husten ausgelöst und beobachtet werden kann. Die Reizungen werden bis zur 30. min nach der Injektion im Abstand von 2 min ausgelöst; danach wird bis zur 90. min im 10minütigen Abstand, anschließend bis zur 180. min im halbstündigen Abstand gereizt. Während der halbstündigen Pausen werden die Versuchstiere aus der Halterung des Registriergerätes entfernt.

Die Arbeitsweise erlaubt die Registrierung des plethysmatisch meßbaren Luftwechsels einschließlich des Hustenstoßes, des Hustengeräusches und der Dauer des Reizstromflusses. Folgende prüfstoffbedingte Abweichungen von der Norm können ausgewertet werden: Veränderungen der Reizschwelle, der Einordnung des Hustenstoßes in den Atemrhythmus, des kymographischen Bildes des Hustenstoßes und des Hustentones. Sicherung der Versuchsergebnisse durch mathematische Differenzkontrolle zwischen Tieren, die mit physiologischer Kochsalzlösung, und solchen, die mit Prüfstoff behandelt werden.

e) Methode von Domenjoz

An Katzen in Aprobarbitalnarkose (55 mg/kg i.p.) wird der N. laryngeus sup. operativ freigelegt und elektrisch gereizt. Etwa 45 min nach der Injektion des Narkoticums wird mit der Operation begonnen. Der Nerv, der im Bereich des Thyreohyoideus leicht aufzufinden ist, muß sorgfältig, ohne Zerrung präpariert werden.

Die Reizelektrode muß beweglich montiert sein, damit sich auch während der Hustenanfälle keine Zerrung der Nerven ergibt. Gereizt wird durch einen Gleichstromgenerator, der rechteckige Stromstöße beliebiger Frequenz und Stärke liefert. 5 Hz Frequenz, 0,15—3,0 V Reizintensität und 5—15 sec Reizdauer eignen sich zur Hustenprovokation. Zwischen zwei Reizungen soll ein Zeitintervall von 60 und 180 sec eingehalten werden (automatische Schaltvorrichtung). Zur Registrierung des Hustens wird eine Mareysche Kapsel benützt, die mit einer Trachealkanüle in Verbindung steht. Das offene Ende der Kanüle wird per os bis dicht an den Larynx herangeführt, wobei die Stimmritze unberührt bleiben muß. Die Applikationen der Versuchssubstanzen erfolgen intravenös: Injektionsvolumen ca. 0,5 cm^3, Injektionsgeschwindigkeit 1 cm^3/min.

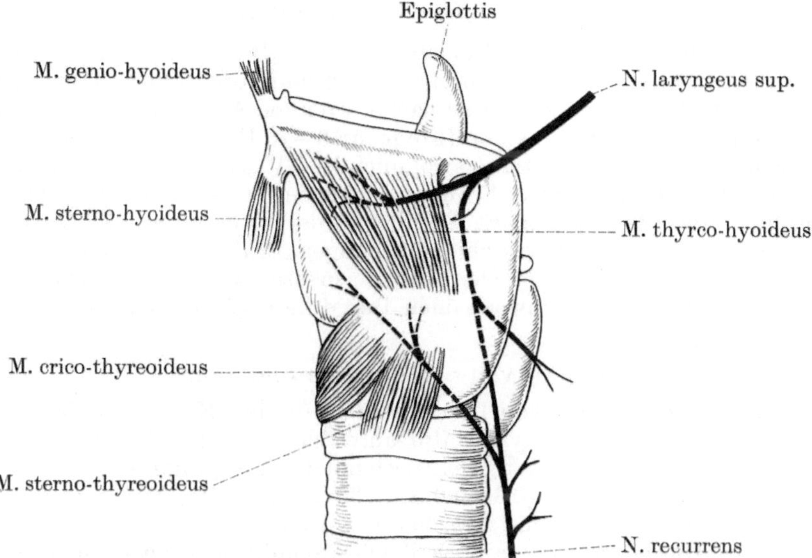

Abb. 12. Topographie des N. laryngeus sup. bei der Katze. (Nach: Jackson: Experimental pharmacology and Materia medica, S. 402. St. Louis: C. V. Mosby Co. 1939)

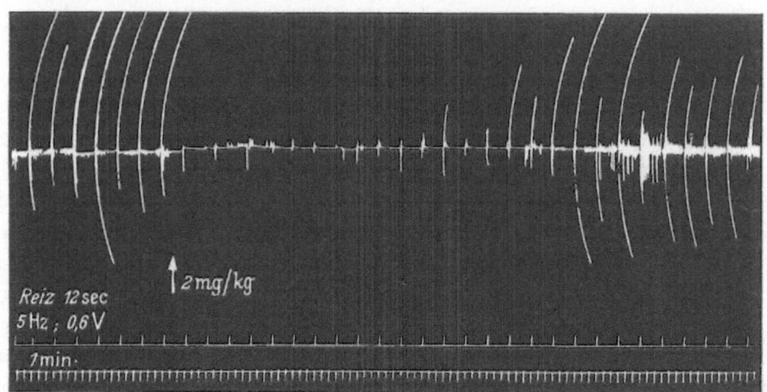

Abb. 13. Husten bei elektrischer Reizung des N. laryngeus superior an der Katze. Wirkung von 2 mg/kg Taoryl, i.v. (Versuch Nr. 54, Katze 2,13 kg, Numal, 55 mg/kg i.p.). [Aus: Domenjoz: Naunyn-Schmiedebergs Arch. exp. Path. Pharmak. **215**, 19 (1952)]

f) Methode von Toner und Macko

Modifikation der Methode von Domenjoz (S. 46). Katzen werden mit Pentobarbital-Na narkotisiert, der linke oder rechte N. laryng. sup. wird freigelegt und der Nerv über eine Porter-Elektrode gelegt. Um Austrocknen zu vermeiden und zur Sicherung des Kontaktes wird geschmolzenes Paraffin von niedrigem Schmelzpunkt über diese Stelle gegossen, auf der es erstarrt. Zur Reizung wird ein Eberbach-Elektrostimulator verwendet. Husten wird als Zwerchfellbewegung auf einem Kymographion registriert, der Schreibhebel ist durch einen Faden mit der vorderen Bauchwand verbunden.

Durchführung der Versuche: Der Nerv wird während einer 15 min dauernden Kontrollperiode im 2 min-Intervall jeweils 5 sec lang stimuliert. Gleichartige Reizungen folgen jeder Prüfstoffgabe. Injektionen in die rechte V. femoralis.

g) Methode von Green und Ward

Modifikation der Methode von Domenjoz (S. 46). Bei Katzen wird in Pentobarbitalnarkose der N. laryng. sup. freipräpariert und durchtrennt. Das zentrale Ende wird in eine Flüssigkeitselektrode nach Porter und Allamon gelegt. Stimulation durch wellenförmige Stromstöße (Frequenz 6—10 Hz, Reizperioden von 3,5 oder 10 sec Dauer), deren Potential (gewöhnlich 1—5 V) so eingestellt wird, daß sie eine Reihe von inspiratorischen Schnappatmungen verursachen. Die Thoraxbewegungen werden durch einen Faden, der an der Haut unterhalb des Brustbeins befestigt ist, auf ein Kymographion übertragen. Prüfstoffe werden in steigenden Dosen intravenös verabfolgt. Die Erholungspause zwischen zwei Dosen muß angemessen groß sein. Nach unwirksamen Dosen beträgt sie 10 min.

h) Methode von Sell, Lindner und Jahn

Modifikation der Methode von Domenjoz (S. 46). Bei Katzen in Pernoctonnarkose (5 sec-Butyl-5β-bromallylbarbitursaures Na) wird der N. laryngicus sup. beiderseits freigelegt und beiderseitig elektrisch mit dem „Stimulator" (Fa. Netheler und Hinz, Hamburg) gereizt (0,3—0,6 mA, 30 bzw. 60 Hz, Reizperioden von 5 bzw. 10 sec). Pausen von 2 min zwischen den Reizperioden. Reizung während der Inspiration. Durch Intubation oder Trachealschnitt wird eine doppelarmige Kanüle in die Trachea gebracht, die zur Registrierung von Atmung und Husten dient. Ein Arm wird mit einer Mareyschen Kapsel verbunden, der andere mit einer Klemme so weit gedrosselt, daß die gleichzeitige Registrierung beider möglich ist.

i) Methode von Chakravarty u. Mitarb.

Husten wird bei Katzen durch unmittelbare Stimulation der Medulla oblongata hervorgerufen. Die Tiere werden in Äthernarkose durch Querdurchtrennung in Höhe der mittleren Hügellinie decerebriert und später in nicht anaesthesiertem Zustand gereizt. Größere Blutverluste werden durch intravenöse Injektionen von Dextran (6%ige Lösung, bis zu 10 ml/kg) ausgeglichen. Hustenreaktionen werden bei Reizung der dorsolateralen Region der Medulla erhalten. Gute Präparate behalten ca. 4 Std eine gleichbleibende Empfindlichkeit. Stimulierung durch monopolare Rechteckimpulse (0,5—5 V, 10—20 Hz, 0,5 m sec) über bipolare Nadelelektroden, die unter Leitung eines stereotaktischen Instrumentes eingeführt werden. Der Husten wird pneumographisch auf Rußpapier registriert, die Atmung über einen kleinen Sphygmomanometer, der um die untere Hälfte der Brust angelegt wird. Es ist aber auch möglich, die Lungenventilation und den Husten über eine Trachealkanüle aufzuschreiben, die abwechselnd mit dem Larynx und einem Spirometer verbunden werden kann. Prüfstoffe werden durch einen Polyäthylenkatheter in die Femoralvene injiziert.

V. Besprechung der Methoden

Die Reizantworten, die nach verschiedenartiger Reizung — mechanischer, chemischer oder elektrischer Stimulation — erhalten werden, sind einander recht ähnlich (Green und Ward). Im Prinzip kann jede zum Studium des Hustens und der antitussiven Wirkung verwendet werden. Untersucht man, inwieweit die einzelnen Methoden den drei Forderungen von Schroeder entsprechen (Untersuchung am wachen Tier, dosierte Reizung, Vermeidung von Schädigung) und andererseits leicht zugänglich, einfach durchzuführen und nicht zu kostspielig sind, so wird man trotz der Fülle der Vorschläge keine ideale Arbeitsweise finden.

Man ist vielmehr gezwungen, die für den jeweiligen Zweck am besten geeignete Methode auszuwählen.

Bei der Auswahl verdienen einige Gesichtspunkte besondere Beachtung:

a) Tierart

Husten kann offensichtlich bei allen üblichen Laboratoriumstieren provoziert werden. Verwendet wurden bisher: Hund (Kasé, 1952, 1954, 1955; Tedeschi u. Mitarb.; Winter und Flataker, 1952; de Vleeschhouwer; Rosiere u. Mitarb.; Stefko und Benson), Katze (May und Widdicombe; Stefko und Denzel; Kroepfli; Domenjoz; Toner und Macko; Green und Ward; Chakravarty u. Mitarb.), Kaninchen (Larsell und Burget), Meerschweinchen (Eichler u. Smiatek, 1940, Friebel u. Mitarb., 1955, 1962, 1964, 1966; Winter und Flataker, 1954; Silvestrini und Maffii; Gösswald; Krause), Ratte (Reichle und Friebel) und Maus (Kelentey u. Mitarb., 1957). Die Bereitschaft der einzelnen Tierarten, die Inhalation von chemischen Stimulantien mit Husten zu beantworten, ist unterschiedlich. Reichle und Friebel mußten Ratten höheren SO_2-Konzentrationen aussetzen als Meerschweinchen, um Husten in vergleichbarer Stärke zu erhalten. Die Laboratoriumstierarten differieren auch darin, daß einige von ihnen auf Reizstoffinhalation stärker mit Husten, andere mit Niesen reagieren. SO_2-Inhalation wird von Meerschweinchen vorwiegend mit Husten beantwortet, Ratten niesen und husten etwa gleich häufig (Reichle und Friebel), Katzen niesen vorwiegend (Friebel, unveröffentlicht). Die Inhalation löst bei den genannten Tierspecies auch erheblichen Speichelfluß aus, bei Katzen ist er am stärksten ausgeprägt. Die Höhe der Hustenreizschwelle wird von Spontanerkrankungen der Atmungsorgane beeinflußt. Derartige Erkrankungen und ihre Auswirkungen auf die Hustenbereitschaft wurden bei Meerscheinchen häufiger angetroffen als bei Ratten (Friebel, Reichle und v. Graevenitz; Reichle und Friebel).

Der Einfluß speciesbedingter Faktoren auf das Ergebnis der Arzneimittelprüfung ist von Friebel und Reichle an Meerschweinchen und Ratten studiert worden. Sie fanden zum Teil wesentliche artbedingte Differenzen zwischen den Testergebnissen, was verständlich ist, da bei der vergleichenden Prüfung der Arzneimittelwirkung neben den artbedingten Differenzen in der Reaktionsweise auf die Hustenprovokation auch speciesgebundene Unterschiede im Arzneimittelstoffwechsel das Untersuchungsergebnis beeinflussen. So metabolisieren z. B. Meerschweinchen das Codein nicht in gleicher Weise wie Ratten (Kuhn und Friebel, 1962).

Mäuse sind bisher nur selten und nur im Inhalationstest verwendet worden. Sie eignen sich wegen ihrer geringen Ventilationsgröße, wegen des schwachen und schlecht registrierbaren Hustens und wegen der schlechten Unterscheidbarkeit von Husten und Niesen weniger gut als größere Laboratoriumstiere.

Ratten, ebenfalls nur im Inhalationstest erprobt, beantworten die Hustenprovokation mit einem SO_2-Luftgemisch in ähnlicher Weise wie Meerschweinchen mit Husten und Niesen. Die visuelle Unterscheidung der beiden Reizungsfolgen erfordert mehr Übung als bei Meerschweinchen, der Husten ist weniger lautstark. Wie Meerschweinchen zeigen sie jahreszeitlich bedingte Veränderungen der Hustenbereitschaft, doch machen sich witterungsbedingte Einflüsse weniger störend bemerkbar als bei Meerschweinchen. Die Auswahl geeigneter Tiere, d.h. von Tieren mit ausreichender und konstanter Hustenbereitschaft in Vorversuchen ist notwendig, die wiederholte Verwendung während eines Zeitraumes von 3 Monaten möglich (Reichle und Friebel), danach wurde eine Abnahme der Hustenbereitschaft beobachtet (Friebel und Kuhn, 1964).

Meerschweinchen bieten die Vorzüge des kleineren Versuchstieres, z. B. leichte Haltung und Hantierbarkeit sowie die Möglichkeit, mit größeren Versuchstiergruppen arbeiten zu können. Bei ihnen kann der Husten durch mechanische, chemische oder elektrische Provokation ausgelöst werden. Der Husten ist kräftig; er kann visuell, akustisch oder instrumentell (als Druckwelle oder plethysmographisch) registriert werden (Abb. 14).

Die Hustenreizschwelle des Einzeltieres, das im ein- oder mehrtägigen Abstand wiederholt in den Versuch genommen wird, erweist sich nicht immer als konstant, sie muß jeweils im Vorversuch ermittelt werden. Bei mehreren an demselben Tage ausgeführten Versuchen erwies sie sich aber als zuverlässig reproduzierbar (Friebel, Reichle und v. Graevenitz). Tiere, deren Käfige im Freien standen, zeigten während der Sommermonate eine erfreuliche Konstanz ihrer Hustenbereitschaft, weniger regelmäßig reagierten sie im Winter. Im Winter wurde aber auch bei Tieren, die in geheizten Räumen gehalten wurden, eine höhere Quote von Abweichungen gefunden (Friebel, Reichle und v. Graevenitz).

In einwöchigen Intervallen wiederholte chemische Hustenprovokation wurde von den Atemwegen vertragen (Friebel und Kuhn, 1962). Die Reizempfindlichkeit erwies sich in einem über 48 Wochen laufenden Versuch als konstant, so daß Alter und Gewicht in einem weiten Bereich ohne Einfluß auf die Sensibilität gegen das Provokationsmittel SO_2 zu sein scheinen (Friebel und Kuhn, 1964). Meerschweinchen eignen sich außerdem für wiederholte und über längere Zeiträume laufende Versuche, weil ihr Lernvermögen offensichtlich geringer als das höher entwickelter Laboratoriumstiere ist und deshalb die Versuchsergebnisse weniger von Dressureffekten beeinflußt werden.

Kaninchen: Die mit dieser Tierart gewonnenen Erfahrungen sind vergleichsweise wenig umfangreich. Sie beschränken sich auf Versuche, bei denen Husten durch mechanische Reizung der Trachealschleimhaut ausgelöst wurde.

Katzen sind häufig in den Versuch genommen worden. Der Husten kann durch mechanische, chemische oder elektrische Stimulation ausgelöst werden. Zur wiederholten Verwendung eignen sie sich weniger, weil die an Katzen anwendbaren Methoden in der Regel Narkose und operative Eingriffe erfordern, die das Opfern der Tiere bedingen. Eine Ausnahme macht die Methode von Ernst (1938), bei der durch die Injektion von Lugolscher Lösung eine chronische Pleuritis erzeugt und die Hustenreizschwelle für längere Zeit so weit gesenkt wird, daß einfaches Beklopfen der Tiere Husten auslöst. Die wiederholte Anwendung von reizenden Gasen stößt auf Schwierigkeiten, weil die Tiere schnell lernen, der Provokation durch Abflachung und Verlangsamung der Atmung zu begegnen, so daß es schwer ist, eine konstant bleibende Reizschwelle zu finden (Friebel, unveröffentlicht). Ihre besondere Eignung haben Katzen in Versuchen gezeigt, in denen der Husten durch elektrische Reizung ausgelöst wurde. Breite Anwendung haben die Methoden von Kroepfli und von Domenjoz gefunden, insbesondere die letztgenannte.

Bei Hunden kann Husten mit mechanischer, chemischer und elektrischer Stimulation provoziert werden. Hunde bieten wegen ihrer Größe gute Voraussetzungen für operative Eingriffe wie Vorlagerung des Vagus, Fensterung der Trachea oder Implantation von Schwingkörpern in die Trachea, nach denen eine Stimulierung im postoperativen, nicht narkotisierten Zustand möglich wird, zugleich auch die wiederholte Verwendung der Versuchstiere. Weiterhin lassen sich Hunde dressieren, das Schlucken des Magenschlauches oder i.v. Injektionen von Prüfstoffen ohne Widerstand hinzunehmen. So kann man bei der Verwendung von Hunden die Hustenprovokationen dem physiologischen Husten des Menschen verhältnismäßig gut anpassen. Limitierend wirken sich gute Hund-Pfeger-Beziehungen, die notwendige Voraussetzung für das Arbeiten mit nicht narkotisierten

Tieren, aus, weil die daraus resultierende Neigung des Versuchstieres, dem Versuchsleiter entgegenzukommen, Fehlergebnisse induzieren kann. Stefko und Benson haben auf diesen wichtigen Faktor vorsichtig hingewiesen. Deutlicher wird er von Koll bei der Beschreibung seiner Analgesieversuche erwähnt. Schlez fand, daß die psychogen bedingten Verhaltensänderungen ihrer Vagusschlingenhunde die erfolgreiche Verwendung der Tiere im Arzneimittelversuch unmöglich machten. Mit zunehmender Versuchszahl und damit Versuchserfahrung wurde von Hunden mit freundschaftlichen Beziehungen zum Versuchsleiter Spontanhusten provoziert, von Schlez als „entgegenkommender Dressureffekt" gedeutet. Derartige Reaktionen störten den Versuchsablauf stärker als z. B. eine fehlerhafte Lage der Elektroden an der Schlinge, als unterschiedliche Wandbeschaffenheit der Schlinge oder irritierende Manipulationen bei der Prüfstoffapplikation.

b) Reizarten

Mechanische Reizung: Bei mechanischer Reizung werden Mechanoreceptoren erregt, die vorwiegend im Trachealbereich zu finden sind. Die empfindlichste Stelle liegt an der Gabelung der Trachea (Kasé, 1952; Larsell und Burget). Zur mechanischen Reizung werden relativ primitive Geräte, Bürsten, Pinsel, Katheter vorgeschlagen. Die Anwendung muß vorsichtig erfolgen, damit Schleimhautverletzungen und dadurch bedingte Sensibilitätsänderungen vermieden werden (Larsell und Burget). Mit diesen Methoden wird man der Forderung von Schroeder, den Hustenreiz genau zu dosieren, weniger vollkommen entsprechen können als mit chemischer oder elektrischer Reizung. Die Anwendung von hustenreflexhemmenden Narkotica läßt sich nicht vermeiden, sofern nicht chronische Trachealfisteln angelegt werden, die mit dem Risiko der leichteren Anfälligkeit für spontane Infektionskrankheiten der Atemwege belastet sind. Die Nachteile der genannten Methoden werden wenigstens zum Teil durch ihre einfache Durchführbarkeit und das Fehlen von apparativem Aufwand ausgeglichen.

Narkose und akute Schleimhautschädigungen bei der Prüfung von hustenhemmenden Arzneimitteln werden bei der Anwendung der Methode von Tedeschi u. Mitarb. vermieden. Diesen Vorteilen steht der operative und apparative Aufwand, die Gefahr von dressurbedingten Fehlergebnissen und einer allmählichen morphologischen Veränderung der Trachealschleimhaut im stimulierten Areal gegenüber (Tedeschi, persönl. Mitteilung).

Mechanische Stimulation verursacht rasch eintretende, temporäre Adaption der Receptoren an den Reiz. Die Wiederholung der Reizung an derselben Stelle sollte nur nach Einschalten ausreichender Intervalle erfolgen (Larsell und Burget; Widdicombe, 1954).

Chemische Reizung: Hustenreizempfindliche Receptoren, die auf chemische Reizmittel reagieren, liegen in der Trachea und den tieferen Atemwegen (Larsell und Burget; Widdicombe, 1954). Bei der Inhalation reizender Chemikalien durch die Nase werden primär die dort liegenden niesreizempfindlichen Receptoren stimuliert, erst danach hustenreizvermittelnde Receptoren in den tieferen Atemwegen. Niesen und Husten treten somit etwa gleichzeitig oder alternierend auf und es ist nicht immer leicht, bei der Beobachtung der Versuchstiere die beiden Reaktionen voneinander zu unterscheiden. Will man Niesreaktionen ausschließen, so muß man den Reizstoff unter Umgehung der Nase direkt in die Trachea leiten (Rosiere u. Mitarb.; Kroepfli; Larsell und Burget), wobei das Arbeiten mit narkotisierten oder mit chronischer Trachealfistel versehenen Tieren in Kauf genommen werden muß.

Die Reizmittel Citronensäure, Essigsäure, Äther, Acrolein, Ammoniak und Schwefelsäure sind in ihrer aggressiven Potenz und in der Nachhaltigkeit der

Wirkung nicht gleichwertig. Bei Meerschweinchen erfordert das Unterdrücken des durch SO_2 provozierten Hustens wesentlich höhere Codeindosen als die Hemmung des durch Ammoniak erzeugten Hustens. Beim Hund sind derartige Unterschiede nicht evident, doch liegen noch keine speziellen Untersuchungen dieses Problems vor. Im Hinblick auf die Vergleichbarkeit und Bewertung der von verschiedenen Autoren mit unterschiedlichen Methoden erhaltenen Ergebnisse von Arzneimittelprüfungen sind sie wünschenswert (s. Tabelle 2).

Bei der Dosierung der chemischen Reizung müssen neben der Aggressivität der Reizmittel ihre Konzentration, Tröpfchen- bzw. Teilchengröße und Dauer der Zuführung berücksichtigt werden. Amdur hat gezeigt, daß die Wirkung von H_2SO_4-Aerosolen auf die Lunge nicht dieselbe ist wie die von SO_2-Gas. Bei gleicher Säurekonzentration verursachten relativ große (7 μ) und sehr kleine (0,8 μ) H_2SO_4-Tröpfchen ein geringeres Anwachsen des Bronchialwiderstandes als 2,5 μ große Tröpfchen, denn die großen Tröpfchen erreichen die Bronchien nur zum Teil, weil sie schon in den oberen Luftwegen niedergeschlagen werden, die kleinsten werden im Bronchialbereich nicht wirksam, weil sie bis in die Alveolen vordringen, nur die 2,5 μ großen Tröpfchen werden in größerer Menge im Bronchialbereich abgelagert, wo sich die sensiblen Receptoren für die Erhöhung des Bronchialwiderstandes befinden. Eine Wirkungsähnlichkeit zwischen H_2SO_4-Aerosolen und SO_2-Gas war nur dann gegeben, wenn das Tröpfchenspektrum des H_2SO_4-Aerosols die Reizung desselben receptorenhaltigen Areals ermöglichte, das auch von inhaliertem SO_2-Gas erreicht wurde. Amdur fand weiter, daß das Abklingen der Reizfolgen nach der Einwirkung feintropfiger Aerosole schneller erfolgt als nach gröberen Aerosolen.

Reizhusten, der mit Chemikalien provoziert wird, ist am gleichen Tage mehrmals reproduzierbar. Friebel, Reichle und v. Graevenitz fanden bei SO_2-gereizten Meerschweinchen eine Versagerquote von 3,8%, wenn die zweite Prüfung der ersten im Abstand von 30 min folgte. Änderungen der Reizschwelle und damit auch der Reaktionsbereitschaft für Arzneimittelwirkungen sind zu befürchten, wenn die Reizstoffkonzentration so hoch und die Erholungspausen so kurz gewählt werden, daß chronische Schädigungen der Atemwege auftreten. Auch Spontanerkrankungen der Atemwege verändern beides, die Hustenreizschwelle und ihre therapeutische Beeinflußbarkeit.

Chemische Stimulation bietet vor anderen Methoden, experimentellen Husten zu provozieren, den Vorteil, daß auf Narkose und operative Eingriffe vor bzw. während des Versuchs verzichtet werden kann. Neben großen Laboratoriumstieren können auch kleinere verwendet werden, was den Einsatz größerer Kollektive und die Beurteilung der Versuchsergebnisse unter Anwendung mathematischer Kriterien erleichtert.

Reizung durch elektrische Stromstöße: Zur elektrischen Reizung werden rhythmische Spannungsstöße unterschiedlicher Geometrie, Voltzahl und Frequenz verwendet (Tabelle 1). Die Form des Stromstoßes kann spitz, rechteckig oder wellenförmig sein. Voltzahlen von 0,05—5 und mA-Zahlen von 0,3—15 werden angegeben. Die Frequenz variiert zwischen 5 und 100 Impulsen pro sec, die Impulsdauer zwischen 0,5 und 5 msec, die Dauer der Reizung zwischen 1 und 15 sec. Das zentrale reizaufnehmende Substrat kann offenbar recht variable elektrische Reizqualitäten dahingehend verarbeiten, daß Hustenstöße ausgelöst werden (Friebel und Hahn).

Die Beziehungen zwischen Reizspannung und -frequenz sind wiederholt (Schroeder; Stefko und Benson), aber mit unterschiedlichen Ergebnissen untersucht worden. Übereinstimmung zwischen den Resultaten von Schroeder, Stefko und Benson besteht insoweit, als innerhalb des Bereiches von 30—50 Hz bei höherer Reizspannung eine geringere Frequenz bzw. bei höherer Frequenz eine geringere Spannung ausreicht, um Husten zu erzeugen.

Bei einer systematischen Untersuchung der Variierbarkeit hustenerzeugender Reizströme an wachen Meerschweinchen, denen vorausgehend Elektroden in die Trachea implantiert worden waren, wurde von Friebel und Hahn folgender Verlauf der Reizschwellen bestimmt: Die bei konstanter Impulsfrequenz erhaltenen Reizschwellenkurven verliefen im doppelt logarhythmischen System in einem weiten Bereich annähernd als geneigte Gerade, und zwar nahm mit steigender Impulsdauer der Schwellenwert der Stromstärke exponentiell ab. Mit weiterer Zunahme der Impulsdauer setzte ein bogenförmiger Verlauf mit flachem Minimum und danach wieder ansteigendem Schenkel ein. Alle Kurven hatten denselben bogenförmigen Verlauf. Sie unterschieden sich hinsichtlich der Lage der Wendepunkte, die mit abnehmender Frequenz in Richtung zunehmender Impulsdauer verlagert waren. Für das Verhältnis von Frequenz zu Impulsdauer am Wendepunkt wurde die Funktion:

$$\text{Frequenz} \cdot \text{Impulsdauer}^{1,4} = 380$$

ermittelt.

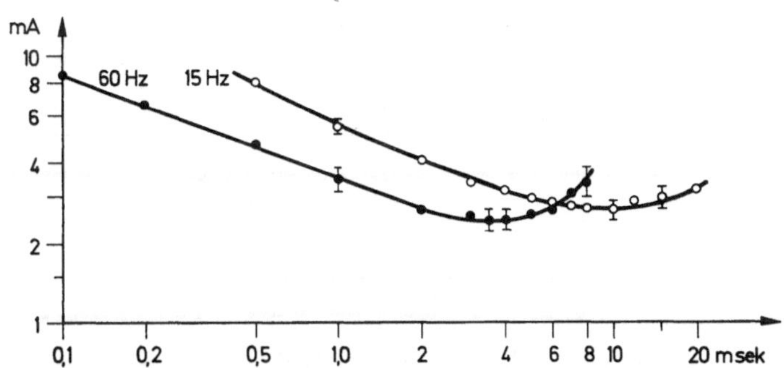

Abb. 14. Reizschwellenkurven für die Stromstärke in mA bei Reizung mit variierter Dauer des Einzelimpulses bei konstanter Frequenz von 15 und 60 Hz. Die Meßwerte sind Mittelwerte aus Messungen an je 8 Tieren. Als Streuung ist der mittlere Fehler des Mittelwertes angegeben. (Aus: Friebel u. Hahn, 1966)

Eine Bestätigung des bogenförmigen Verlaufs ergab sich mit Reizungen bei konstanter Stromstärke (2,5 mA) unter Variation der Frequenz und Impulsdauer. Hier wurden zwei Reizschwellen gefunden, die den beiden Schenkeln der oben beschriebenen Kurven entsprechen.

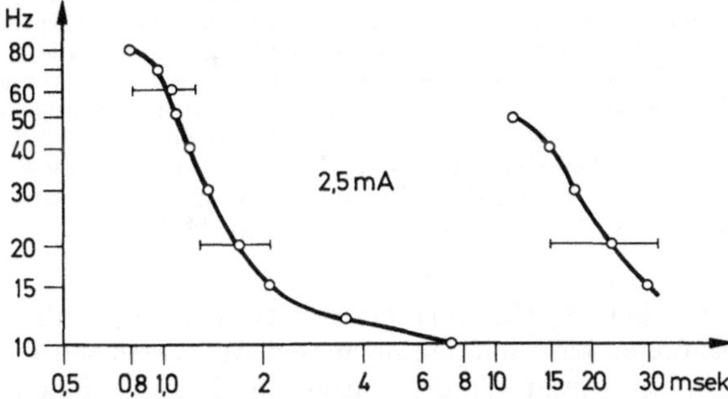

Abb. 15. Reizschwellenkurven für die Dauer des Einzelimpulses in msec bei Reizung mit variierter Frequenz bei konstanter Stromstärke von 2,5 mA. Die Meßwerte sind Mittelwerte aus Messungen an 5 Tieren. Als Streuung ist der mittlere Fehler des Mittelwertes angegeben. Aus: Friebel u. Hahn, (1966)

Die bei konstanter Impulsdauer von 8 msec erhaltene Schwellenkurve hatte ihr Minimum für den mA-Wert bei 20 Hz, wie es nach der oben genannten Funktion erwartet werden mußte.

Überschwellige Reize lösten, unabhängig von ihrer Zusammensetzung, in 90% der Fälle gleichartige Hustenstöße aus. Erst ein Überschreiten des durchschnittlichen Schwellenwertes für Stromstärken von 2,3 mA ± 0,6 um das 3—4-fache wurde mit Zappeln, Schreien und irreversiblem Anstieg der Reizschwellen beantwortet.

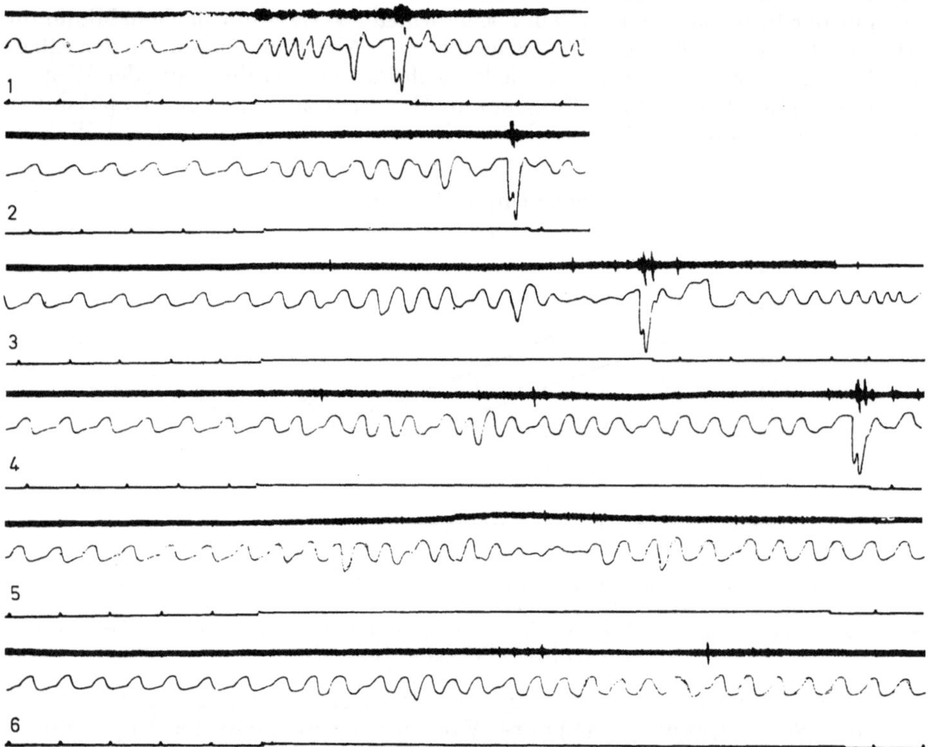

Abb. 16. Ausschnitte aus kymographisch registrierten Hustenprovokationsversuchen mit einem Reizstrom von 30 Hz und 2 msec und abnehmender Stromstärke von 5 mA in Versuch 1; 4 mA in Versuch 2; 3,5 mA in Versuch 3; 3,2 mA in Versuch 4; 3 mA in Versuch 5 und 2,6 mA in Versuch 6. In allen Kurvenausschnitten gibt die obere Linie die vom Mikrophon aufgenommenen Geräusche oder Hustentöne, die mittlere Linie atmungs- und hustenbedingte Veränderungen des Körpervolumens, die untere Linie die Zeitmarkierung in Sekunden sowie die Dauer der Reizperioden an. Senkung der Stromstärke von 5 auf 3,2 mA bedingt eine Zunahme der Latenzzeit zwischen Reizbeginn und Hustenstoß von 2 auf 9 sec (Versuche 1—4). Bei weiterer Verminderung der Stromstärke löst die Reizung keinen Husten mehr aus. [Aus: Friebel u. Hahn: Med. Pharmacol. exp. **14**, 78 (1966)]

Bei Frequenzen über 80 Hz verhinderte Glottisverschluß sowohl hustenbedingte Luftentladungen als auch den normalen Atemwechsel. Die Verhinderung der Hustenreaktion an dieser Stelle wurde an Tieren, denen verschließbare Trachealkanülen implantiert waren, bewiesen.

Für die Impulsdauer ergab sich keine von den Faktoren Frequenz und Stromstärke unabhängige Begrenzung.

Latenzzeit: Vom Einschalten des Reizstromes bis zum Husten vergingen durchschnittlich 2,8 ($\pm 1,9$) sec. Wenn aber in unmittelbarer Nähe der Reizschwelle bei aufeinanderfolgenden Reizungen mit abnehmender Reizintensität einer der 3 Faktoren des Reizstromes so lange in kleinen Stufen verringert wurde, bis der Reiz unterschwellig wurde, so trat kurz vor Erreichen der Reizschwelle eine mit der Annäherung zunehmende Verlängerung der Latenzzeit (bis auf 16 sec) auf. Schließlich wurde überhaupt nicht mehr gehustet. Bei verlängerter Latenzzeit hatte der Husten dieselbe Charakteristik und Stärke wie bei normaler Latenzzeit. Reizströme, die geringfügig unterschwellig waren, riefen gelegentlich Veränderungen der Atemfrequenz und -tiefe hervor. Mit zunehmender Unterschreitung der Reizschwelle blieb auch die Atmung unbeeinflußt (Abb. 14).

Die von Friebel und Hahn erhaltenen Befunde zeigen, daß die Variierbarkeit hustenerzeugender Reizströme nicht auf den Schwellenbereich begrenzt ist. Das Areal zwischen Strömen, die gerade überschwellig sind, und solchen, die Unverträglichkeitserscheinungen hervorrufen, ist vielmehr recht groß und läßt für Variationen der einzelnen Reizstromgrößen einen weiten Spielraum. Die Befunde machen verständlich, daß in der Literatur so verschiedenartige Reizstromformeln als hustenauslösend angegeben werden (Tabelle 1).

Elektrische Reizung zum Husten findet unter den Mechanismen, die unter physiologischen oder pathophysiologischen Bedingungen Husten auslösen, kein Äquivalent. Die Anwendung der elektrischen Reizmethoden erfordert die operative Vorbereitung der Versuchstiere und, sofern Operation und Versuch unmittelbar aufeinanderfolgen, die Behandlung mit Narkotica. Dennoch haben viele Untersucher diese Methoden verwendet. Sie erlauben eine wesentlich genauere Definierung und Quantifizierung von Reizstärke und Reizqualität als es bei der Anwendung von chemischen und mechanischen Stimulantien möglich ist.

c) Narkose

Beim Studium der Organisation und Funktion der Hustenreflexbahn lassen sich operative Eingriffe und damit Narkose oft nicht vermeiden. Man muß in diesen Fällen prüfen, ob und in welcher Weise die pharmakodynamischen Eigenschaften des Narkosemittels das Versuchsergebnis beeinflussen. Narkotica können hochdosiert nicht nur die Atmung dämpfen, sondern auch den Hustenreflex unterdrücken.

Friebel und Kuhn (1962) bestimmten an Meerschweinchen die hustenhemmende ED_{50} (Erhöhung der Hustenreizschwelle um durchschnittlich 3,4 mA) von Hexobarbital-Natrium mit 77,0 (70,5—84,0) mg/kg, Hahn und Friebel mit 70 mg/kg. Sie fanden, daß die zur Hustenhemmung erforderliche Dosis höher als die zur Narkose ausreichende Dosis liegt. Das ist nicht bei allen Narkotica der Fall. So unterbricht Chloralose bei Katzen in der zur Narkose erforderlichen Dosis den Hustenreflex (Domenjoz) und bei Hunden unterdrückt Pentobarbital Na den Husten noch vor dem Erlöschen der motorischen Aktivität (Tedeschi u. Mitarb.). Auch die Tierart muß in diesem Zusammenhang berücksichtigt werden, denn die Aprobarbitalnarkose, die bei Katzen den Hustenreflex nicht auslöscht, macht Hunde unfähig, elektrische Stimulation mit Husten zu beantworten (Domenjoz).

Die Tiefe der Narkose und damit wahrscheinlich auch die Hustenbereitschaft bleibt bei längerer Versuchsdauer nicht konstant. In Versuchen von Hahn und Friebel riefen 70 mg/kg Hexobarbital-Natrium bei Meerschweinchen zuerst Somnolenz, dann Narkose hervor. Mit dem Eintritt ins Narkosestadium kam es zu einer zunehmenden Verzögerung des Hustenreflexablaufs. Die Hustenstöße traten in 57% der Fälle erst nach dem Abschalten des Reizstromes auf. Vereinzelt wurde noch 3 sec nach der Stromflußunterbrechung gehustet. Gleichzeitig trat allmählich eine Erhöhung der Hustenreizschwelle bis um durchschnittlich 3,4 mA und eine Abschwächung der Hustengeräusche bis zu ganz geräuscharmen Exspirationen, die nicht mehr als Husten gewertet werden konnten, auf. Abweichend von der Norm ging weiterhin den Hustenstößen ausnahmslos eine Inspiration voran. Diese Veränderungen wurden 6 min nach der s.c. Injektion von Hexobarbital erstmals und beginnend sichtbar, sie erreichten ca. 30 min nach der Injektion ihren Höhepunkt und bildeten sich zwischen der 60. und 90. min zurück.

Die narkosebedingte Inkonstanz der Hustenbereitschaft behindert die vergleichende Prüfung von hustenhemmenden Pharmaka, denn es muß mit Summationseffekten hinsichtlich der antitussiven, atemdepressorischen und narkotischen Wirkung gerechnet werden. Allgemeingültige Voraussagen über deren Art und Stärke sind nicht möglich. So wird z. B. beim Meerschweinchen die antitussive Wirkung von Codein durch Hexobarbital-Natrium verstärkt und gleichzeitig werden Atemvolumen und -frequenz reduziert, während die hustenhemmende Wirkung eines Thipendylcarbonsäureesters (Pipazethate) nicht verstärkt wird, obwohl an der Dämpfung der Atmung ein Synergismus sichtbar wird (Friebel und Kuhn, 1962).

Die von Schroeder ausgesprochene Ablehnung der Narkose beim experimentellen Husten erscheint nach diesen Befunden nicht unbegründet. Andererseits sind zahlreiche und grundlegende Befunde zur Kenntnis der Hustenreflexbahn, ihrer Funktion und Beeinflußbarkeit an narkotisierten Tieren erarbeitet worden und haben der Nachprüfung an nicht narkotisierten Tieren standgehalten.

d) Chirurgische Eingriffe

Trachealfistel: Nach dem Anlegen einer Trachealfistel wird die Lunge in unphysiologischer Weise beatmet. Anstelle der im Nasen-Rachen-Raum mit Wasserdampf gesättigten Atemluft wird trockene Laboratoriumsluft inhaliert. Unter diesen Bedingungen verdampft mehr als 95% des in die Atemwege ausgeschiedenen Sekretwassers. Die Folgen sind Schädigung der Flimmertätigkeit und Sistieren des Sekrettransports (Perry und Boyd; Dalhamn). Selbst bei Inhalation einer Luft mit etwa 30% Feuchtigkeitsgehalt wurde 3—5 min nach Eröffnung der Trachea die Beendigung der Ciliarbewegung beobachtet. Der Ausfall der Transportfunktion begünstigt die Bildung eines unbeweglichen Sekretfilms auf der Trachealschleimhaut und damit eine Änderung der Hustenreizschwelle (Pellmont und Bächtold).

Wird eine Fistel in einer den Hustenprovokationsversuchen vorausgehenden Operation angelegt und dann längere Zeit getragen, wie es Kasé (1952, 1954, 1955) sowie Rosiere u. Mitarb. vorschlagen, so muß auch bei gut gelungener Operation mit einer vermehrten Anfälligkeit gegenüber chronischer Bronchitis und Pneumonitis gerechnet werden (Rosiere u. Mitarb.). Derartige entzündliche Veränderungen erniedrigen die Reizschwelle für husteninduzierende Reize. Man wird daher der Gesunderhaltung der Atemwege dieser Tiere besondere Aufmerksamkeit widmen müssen. Operierte Tiere benötigen besondere Pflege, häufige Reinigung der Trachealkanüle und des umgebenden Gewebes, klimatisierte Ställe u. a.

e) Implantieren von Trachealelektroden

Stefko und Benson beschreiben eine Reizschwellenänderung, die keine pathogene Ursache hat. Sie fanden bei den nach ihrer Methode operierten Hunden eine allmählich zunehmende Unempfindlichkeit gegenüber elektrischer Stimulation. Sie nehmen an, daß die zwei Metallelektroden, die als Fremdkörper in die Trachealwand eingelegt sind, von fibrotischen Niederschlägen bedeckt und isoliert werden. Friebel und Hahn konnten Meerschweinchen nur während der ersten 3 Tage nach der Elektrodenimplantation verwenden, da die Reizempfindlichkeit danach schnell abnahm. Die Erhöhung der Reizschwelle war offenbar nicht durch Widerstandserhöhung zwischen den Elektroden bedingt, denn ein Ansteigen des normalen Widerstandes von 1,4—6 kΩ wurde nicht beobachtet.

Freilegen des N. laryngeus: Der Nerv soll schonend präpariert und anschließend vor dem Austrocknen geschützt werden (Toner und Macko).

Herstellen der Vagusschlinge: Verbesserungen der Methode von Schroeder werden von Schlez angegeben.

f) Applikation von Antitussiva

Prüfstoffe werden üblicherweise peroral, subcutan oder intravenös verabfolgt. Bei narkotisierten Tieren wird der intravenöse Weg bevorzugt, bei wachen Tieren überwiegen die übrigen Zuführungsarten. Perorale Applikation entspricht dem humantherapeutischen Gebrauch der Antitussiva am besten. Intravenöse Zufuhr bietet den Vorteil der geringeren Dosierung und des schnellen Abklingens der Wirkung. Bei intravenöser Gabe sind daher Dosiswiederholungen möglich bzw. während eines orientierenden Versuches an einem Tier können mehrere Stoffe miteinander verglichen werden. Eine Summation von unterschwelligen Wirkungen und Tachyphylaxie ist bei diesem Vorgehen aber nicht ausgeschlossen.

Bei Tieren, die wiederholt zur Arzneimittelprüfung herangezogen werden, muß auf Gewöhnung geachtet werden. Gewöhnung an die antitussive Wirkung von Codein, Morphin und morphinähnlichen Analgetica kann von Hunden recht schnell erworben werden (Schroeder; Rosiere u. Mitarb.; Kasé, 1955). Friebel und Kuhn (1964) studierten die Gewöhnung und Rückbildung von Gewöhnung an die antitussive Wirkung von Codein an Meerschweinchen und Ratten. Die Tiere wurden ein- oder dreimal täglich 6—7 Wochen lang subcutan behandelt. Die antitussive ED_{50} wurde in 14tägigen Abständen bestimmt, die Dosierung der Toleranzentwicklung angepaßt. Die antitussive ED_{50} stieg im Verlauf der toleranzerzeugenden Behandlung bei beiden Tierarten auf ein Mehrfaches des Ausgangswertes an und bildete sich anschließend langsam zurück. Meerschweinchen benötigten für die Entwöhnung etwa 27 Wochen oder $4^1/_2$mal soviel Zeit wie für die Gewöhnung. Wiedererwerb von Toleranz nach abgeschlossener Entwöhnung ist möglich. Bei diesem Vorgang schritt die Entwicklung der Toleranz etwas langsamer als beim ersten Versuch voran. Sie erreichte auch einen geringeren Grad. Aber die Tiere waren beim zweiten Toleranzversuch auch wesentlich älter als beim ersten. Die Schnelligkeit, mit der Gewöhnung sich entwickelte, verlief offensichtlich in partieller Unabhängigkeit von kleineren oder vorübergehenden Änderungen des Dosierungsschemas, also in primärer Abhängigkeit von zell- oder systemgebundenen Gegebenheiten. Das Fortschreiten der Toleranz verlief nach Art einer Exponentialfunktion. Auch die Rückbildung lieferte bei logarhythmischer Darstellung eine Gerade. In entsprechender Weise entwickelte sich bei Meerschweinchen Gewöhnung an die antitussive Wirkung von Morphin. Auch hier dauerte die Entwöhnung wesentlich länger als die Toleranzentwicklung (Friebel, Jacob und Cros).

Die Frage, ob Gewöhnung an die antitussive Wirkung ausschließlich von „morphinähnlichen“ Pharmaka hervorgerufen werden kann, ist noch nicht ausreichend untersucht worden.

Vor unerwünschter Toleranzentwicklung schützen breite Versuchsintervalle (einmalige Prüfstoffapplikation pro Woche).

g) Beurteilung von antitussiver Wirkung

Experimenteller Husten wird als forcierter exspiratorischer Luftstrom unterhalb (Kroepfli) und oberhalb (Domenjoz) der Glottis kymographisch registriert. Er wird durch die Tätigkeit der exspiratorischen Muskulatur objektiviert (Krause). Er kann visuell oder akustisch wahrgenommen werden (Friebel, Reichle und v. Graevenitz; Rosiere u. Mitarb.; Stefko und Benson).

Eine Verhütung oder Abschwächung des Hustens kann an der Abnahme von Volumen oder Stärke des exspiratorischen Luftstromes (Domenjoz; May und Widdicombe), an der Arbeit der exspiratorisch bewegten Muskulatur oder an der Tiefe der ersten Inspiration nach einem Hustenstoß (May und Widdicombe), an der Reduktion der Zahl der Hustenstöße (Stefko und Benson; Winter und Flataker), an der Zunahme der Latenzzeit bis zum Auftreten des Hustens nach Reizbeginn (Chakravarty u. Mitarb.), an der Notwendigkeit, Reizstärke und -frequenz zu erhöhen (Schroeder; Hahn und Friebel), schließlich am völligen Ausbleiben des Hustenreflexes (Friebel, Reichle und v. Graevenitz; Reichle und Friebel; Krause) erkannt werden. Man darf erwarten, daß eine so differente Objektivierung von „antitussiver Wirkung" die Vergleichbarkeit von experimentellen Ergebnissen verschiedener Autoren erschwert.

Bei der quantitativen Bewertung der antitussiven Wirkung müssen zusätzlich Besonderheiten der verwendeten Tierart und der tierexperimentellen Methodik berücksichtigt werden.

Auch aus dieser Sicht sollten Ergebnisse, die mit verschiedenen Tierarten, Reizmitteln oder anderen methodischen Differenzen erarbeitet wurden, nicht uneingeschränkt vergleichend bewertet werden. Man darf erwarten, daß schwach wirksame Antitussiva oder Pharmaka mit geringer antitussiver Spezifität (Domenjoz; Enders und Schmidt) sich an narkotisierten, schwach gereizten oder intravenös mit Prüfstoff behandelten Tieren eher als wirksam erweisen als bei kräftig und nachhaltig gereizten wachen Tieren sowie bei peroraler oder subcutaner Prüfstoffapplikation. Für das spezifisch und kräftig wirkende Codein ist die Abhängigkeit der antitussiven ED_{50} von der hustenproduzierenden Reizgaskonzentration nachgewiesen worden (Friebel und Kuhn, 1962). Sie betrug bei nicht narkotisierten Meerschweinchen, die 2 min lang 10,6 ml SO_2 in 15 Liter Luft inhalierten, 8,0 (6,1—10,4) mg/kg Codeinphosphat, bei Inhalation von 11,2 ml SO_2/15 Liter Luft 11,5 (8,8—14,9) mg/kg und von 13,4 ml SO_2/15 Liter Luft 15,4 (11,0—21,6) mg/kg.

h) Spezifität der antitussiven Wirkung

Die Entwicklung spezifischer Antitussiva kam in Fluß, nachdem tierexperimentelle Methoden entwickelt worden waren, mit denen eine prüfstoffbedingte Hemmung des Hustenreflexes neben und unabhängig von der Hemmung der Atmung nachgewiesen werden konnte.

Cushny führte 1913 die Hustenstillung durch Morphin auf dessen lähmende Wirkung auf das Atemzentrum zurück. Schmitt und Harer hielten 1923 die Unterdrückung des Hustenreflexes für eine Hemmung der exspiratorischen Phase der Atmung. Eddy wählte 1932 die Verlangsamung der Atmung des Kaninchens als Modell für hustendepressorische Wirkung. Bucher bezeichnete 1952 Husten als Ergebnis einer reflektorischen Modulation der normalen Atmungstätigkeit. Bis dahin war es naheliegend, husten- und atemdepressorische Wirkung als gleichartig oder parallelgehend anzusehen. Schaumann faßte 1952 darüber hinaus den Hustenreflex, den Schmerzreflex und einige andere funktionelle Einheiten zu einem System zusammen, das auf morphinähnlich wirkende Pharmaka pharmakologisch gleichartig reagiere.

In den folgenden Jahren setzten sich in rascher Folge andere Auffassungen durch. Friebel, Reichle und v. Graevenitz wiesen an zwei Tierarten (Meerschweinchen und Ratte) nach, daß die antitussive und die analgetische Wirksamkeit der morphinähnlichen Verbindungen nicht parallel verläuft. Kurz vorher war von Domenjoz, von Pellmont und Bächtold, und von Winter und Flataker gezeigt worden, daß Verbindungen wie Benadryl, Dextromethorphan und Noscapine den Husten, aber nicht den Schmerz hemmen.

Aus Versuchen von Eichler und Smiatek, Haas, Kuhn und Friebel (1960) an Meerschweinchen und Katzen geht hervor, daß man zwischen dämpfender Wirkung auf das Hustenzentrum und auf das Atemzentrum unterscheiden kann. Friebel und Kuhn (1962) fanden im 2-Aminoindan eine Verbindung, die das Hustenzentrum hemmt und die Atmung zugleich stimuliert. Damit war die prinzipielle Selbständigkeit des Hustenreflexmechanismus im physiologischen und pharmakologischen Sinne dokumentiert.

In jüngeren Arbeiten wird daher nach dem Angriffspunkt der Antitussiva im Hustenzentrum selbst gefragt. Hahn und Friebel verglichen fünf antitussiv wirkende Substanzen (Codein, Dextromethorphan, Pipazethat, 2-Aminoindan und Hexobarbital) an Meerschweinchen, die über Trachealelektroden zum Husten gereizt wurden. Bezugspunkt für prüfstoffbedingte Veränderungen der Hustenreizschwelle war der im unbehandelten Zustand ermittelte Schwellenwert der Stromstärke. Nach Ermittlung der Ausgangsempfindlichkeit und subcutaner Injektion der Prüfstoffe wurden die Veränderungen der Hustenreizschwelle fortlaufend durch Anpassen der Reizstromstärke in Stufen von 1 mA gerade soweit ausgeglichen, daß auch unter dem Einfluß von Prüfstoffen noch Husten ausgelöst werden konnte. Die Registrierung der Schwellenänderungen wurde über einen Zeitraum von 3 Std ausgedehnt. Registriert und ausgewertet wurden Veränderungen der Reizschwelle, Einordnung des Hustenstoßes in den Atemrhythmus, Veränderungen des kymographischen Bildes des Hustenstoßes und Hustentons. Jede der geprüften Verbindungen verursachte eine Reihe von Abweichungen vom Normalverhalten. In der Zusammensetzung der Abweichungen glich keine Verbindung einer anderen. Nur eine Wirkung war allen gemeinsam: Die Erhöhung der Hustenreizschwelle. Die Herabsetzung der Sensibilität des Hustenreflexmechanismus konnte immer durch Anheben der Reizstromstärke, d.h. durch Vermehrung der pro Zeit im Hustenzentrum einlaufenden Potentiale ausgeglichen werden. Offensichtlich verursachen die Antitussiva im Speicherungssystem einen über das Normale hinausgehenden Verlust von husteninduzierenden Potentialen; die Speicherfähigkeit oder die Fähigkeit zur Bahnung war herabgesetzt. Die zentrale antitussive Wirkung wird daher für eine Hemmung der Reizspeicherung oder -bahnung im zuständigen Neuronengeflecht gehalten.

Dieser Angriffspunkt war nicht der einzige, den die Prüfstoffe im Bereich des Hustenzentrums erkennen ließen. Vereinfachungen und Komplizierungen der W-förmigen Zeichnung des exspiratorischen Luftstoßes, die durch Prüfsubstanzen hervorgerufen wurden, sprechen für eine Hemmung (Hexobarbital, Codein in höherer Dosierung) oder Stimulation (2-Aminoindan, Pipazethat, Dextromethorphan) der die Glottis steuernden Neurone im pneumotaktischen Apparat. Verzögerung des Reflexablaufs, wie ihn Hexobarbital bedingt, dokumentiert eine allgemeine, wahrscheinlich unspezifische Hemmung oder Verlangsamung der Reizübertragung im Reflexbogen. Abweichungen vom Normalen, die bei der Einordnung des Hustenstoßes in den Atemcyclus beobachtet wurden (Hexobarbital, 2-Aminoindan, Dextromethorphan), weisen auf Angriffspunkte an Neuronen hin, die für die Korrelation von Hustenreaktion und Atmungsrhythmik zuständig sind.

Tabelle 2. *Pharmakodynamische Wirkungsspektren einiger Antitussiva (in Anlehnung an Eddy, Friebel, Hahn und Halbach)*

	Antitussive Dosierung	Analgetische Dosierung	Sedative Wirkung	Respiratorische Wirkung
Normethadon	$<$ C	$<$ C	$=$ C	depress.
Pholcodin	$<$ C	?	?	$=$ C, oder $>$
Caramiphen	$=$ C (i.v.)	—		?
Dihydrocodein	$=$ C	$=$ C	$=$ C, oder $>$	$=$ C, oder $>$
Dextromethorphan	$=$ C, oder $>$	—		
Äthylmorphin	$>$ C	$=$ C	$=$ C	?
Codein	$>$ M	$>$ M	$<$ M	depress.
Dimethylamino-dithienylbuten	$=$ C	—		
Carbetapentan	$=$ C	—		?
Dimethoxanat	$=$ C	—	—	—
Pipazethat	$=$ C, oder $>$		—	depress.
Dibunat-Na.	$=$ C			stimul.
Noscapin	$=$ C, oder $>$	—	—	stimul.
Clophedianol	$>$ C	—	—	?
Silomat	$=$ C	—	—	?
Isoaminil	$>$ C	?	—	$<$ C
l-Propoxyphen	$>$ C	—		—
Benzonatate	$=$ C	—	—	?
Oxolamin	$<$ C	$>$ C		—

Der wesentlichste Befund der Untersuchungen, die intrazentrale, neuronale Hemmung wird durch Ergebnisse von Engelhorn und Weller (**1966**) bestätigt. Diese Autoren leiteten an Katzen in leichter Numalnarkose die Aktionsströme exspiratorischer Neurone der Medulla oblongata mit Hilfe von Wolfram-Mikroelektroden ab. Dabei konnten die autonomen E_α-Neurone und die als zentrale Repräsentanten hustenwirksamer sensibler Afferenzen angesehenen E_β-Neurone getrennt erfaßt werden. Der Hustenreflex wurde durch mechanische Reizung in der Trachea oder durch elektrische Reizung am N. laryngeus superior beiderseits ausgelöst. Als Vertreter verschiedenartiger antitussiver Wirkungstypen wurden Codein, Dextromethorphan und Noscapine verwendet. Zur Hemmung des Hustenreflexes und der für den Husten charakteristischen E_α- und E_β-Entladungen reichten 2,0 mg/kg Codein oder Dextromethorphan oder 8,0—16 mg/kg Noscapine intravenös zugeführt aus. Alle Stoffe verkürzten vorübergehend die Pause zwischen den E_α-Serien bei Normalatmung. Codein und Dextromethorphan verursachten unter diesen Bedingungen eine Verlangsamung der Normalatmung und eine Verlängerung der E_α-Serien sowie eine Abnahme der mittleren Spike-Frequenzen. Nach antitussiv wirkenden Mengen von Noscapine war die Atmung beschleunigt und die Aktivität der E_α-Neurone herabgesetzt und verkürzt. Die stärksten Effekte auf das E_α-System waren innerhalb $^1/_2$ Std nach der intravenösen Injektion abgeklungen. Sie hielten nicht solange an wie die hustenstillende Wirkung. Alle Substanzen bewirkten, in ausreichender Dosierung gegeben, eine Hemmung der E_β-Aktivität über den gleichen Zeitraum, in dem auch der Hustenreflex herabgesetzt war. Dabei bestand ein Zusammenhang zwischen Dosis und Wirkungsgrad sowie zwischen Reizstärke und Wirkungsdauer.

C = Codein, M = Morphin, P = Procain, Coc. = Cocain; + = aktiv, — = inaktiv, ? = Wirksamkeit nicht gesichert. Die Angaben sind im wesentlichen aus tierexperimentellen Arbeiten zusammengetragen. Einzelheiten in der o. a. Monographie.

Zirkulatorische Wirkung	Gastrointestinale Wirkung	Bronchomotorische Wirkung	Bronchosekretorische Wirkung	Lokalanaesthetische Wirkung	Antiphlogistische Wirkung
	?	= C	depress.	> P	
= C	antispasm.	antispasm.	stimul.	< Coc.	
= M					
			?		+
			?		
?	peristalt.	constrict.	depress.		+
vascul.	depress.		?	> P	
depress.	antispasm.				
depress.	antispasm.	antispasm.	depress.	> P	
depress.	antispasm.			< P	
—		antispasm.		< P	
—		—	—		
vascul.		antispasm.	stimul.		
depress.					
?	—		depress.	> P	
?	—	antispasm.	stimul.	—	
depress.	antispasm.		—	< P	
	—		?	> P	
depress.	antispasm.	antispasm.		= P	+

Alle zur Prüfung auf antitussive Wirkung geeigneten Methoden sind auch zur Aufklärung der antitussiven Spezifität der Wirkung mit herangezogen worden. Die diesbezügliche Aussagefähigkeit der Ergebnisse ist methodisch bedingt unterschiedlich. Sie ist begrenzter, wenn sedierte oder narkotisierte Versuchstiere verwendet werden, denn der Hustenreflexapparat wird — wie andere zentrale Mechanismen auch — von den zur Vorbehandlung verwendeten Substanzen „unspezifisch" gedämpft; s. V, c), Narkose, S. 55. Entsprechendes gilt nach Ansicht von Boissier und Pagny (1960, 2) für die Behandlung mit neuroleptisch wirkenden Verbindungen, die eine Verstärkung der aus der Vorbehandlung stammenden Depression bewirken können.

Viele Antitussiva beeinflussen nicht nur den Hustenreflexmechanismus, sondern auch weitere physiologische Funktionen. Die Zahl und Art der zusätzlichen Angriffspunkte variieren von Substanz zu Substanz. Morphinähnlich wirkende Antitussiva haben analgetische, sedierende, atmungshemmende Eigenschaften und erzeugen Abhängigkeit. Caramiphen, Carbetapentan, Dimethoxanat, Pipazethat und andere haben eine spasmolytische Wirkungskomponente. Benzonatate kann als Lokalanästheticum verwendet werden. Substanzen wie Dextromethorphan und Noscapin, die kaum andere als antitussive Wirkungen erkennen lassen, befinden sich in der Minderzahl (Tabelle 2). Wenn bei einer Substanz neben der antitussiven auch sedative, hypnotische, neuroleptische oder atmungshemmende Eigenschaften nachweisbar sind, wird zu prüfen sein, wieweit das Ergebnis der Untersuchung auf antitussive Wirkung von den zusätzlichen Wirkungen beeinflußt wird. Ein Vergleich von Dosis-Wirkungskurven für die verschiedenen Teilwirkungen — möglichst an derselben Tierart und unter vergleichbaren Bedingungen erarbeitet — wird die notwendigen Kriterien bringen. In diesen Fällen ist es also zweckmäßig, bei der Auswahl der Methode zum Nachweis antitussiver Wirkung für eine Abstimmung mit den weiteren pharmakologischen Untersuchungsmethoden zu sorgen.

D. Experimenteller Husten beim Menschen

I. Allgemeines

Höglund und Michaelsson veröffentlichten als erste 1950 einen Bericht über experimentellen Husten, der durch die Inhalation eines irritierenden chemischen Stoffes bei gesunden Freiwilligen erzeugt wurde. Die Versuchspersonen inhalierten die Atemluft durch ein Rohrsystem, in das mit einer Injektionsspritze 2%iger Ammoniakdampf in der erforderlichen Quantität eingeblasen wurde. Das Irritans verursachte einen reflektorischen Glottisschluß (nicht Husten), der mit Hilfe eines um den Thorax gelegten Pneumographen registriert wurde. Mehr oder weniger modifiziert ist diese Methode auch von Trendelenburg, Blix, Hahn und Wilbrand sowie Gravenstein, Devloo und Beecher verwendet worden. Mit Ausnahme der letztgenannten Gruppe konnten alle Autoren mit diesem Verfahren ein Ansteigen der Reizschwelle nach Codeingaben beobachten.

Gegen diese Methode und die mit ihr erarbeiteten Ergebnisse sind Bedenken vorgetragen worden: Trendelenburg und andere haben das von Höglund und Michaelsson eingeführte Registrierungssystem nicht verwendet, sondern sich auf die subjektive Wahrnehmung des vermutlichen Glottisverschlusses verlassen in der Erwartung, daß Übereinstimmung mit den bei mechanischer Registrierung anfallenden Ergebnissen bestehe. Glottisverschluß war das entscheidende Kriterium für Reaktion, unabhängig davon, ob ihm ein Hustenstoß nachfolgte oder nicht; am Glottisverschluß wurde daher sowohl die schwellenüberschreitende Ammoniakmenge als auch die Schwellenerhöhung durch Antitussiva bestimmt. Gravenstein, Devloo und Beecher konnten nicht eruieren, warum es ihnen nicht gelang, die Ergebnisse ihrer Vorgänger zu bestätigen. Sie weisen auf zwei Punkte hin: Höglund und Michaelsson verwandten weder Placebos noch arbeiteten sie unter Doppeltblindbedingungen. Gravenstein u. Mitarb. bemerkten außerdem, daß der empfohlene Ammoniakbehälter schnell Ammoniak verlor, so daß die Ammoniakkonzentration im inhalierten Reizgas im Verlaufe eines länger dauernden Versuchs oder bei aufeinanderfolgenden Versuchen nicht dieselbe blieb. Trendelenburg sowie Hahn und Wilbrand bemerkten, daß die Höhe der Reizschwelle weitgehend von meteorologischen Bedingungen und psychologischen Faktoren beeinflußt wurde. Gravenstein, Devloo und Beecher fanden sie wesentlich konstanter und reproduzierbarer, konnten aber durch Behandlung mit Antitussiva keine signifikante Erhöhung erzielen.

Der Reizstoff Ammoniak wurde verlassen, nachdem Bickerman und Barach gezeigt hatten, daß Citronensäure als zuverlässiges und gut verträgliches hustenerzeugendes Irritans verwendet werden kann.

II. Chemische Stimulation

a) Methode von Bickerman u. Mitarb. (1956, 1957)

Der Inhalationsapparat besteht aus einem Atmungsluft liefernden System, das über eine Gesichtsmaske fest mit der Versuchsperson verbunden wird. Über einen Nebenschluß kann citronensäurehaltiges Aerosol zeitweise der Atemluft beigemischt werden. Die Exspirationsluft wird durch einen Pneumotachographen geleitet, in dessen Nebenschluß sich ein Kondensatormikrophon befindet. Die (gesunden) Versuchspersonen inhalieren Luft, der in steigender Konzentration 1,25%, 2,5%, 5%, 7,5%, 10,0%, 15,0%, 20,0% oder 25% Citronensäure in Form eines stabilen Aerosols von überwiegend 2,5 μ großen Tröpfchen beigemischt wird. Kymographisch werden das inhalierte Gasvolumen und die Dauer der Inspiration aufgezeichnet. Der Husten wird mit einem 2-Kanal-Schreiber als „Ton-Druck" und als Luftdurchfluß in Liter/sec aufgezeichnet. Die Versuchspersonen müssen frei von Infekten des Atmungstraktes sein. Ihre jeweilige Reizschwellenhöhe wird ermittelt. Anschließend wird die Citronensäurekonzentration verwendet, die bei 5 Inhalationen, von 1—2 min dauernden Intervallen unterbrochen, wenigstens viermal Husten auslöst. Von den Versuchspersonen, die Bickerman u. Mitarb. (1957) verwendeten, reagierten die meisten auf 5—10% Citronensäure enthaltende Lösungen. Nach jeder Inhalation muß die in der Mundhöhle zurückbleibende Säure mit einem Schluck Wasser herausgespült werden.

Nach der Ermittlung der Reizschwelle wird die Versuchssubstanz unter Doppeltblindbedingungen eingenommen und in stündlichen Abständen 4 Std lang auf Wirksamkeit untersucht. Bickerman u. Mitarb. (1957) zogen zur Bestimmung jeder Arzneimitteldosis 8 im Umgang mit der Methode erfahrene Versuchspersonen heran. Entscheidendes Kriterium für die Wirksamkeit der Prüfstoffe war in diesen Versuchen die durchschnittliche Zahl der Hustenstöße nach Inhalation einer Citronensäuredosis.

Bickerman u. Mitarb. haben mit diesem Verfahren länger als 5 Jahre gearbeitet und eine große Zahl von Antitussiva vergleichend geprüft (Bickerman und Itkin). Es ist auch von Rasch, von Archibald, Slipp und Shane, Morris und Shane, Großman, Birker und Casimir, Calesnick, Christensen und Munch, Tannenbaum und von Silson verwendet worden. Alle diese Autoren konnten eine Reduktion der Zahl der Hustenstöße nach der Gabe von Antitussiva registrieren. Gravenstein, Devloo und Beecher sowie Sevelius, Lester und Colmore konnten keine Arzneimittelwirkung nachweisen. Gravenstein, Devloo und Beecher kritisieren, daß von Bickerman nicht zwischen einem lauten explosiven Hustenstoß und einem von geringer Intensität unterschieden wird, daß die Aerosolquantität, die die Lunge erreicht, nicht akkurat kontrolliert bzw. determiniert werden kann, und daß es nicht immer gelingt, Doppeltblindbedingungen einzuhalten, weil die Versuchspersonen unspezifische Arzneimittelwirkungen (z.B. sedative oder andere Effekte) wahrnehmen. Sevelius, Lester und Colmore änderten das Verfahren von Bickerman etwas ab. Sie suchten die Citronensäurekonzentration auf, welche gleichbleibend eine maximale Hustenreaktion auslöste. Trotz sorgfältiger Auswahl und Übung von Versuchspersonen veränderte sich die Hustenreaktion im Leerversuch nach gleichbleibenden Citronensäurekonzentrationen von Stunde zu Stunde bis zu 50%. Schließlich gewöhnten sich die Versuchspersonen an die Irritation und husteten von Versuch zu Versuch seltener. Bei Arzneimittelversuchen konnten 15 und 30 mg Codein nicht von Placebo unterschieden werden. Die Frage, ob die von Sevelius u. Mitarb. beobachtete Gewöhnung an die Citronensäure eine Folge der von ihnen verwendeten höheren Citronensäurekonzentrationen ist, bleibt unbeantwortet.

b) Methode von Calesnick und Christensen

Die Autoren modifizierten die Methode von Bickerman u. Mitarb. (1956). Sie werten das Zeitintervall aus, das vom Beginn der Citronensäureinhalation bis zum Hustenstoß vergeht. Verlängerung der Latenz nach Prüfstoffgaben zeigt antitussive Wirkung an. Bei diesem Vorgehen muß auf guten Maskensitz geachtet werden. Die Autoren empfehlen, nur männliche Versuchspersonen zu verwenden, weil weibliche Personen leichter mit initialem Glottisverschluß reagieren und damit die Inhalation einer ausreichenden Menge von Citronensäureaerosol fraglich wird. Es wird 25% Citronensäurelösung vernebelt. Es werden nicht nur Versuchspersonen ausgeschieden, die auf Citronensäureinhalation unzureichend husten, sondern auch solche, die nach einer Testdosis von 40 mg Codein oral keine antitussive Wirkung erkennen lassen.

c) Methode von Tiffeneau

Acetylcholin in Form von Aerosolen hat, wenn es über die Atemwege zugeführt wird, außer der Wirkung auf die Ventilation eine Reizwirkung auf die sensiblen Nervenenden in der Lunge. Acetylcholin löst Husten aus, wenn die Receptoren besonders reizbar sind, wie bei Personen mit chronischen Affektionen der Luftwege.

Tiffeneau läßt Acetylcholinlösungen von einem Vernebler aerolisieren, der, mit Preßluft bei einem wirksamen Druck von 800 g betrieben, 0,2 ml bei einem Gasverbrauch von 20 l/min verbraucht. Die Versuchsperson inhaliert das Aerosol jeweils 90 sec lang. Die Zahl der Hustenstöße wird während der Inhalation und während der folgenden 90 sec gezählt. Der Versuch kann mehrmals wiederholt werden, wenn Intervalle von 5—10 min eingehalten werden. Ausgewertet wird die Zahl der Hustenstöße nach der Inhalation einer 1%igen Acetylcholinlösung, oder die minimale Acetylcholinkonzentration, die bei Prüfung einer aufsteigenden Reihe von Aerosolen mit 10, 25, 50, 100, 250 und 500 μg Acetylcholin pro Liter Aerosol tussigen wirkt.

Die Probe wird als unschädlich bezeichnet. Sie ist einfach und kurz und erfordert keinen wesentlichen Aufwand. Überschießender Husten kann durch Inhalation von Hexamethonium gestillt werden. Gelegentlich, besonders bei Asthmatikern kann ein Anfall von Dyspnoe hervorgerufen werden. Dieser ist von kurzer Dauer oder kann durch Atropin oder Adrenalin gelöst werden.

Beim Gesunden sind Acetylcholinhustenproben immer negativ. Sie sind oft positiv bei Personen mit chronischen Erkrankungen der Atemwege. Sie werden zu diagnostischen Zwecken angestellt. Tiffeneau hat aber auch die Wirkung einiger Pharmaka mit seinem Test geprüft. Das Ergebnis dieser orientierenden Versuche wird folgendermaßen beschrieben: Der Acetylcholinhusten kann abgeschwächt werden durch zentral angreifende Hustenmittel (Codein) und, wenigstens bei respiratorischer Insuffizienz, durch Eupnoica (Adrenergica, Xanthine). Er wird in auffälliger Weise unterdrückt durch die Ganglioplegica (Penta- und Hexamethonium).

d) Methode von Haslreiter

Haslreiter modifizierte die Methode von Tiffeneau nur wenig. Acetylcholinlösung wird an einem Pari-Optimal Aerosolgerät (600—700 mg/min) 90 sec in ansteigender Konzentration von 0,1, 0,25, 0,5, 1,0% inhaliert. Mehrfache Hustenstöße, die nach einer solchen Inhalation auftreten, werden als positiver Test bezeichnet; die entsprechende Konzentration wird als Reizschwelle notiert. Die Hustenstöße werden graphisch registriert, es ist dies mit einem Tastenschreiber auf einem Kymographion, aber auch lediglich mit reiner Strichführung möglich. Es muß sowohl die Häufigkeit, die Dauer und die Intensität des Hustens daraus hervorgehen, als auch der Zeitpunkt des Einsetzens der Beschwerden. Als Kontroll-Aerosol wird vor jedem Test Aqua dest. inhaliert. Patienten, die auf dieses Aerosol mit Husten reagieren, werden von weiteren Versuchen ausgeschlossen.

Haslreiter verwendet — wie Tiffeneau — den Test zu diagnostischen Zwecken und zur Wirksamkeitsprüfung von Antitussiva. Er bestätigt die Angaben von Tiffeneau über die Unempfindlichkeit von Gesunden, über die Harmlosigkeit, die positive Reaktion von etwa 80% der Patienten mit chronisch entzündlichen Atemwegserkrankungen sowie die Dyspnoe der Asthmatiker. Abweichend von Tiffeneau beobachtet er eine gute Beeinflußbarkeit des Hustens durch Codein im Doppeltblindversuch. In mehr als 50% seiner Fälle unterdrückt Codein (30 mg oral) den Husten vollkommen.

Mit geringer Abweichung verwandte auch Prime den Acetylcholinhusten zur Arzneimittelprüfung. Seine Versuchspersonen waren Zigarettenraucher mit einem Zigarettenverbrauch von 20 und mehr Zigaretten täglich. Alle husteten nach der Inhalation einer 1%igen Acetylcholinlösung (Inhalationsdauer 90 sec). Die Zahl der Hustenstöße, die in den dem Test folgenden 20 min produziert wurden, sind gezählt worden. Bei dem Versuch den Acetylcholinhusten nach dem Verfahren von Haslreiter zu quantifizieren war Prime nicht erfolgreich. Wie Haslreiter hält er den Acetylcholinhusten für eine Methode, mit der die antitussive Wirkung von Codein (16 mg oral) nachgewiesen werden kann. Sevelius, Lester und Colmore arbeiteten die Versuche von Prime nach. Sie konnten seine Ergebnisse nicht bestätigen. Ihre 9 Versuchspersonen konnten nicht zwischen 30 mg Codeinphosphat und Placebo unterscheiden. Ein anschließender Briefwechsel mit Prime ergab, daß auch dieser seine früheren Ergebnisse nicht reproduzieren konnte.

e) Hustenprovokation mit Paraldehyd

Gravenstein, Devloo und Beecher fanden, daß die Dosis, die gesunden Versuchspersonen intravenös injiziert, kräftigen Husten auslöst, individuell unterschiedlich zwischen 0,25 und 0,5 ml liegt. Konar injizierte 1 ml in eine Unterarmvene (als 5%ige Dextroselösung in Form eines Dauertropf). Bei der Versuchsperson trat das Gefühl auf, als würde die Brust zusammengeschnürt, schließlich trat mit einem explosiven Hustenanfall Befreiung ein. Der Husten dauerte 30—60 sec und war gelegentlich von einem zweiten Anfall gefolgt. Wenn die wirksame Paraldehyddosis ermittelt und nach 30 min wiederholt worden war, wurde das Antitussivum gegeben und die Paraldehydinjektion in halbstündigem Abstand während der nächsten $2^1/_2$ Std wiederholt.

Gravenstein, Devloo und Beecher bemerkten einen Unterschied in der Reaktion auf Paraldehyd zwischen Heroin (2,5 mg/sec) und Placebo, wenn die Versuchspersonen als ihre eigenen Kontrollen verwendet wurden; sie fanden keinen Unterschied zwischen Codein und Placebo. Auch Konar konnte die Codeinwirkung bei paraldehydbehandelten Versuchspersonen nicht nachweisen. Gravenstein, Devloo und Beecher brachen ihre Versuche nicht nur wegen der unbefriedigenden Resultate ab, sondern auch, weil Paraldehyd an der Injektionsstelle Schmerz und Phlebitis verursacht, weil die Versuchspersonen das zusammenschnürende Gefühl fürchten und weil große individuelle Schwankungen zwischen den Versuchsergebnissen bestehen.

f) Hustenprovokation mit Lobelin

Intravenös injiziertes Lobelin erregt nach Ansicht von Chabrier, Giudicelli und Thuillier möglicherweise durch direkte Einwirkung auf den zentralen Teil der Hustenreflexbahn Husten. Die Autoren geben 3,0—10,0 mg als wirksame Dosen an. Der Hustenanfall dauert 10—20 sec. Ihm folgt eine etwa 60 sec dauernde Polypnoe. Sie weisen darauf hin, daß Lobelin wegen toxischer Reaktionen vorsichtig angewendet werden muß. Sie fanden, daß 80—100 mg Pholcodin die Lobelinreaktion abschwächten.

Hillis und Kelly waren aber bei Versuchen, den durch 5 mg α-Lobelin ausgelösten Husten mit Codein, Morphin und Heroin zu beeinflussen, nicht erfolgreich. Der Husten konnte durch Hexamethoniumjodid verhindert werden.

g) Zusammenfassende Beurteilung der Methoden

Bickerman und Barach sagen, daß artifizieller Husten folgende Bedingungen erfüllen sollte:

1. Gleichbleibendes und anhaltendes Reaktionsvermögen der Versuchsperson gegenüber demselben Schwellenreiz.
2. Der hustenprovozierende Stoff muß untoxisch sein, und seine Anwendung so einfach, daß Beobachtungen an vielen Versuchspersonen möglich sind.
3. Die Versuchsergebnisse sollten reproduzierbar sein. Keine der beschriebenen Methoden erfüllt diese Bedingungen vollkommen. Die Citronensäuremethode kann wohl als die am meisten versprechende Methode, die am subtilsten ausgearbeitete Arbeitstechnik und schließlich als die harmloseste angesehen werden. Aber sie ist nicht vollkommen.

Die Ergebnisse, die bei ihrer Verwendung erhalten werden, korrelieren nicht immer befriedigend mit Untersuchungsergebnissen, die am Krankenbett gewonnen wurden. Bickerman und Itkin konnten die antitussive Wirkung von Normethadon nicht nachweisen, obwohl sie tierexperimentell und klinisch gut gesichert erscheint. Umgekehrt fanden Bickerman u. Mitarb. (1957) und Calesnick, Christensen und Munch Lävopropoxyphen beim artifiziellen Husten wirksam, während Woolf und Rosenberg die Substanz als klinisch unwirksam beurteilten; sie verwendeten zur Objektivierung ihrer Resultate ein Tape-Recorder-System.

Die Methoden, die verwendet werden, um beim gesunden oder kranken Menschen experimentell Husten zu erzeugen, sollten noch weiter entwickelt werden. Als Ergänzung zur tierexperimentellen Methodik und als Brücke zur klinischen Situation wird man sie auch in Zukunft benötigen.

E. Beziehungen zwischen dem experimentellen Husten und dem spontanen Husten des Kranken

Die experimentell erzeugte Hustenreaktion verläuft uniform, unkompliziert, denn die Variablen werden begrenzt. Die Versuchsergebnisse sollen reproduzierbar sein. Die Symptomatik, die der Kranke bietet, ist vielfältiger. Sein Husten ist ein Produkt verschiedenartiger morphologischer und funktioneller Zustandsänderungen im sensiblen und afferenten Bereich der Hustenreflexbahn. Er kann auch von Afferenzen hervorgerufen und modifiziert werden, die dem medullären Teil der Reflexbahn von benachbarten Funktionseinheiten oder höheren Abschnitten des ZNS her zufließen. Die Variablen sind daher kaum begrenzbar.

Beim experimentellen Husten sollen reproduzierbare Ergebnisse anfallen. Daher wird bei wiederholter Reizung für qualitativ und quantitativ gleichbleibende Stimulation gesorgt und eine Gewöhnung des gereizten Reflexmechanismus an den Reiz ausgeschlossen. Der Stimulus wirkt nur kurzfristig, bei wiederholter Stimulation nur nach größeren Intervallen auf sein Substrat ein. Das wesentlichste Charakteristikum des pathologischen Hustens ist, daß er den Stimulus, der ihn provoziert, nicht eliminieren kann. Husten dieser Art verläuft in der Regel weder gleichartig noch gleichbleibend. Der Organismus kann bei Unvermögen, das irritierende Agens zu beseitigen, Faktoren ins Spiel bringen, die den Reflexmechanismus und das Individuum vor der Erschöpfung bewahren: z.B. Gewöhnung an das Irritans. Hinzu kommt eine unterschiedliche Neigung

Tabelle 3. *Codeindosen, die im Tierexperiment antitussiv wirken*

Tierart	Reizart	Narkose	Codein-dosis mg|kg	Appli-kation	ED_{50}	Autor
Maus	H_2SO_4	—	10,0	s.c.		Kelentey u. Mitarb. (1958)
	H_2SO_4	—	10,0	s.c.		Kelentey u. Mitarb. (1957)
Ratte	SO_2	—	10,0	s.c.	+	Friebel, Kuhn (1964)
	SO_2	—	10,0	s.c.		Reichle, Friebel
	SO_2	—	13,5	s.c.	+	Hengen, Kasparek
	SO_2	—	26,0	s.c.		Weidemeyer u. Mitarb.
Meer-schwein-chen	SO_2	—	15,4	s.c.		Friebel, Kuhn (1962)
	SO_2	—	20,0	s.c.		Boissier, Pagny (1960, 1)
	SO_2	—	25,0	s.c.	+	Friebel, Kuhn (1964)
	SO_2	—	30,0	i.p.		Cahen
	SO_2	—	10,0	i.v.		Green, Ward
	NH_3	—	12,0	p.o.		Sallé, Brunaud
	NH_3	—	0,3	s.c.	+	Graham
	NH_3	—	0,5—2,0	s.c.		Winter, Flataker (1954)
	NH_3	—	1,0	s.c.		Silvestrini, Maffii
	Acrolein	—	3,5	s.c.		Silvestrini, Maffii
	Acrolein	—	9,6—11,8	i.p.		Silvestrini, Pozzatti
Kanin-chen	mechanisch	—	100,0	p.o.		Furakawa, Okabe
	mechanisch	—	3,0—4,0	i.v.		Furakawa, Okabe
	mechanisch	—	13,5	i.v.		Graham
Katze	Seifenpulver	+	1,5	i.v.		Pellmont, Bächtold
	NH_3	+	1,5	i.v.		Silvestrini, Maffii
	NH_3	+	3,5	i.v.		Pellmont, Bächtold
	NH_3	(+)	10,0	i.v.		Mulinos
	NH_3	(+)	0,61	s.c.	+	Engelhorn
	NH_3		15,0	i.p.		Cahen
	J-Pleuritis	—	2,5—3,0	s.c.		Van Dongen
	mechanisch	(+)	0,74	i.v.	+	Engelhorn
	mechanisch	+	3,0	i.v.		Silvestrini, Maffii
	mechanisch	(+)	10,0	i.v.		Mulinos
	mechanisch	+	16,3	i.v.		May, Widdicombe
	N. laryng.	(+)	8,1	p.o.	+	Engelhorn
	N. laryng.	(+)	0,52	i.v.	+	Engelhorn
	N. laryng.		1,0	i.p.		Cahen
	N. laryng.	+	1,0	i.v.		Plisnier
	N. laryng.	+	1,5	i.v.		Kohli u. Mitarb.
	N. laryng.	+	1,5	i.v.		Levis u. Mitarb.
	N. laryng.	+	1,5	i.v.		Klein
	N. laryng.	+	0,5—2,0	i.v.		Boissier, Pagny (1960, 1)
	N. laryng.	+	0,1—3,0	i.v.		Domenjoz
	N. laryng.	+	2,0—3,0	i.v.		Haas
	N. laryng.	+	4,0	i.v.	+	Green, Ward
	Medull. obl.	+	1,0—6,0	i.v.		Matallana, Borison
	Medull. obl.	+	4,0—10,0	i.v.		Chakravarty u. Mitarb.
	elektrisch	+	1,0	i.v.		Toner, Macko
	elektrisch	+	1,5	i.v.		Silvestrini, Maffii
	elektrisch	+	2,3	i.v.		Green, Ward
Hund	H_2SO_4	—	0,5	p.o.		Winter, Flataker (1952)
	H_2SO_4	—	1,0	s.c.		Silvestrini, Maffii

Tabelle 3 (Fortsetzung)

Tierart	Reizart	Narkose	Codeindosis mg/kg	Applikation	ED_{50}	Autor
Hund	SO_2	—	1,0			Chen u. Mitarb.
	SO_2	+	ca. 1,0	i. v.		Green, Ward
	NH_3	—	2,0	s. c.	+	Rosiere, Winder (1955)
	NH_3	—	2,8	s. c.		Winder u. Mitarb.
	NH_3	—	5,0	s. c.		Winder, Rosiere (1954)
	NH_3	—	1,0—5,7	s. c.		Rosiere, Winder (1956)
	NH_3	—	1,0—7,0	s. c.		Winder, Rosiere (1955)
	mechanisch	—	3,31	s. c.	+	Tedeschi u. Mitarb.
	mechanisch		7,5	i. p.		Cahen
	mechanisch	+	ca. 1,0	i. v.		Green, Ward
	mechanisch	—	2,0—4,0	i. v.		Kasé (1952)
	elektr. tracheal	—	1,1	p. o.	+	Stefko u. Mitarb.
	elektr. tracheal	—	3,5	s. c.		Silvestrini, Maffii
	elektr. tracheal	—	1,0—4,0	s. c.		Stefko, Benson
	elektr. tracheal	—	2,0—4,0	i. v.		Granier-Doyeux u. Mitarb.
	elektr. tracheal	—	2,5—3,5			Hara, Yanaura
	elektr. tracheal	+	5,0			Graham
	N. laryng.	—	1,5	i. v.		Klein

Tabelle 4. *Codeindosen, die bei humanexperimentellem*

Zahl der Probanden	Art der Probanden	Stimulans	Codeindosis mg
21	ausgewählte Gesunde	10% Citronensäureaerosol	30
17	Bronchialasthma-Patienten	10% Citronensäureaerosol	30
13	Gesunde	5—15% Citronensäureaerosol	10—60
20	Patienten	15% Citronensäureaerosol	32,5
20	Gesunde	10% Citronensäureaerosol	25
19	trainierte Gesunde	10% Citronensäureaerosol	5, 15, 30
14	ausgewählte Gesunde	10, 15% Citronensäureaerosol	30
24	Tuberkulöse Patienten	10, 15% Citronensäureaerosol	30
70	Gesunde	25% Citronensäureaerosol	15
6	ausgewählte Gesunde	10% Citronensäureaerosol	{ 15 30
6	Gesunde	5—25% Citronensäureaerosol	15, 30
9	Gesunde	Citronensäureaerosol	30
32	ausgewählte Gesunde	25% Citronensäureaerosol	5—120
15	Gesunde	Ammoniakinhalation	10—30
6	Gesunde	Ammoniakinhalation	10—40
	Gesunde	Ammoniakinhalation	
30	Gesunde	Ammoniakinhalation	20
24	Gesunde	Ammoniakinhalation	10—60
	Pat., Erkrankungen der Atmungsorgane	1% Acetylcholinaerosol	40
120	Pat., Erkrankungen der Atmungsorgane	0,1—1% Acetylcholinaerosol	30
12	Pat., Erkrankungen der Atmungsorgane	1% Acetylcholinaerosol	16
12	chronische Raucher	1% Acetylcholinaerosol	30
1	Gesunder	Pfefferminz-Wasser-Aerosol	{ 40 180
	Gesunde	α-Lobelin i. v.	hoch
5	Gesunde	0,025—0,5 ml Paraldehyd i. v.	10—60
	Gesunde	1 ml Paraldehyd i. v.	

der Kranken, sich psychisch an den Husten zu adaptieren oder ihn zunehmend als quälend zu empfinden. Hieraus resultiert: Zwischen der Intensität des Hustens, der Wahrnehmung des Hustens und der Schwere der Erkrankung besteht keine Korrelation. Vom einzelnen Kranken können folglich keine reproduzierbaren Versuchsergebnisse erwartet werden.

Ergebnisse der Arzneimittelprüfung am experimentellen Husten orientieren über die reflexhemmende Potenz eines Pharmakons. Ergebnisse der klinischen Prüfung geben über diese Wirkungskomponente Auskunft, wenn der Husten der Kranken durch Beobachter oder mechanisch registriert wird. Nicht berücksichtigt bleiben bei diesem Vorgehen die subjektiven Empfindungen der Kranken. Bezieht man sie aber in die Auswertung der Versuche mit ein, so erschwert man die Vergleichbarkeit der klinischen Ergebnisse mit denen, die beim experimentellen Husten gewonnen wurden und diese Wirkungskomponente nicht enthalten können.

Husten kann vom Kranken als belanglos oder als quälend empfunden werden. Diesem Faktor messen Gravenstein, Devloo und Beecher große Bedeutung bei. Sie konnten durch Behandlung des pathologischen Hustens mit Codein, Heroin, Dextromethorphan oder Placebo zwar keine objektiv feststellbare Senkung der Hustenfrequenz erreichen, erhielten aber die subjektive Aussage der Behandelten, daß nach Codein und Heroin, nicht nach Dextromethorphan und Placebo eine Besserung eingetreten sei. Sie glauben daher, daß Codein und Heroin den Patienten lediglich den Eindruck verschaffen, daß ihr Husten objektiv gebessert sei. Somit würde bei der Behandlung des spontanen Hustens mit diesen Arzneimitteln etwas ganz anderes erreicht als bei der Behandlung des experimentellen Hustens.

Husten antitussiv wirken bzw. unwirksam sind

Applikation	Behandlungserfolg	Erfolgskriterium	Autoren
p.o.	+	Reduktion der Hustenstoßzahl	Bickerman, Barach
p.o.	+	Reduktion der Hustenstoßzahl	Bickerman, Barach
s.c.	–	Reduktion der Hustenstoßzahl	Gravenstein, Devloo, Beecher
p.o.	+	Reduktion der Hustenstoßzahl	Shane, Krzyski, Copp
p.o.	+	Reduktion des Hustens in %	Rasch
p.o.	+	Reduktion des Hustens in %	Bickerman u. Mitarb. (1957)
p.o.	+	Reduktion der Hustenstoßzahl	Archibald, Slipp, Shane
p.o.	(+)	Reduktion der Hustenstoßzahl	Großman, Birker, Kasimir
p.o.	+	Reduktion der Hustenstoßzahl	Calesnick, Christensen, Munch
p.o. p.o.	– +	Reduktion der Hustenstoßzahl	Tannenbaum
p.o.	–	Reduktion der Hustenstoßzahl	Sevelius, Lester, Colmore
p.o.	+	Anstieg der Hustenlatenz	Silson
p.o.	+	Anstieg der Reizschwelle	Calesnik, Christensen
p.o.	+	Anstieg der Reizschwelle	Höglund, Michaelsson
p.o.	+	Anstieg der Reizschwelle	Trendelenburg
	+		Hahn, Wilbrand
p.o.	+	Anstieg der Reizschwelle	Blix
s.c.	–	Anstieg der Reizschwelle	Gravenstein, Devloo, Beecher
p.o.	(+)	Reduktion der Hustenstoßzahl	Tiffeneau
p.o.	+	Unterdrücken von Husten	Haslreiter
p.o.	+	Reduktion der Hustenstoßzahl	Prime
p.o.	–	Reduktion der Hustenstoßzahl	Sevelius, Lester, Colmore
s.c. p.o.	– –	Reduktion des Hustens in %	Hillis
i.v.	–	Unterdrücken von Husten	Hillis, Kelly
i.v.	–	Reduktion der Hustenstoßzahl	Gravenstein, Devloo, Beecher
	–	Unterdrücken von Husten	Konar

Tabelle 5. *Codeindosen, die oral Patienten verabfolgt subjektiv oder objektiv antitussiv wirken*

Zahl der Patienten	Diagnose	Codeindosis mg	Wirkung	Signifikante Wirkung	Autoren
12	Tuberkulose	10	subjektiv +		Himmelsbach u. Mitarb.
26	Tuberkulose	10	subjektiv +		Mulinos u. Mitarb.
26	Tuberkulose	20	subjektiv +		Mulinos u. Mitarb.
34	chronische Bronchitis	30	objektiv +	+	Nicolis, Pasquariello
21	chronische Bronchitis	60	objektiv +		Cavalieri u. Mitarb.
40	chronische Bronchitis	60	objektiv +	+	Pasquariello, Nicolis
28	chronische Bronchitis	3 × 10	objektiv +		Gravenstein, Devloo, Beecher
69	chronische Bronchitis	3 × 15	subjektiv +		Cass, Frederik (1954)
28	chronische Bronchitis	3 × 15	subjektiv +	+	Gravenstein, Devloo, Beecher
12	chronische Bronchitis	3 × 15	objektiv +		Sevelius, Colmore
60	chronische Bronchitis	3 × 30	subjektiv +		Haslreiter
65	chronische Bronchitis	3 × 30	subjektiv +		De Gregorio
43	chronische Bronchitis	3 × 30	subjektiv +		De Gregorio
25	akute Bronchitis	3 × 30	subjektiv +		De Gregorio
196	akute Bronchitis	3 × 40	subjektiv +	+	Renovanz und Liebrich
37	chronische Bronchitis	4 × 15	subjektiv +		Cass, Frederik (1964)
63	chronische Bronchitis	4 × 15	subjektiv +		Cass, Frederik (1956)
65	chronische Bronchitis	4 × 17	subjektiv +		Cass, Frederik (1953)
13	chronische Bronchitis	4 × 30	subjektiv +		Cavalieri u. Mitarb.
56	chronische Bronchitis	4 × 30	subjektiv —		Nicolis, Pasquariello
30	chronische Bronchitis	5 × 32,4	subjektiv +		Woolf, Rosenberg (1962)
30	chronische Bronchitis	5 × 32,4	objektiv +	+	Woolf, Rosenberg (1964)

Aus diesen Gründen können die im Tierexperiment erhaltenen Ergebnisse über den antitussiven Effekt von Pharmaka nicht uneingeschränkt zur Urteilsbildung über den humantherapeutischen Wert der Substanzen verwendet werden.

Eddy, Friebel, Hahn und Halbach haben kürzlich die ihnen zugänglichen Resultate tier- und humanexperimenteller Prüfung von Antitussiva gesammelt und mit Ergebnissen der klinischen Erfahrung verglichen. In der Tabelle 3 sind Angaben über Codeindosen zusammengestellt, die im Tierversuch den Husten hemmen. Die Größe der wirksamen Dosen differiert in weitem Ausmaß; und die Wahl der Tierart, des Reizmittels, der Vorbehandlung und der Applikationsweise kann diese großen Differenzen offensichtlich nicht begründen. Aber jeder der Autoren fand eine Codeindosis, die den tierexperimentellen Husten dämpft oder verhütet. In der Tabelle 4 sind Resultate der Codeinprüfung am humanexperimentellen Husten gesammelt. Bei Freiwilligen wirkt Codein nicht mit gleicher

Zuverlässigkeit wie im Tierversuch antitussiv. Die Gründe sind nicht ersichtlich. Die Tabelle 5 enthält die Ergebnisse einiger kontrollierter klinischer Prüfungen. Trotz heterogener Patientenkollektive und unterschiedlicher Ätiologie des Hustens liegen die hustendämpfenden Codeindosen in einem relativ engen Dosisbereich. Codein war in jeder Beobachtungsreihe wirksam.

Der Vergleich der in den Tabellen 3—5 gesammelten Daten zeigt noch einmal, daß Erkenntnisse, die am tier- oder humanexperimentellen Husten gewonnen werden, im Bereich des pathologischen Hustens eine nur begrenzte Gültigkeit haben.

Literatur

Adrian, E. D.: Afferent impulses in the vagus and their effect on respiration. J. Physiol. (Lond.) **79**, 332 (1933).

Amdur, M. O.: The influence of aerosols upon the respiratory response of guinea pigs to sulfur dioxide. Amer. industr. Hyg. Ass. Quart. **18**, 149 (1957).

Archibald, D. W., L. B. Slipp, and S. J. Shane: The evaluation of a cough suppressant: An exercise in clinical pharmacology. Canad. med. Ass. J. **80**. 734 (1959).

Banyai, A. L., and M. Joannides Jr.: Cough hazard. Dis. Chest **29**, 52 (1956).

Benson, W. M., P. L. Stefko, and L. O. Randall: Comparative pharmacology of levorphan, racemorphan and dextrorphan and related methyl ethers. J. Pharmacol. exp. Ther. **109**, 189 (1953).

Bickerman, H. A.: The choice of antitussive agents. In: W. Modell, Drugs of choice 1960—1961, p. 493. St. Louis: C. V. Mosby Co. 1960a.

— Bronchial drainage and the phenomena of cough in clinical cardiopulmonary physiology, p. 495. New York: Grune & Stratton, Inc. 1960b.

— A. L. Barach, S. Itkin, and F. Drimmer: The experimental production of cough in human subjects induced by citric acid aerosols. Amer. J. med. Sci. **228**, 156 (1954).

— B. M. Cohen, E. German, and S. Itkin: The cough response of normal human subjects stimulated experimentally by citric acid aerosol: Alterations produced by antitussive agents. Part I: Methodology. Amer. J. med. Sci. **232**, 57 (1956).

— E. German, B. M. Cohen, and S. E. Itkin: The cough response of healthy human subjects stimulated by citric acid aerosol. Part II: Evaluation of antitussive agents. Amer. J. med. Sci. **234**, 191 (1957).

—, and S. E. Itkin: Further studies on the evaluation of antitussive agents employing experimentally induced cough in human subjects. Clin. Pharmacol. Ther. **1**, 180 (1960).

Bidder: Virchows Arch. path. Anat. (1865).

Blix, M.: Persönliche Mitteilung 1952. Siehe N. B. Eddy, H. Friebel, K.-J. Hahn u. H. Halbach.

Bobb, J. R. R., and S. Ellis: Production of cough and its suppression in the unanesthetized dog. Amer. J. Physiol. **167**, 768 (1951).

Boissier, J.-R., et J. Pagny: Action expérimentale comparée de trois antitussifs dérivés du phénylaminopropane. Thérapie **15**, 93 (1960a).

— — Action antitussive de quelques phénothiazines. Thérapie **15**, 97 (1960b).

Borison, H. L.: Electrical stimulation of the neural mechanism regulating spasmodic respiratory acts in the cat. Amer. J. Physiol. **154**, 55 (1948).

Bucher, K.: Reflektorische Beeinflußbarkeit der Lungenatmung. Wien: Springer 1952.

— Tessalon, ein hustenstillendes Mittel von neuartigem Wirkungsmechanismus. Schweiz. med. Wschr. **86**, 94 (1956).

— Pathophysiology and pharmacology of cough. Pharmacol. Rev. **10**, **43** (1958).

— Antitussive drugs. In: Physiological pharmacology, vol. II. New York and London: Academic Press 1965.

—, u. C. Jacot: Zum Mechanismus des Hustens. Helv. physiol. pharmacol. Acta **9**, 454 (1951).

Cahen, R., et A. Boucherle: Etude pharmacologique de la nicotinyldihydrocodéine. C. R. Soc. Biol. (Paris) **158**, 1021 (May 1964).

Calesnick, B., J. A. Christensen, and J. C. Munch: Antitussive action of L-propoxyphene in citric acid-induced cough response. Amer. J. med. Sci. **242**, 560 (1961).

Cass, L. J., and W. S. Frederik: Evaluation of a new antitussive agent. New Eng. J. Med. **249**, 139 (1953).

— — Clinical evaluation of antitussive agents. Bull. Drug. Addict. Narc. 725 (1954).

— — Quantitative comparison of cough-suppressing effects of romilar and other antitussives. J. Lab. clin. Med. **48**, 879 (1956).

— — The clinical evaluation of silomat as an antitussive. Curr. ther. Res. **6**, 14 (1964).

Cavalieri, U., F. B. Nicolis, G. Paquariello, A. Quadri e A. E. Tammaro: Valutazione del l'attivita terapeutica degli antitosse in geriatria. G. Geront. **8**, 981 (1960).
Chabrier, P., R. Giudicelli et J. Thuillier: Etude chimique, pharmacologique et clinique d'un nouveau *sédatif* de la toux: la morpholyléthylmorphine (M.E.M.). Anal. Pharmaceut. franc. **8**, 261 (1950).
Chakravarty, N. K., A. Matallana, R. Jensen, and H. L. Borison: Central effects of antitussive drugs on cough and respiration. J. Pharmacol. exp. Ther. **117**, 127 (1956).
Chen, J. Y. P., H. F. Biller, and E. G. Montgomery, Jr.: Pharmacologic studies of a new antitussive, alpha (dimethyl-aminoethyl)-ortho-chlorobenzhydrol hydrochloride (SL-501, Bayer B-186). J. Pharmacol. exp. Ther. **128**, 384 (1960).
Christoffel, P., u. H. Kolberg: Die antitussive Wirkung eines Aminonitrils. Med. Klin. **53**, 1507 (1958).
Craigie, E. H.: The reflex produced by chemical stimulation of the deeper respiratory passages. Amer. J. Physiol. **59**, 346 (1922).
Cromer, S. P., R. H. Young, and A. C. Ivy: On the existence of afferent respiratory impulses mediated by the stellate ganglia. Amer. J. Physiol. **104**, 468 (1933).
Cushny, A. R.: The reversible action of adrenaline and some kindred drugs on the bronchioles. J. Pharmacol. exp. Path. **4**, 363 (1913).
Dalhamn, T.: The determination in vivo of the rate of ciliary beat in the trachea. Acta physiol. scand. **49**, 242 (1960).
Dawes, G. S., J. C. Mott, and J. G. Widdicombe: Respiratory and cardio-vascular reflexes from the heart and lungs. J. Physiol. (Lond.) **115**, 258 (1951).
Domenjoz, R.: Zur Auswertung hustenstillender Arzneimittel. Arch. exp. Path. Pharmak. (Lpz.) **215**, 19 (1952).
Dongen, K. van: The effect of narcotine, ticarda and romilar on coughs and on the movements of cilia in the air passages. Acta physiol. pharmacol. neerl. **4**, 500 (1956).
Dubi, A.: Zur Bedeutung pontiner Atmungssubstrate für den Husten. Helv. physiol. pharmacol. Acta **17**, 166 (1959).
Eddy, N. B.: Studies of morphine, codeine and their derivatives. I. General methods. J. Pharmacol. exp. Ther. **45**, 339 (1932).
— H. Friebel, K.-J. Hahn, and H. Halbach: Codeine and its alternates for pain and cough relief. Bull. Wld Hlth Org. **38**, 673 (1968) und folgende Mitteilungen.
Eichler, O.: Anordnung zur Herstellung von Nebel aus Schwefelsäure und anderen geeigneten Substanzen. Arch. int. Pharmacodyn. **133**, 10 (1961).
—, u. H. G. Scholtze: Klin. Wschr. **19**, 517 (1940).
—, u. A. Smiatek: Versuche zur Auswertung von Mitteln zur Bekämpfung des Reizhustens. Arch. exp. Path. Pharmak. (Lpz.) **194**, 621 (1940).
Elftman, A. G.: The afferent and parasympathetic innervation of the lungs and trachea of the dog. Amer. J. Anat. **72**, 1 (1943).
Enders, A., u. L. Schmidt: Die reflektorische Tätigkeit des Husten- und Atemzentrums unter dem Einfluß von Papaverinhydrochlorid. Arch. int. Pharmacodyn. **114**, 446 (1958).
Engelhorn, R.: Pharmacological investigation of a new antitussive drug, 1-p-chlorophenyl-2:3-dimethyl-4-dimethylamino-2-butanol. Arzneimittel-Forsch. **10**, 785 (1960).
—, u. E. Weller: Aktionspotentiale atmungssynchron entladender Neurone der Medulla oblongata der Katze. Pflügers Arch. ges. Physiol. **273**, 614 (1961).
— — Zentrale Repräsentation hustenwirksamer Afferenzen in der Medulla oblongata der Katze. Pflügers Arch. ges. Physiol. **284**, 224 (1965).
— — Der Einfluß von Codein, Dextromethorphan und Narkotin auf exspiratorisch entladende Neurone der Medulla oblongata der Katze. Naunyn-Schmiedebergs Arch. Pharmak. exp. Path. **254**, 170 (1966).
Ernst, A. M.: Pharmakologische Untersuchungen und Wertbestimmung von hustenstillenden Mitteln. Arch. int. Pharmacodyn. **58**, 363 (1938).
— Morphin, Kodein und Hustenreiz. Arch. int. Pharmacodyn. **61**, 73 (1939).
Finney, D. J.: Probit analysis, 2nd ed. London: Cambridge University Press 1952.
Floersheim, G. L.: Über die Rolle der Glottis beim Husten. Helv. physiol. pharmacol. Acta **17**, 153 (1959).
Friebel, H., u. K.-J. Hahn: Über die Variierbarkeit hustenerzeugender Reizströme. Med. Pharmacol. exp. **14**, 78 (1966).
— R. Jacob u. J. Cros: Gewöhnung von Meerschweinchen an die husten- und schmerzstillende Wirkung von Morphin. Med. Pharmacol. exp. **12**, 97 (1965).
—, u. H.-F. Kuhn: Über husten- und atemdepressorische Wirkung. Arch. exp. Path. Pharmak. (Lpz.) **243**, 162 (1962).
— — Gewöhnung an die hustenhemmende Wirkung von Codein. Arch. exp. Path. Pharmak. (Lpz.) **246**, 527 (1964).

Friebel, H., u. C. Reichle: Versuchstierart und Testergebnis bei Prüfung schmerz- und hustenstillender Arzneimittel. Arch. exp. Path. Pharmak. (Lpz.) **229**, 400 (1956).

— — u. A. v. Graevenitz: Zur Hemmung des Hustenreflexes durch zentral angreifende Arzneimittel. Arch. exp. Path. Pharmak. (Lpz.) **224**, 384 (1955).

Furakawa, T., and M. Okabe: Antitussive action of dextromethorphan HBr. Igaku Kenkyu **28**, 1643 (1958).

Gösswald, R.: 1-Phenyl-1-1(o-chlorphenyl)-3-dimethylamino-propanol-(1), ein neuer hustenhemmender Stoff. Arzneimittel-Forsch. 8, 550 (1958).

Graham, J. D. P.: Evaluation of isoaminile citrate as an antitussive. J. New Drugs **2**, 43 (1962).

Granier-Doyeux, M., M. Horande et W. Kucharski: Méthode d'evaluation quantitative des agents antitussigènes. Arch. int. Pharmacodyn. **121**, 287 (1959).

Gravenstein, J. S., R. A. Devloo, and H. K. Beecher: Effect of antitussive agents on experimental and pathological cough in man. J. appl. Physiol. **7**, 119 (1954).

Green, A. F., and N. B. Ward: The action of analgesics and nalorphine on the cough reflex. Brit. J. Pharmacol. **10**, 418 (1955).

De Gregorio, M.: Attività bechica nell'uomo e caratteristiche farmaco-terapiche dell'oxolamina (Perebron). Minerva med. **51**, 4086 (1960).

Grosse-Brockhoff, E.: Pathologische Physiologie. Berlin-Göttingen-Heidelberg: Springer 1950.

Großman, M., J. O. Birker, and F. Casimir: An evaluation of an antitussive agent preparation, Ciba 10611 (Mellipan). Appl. Ther. **3**, 95 (1961).

Haas, H.: Vergleichende Untersuchungen über Analgetika. Arch. exp. Path. Pharmak. (Lpz.) **225**, 442 (1955).

Hahn, K.-J., u. H. Friebel: Wirkungen hustenhemmender Pharmaka im zentralen Anteil der Hustenreflexbahn. Med. Pharmacol. exp. **14**, 87 (1966).

Hahn, L. A., and H. Wilbrand: The cough alleviating effect of β-(diphenyl-methoxy)-ethyltrimethylammoniumbromide. Arch. int. Pharmacodyn. **91**, 144 (1952).

Hansen, F., u. A. Dortmann: Über die Provokation typischer Keuchhustenanfälle durch intravenöse Lobelingaben. Arch. Kinderheilk. **152**, 121 (1956).

Hara, S., and S. Yanaura: A method of inducing and recording cough and examination of the action of some drugs with this method. Jap. J. Pharmacol. **9**, 46 (1959).

Haslreiter, E.: Acetylcholin-Hustentest im Rahmen der Prüfung einer neuen hustenstillenden Substanz. Arzneimittel-Forsch. **9**, 769 (1959).

Hengen, O., u. H. Kasparek: Husten-hemmende Wirkung einer neuen Substanz. Arneimittel-Forsch. 8, 620 (1958).

Herzog, H.: Klinik und Therapie der chronischen Bronchitis. Therapiewoche **17**, 532 (1967).

Hildebrandt, F.: Die Prüfung der Analgetika im Tierexperiment mittels einer neuen Methode. Arch. exp. Path. Pharmak. (Lpz.) **174**, 405 (1934).

Hillis, B. R.: The assessment of cough-suppressing drugs. Lancet **1952 I**, 1230.

—, and J. C. C. Kelly: Effect of hexamethonium iodide on lobeline-stimulated coughing. Glasg. med. J. **32**, 72 (1951).

Himmelsbach, C. K., H. L. Andrews, R. H. Felix, F. W. Obeist, and L. F. Davenport: Studies on codeine addiction. U.S. Publ. Hlth Rep., Suppl. 158 (1940).

Höglund, N. J., and M. Michaelsson: A method for determining the cough threshold with some preliminary experiments on the effect of codeine. Acta physiol. scand. **21**, 168 (1950).

Isbell, H., and H. F. Fraser: Actions and addiction liabilities of dromoran derivatives in man. J. Pharmacol. exp. Ther. **107**, 524 (1953).

Job, C., u. W. Schaumann: Bronchokonstriktorische Fasern im Halsvagus des Meerschweinchens. Arch. exp. Path. Pharmak. (Lpz.) **231**, 388 (1957).

Kandarazki, M.: Über den Husten nebst einigen Bemerkungen über den Einfluß des Chloroforms auf die Atmung der Tiere. Pflügers Arch. ges. Physiol. **26**, 470 (1881).

Kasé, Y.: New methods of estimating cough depressing action. Jap. J. Pharmacol. **2**, 7(1952).

— The "coughing dog". — An improved method for the evaluation of an antitussive. Chem. Pharm. Bull. Jap. **2**, 298 (1954).

— Pharmacological studies on cough reflex, Part 3, "coughing dog" and its application. Jap. J. Pharmacol. **4**, 130 (1955).

Kelentey, B., F. Czollner, E. Stenszky, Z. Mészáros u. J. Szlávik: Darstellung und pharmakologische Untersuchung einiger morpholyläthylisierter Morphin-Derivate. Arneimittel-Forsch. 8, 325 (1958).

— E. Stenszky u. F. Czollner: Neue Untersuchungen zur Pharmakologie des Narceins. Arch. exp. Path. Pharmak. (Lpz.) **233**, 550 (1958).

— — — J. Szlávik u. Z. Mészáros: Darstellung und pharmakologische Untersuchungen der N-Oxyde der Opium-Alkaloide. Arzneimittel-Forsch. **7**, 594 (1957).

Klein, B.: The cough sirup as palliative therapy. A clinical evaluation of dimethoxanate. Antibiot. Med. **5**, 462 (1958).

Kohli, R. P., G. P. Gupta, and K. P. Bhargava: Effect of some newer compounds on experimental cough. Indian J. med. Res. **48**, 193 (1960).
Kohts, O.: Experimentelle Untersuchungen über den Husten. Virchows Arch. Anat. u. Physiol. **60**, 191 (1874).
Koll, W.: Analgetica und Analgesie. Pharmazie **15**, 290 (1960).
Konar, N. R., and S. Dasgupta: A chemical method for exciting cough reflex in human beings and its use in assessing the effectiveness of cough sedatives. J. Indian med. Ass. **32**, 189 (1959).
Krause, D.: Pharmakologie des α-(Isopropyl)-α-(β-dimethyl-aminopropyl)-phenylacetonitril-citrat. Arzneimittel-Forsch. **8**, 553 (1958).
Krimer, W.: Untersuchungen über die nächste Ursache des Hustens etc. Leipzig 1819.
Kroepfli, P.: Über das Verhalten einiger Atmungsgrößen beim Husten. Helv. physiol. pharmacol. Acta **8**, **33** (1950).
Kuhn, H.-F., u. H. Friebel: Zur Einordnung des Hustenstoßes in den Atemrhythmus. Med. exp. **3**, 329 (1960).
— — Die Ausscheidung von Codein und Codeinmetaboliten im Harn codeingewöhnter Ratten und Meerschweinchen. Med. exp. **7**, 255 (1962).
La Barre, et H. Plisnier: A propos des propriétés antitussigènes et bronchodilatatrices du chlorhydrate de narcotine. Arch. int. Pharmacodyn. **119**, 205 (1959).
Larsell, O.: Nerve endings in the human pleura pulmonalis. J. comp. Neurol. **61**, 407 (1935).
—, and G. E. Burget: The effects of mechanical and chemical stimulation of the tracheobronchial mucous membrane. Amer. J. Physiol. **70**, 311 (1924).
—, and R. S. Dow: The innervation of the human lung. Amer. J. Anat. **52**, 125 (1933).
Levis, S., S. Preat, and F. Moyersoons: Evaluation of the antitussive activity of some esters of phenyl-cycloalkane carbocyclic acids and study of different pharmacological properties of the most effective among them: The hydrochloride of diethyl-aminoethoxyethyl-1-phenyl-1-cyclopentane carboxylate. Arch. int. Pharmacodyn. **103**, 200 (1955).
Lindner, E., u. L. Stein: Abkömmlinge des Diphenyl-piperidino-propans — eine neue Reihe hustenstillender Mittel. Arzneimittel-Forsch. **9**, 94 (1959).
Litchfield Jr., J. T., and F. Wilcoxon: Simplified method of evaluating dose-effect experiments. J. Pharmacol. exp. Ther. **96**, 99 (1949).
Mattallana, A., and H. L. Borison: Antitussive agents and centrally induced cough. Fed. Proc. **14**, 367 (1955).
May, A. J., and J. G. Widdicombe: Depression of the cough reflex by pentobarbitone and some opium derivatives. Brit. J. Pharmacol. **9**, 335 (1954).
Mayer, Magne et Plantefol: C. R. Acad. Sci. (Paris) **170**, 1347 (1920).
Morris, D. J., and S. J. Shane: Human bioassay of a new antitussive agent. Canad. med. Ass. J. **83**, 1093 (1960).
Morton, D. R., K. P. Klassen, and G. M. Curtis: The effect of high vagus section upon the clinical physiology of the bronchi. J. Lab. clin. Med. **34**, 1730 (1949).
Müller, B.: Zum Mechanismus des Hustens. Helv. physiol. pharmacol. Acta **12**, 137 (1954).
Mulinos, M. G.: Antitussive properties of morpholin-ethylmorphine (Pholcodine). Toxicol. Appl. Pharmacol. **2**, 635 (1960).
— K. G. Nair, and J. G. Epstein: Clinical investigation of antitussive properties of pholcodine. N. Y. St. J. Med. **62**, 2373 (1962).
Nicolis, F. B., and G. Pasquariello: Controlled clinical trials of antitussive agents: An experimental evaluation of different methods. J. Pharmacol. exp. Ther. **136**, 183 (1962).
Nothnagel, H.: Lehre vom Husten. Virchows Arch. path. Anat. **44**, 95 (1868).
Pasquarriello, G., e F. B. Nicolis: Esperience cliniche controllate con nuovi farmaci antitossive. II. Attivita antitosse della benzobutamina. Clin. ter. **23**, 226 (1962).
Pellmont, B., u. H. Bächtold: Pharmakologie des „Romilar“ Roche, einer hustenhemmenden Substanz mit zentralem Angriffspunkt. Schweiz. med. Wschr. **84**, 1368 (1954).
Perry, W. F., and E. M. Boyd: A method for studying expectorant action in animals by direct measurement of the output of respiratory tract fluids. J. Pharmacol. exp. Ther. **73**, 65 (1941).
Phillips, A. M., R. W. Phillips, and J. L. Thompson: Ann. intern. Med. **45**, 216 (1956).
Plisnier, H.: A propos des propriétés antitussigènes d'un bromure d'ammonium quarternaire (bromure de 2-triméthylamino-1,2-diphényldiéthyléther) (TDBr). C. R. Soc. Biol. (Paris) **152**, 1267 (1958).
Porter, E. L., and E. L. Allamon: Barbiturate-strychnine antagonism in the spinal cat. A quantitative study. J. Pharmacol. exp. Ther. **58**, 178 (1936).
Porter, R.: Unit responses evoked in the medullary nuclei of the vagus nerves. J. Physiol. (Lond.) **163**, 26 (1962).
— Unit responses evoked in the medulla oblongata by vagus nerve stimulation. J. Physiol. (Lond.) **168**, 717 (1963).

Prime, F. J.: The assessment of antitussive drugs in man. Brit. med. J. **1961** I, 1149.
Rasch, M.: Dextrometadons hostlindrande effekt. Nord. Med. **57**, 629 (1957).
Reichle, C., u. H. Friebel: Zur Hemmung des Hustenreflexes durch zentral angreifende Arzneimittel. Arch. exp. Path. Pharmak. (Lpz.) **226**, 558 (1955).
Rein, H., u. M. Schneider: Physiologie des Menschen, 11. Aufl. Berlin-Göttingen-Heidelberg: Springer 1955.
Renovanz, H.-D., u. K. G. Liebrich: Prüfung von Hustenmitteln, dargestellt am Beispiel von 1-p-Chlorphenyl-2,3-dimethyl-4-dimethylamino-butanol-2 HCl. Arzneimittel-Forsch. **15**, 1393 (1965).
Rienzo, S. di: Physiopathologie des Hustens. Fortschr. Röntgenstr. **78**, 1 (1953).
Rohrer, F.: Der Strömungswiderstand in den menschlichen Atemwegen und der Einfluß der unregelmäßigen Verzweigung des Bronchialsystems auf den Atmungsverlauf in verschiedenen Lungenbezirken. Pflügers Arch. ges. Physiol. **162**, 225 (1915).
Rosiere, C. E., and C. V. Winder: Tussal studies with ammonia in unanesthetized dogs with chronic tracheal side-tubes. J. Pharmacol. exp. Ther. **113**, 46 (1955) Proc.
— —, and J. Wax: Ammonia cough elicited through a tracheal side tube in unanesthetized dogs. Comparative antitussive bioassay of four morphine derivatives and methadone in terms of ammonia tresholds. J. Pharmacol. exp. Ther. **116**, 296 (1956).
Ross, B. B., R. Gramiak, and H. Rahn: Physical dynamics of the cough mechanism. J. appl. Physiol. **8**, 264 (1955).
Sallé, J., et M. Brunaud: Nouvelle technique d'enregistrement des mouvements de toux provoqués par l'inhalation de vapeurs irritantes chez le cobaye. Arch. int. Pharmacodyn. **126**, 120 (1960).
Sanzari, N. P., F. B. Fainman, and S. F. Emde: Cough induced by 1,1-dimethyl-4-phenylpiperazinium jodide: A new antitussive method. J. Pharmacol. exp. Ther. **162**, 190 (1968).
Schaumann, O.: Über eine neue Klasse von Verbindungen mit spasmolytischer und zentral analgetischer Wirksamkeit unter besonderer Berücksichtigung des 1-Methyl-4-phenylpiperidin-4-carbonsäure-äthylesters (Dolantin). Arch. exp. Path. Pharmak. (Lpz.) **196**, 109 (1940).
— Die medikamentöse Schmerzbekämpfung. Wien. klin. Wschr. **65**, 133 (1953).
— Analgetika und „protektives" System. Naturwissenschaften **41**, 96 (1954).
Schlez, K.: Über die Verwendung des Vagusschlingenhundes für die Wertbestimmung hustenstillender Substanzen. Diss. Heidelberg 1965.
Schmidt, C. F., and W. B. Harer: The action of certain drugs on respiration. J. Pharmacol. exp. Ther. **19**, 269 (1923).
Schroeder, W.: Die Verwendung des Vagusschlingenhundes für die Wertbestimmung hustenstillender Substanzen. Arch. exp. Path. Pharmak. (Lpz.) **212**, 433 (1951).
Sell, R., E. Lindner u. H. Jahn: Untersuchungen über die Anaesthesie der Dehnungs- und Berührungsreceptoren durch einige Lokalanaesthetica im Vergleich zur hustenstillenden Wirkung. Arch. exp. Path. Pharmak. (Lpz.) **234**, 164 (1958).
Sevelius, H., and J. P. Colmore: Antitussive effect of ethyl dibunate in patients with chronic cough. Clin. Pharmacol. Ther. **8**, 381 (1967).
— P. D. Lester, and J. P. Colmore: Objective evaluation of antitussive agents. Clin. Pharmacol. Ther. **6**, 146 (1965).
Shane, S. J., T. K. Krzyski, and S. E. Copp: Clinical evaluation of a new antitussive agent. Canad. med. Ass. J. **77**, 600 (1957).
Silson, J. S.: A new method for evaluating antitussive medications using the citric acid challenge technique. J. New Drugs **5**, 94 (1965).
Silvestrini, B., e G. Maffii: Rilievo dell'azione antitosse negli animals di Laboratorio e rapporti tra azione bechica et altre proprieta farmacologiche jl farmaco. Ed. Sci. Pavia **14**, 440 (1959).
—, e C. Pozzatti: Pharmacological properties of 3-phenyl-5α-diethylamino-ethyl-1,2,4-oxadiazole. Brit. J. Pharmacol. **16**, 209 (1961).
Sollmann, T.: A manual of pharmacology, 8. ed., Philadelphia: W. B. Saunders Co. 1957.
Staehelin, R.: Respirationskrankheiten. Jkurse ärztl. Fortbild. **5**, 32 (1914).
Stefko, P. L., and W. M. Benson: A method for the evaluation of antitussive agents in the unanesthetized dog. J. Pharmacol. exp. Ther. **108**, 217 (1953).
—, and J. Denzel: A simple method for the evaluation of antitussive preparations in the unanesthetized cat. J. Pharmacol. exp. Ther. **119**, 185 (1957).
— —, and I. Hickey: Experimental investigation of nine antitussive drugs. J. pharm. Sci. **50**, 216 (1961).
Tannenbaum, P. J.: The utility of the Bickerman technique for the study of antitussive agents in man. Pharmacologist **7**, 77 (1965).
Tedeschi, R. E., D. H. Tedeschi, J. H. Hitchens, L. Cook, P. A. Mattis, and E. J. Fellows: A new antitussive method involving mechanical stimulation in unanesthetized dogs. J. Pharmacol. exp. Ther. **126**, 338 (1959).

Tiffeneau, R.: Die tussigene Wirkung von Acetylcholin-Aerosolen. Kriterien der pathologischen Reizbarkeit der sensiblen Nervenenden in der Lunge. Z. Aerosol-Forsch. **4**, 116 (1955).

Toner, J. J., and E. Macko: Pharmacology studies on Bis-(1-carbo-β-diethyl-amino-ethoxy)-1-phenyl-cyclopentane)-ethane disulfonate. J. Pharmacol. exp. Ther. **106**, 246 (1952).

Trendelenburg, U.: Über die Wirkung einiger Hustenmittel auf Hustenreizschwelle und Atmung. Acta physiol. scand. **21**, 174 (1950).

Vleeschhouwer, G. R. de: Contribution a l'étude pharmacologique et toxicologique du diterbutyl naphtalène sulfonate sodique. Arch. int. Pharmacodyn. **97**, 34 (1954).

Wagner, R., u. E. Wetterer: Ein elektrisches Gerät zur Erzeugung rhythmischer linear ansteigender und abfallender Reizspannungen einstellbarer Steilheit sowie rechteckiger und anderer Reizspannungsformen. Pflügers Arch. ges. Physiol. **251**, 585 (1949).

Watt, J.: Streiflichter aus dem Commonwealth. Pharm. Industrie **21**, 386 (1959).

Weidemeyer, J. C., H. W. Kremer, and D. K. de Jongh: A screening method for antitussive compounds. Acta physiol. pharmacol. neer. **9**, 501 (1960).

Weidmann, H., B. Berde u. K. Bucher: Die Lage der vagalen Dehnungsreceptoren in der Lunge. Helv. physiol. pharmacol. Acta **7**, 476 (1949).

Weisser, K.: Zum Mechanismus des Hustens. Helv. physiol. pharmacol. Acta **11**, 55 (1953).

Widdicombe, J. G.: Respiratory reflexes from the trachea and bronchi of the cat. J. Physiol. (Lond.) **123**, 55 (1954a).

— Receptors in the trachea and bronchi of the cat. J. Physiol. (Lond.) **123**, 71 (1954b).

— Action potentials in vagal afferent nerve fibres to the lungs of the cat. Arch. exp. Path. Pharmak. (Lpz.) **214**, 415 (1961).

Winder, C. V.: The nociceptive contraction of the cutaneous muscle of the guinea pig as elicited by radiant heat. Arch. int. Pharmacodyn. **72**, 329 (1946).

—, and C. E. Rosiere: Preliminary antitussive studies on the unanesthetized dog with chronic tracheal tube. Bull. Drug. Addict. Narc. **1954**, 696.

— — Comparative antitussive bioassay of four morphine derivatives and methadone, employing ammonia in unanesthetized dogs with tracheal side-tubes. J. Pharmacol. exp. Ther. **113**, 55 (1955) Proc.

— J. Wax, B. Serrano, L. Scotti, S. P. Stackhouse, and R. H. Wheelock: Pharmacological studies of 1,2-dimethyl-3-phenyl-3-propionoxypyrrolidine (Cl-427) an analgetic agent. J. Pharmacol. exp. Ther. **133**, 117 (1961).

Winter, Ch. A., and L. Flataker: Antitussive action of d-isomethadone and d-methadone in dogs. Proc. Soc. exp. Biol. (N.Y.) **81**, 463 (1952).

— — Antitussive compounds: Testing methods and results. J. Pharmacol. exp. Ther. **112**, 99 (1954).

Woolf, C. R., and A. Rosenberg: The cough suppressant effect of heroin and codeine: A controlled clinical study. Canad. med. Ass. J. **86**, 810 (1962).

— — Objective assessment of cough suppressants under clinical conditions using a tape recorder system. Thorax **19**, 125 (1964).

Erzeugung von tierexperimentellen Asthmareaktionen

Joachim E. Alberty

Mit 22 Abbildungen

Einleitung

Im klinischen Sprachgebrauch bezeichnet „Asthma“ oder „Asthmaanfall“ in der Regel das Asthma bronchiale. Es ist gekennzeichnet durch eine akute anfallsartig auftretende vorwiegend exspiratorische Dyspnoe. Ihre Ursache ist eine Bronchialstenose, an der sich Bronchialmuskelspasmus, Schleimhautödem und Schleimsekretion der Bronchien in wechselndem Maße beteiligen. Von manchen (Wyss und Schmid [195]) wird einem Zwerchfellspasmus entscheidende Bedeutung am Zustandekommen der Dyspnoe zugeschrieben.

Das Asthma ist primär ein funktionelles Geschehen. Häufige Wiederholungen der Anfälle führen zu typischen, überwiegend durch die Funktionsstörungen, weniger durch die auslösende Ursache selbst bestimmten, morphologischen Veränderungen der anatomischen Strukturen der Lunge.

Nach heutigen Erkenntnissen wird das Asthma bronchiale des Menschen in der Mehrzahl der Fälle als allergische Erkrankung angesehen. Das heißt, der grundlegende Auslösungsmechanismus des Asthmaanfalls ist die Antigen-Antikörper-Reaktion, auch wenn besonders im Verlaufe längerer Dauer der Erkrankung eine Reihe weiterer Faktoren physischer wie auch psychischer Art gegebenenfalls starken Einfluß gewinnen können.

Die experimentelle Asthmaforschung begann mit der Erkennung der Parallelen zwischen Asthma bronchiale bzw. Status asthmaticus des Menschen und Volumen pulmonum auctum im anaphylaktischen Schock des Meerschweinchens (Meltzer [136], s. auch Doerr [66]). Ihr Schwergewicht lag zunächst vorwiegend bei grundsätzlichen Fragen der Pathogenese und Erzeugung des tierexperimentellen Asthmas und seiner Eignung als Modell des menschlichen Asthma bronchiale (s. Übersichten bei Ratner [163], Doerr [66], Friebel [85]). Untersuchungen, die derartige Probleme von verschiedenen Seiten her angriffen, wurden bis in die neuere Zeit fortgesetzt. Die als Basis der vorliegenden Abhandlung wesentlichen Erkenntnisse seien im folgenden herausgestellt:

1. Das Meerschweinchen ist die einzige Versuchstierspecies, bei der es sicher gelingt, ein allergisches Asthma zu erzeugen.

Die Anaphylaxie ist ein Sonderfall der Allergie. Die Bezeichnung „anaphylaktisches Asthma“ kann daher m. E. ohne Mißverständnisse durch die allgemeingültigere Bezeichnung „allergisches Asthma“ ersetzt werden.

2. Das allergische Asthma des Meerschweinchens ist ein geeignetes Modell des menschlichen Asthma bronchiale, die Basis beider Reaktionen ist gleich.

Hierbei sollen natürlich u. U. schwerwiegende Unterschiede nicht negiert werden, wie z. B. die Verschiedenheit der Species sowie der Entstehungsgeschichte und des Verlaufs des experimentell induzierten im Gegensatz zum „natürlich“, „schicksalshaft“ entstandenen Asthmas.

3. Ein dem allergischen Asthma ähnlicher Asthmazustand läßt sich bei verschiedenen Versuchstierspecies durch zahlreiche Pharmaka erzeugen, wie z. B. Histamin, Cholinergica wie Acetylcholin, Pilocarpin, ferner 5-Hydroxytryptamin, Kinine wie Bradykinin, Kallidin, und andere Stoffe, die Asthma in erster Linie durch ihre bronchoconstrictorische Wirkung verursachen. Solche experimentellen Asthmareaktionen dienen ebenso der Erforschung der Pathophysiologie des allergischen Asthmas wie auch als brauchbare pharmakologische Asthmamodelle. Sie sind jedoch vom „echten" allergischen Asthma zu unterscheiden und sollen als „pharmakonbedingtes Asthma" oder experimenteller Bronchospasmus bezeichnet werden.

Eine dem Englischen „drug-induced" entsprechende ebenso kurze wie umfassende deutsche Bezeichnung findet sich nicht. Droge wird sprachlich in engerem Sinne verstanden als drug und viele Asthmogene wie z.B. 5-Hydroxytryptamin oder Bradykinin sind keine Arzneimittel.

Das Asthma, sei es allergisch oder pharmakonbedingt, ist ein komplexes Symptom. Seine Registrierung, insbesondere die quantitative Erfassung der Funktionsstörung und/oder ihrer Teilkomponenten kann mehr Schwierigkeiten bereiten als die Erzeugung eines geeigneten Asthmaanfalls selbst. Auch hängen die Möglichkeiten der Registrierung bestimmter Größen u. U. entscheidend vom Zustand des Versuchstieres und der jeweiligen Technik der Auslösung und Steuerung des experimentellen Asthmas ab. Die Registrierungsmethoden, ebenso wie die experimentellen Zielsetzungen bzw. Ergebnisse, müssen daher in dieser Darstellung eingehend berücksichtigt werden.

Eine Beschreibung der Methoden zur Erzeugung von Asthma läßt sich angesichts der Komplexizität von Symptomauslösung, Erfassung des Asthmas und experimenteller Zielsetzung in sehr verschiedener Weise gliedern, von denen keine befriedigt und Wiederholungen ausschließt. Im folgenden wird versucht, zwischen logisch-systematischen und praktischen Gesichtspunkten einen Kompromiß zu finden.

A. Allgemeine methodische Grundlagen

I. Allergisches Asthma

1. Versuchstier

Meltzer [136] wies wohl als erster auf die Parallelen zwischen dem Asthma im anaphylaktischen Schock des Meerschweinchens und dem Asthma bronchiale des Menschen hin. Das Meerschweinchen erwies sich in der Folge als einziges Versuchstier, bei der ein allergisches Asthma zuverlässig hervorgerufen werden kann.

Die Frage nach Übereinstimmungen und Differenzen zwischen Meerschweinchenasthma und menschlichem Asthma ist Gegenstand zahlreicher Untersuchungen, Polemiken und Kontroversen bis in die neuere Zeit gewesen (s. insbesondere Kallós und Pagel [118], Ratner [163], Doerr [66], Friebel [85], Noelpp-Eschenhagen *et al.* [152] u.a.). Sie kann im wesentlichen als beantwortet angesehen werden: Die fundamentalen Mechanismen des allergischen Asthmas von Meerschweinchen und Mensch stimmen überein. Das gleiche gilt für die wesentlichen pathologisch-physiologischen und pathologisch-anatomischen Befunde sowie für die pharmakologische Beeinflußbarkeit. Unterschiede, die durch die Verschiedenheit der Species und der „Krankheitsgeschichte" bedingt und als solche von vornherein zu erwarten sind, fallen demgegenüber nicht entscheidend ins Gewicht, dürfen aber natürlich nicht übersehen werden. Das gilt besonders für die Übertragung tierexperimenteller Befunde auf die Verhältnisse beim Menschen.

2. Sensibilisierung

Fragen nach der Verwendbarkeit verschiedener Antigene und nach der Bedeutung von Darreichungsform und Zufuhrweg haben in den ersten Jahrzehnten der experimentellen Asthmaforschung zahlreiche Untersucher beschäftigt. Insbesondere wurde die pulmonale Zufuhr vernebelter oder staubförmiger Antigene beim Meerschweinchen untersucht, in Anlehnung an die Vorstellungen über die „natürliche" Sensibilisierung des Asthmatikers (s. Übersicht von Ratner [163]). Diese Probleme können ebenfalls als gelöst angesehen werden. Prinzipiell ist auch eine inhalative Sensibilisierung mit nebel- oder staubförmigen Antigenen beim Meerschweinchen möglich. Sie ist jedoch mühsam und unsicher und bietet keine grundsätzlichen Vorzüge. Am sichersten und für alle experimentellen Zwecke geeignet ist die parenterale Gabe eines hochwertigen Antigens, wie z.B. Ovalbumin. Die Verwendung möglichst reinen Antigeneiweißes ist empfehlenswert. Gute Sensibilisierung wird erreicht durch 1—3malige intraperitoneale oder intramuskuläre Injektion, in Abständen von 1—2 Tagen, von 0,5—1,0 ml einer 5—10%igen Lösung von kristallisiertem Ovalbumin oder einer 10—20%igen Lösung von Hühnereiklar in physiologischer Salzlösung. Die Auslösung des Asthmas erfolgt frühestens 2—3 Wochen danach.

Die passive Sensibilisierung führt schneller zum Ziel und erlaubt eine gewisse wenn auch begrenzte quantitative Aussage über die zugeführte Antikörpermenge, z.B. als Menge Antikörper-Stickstoff, was bei aktiver Sensibilisierung nicht möglich ist. Demgegenüber ist die Präparierung von hochaktivem Antiserum und dessen Konzentrierung erheblich aufwendiger. Passive Sensibilisierung wird deshalb seltener und nur für besondere Fragestellungen verwendet. Für methodische Angaben über Gewinnung und Verwendung von Antiserum s. Kabat und Landow [115], Feinberg und Malkiel sowie Feinberg, Malkiel und McIntire [73], Carr und Curry [39].

3. Auslösung

a) Inhalative Antigenzufuhr

Versuche, das tierexperimentelle allergische Asthma inhalativ durch Zufuhr vernebelten oder verstäubten Antigens zur Atmungsluft auszulösen, gehen wohl ursprünglich auf die Annahme zurück, daß der Asthmaanfall beim Menschen hauptsächlich durch Inhalationsantigene ausgelöst wird. Die Aerosolmethode zur Asthmaauslösung im Tierexperiment wurde zuerst verwendet von Busson [33, 34]. Sie wurde in der Folgezeit entwickelt und ausgebaut, insbesondere durch die Untersuchungen von Alexander, Becke und Holmes [8], Manteufel und Preuner [132], und Kallós und Pagel [118], nachdem W. Heubner [106] in seiner Arbeit über die Inhalation zerstäubter Flüssigkeiten auf die entscheidende Bedeutung der Teilchengröße des Aerosols hingewiesen hatte.

Die inhalative Antigenzufuhr zur Asthmaauslösung ist die Methode der Wahl vor allem für Versuche am nichtnarkotisierten frei atmenden Tier, denn sie erlaubt die kontinuierliche Zufuhr kleiner Antigenmengen ohne Manipulierung des Versuchstieres. Viele Autoren führen als weiteren Vorzug an, daß das Antigen am Wirkungsort zur Anwendung gebracht wird. Ob diese Annahme zu Recht besteht, mag dahingestellt bleiben. Strenggenommen bezieht sie sich in erster Linie auf die Bronchialschleimhaut, durch die das Antigen erst gelangen muß, bevor es den Bronchialmuskel als wesentlichen Wirkungsort erreicht. Nach den Untersuchungen von Dautrebande *et al.* [60] muß zum mindesten mit einer starken Beteiligung pulmonal resorbierten und über den Kreislauf an die bronchialen Reaktionsorte gelangenden Antigens gerechnet werden.

Nachteile der Aerosolmethode liegen vor allem in der Unkenntnis und Inkonstanz der Antigendosierung: Die aufgenommene Antigenmenge hängt ab vom Atemvolumen und dem Spektrum der Teilchengröße des Aerosols. Das Atemvolumen ändert sich mit dem Grad der asthmatischen Bronchostenose. Die Teilchengröße wird durch Temperatur und Feuchtigkeitsgehalt der Umgebungsluft beeinflußt, welche kaum konstant zu halten sind. Andererseits erfolgt durch die Drosselung der Atemluftzufuhr bei zunehmender Bronchostenose auch eine gewisse Selbststeuerung der Antigenzufuhr. In der Versuchsanordnung von Friebel und Basold [87] gelingt es, ein steuerbares Asthma beim Meerschweinchen durch Zufuhr des Antigens oder von Pharmaka als Aerosol hervorzurufen (s. S. 92).

Technik der Aerosolzufuhr

Eine Teilchengröße des antigenhaltigen Aerosols von vorwiegend 1—5 μ ist Grundbedingung für die Beförderung der Antigenteilchen in die Bronchiolen und Alveolen und damit für die Auslösung des allergischen Asthmas beim sensibilisierten Meerschweinchen. Zu große Teilchen gelangen nicht in die tiefen Luftwege, zu kleine Teilchen werden wieder ausgeatmet (Heubner [106], s. auch Findeisen [74]). Bei dem derzeitigen Stand der Aerosoltechnik bereitet die Beschaffung geeigneter Zerstäuberaggregate keine Schwierigkeiten. Hersteller von Aerosolaggregaten sind den einschlägigen Katalogen zu entnehmen. Die Leistungsfähigkeit des Aggregates (Luftdurchtritt pro Minute) muß den Abmessungen des Versuchsraumes entsprechen. Eine bequeme Methode zur Herstellung eines gleichbleibenden Aerosols mit Teilchen von im Mittel 1—2 μ Durchmesser findet sich bei Eichler *et al.* [69]. Eine genaue Dosierung ist möglich.

Die zu zerstäubende Flüssigkeit enthält das spezifische Antigen in geeigneter Konzentration. Diese muß passend zur Kapazität des Zerstäubers, Größe des Versuchsraumes und sonstigen Versuchstechnik empirisch ermittelt werden. Bei Verwendung von kristallisiertem Ovalbumin werden von den meisten Autoren Konzentrationen zwischen 1 und 20%, meist 5—10% verwendet.

Der Versuchsraum, in dem sich das Tier befindet, muß eine Luftabfuhr haben. Diese ist zweckmäßig in einen Abzug zu leiten, um Sensibilisierung oder allergische Reaktionen beim Experimentator zu vermeiden. Für detaillierte apparative Angaben s. die Darstellung der verschiedenen Versuchstechniken.

b) Parenterale Antigenzufuhr

Von parenteralen Zufuhrwegen ist die intravenöse Injektion praktisch nur zur Anwendung am narkotisierten Tier geeignet. Mit subcutaner oder intramuskulärer Injektion lassen sich offensichtlich auch Asthmareaktionen auslösen (Noelpp-Eschenhagen und Noelpp [152]), die Reaktionsstärken wechseln aber und oft kommt es zum protrahierten Schock, bei dem das Asthma nicht das beherrschende Symptom darstellt oder ganz fehlt.

Es ist eine Besonderheit des Meerschweinchens, daß sich bei diesem Tier so leicht Asthmareaktionen hervorrufen lassen und daß es im akuten anaphylaktischen Schock in der Regel an einem totalen Bronchialverschluß, einem „Status asthmaticus absolutus" eingeht. Die Reversiblität der allergischen Asthmareaktion ist offenbar eine Frage der Antigendosierung, die bei der inhalativen Zufuhr niedrig gehalten werden kann, wenn auch hier schon besondere Vorsichtsmaßregeln erforderlich sind. Da über den Grad der allergischen Reaktivität keine Voraussage möglich ist, führt die intravenöse oder intrakardiale Reinjektion sehr leicht zur maximalen letalen Bronchostenose. Die meisten Untersucher verwenden daher auch beim narkotisierten und künstlich beatmeten Tier anstelle der intravenösen die inhalative Antigenzufuhr. Auch mit intravenöser

Antigeninjektion gelingt jedoch die Auslösung wiederholter, nicht maximaler reversibler Asthmaanfälle am narkotisierten Meerschweinchen (Alberty [5, 6]): Man stellt eine um den Faktor 2 ansteigende Verdünnungsreihe des Antigens her und beginnt die Antigeninjektionen mit einer sehr niedrigen Dosis, z.B. kristallisiertem Ovalbumin 10^{-8} g·kg^{-1}. In Abständen von jeweils 10—20 min wird dann die nächst größere Antigendosis injiziert, bis ein Asthmaanfall auftritt. Nach dessen Abklingen werden die Antigeninjektionen von der zuletzt wirksamen Dosierungsstufe an fortgesetzt, und so fort. Hierbei kommt es zu schrittweiser Desensibilisierung auf jeder Dosierungsstufe (s. S. 110). In prinzipiell gleicher Weise gingen auch Hicks und Leach [107] vor. Sie untersuchten quantitative Beziehungen zwischen Antigendosis und Intensität der Asthmareaktion systematisch.

II. Pharmakonbedingtes Asthma

Grundsätzlich können mit allen bronchoconstrictorisch wirksamen Substanzen Asthmareaktionen erzeugt werden. Bei dem am meisten verwendeten durch Histamin hervorgerufenen experimentellen Asthma spielen Schleimhautödem und vermehrte Bronchialsekretion als Teilkomponenten der Bronchostenose je nach den Versuchsbedingungen eine gewisse Rolle. Die meisten der anderen verwendeten Substanzen erzeugen einen praktisch reinen Bronchospasmus.

Durch Pharmaka erzeugte Asthmareaktionen haben u. a. breite Anwendung gefunden zu vergleichenden Untersuchungen mit dem allergischen Asthma und als Asthmamodell zum Studium zahlreicher Probleme der pharmakologischen Grundlagenforschung ebenso wie der angewandten Pharmakologie.

Auch hier wird die inhalative Auslösung als Methode der Wahl am frei atmenden nicht narkotisierten Tier angewandt. Am narkotisierten Versuchstier wird das Asthmogen intravenös injiziert oder infundiert. Als Versuchstiere werden neben dem Meerschweinchen besonders Hund und Katze verwendet.

1. Inhalative Zufuhr des Asthmogens

Das Standard-Versuchstier für diese Applikationsmethode ist das Meerschweinchen. Die Technik der Zufuhr asthmaerzeugender Substanzen ist die gleiche wie bei der Zufuhr von Antigenaerosol. Die Konzentration des wirksamen Stoffes in der Vernebelungsflüssigkeit hängt in gleicher Weise von den technischen Eigenschaften des Zerstäubers, der Größe des Versuchsraumes und der gewünschten Reaktionsstärke ab und muß den jeweiligen Verhältnissen entsprechend empirisch ermittelt werden. Im folgenden werden Konzentrations-Größenordnungen angegeben, wie sie von verschiedenen Untersuchern verwendet wurden:

Histamin (als Bihydrochlorid oder Phosphat) 10^{-2} bis 10^{-4} g·ml^{-1}, von den meisten Autoren $5—1 \times 10^{-3}$ g·ml^{-1} und weniger. Manche verwenden einen Zusatz von 10^{-1} ml Glycerin oder 10^{-1} bis 5×10^{-1} ml Propylenglykol pro ml Vernebelungsflüssigkeit.

Acetylcholin oder Methacholin (als Hydrochlorid oder Hydrobromid) 5×10^{-4} bis 5×10^{-3} bis 3×10^{-2} g·ml^{-1}.

5-Hydroxytryptamin (als Kreatininsulfat) 10^{-2} g·ml^{-1}.

2. Parenterale Zufuhr des Asthmogens

Methode der Wahl für die Erzeugung von Asthmareaktionen am narkotisierten Versuchstier ist die intravenöse Injektion oder Infusion des Asthmogens. Die wirksame Dosis des verwendeten Pharmakons hängt, abgesehen von Species und

Tabelle 1. *Asthmareaktionen am narkotisierten Versuchstier durch intravenöse Verabreichung verschiedener Pharmaka (Dosierungsbeispiele)*

Tierart	Dosierung ($\mu g \cdot kg^{-1}$)	Versuchstechnik	Literatur
	Histamin		
Meerschweinchen	2	Konzett-Rössler	[24, 52]
Meerschweinchen	10	Konzett-Rössler	[153]
	2—25	Konzett-Rössler	[93]
	2—15 $\cdot$ min^{-1} (Dauerinfusion)	Konzett-Rössler	[6]
	50—60	Konzett-Rössler	[94, 169]
	3—30	Spirometer	[39]
Katze	10	Konzett-Rössler	[145]
Katze	100—800	Spirometer	[119]
Hund	1—10	Konzett-Rössler	[42]
Hund	6	Plethysmographie	[172]
Hund	15—50	Plethysomographie	[196]
	Acetylcholin		
Meerschweinchen	6	Konzett-Rössler	[72]
Meerschweinchen	8—22	Konzett-Rössler	[108]
Meerschweinchen	50	Konzett-Rössler	[64]
Meerschweinchen	50—100	Konzett-Rössler	[93, 169]
Hund	3—10	Konzett-Rössler	[90, 91]
Hund	10	Konzett-Rössler (modif.)	[42]
Hund	10—20	Konzett-Rössler	[14]
	Carbacholin		
Katze	2—150	Konzett-Rössler	[145]
	Pilocarpin		
Katze	1000—6000	Spirometer u.a.	[15, 119, 125]
Hund	1000 3,5—4,3 $\cdot$ min^{-1}	Konzett-Rössler	[90, 91]
	5-Hydroxytryptamin		
Meerschweinchen	1—4	Konzett-Rössler	[111]
Meerschweinchen	2—8	Konzett-Rössler	[190]
Meerschweinchen	3—22	Konzett-Rössler	[121]
Meerschweinchen	50	Konzett-Rössler	[94]
Katze	3—35	Konzett-Rössler	[121]
Katze	5—200	Plethysmographie	[123]
	Bradykinin		
Meerschweinchen	1—10 u. mehr	Konzett-Rössler	[24, 50—53, 167]
	Kallidin-10		
Meerschweinchen Ratte Kaninchen	3—6	Konzett-Rössler	[24]
	Substanz P		
Meerschweinchen Ratte Kaninchen	50—75 E $\cdot$ kg^{-1}	Konzett-Rössler	[24]
	Angiotensin		
Meerschweinchen Ratte Kaninchen	20—30	Konzett-Rössler	[24]

Zustand des verwendeten Versuchstieres, offenbar auch stark von der Empfindlichkeit der Registrierung der Erfolgsreaktion ab. In der folgenden Übersichtstabelle (Tabelle 1) sind repräsentative Dosierungsbeispiele für die meisten zur Erzeugung von Asthmareaktionen verwendeten Pharmaka aufgeführt.

B. Methoden zur Erzeugung und Registrierung von Asthma-Reaktionen

I. Methoden am nicht-narkotisierten Tier mit inhalativer Auslösung der Asthmareaktion

Wie schon vorstehend erörtert, ist die inhalative Auslösung der Asthmareaktion die Methode der Wahl für Versuche am nichtnarkotisierten Meerschweinchen. Quantitative Aussagen über die experimentellen Beobachtungen erfordern, daß die Stärke des Asthmas bzw. einzelner Atmungsgrößen erfaßt und möglichst auch gesteuert werden kann. Jede Manipulation des nichtnarkotisierten Tieres stört dessen Reaktionen beträchtlich. In der Regel müssen Veränderungen der Atmung deshalb indirekt registriert werden.

Die Steuerung des Asthmas ist eine Frage der Dosierung des asthmaerzeugenden Agens, die bei inhalativer Zufuhr nicht ohne weiteres annähernd konstant zu halten ist. Die bronchiale Reaktivität des Meerschweinchens ist zudem sehr stark ausgeprägt. Es kommt sehr leicht zu einem totalen Bronchialverschluß. Das allergische Asthma ist außerdem ein eigengesetzliches Geschehen, dessen Stärke und Verlauf außer von der Antigendosierung noch von zusätzlichen, individuell nicht vorauszusagenden Faktoren bestimmt wird. Steuerung und Registrierung der Asthmareaktion bilden in dieser Versuchsanordnung deshalb besondere Probleme.

1. Qualitative Beurteilung der Asthmaintensität

Im Zusammenhang mit ihren grundlegenden Untersuchungen über das experimentelle allergische Asthma bronchiale des Meerschweinchens verglichen Kallós und Pagel [118] die Wirkung von Calcium, Adrenalin und Bellafolin. Später erweiterten Kallós und Kallós-Deffner [116, 117] diese Untersuchungen. Sie erreichten durch Zufuhr von Antigenaerosol länger dauernde reversible Asthmareaktionen. Kallós und Pagel [118] zeigten, daß man durch Vernebelung von $10^{-3}\,g \cdot ml^{-1}$ Histamin oder Acetylcholin enthaltender Lösungen beim Meerschweinchen Asthmaanfälle auslösen konnte, die das gleiche äußere Symptombild zeigten wie das allergische Asthma durch Antigenexposition an sensibilisierten Tieren.

Colldahl [45] führte eine breit angelegte Untersuchung über Gaswechsel und Gewebsatmung beim experimentellen Asthma des Meerschweinchens aus. Er applizierte nach dem Vorgehen von Kallós und Pagel [118] Antigen oder Histamin als Aerosol und führte Stoffwechseluntersuchungen im geschlossenen und offenen Respirationssystem vorwiegend an nichtnarkotisierten, in geringerem Maße auch an narkotisierten Meerschweinchen durch. Hinsichtlich der relativ aufwendigen Technik wird auf die Originalarbeit verwiesen. Colldahl wies nach, daß die mechanische Behinderung bei der asthmatischen Stenoseatmung die Lungenventilation erheblich verschlechtert, so daß der Organismus in einen hypoxämischen Zustand gerät. Bei längerer Dauer kommt es zu einer Schädigung des Gewebsstoffwechsels. Colldahl führte keine scharfe Trennung von allergischem und histaminbedingtem Asthma durch.

Die Fragestellungen der Untersuchungen von Kallós und Pagel und von Colldahl erforderten keine genaue quantitative Beurteilung der Asthmaintensität.

Durch Zufuhr von Histaminaerosol erzeugtes Asthma verwendeten Schaumann [170] und Halpern [93] frühzeitig zur Wirksamkeitsprüfung von Arzneimitteln. Schaumann verwendete einen Tancré-Inhalator mit Doppelkugel. Bei einem Druck von 1 kg · cm^{-1} betrug der Luftdurchgang 8,8 l · min^{-1}. Dabei wurden 0,134 ml · min^{-1} Flüssigkeit vernebelt, welche 10^{-3} g · ml^{-1} Histamin enthielt. Die Nebeldichte betrug 0,015 ml mit 0,015 mg Histamin pro Liter Luft. Schaumann wählte in Vorversuchen Tiere aus, die innerhalb von 5 min schwere Asthmasymptome zeigten. Pethidin (Dolantin) in einer Konzentration von 10^{-2} g · ml^{-1} in der Vernebelungsflüssigkeit gleichzeitig mit Histamin versprayt oder 10 mg · kg^{-1}

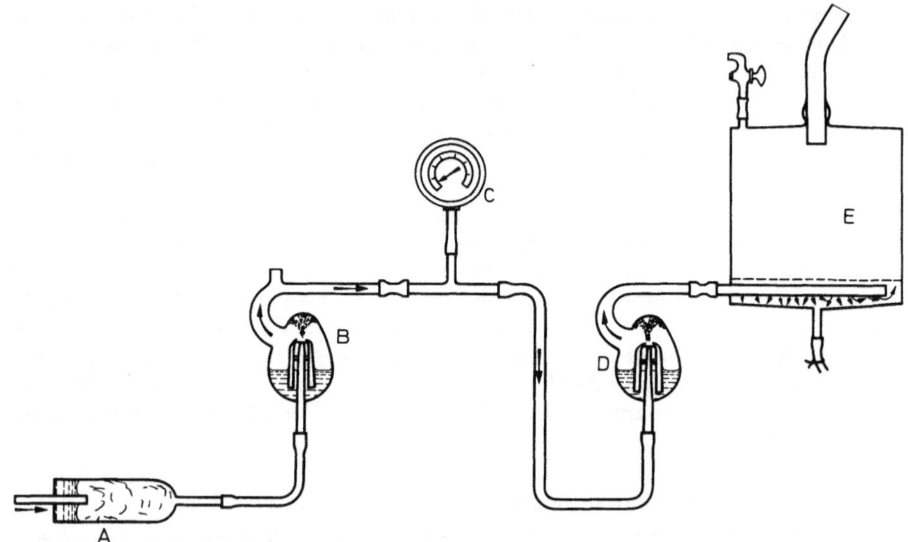

Abb. 1. Zufuhr des asthmaerzeugenden Agens als Aerosol. Versuchsanordnung nach B. N. Halpern, Arch. int. Pharmacodyn. 68,—339 408 (1942). Erklärung s. Text

subcutan mindestens 10 min vor Aerosolexposition gegeben verhinderten den Asthmaanfall „fast völlig". Atropin oder Papaverin in gleicher Konzentration von 10^{-2} g · ml^{-1} in der Aerosolflüssigkeit hatte keine Wirkung.

Halpern [93] prüfte die Wirksamkeit einer Reihe neuartiger spezifischer Antihistaminica u. a. am durch Histaminaerosol erzeugten Asthma des Meerschweinchens. Er registrierte drei Intensitätsstufen der Reaktion:

++: Intensive Dyspnoe mit Bradypnoe und Einziehen der Flanken.
+: Weniger starke Dyspnoe.
(+): Kaum bemerkbare Dyspnoe.

Halpern verabreichte den zu prüfenden Stoff parenteral oder peroral und betrachtete diejenigen Tiere als geschützt, die bei nachfolgender Aerosolexposition innerhalb von 10 min keine schwere Dyspnoe zeigten. Die von Halpern für seine Versuche beschriebene Versuchsanordnung sei als Beispiel des Prinzips der Histaminaerosol-Versuchstechnik im folgenden wiedergegeben (Abb. 1).

Die Preßluft wird bei *A* durch Watte filtriert und passiert zwei in Serie geschaltete Zerstäuber *B* und *D*. Der erste enthält Wasser als Vernebelungsflüssigkeit. Die nach Durchgang durch *B* mit Wasser gesättigte Luft passiert den zweiten Zerstäuber *D*, enthaltend 2×10^{-3} g · ml^{-1} Histaminbihydrochlorid und 10 g · ml^{-1} Glycerin in wäßriger Lösung. Der Luftdurchgang betrug 55 l · min^{-1}, der Luftdruck an Düse *D* 0,45 kg, die vernebelte Flüssigkeitsmenge 20 ml pro

Stunde. Das Aerosol gelangt in die Versuchskammer *E* von ungefähr 10 Liter Inhalt unter die perforierte Bodenplatte. Die Versuchskammer hat Auslässe zur Entfernung von kondensierter Flüssigkeit und Urin, Ableitung des Aerosols und Luftausgleich.

Preuner [156, 157] setzte Meerschweinchen für die Dauer von 10 min dem Antigenaerosol aus und verwendete zur Beurteilung der Intensität des Asthmas folgende Zahlenwerte als willkürliche subjektive Intensitätsstufen:

0: Keine oder nur undeutliche Erscheinungen.
1: Geringgradige Reaktion, wie Putzen der Schnauze, leichte Hustenstöße, motorische Unruhe.
2: Stark erhöhte Atemfrequenz mit Beteiligung der Hilfsmuskulatur.
3: Schwere Atemnot mit wieder geringerer Frequenz, erhobenem Kopf und maximaler Beteiligung der Hilfsmuskulatur.
4: Anhaltender Husten bei schwerer Atemnot mit steif gestreckten Extremitäten oder beginnende anaphylaktische Erscheinungen mit Auftreten klonischer Krämpfe.
5: Das Tier legt sich nach vorhergegangenen Krämpfen vorübergehend auf die Seite.
6: Tod nach vorangegangenem Anfall mit für Anaphylaxie typischem Sektionsbefund.

Reichel [164] objektivierte diese Stadien plethysmographisch (s. Abb. 2). Die Intensitätsstufen 1, 2 und 5 unterschieden sich durch Frequenz und Amplitude der Atmung, Stadium 3 und 4 durch die Kurvenform des Ex- und Inspiriums. Ähnliche Bilder erhielten Noelpp *et al.* [147] mit thorakographischer Methode (s. S. 97). Friebel [87] erweiterte diese Registriermethode für seine später zu beschreibende Versuchstechnik (s. S. 92). Preuner *et al.* [160] vereinfachten die Intensitätsstufen später durch folgende Einteilung in drei Stärken.

1: Hustenstöße, Niesen, Naseputzen usw.
2: Flache, gegenüber der normalen frequente Atmung mit oder ohne Husten und ohne oder mit nur geringem Einsatz der Hilfsmuskulatur.
3: Langsame, mühselige, exspirationsbehinderte Atmung unter Einsatz der gesamten Hilfsmuskulatur, häufig unterbrochen von quälendem Husten ohne Expektoration.

Preuner u. Mitarb. [160] verwendeten diese Beurteilung der Asthmaintensität zur Bestimmung der therapeutischen Wirksamkeit einiger Pharmaka am Meerschweinchen in folgender Weise:

Sensibilisierung durch einmalige Injektion von 0,5 ml Hühnereiklar 1:10 mit isotonischer NaCl-Lösung verdünnt intraperitoneal. Nach Ablauf der Sensibilisierungszeit Testung durch Zufuhr von Antigenaerosol. In orientierenden Vorversuchen wurde das Antigen so verdünnt, daß allzu heftige Reaktionen möglichst vermieden wurden, gewöhnlich 1:50. Jedes Tier wurde durch mehrere in kurzen Abständen aufeinanderfolgende Asthmaanfälle „zum Asthmatiker gemacht", anschließend in regelmäßigem Wechsel als Kontrolltier und als Versuchstier verwendet. Die Antigeninhalation im eigentlichen Versuch dauerte insgesamt 20 min. Die Reaktionsstärke wurde alle 2 min bewertet. Eliminiert wurden alle Tiere, die bis zum Ablauf der ersten 8 min geringer als Reaktionsstärke 2 oder stärker als Reaktionsstärke 3 reagierten. Die zu prüfende Substanz wurde der Hälfte der Tiergruppe 10 min nach Inhalationsbeginn injiziert. Die andere Hälfte der Tiere diente als Kontrolle. Die Antigenzufuhr wurde 20 min nach Beginn abgebrochen und Frischluft zugeführt. Das Abklingen des Asthmas wurde weitere 20 min lang

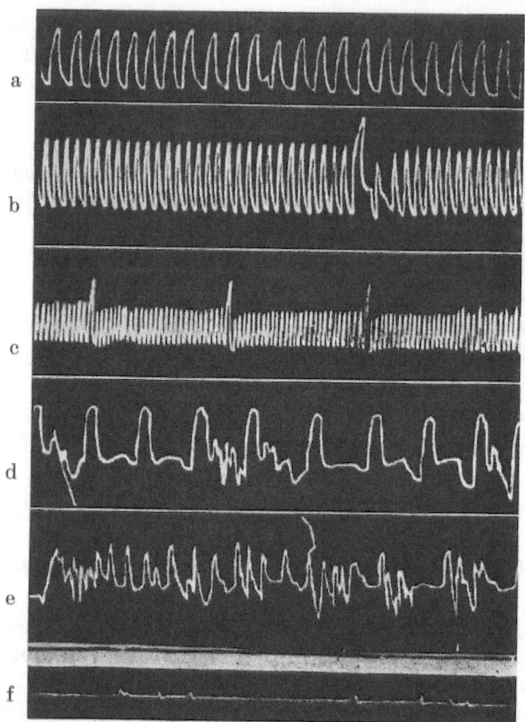

Abb. 2a—f. Plethysmographisches Bild der verschiedenen Intensitätsstufen des allergischen Asthmas des Meerschweinchens nach Preuner [157], aufgezeichnet von F. Reichel [164]. a Normale Atmung, b Bronchialasthma Stärke 1, c Bronchialasthma Stärke 2, d Bronchialasthma Stärke 3, e Bronchialasthma Stärke 4, f Bronchialasthma Stärke 5. [Aus: R. Preuner, Ärztl. Forsch. 5, 64—71 (1951)]

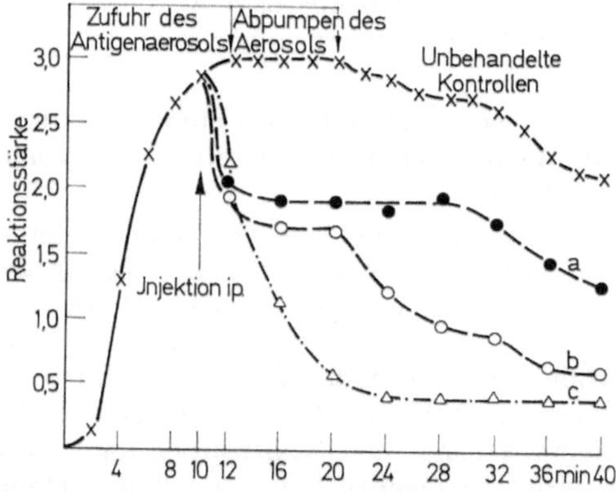

Abb. 3. Die Wirkung verschiedener Kombinationen auf den Asthmaanfall. Kurve a: Khellin 10 mg/kg + Ephedrin 10 mg/kg + Theophyllin 30 mg/kg; b: Khellin 10 mg/kg + Ephedrin. hydrorhod. 15 mg/kg + Theophyllin 30 mg/kg; c: Khellin 10 mg/kg + Ephedrin. hydrorhod. 15 mg/kg + Theophyllin 30 mg/kg + Diphenhydramin 10 mg/kg. Beispiel der Auswertung von Versuchen über die Wirkung verschiedener Arzneimittel auf das allergische Asthma des Meerschweinchens. [Nach R. Preuner, J. von Prittwitz und Gaffron u. W. Brehmer, Arzneimittel-Forsch. 3, 337—341 (1953)]

notiert. Aus den Einzelwerten von Gruppen von je 20 Tieren wurden Mittelwerte gebildet und der Versuchsverlauf graphisch dargestellt (s. Beispiel Abb. 3).

Folgende Pharmaka und ihre Kombinationen verringerten das Asthma:

Dimethylphenylthiazolidin	9—18	$mg \cdot kg^{-1}$ intraperitoneal
Ephedrin	9—18	$mg \cdot kg^{-1}$ intraperitoneal
Dimethylphenylthiazolidin	6,25	$mg \cdot kg^{-1}$
Ephedrin	12,5	$mg \cdot kg^{-1}$
Theophyllin	31,25	$mg \cdot kg^{-1}$ intraperitoneal
Khellin	4	$mg \cdot kg^{-1}$ intraperitoneal
Papaverin	10	$mg \cdot kg^{-1}$ intraperitoneal
Diphenhydramin	5	$mg \cdot kg^{-1}$ intraperitoneal

Neely [142] fand mit der Methode von Preuner keinen Einfluß von Histaminase (3 E intravenös) auf das allergische Asthma des Meerschweinchens, erreichte dagegen Sensibilisierung und Schock mit diesem Enzym.

In seinen Untersuchungen über Sensibilisierung und Asthmaauslösung mit Anaphylatoxin teilte Mendes [137] in ähnlicher Weise wie Preuner die Asthmaintensität in 4 Stadien ein. Van Arman, Miller und O'Malley [10] beurteilten die Stärke des allergischen Meerschweinchenasthmas ebenfalls in 4 Intensitätsstufen. Sie untersuchten die bronchodilatorische und hyperglykämische Wirkung von SC-10049 = L-3-{2-[-2-hydroxy-2-(3,4-dihydroxyphenyl)-äthylamino]-propyl}-indoltartrat.

2. Quantitative Erfassung der Asthmaintensität

a) Präkonvulsionszeit („Kollapszeit“)

Die Latenzzeit vom Beginn der Zufuhr des asthmaerzeugenden Aerosols bis zum Einsetzen eindeutiger Asthmasymptome ist ein quantitativer Meßwert, der offenbar mit Reaktionsbereitschaft und -intensität korreliert ist.

Siegmund, Granger und Lands [173] registrierten „Beginn“ (onset) und „Dauer“ des durch Histamin erzeugten Meerschweinchenasthmas. Sie vernebelten eine 0,2%ige Lösung von Histamindiphosphat. „Beginn“ bedeutete die Dauer der Aerosolzufuhr bis zum Einsetzen auffallender Symptome, wie Zunahme der Atemfrequenz, forcierte Inspiration usw. Als „Dauer“ wurde die gesamte Zeit vom Beginn der Exposition bis zum Einsetzen asphyktischer Konvulsionen bzw. bis zum Kollaps bezeichnet. Siegmund *et al.* [173] untersuchten mit dieser Methode die bronchodilatorische Wirkung von Adrenalinderivaten und fanden Isoprenalin am wirksamsten im Vergleich mit den entsprechenden N-Methyl- und N-sec.-Butylderivaten.

Lish, Robbins und Dungan [128] verwendeten lediglich das Intervall zwischen Beginn der Aerosolzufuhr und Einsetzen von Dyspnoe und Husten („precough intervall“). Die Differenz zwischen den entsprechenden Intervallzeiten von behandelten und unbehandelten Tieren wurde als Maß der protektiven oder antagonistischen Arzneimittelwirkung verwendet. Lish *et al.* [128] untersuchten die bronchodilatorische Wirkung des α-adrenergischen Blockers Phentolamin. Sie kamen zu der Schlußfolgerung, daß diese hauptsächlich auf die Freisetzung von Adrenalin aus dem Nebennierenmark oder anderen Depots zurückzuführen sei.

Bucher [31] registrierte die Zeit vom Beginn der Aerosolzufuhr bis zum Einsetzen eindeutiger Asthmasymptome bei Anwendung von Aerosol enthaltend etwa 0,2 mg Histamin oder 0,8 mg Acetylcholin pro Liter Luft. Er suchte annähernd gleich empfindliche Tiere aus und stellte fest, daß die Meerschweinchen durch tägliche wiederholte Verabreichung des Aerosols an Histamin gewöhnt werden konnten. Wenn Histamin gleichzeitig mit Tripelennamin in einer

Konzentration von 1 mg pro Liter Luft gegeben wurde, entstand keine Gewöhnung, was Bucher als weiteren Beweis für die kompetetive Natur des Antagonismus Histamin-Tripelennamin interpretierte.

Feinberg, Malkiel und MacIntire [73] sensibilisierten Meerschweinchen passiv mit 0,5—2,0 ml · kg^{-1} Meerschweinchen-Antiovalbuminserum intravenös und setzten die Tiere 28 Std später dem Nebel einer 0,2%igen Antigenlösung aus. Geeignete Antiserumdosen und Antigenkonzentrationen waren in Vorversuchen experimentell ermittelt worden. Vorher injiziertes Cortison (50 mg 18 Std vorher) oder ACTH (2×10 mg 8 und 4 Std vorher) verlängerten die Latenzzeit von Antigenexposition bis Asthmabeginn um etwa das Doppelte von 2,5 auf 5,2 min.

Herxheimer [99] verwendete als Maß der Asthmaintensität ebenfalls die Dauer der Antigeninhalation bis zum Erreichen eines bestimmten Stadiums der Dyspnoe. Er bezeichnete diese Zeit als „preconvulsion time", in einer deutschsprachigen Publikation [105] als „Kollapszeit". Da die wörtliche Übersetzung „Präkonvulsionszeit" m. E. die gemessene Reaktion eindeutiger kennzeichnet, wird sie im folgenden verwendet. Herxheimer *et al.* [99—105] erarbeiteten in systematischen Untersuchungen die methodischen Bedingungen zur wiederholten Erzeugung von Asthmaanfällen annähernd gleichbleibender Intensität, „anaphylaktischer Mikroschocks", beim Meerschweinchen, durch folgendes Vorgehen:

Meerschweinchen werden sensibilisiert durch intramuskuläre Injektion von 0,7 ml einer 5%igen Lösung von kristallisiertem Ovalbumin. Das gleiche Antigen wird 3 Wochen danach als 5%ige Zerstäuberflüssigkeit verwendet. Die Abmessungen des Versuchsraumes betrugen 70×35×35 cm. Die Atmung des Tieres während der Aerosolzufuhr wird beobachtet. Endpunkt ist ein Grad der Dyspnoe, bei dem die Respiration schnell und oberflächlich wird und das ganze Tier an den Respirationsbewegungen teilnimmt. Das Tier bewegt den Kopf schnell auf und ab. In diesem Augenblick muß es aus der Aerosolkammer entfernt werden. Da dieses Stadium den asphyktischen Konvulsionen (convulsion point) vorausgeht, bezeichnet Herxheimer die Zeit bis zu seinem Eintreten als Präkonvulsionszeit. Ihre Bestimmung ist subjektiv und erfolgt durch zwei erfahrene Beobachter.

Bei der ersten Exposition ist die Präkonvulsionszeit gewöhnlich $\leqq$ 60 sec. Sie verlängert sich bei täglich wiederholter Exposition schnell bis zu weitgehender Desensibilisierung, bleibt aber kurz bei Wiederholung in 8—10tägigen Intervallen infolge Resensibilisierung im Intervall. Befriedigende Konstanz der Präkonvulsionszeit wird erreicht durch wiederholte Expositionen mit individuellem Intervall, gewöhnlich von 2—3 Tagen. Dabei wird ein Gleichgewicht zwischen De- und Resensibilisierung erreicht (vgl. Tabelle 2).

Tabelle 2. *Relative Konstanz der Präkonvulsionszeit bei Auslösung von Mikroschocks in Abständen von 2—3 Tagen*

Tier Nr.	23. 6. 51	25. 6. 51	27. 6. 51	30. 6. 51	2. 7. 51
53	80	85	75	95	95
54	105	105	135	95	110
56	80	100	80	90	75
66	100	120[a]	140[a]	110[a]	100
67	125	90	130	100	110
69	120	85	115	130	130
Mittelwert	103	97	112	103	103

[a] Krämpfe.

Nach H. Herxheimer, J. Physiol. (Lond.) **117**, 251—255 (1952).

Später untersuchte Stresemann [179] systematisch den Einfluß des Intervalls zwischen den Antigenexpositionen und den Einfluß der Antigenkonzentration in der Aerosolflüssigkeit auf die Länge der Präkonvulsionszeit. Er fand annäherndes Gleichbleiben der allergischen Sensibilität bei wöchentlicher Exposition, dagegen Abnahme bei kürzerem Intervall (Abb. 4). Die Reaktion der Tiere zeigte aller-

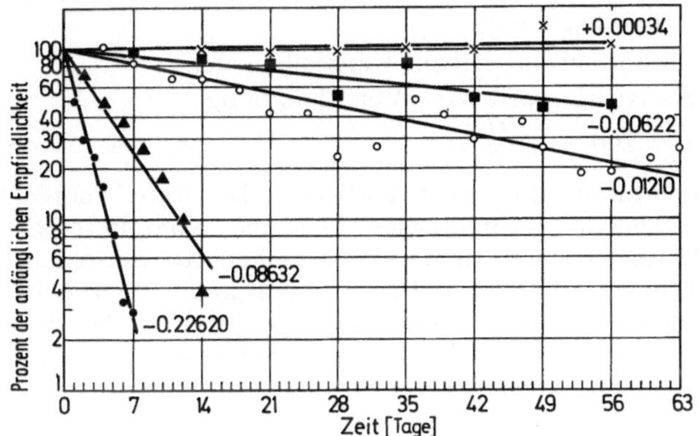

Abb. 4. Effekt der Dauer des Intervalls zwischen den einzelnen Antigenexpositionen. • Tägliche Aerosolanwendung, ▲ jeden zweiten Tag, ○ alle 3—4 Tage, × Intervall von 7 Tagen, ▪ 7-Tage-Intervall, alte Tiere. Am Ende jeder Regressionslinie ist der Wert von *b*, dem Steigungsfaktor der Kurve, angegeben. Semilogarithmisches Koordinatensystem. [Aus: E. Stresemann, J. Physiol. (Lond.) **159**, 384—390 (1961)]

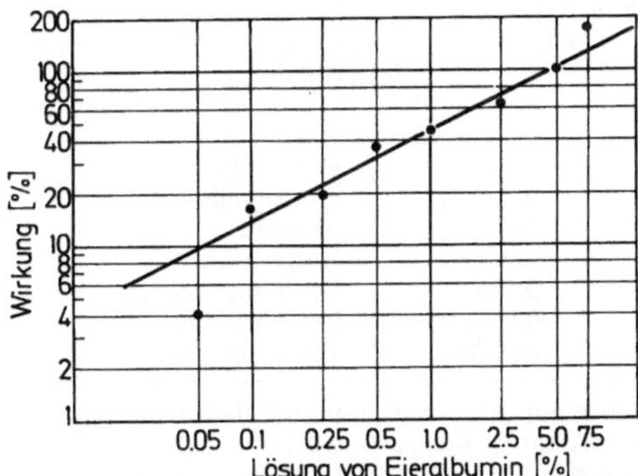

Abb. 5. Wirkung (Ordinate) verschiedener Antigenkonzentrationen (Abszisse) auf die Stärke des „anaphylaktischen Mikroschocks", ausgedrückt in Prozent der Wirkung der Standardlösung von Eieralbumin (5%). Logarithmischer Maßstab. [Nach E. Stresemann, J. Physiol. (Lond.) **159**, 384—390 (1961)]

dings beträchtliche individuelle Variation. Die Präkonvulsionszeit nahm ab mit zunehmender Konzentration des Antigens im Aerosol (Abb. 5). Die hauptsächlichsten Nachteile dieser Methode sind die individuelle Variabilität der Meerschweinchen und die Schwierigkeit der exakten Bestimmung des Endpunktes (Herxheimer [99]).

Armitage, Herxheimer und Rosa [11] untersuchten mit Herxheimers Methode die Wirkung von Antihistaminica auf das allergische Asthma des Meerschweinchens. Sie bestimmten für jedes Versuchstier das angemessene Expositionsintervall, bei dem die Präkonvulsionszeit konstant blieb, und bildeten Gruppen von

Tieren mit gleichem Intervall. Jedes Tier kam abwechselnd in einen Versuch mit und ohne Vorbehandlung mit dem zu prüfenden Stoff. Die Antihistaminsubstanz oder Atropinsulfat wurde intramuskulär 60—90 min vor Antigenexposition, Procain und Procainamid intraperitoneal 20 min vor Antigenexposition gegeben. Die mittlere Präkonvulsionszeit im Kontrollversuch wurde in Beziehung gesetzt zur Präkonvulsionszeit unter Pharmakonwirkung und in „Prozent Schutzwirkung" für jedes Tier berechnet:

C = mittlere Präkonvulsionszeit im Kontrollversuch;

T = mittlere Konvulsionszeit nach Vorbehandlung;

$$\text{Schutzwirkung} = 100\left(1 - \frac{C}{T}\right).$$

Die Ergebnisse wurden statistisch analysiert. Die untersuchten Stoffe verzögerten das Einsetzen der asthmatischen Dyspnoe. Kompletter Schutz wurde nur bei einigen Tieren erreicht. In der Wirksamkeit der einzelnen Substanzen bestanden beträchtliche Differenzen. Die Wirkung konnte durch Erhöhung der Dosis nur bis zu einer bestimmten Grenze gesteigert werden. Die antagonistische Wirkung von Atropin war schwach, die von Procain noch schwächer. Die Ergebnisse sind in Tabelle 3 aufgeführt.

Tabelle 3

a) Niedrigste Dosis, bei der signifikante Schutzwirkung eintritt. (Chlortrimeton wurde aus dieser Tabelle fortgelassen, da keine zwischen 0,05 und 1 mg · kg⁻¹ liegenden Dosen geprüft wurden.)	mg · kg^{-1}	b) Niedrigste Dosis, oberhalb welcher keine signifikante Zunahme der Schutzwirkung mehr eintritt. (Chlortrimeton wurde aus dieser Tabelle fortgelassen, da keine zwischen 0,05 und 1 mg · kg⁻¹ liegenden Dosen geprüft wurden.)	mg · kg^{-1}
Antazolin	0,5	Antazolin	3,0[a]
Atropin	0,325	Chlorcyclizin	1,0
Diphenhydramin	0,2	Atropin	0,65
Chlorcyclizin	0,2	Mepyramin	0,4
Promethazin	0,025	Diphenhydramin	[b]
Mepyramin	0,005 (?)[a]	Promethazin	0,25
Tripelennamin	0,005[a]	Tripelennamin	[c]

[a] Höhere Dosen führen zu einer Abnahme der Schutzwirkung.

[b] Die beobachtete Schutzwirkung bleibt recht konstant zwischen 0,2 und 6,0 mg · kg^{-1} mit signifikanter Zunahme bei der exzessiven Dosis von 12,0 mg · kg^{-1}.

[c] Die beobachtete Schutzwirkung bleibt recht konstant zwischen 0,01 und 3,0 mg · kg^{-1} mit signifikanter Zunahme bei der exzessiven Dosis von 30,0 mg · kg^{-1}.

Nach P. Armitage, H. Herxheimer, and L. Rosa, Brit. J. Pharmacol. 7, 625—636 (1952).

Mit gleicher Methode verglich Herxheimer [100, 101, 103] die Wirkung verschiedener Pharmaka auf den „anaphylaktischen Mikroschock" mit ihrer Wirkung auf den durch andere asthmogene Substanzen hervorgerufenen „bronchoconstrictorischen Schock". Er applizierte Aerosole folgender *Asthmogene:*

Histaminphosphat 5×10^{-3} g · ml^{-1};

Acetylcholinbromid $3{,}125 \times 10^{-2}$ g · ml^{-1};

Methacholinchlorid $2{,}5 \times 10^{-3}$ g · ml^{-1};

Nicotinsulfat 4×10^{-2} g · ml^{-1};

5-Hydroxytryptamincreatininsulfat 10^{-2} g · ml^{-1};

„Furmethide" $2{,}5 \times 10^{-3}$ g · ml^{-1} (5-Methylfurfuryltrimethylammoniumjodid).

Als *Antagonisten* wurden verwendet in folgenden (wirksamen) Dosen:
Hexamethoniumbromid 0,1—20 mg·kg^{-1};
Atropinsulfat 0,013—1,28 mg·kg^{-1} intramuskulär 15—60 min vor Inhalation;
Lysergsäurediäthylamid 0,005—0,4 mg·kg^{-1} intramuskulär 15—60 min vor Inhalation;
Adrenalintartrat 0,01—0,3 mg·kg^{-1} intramuskulär 15—60 min vor Inhalation:
Mepyraminmaleat 0,01—6,0 mg·kg^{-1} intramuskulär 15—60 min vor Inhalation;
Propanthelin 0,1—10,0 mg·kg^{-1} intraperitoneal 20 min vor Inhalation;
Chlorpromazin 3,0—20,0 mg·kg^{-1} intraperitoneal 20 min vor Inhalation;
Papaverinsulfat 20,0—80,0 mg·kg^{-1} intraperitoneal 20 min vor Inhalation;
Aminophyllin 25,0—100,0 mg·kg^{-1} intraperitoneal 20 min vor Inhalation;
Cocainhydrochlorid als Aerosol einer 2,5—5 $\times 10^{-3}$ g·ml^{-1} enthaltenden Lösung 1,5—25 min vor Exposition.

Herxheimer [103] unterschied drei Gruppen von Antagonisten:

1. Substanzen, die gegen alle oder gegen die meisten Asthmogene wirkten, aber gegen einen besonderen Agonisten stärker als gegen die anderen: Atropin und Propanthelin vornehmlich gegen Acetylcholin, Methacholin und Furmethide, Hexamethonium, Cocain und Adrenalin vornehmlich gegen Nicotin, Hexamethonium jedoch stärker als die beiden letztgenannten Substanzen.

2. Substanzen, die gegen alle Asthmogene gleich gut aber nur in hohen Dosen wirkten: Aminophyllin, Papaverin und Chlorpromazin.

3. Substanzen, die nur gegen Histamin und 5-Hydroxytryptamin stark antagonistisch wirkten, gegen die anderen Agonisten jedoch nur schwach oder gar nicht, wie Mepyramin, sowie LSD, welches das durch 5-HT erzeugte Asthma wirksam hemmte, jedoch in allen anderen Fällen die Asthmaintensität verstärkte.

Alle Antagonisten mit Ausnahme von LSD und Papaverin beeinflußten auch das allergische Asthma. Die antiallergische Wirkung von Mepyramin war geringer als die Wirkung gegen histaminbedingtes Asthma. Die antiallergische Wirkung von Atropin und Hexamethonium war geringer als im acetylcholin- bzw. nicotinbedingten Asthma. Herxheimer schließt aus seinen Ergebnissen, daß bei der Wirkung von Histamin eine ganglionäre Komponente beteiligt ist, daß Histamin eine dominierende Rolle beim allergischen Asthma („anaphylaktischen Mikroschock") des Meerschweinchens spielt, und daß die nervösen Elemente der bronchialen Mucosa ebenfalls beteiligt sind.

Herxheimer [101] prüfte mit seiner Methode am allergischen Asthma des Meerschweinchens eine Reihe anderer Substanzen, die nicht zu den bekannten Bronchospasmolytica und Antihistaminica zu zählen waren. Er beobachtete hierbei antagonistische Wirkungen von Methanthelin, Propanthelin, Butylscopolamin und Natriumcyanat. Morphin wirkte erst in Dosen von 50 mg·kg^{-1}, Coffein erst bei 100 mg·kg^{-1}. Wirkungslos waren dagegen die folgenden Substanzen: Ascorbinsäure, Bariumchlorid, Chloralhydrat, Chlorpromazin, Cyanocobalamin, Dibenzylin, Heparin, Khellin, Phenobarbital, Phenylbutazon, Phenylephrin, Salicylsäure.

Über Verlängerung der Präkonvulsionszeit durch Chlordiazepoxid in Dosen von 0,65 bis 1,25 mg·kg^{-1} im allergischen Asthma des Meerschweinchens sowie Hemmung des Bronchospasmus in dieser wie auch in anderen Versuchsanordnungen (s. auch S. 123) berichteten Kovács und Görög [124].

Herxheimer [104] sowie Herxheimer und Langer [105] erzeugten am Meerschweinchen Asthma durch intraperitoneale Injektion von 40 mg·kg^{-1} Propranolol oder durch Applikation eines Aerosols der 12%igen Lösung. Hexamethonium und Atropin schwächten bei ausreichender Dosierung (2,5 bzw. 6 mg·kg^{-1} i.p.) die Propranololwirkung ab. Mepyramin 3 mg·kg^{-1} oder Guanethidin als Aerosol der 10%igen Lösung hatten keinen Einfluß. An Patienten wurden grundsätzlich die gleichen Ergebnisse erhalten (Propranololaerosol der 1—5%igen Lösung, Messung der Vitalkapazität mittels Spirometer).

b) Steuerbares Asthma und plethysmographische Registrierung

Reichel [164] hatte bereits die visuellen Intensitätsstufen Preuners [156, 157] plethysmographisch aufgezeichnet und bestätigt. Friebel *et al.* [87] sowie auch Noelpp *et al.* [147] entwickelten diese Methode weiter und kontrollierten die Asthmaintensität durch fortlaufende objektive Registrierung.

Friebel *et al.* [82, 87, 88] registrierten die Asthmaintensität als gedämpfte Druckschwankungen im Versuchsgefäß. Sie entwickelten ein Vorgehen, Dauer und Stärke des allergischen ebenso wie des durch Pharmaka erzeugten Asthmas

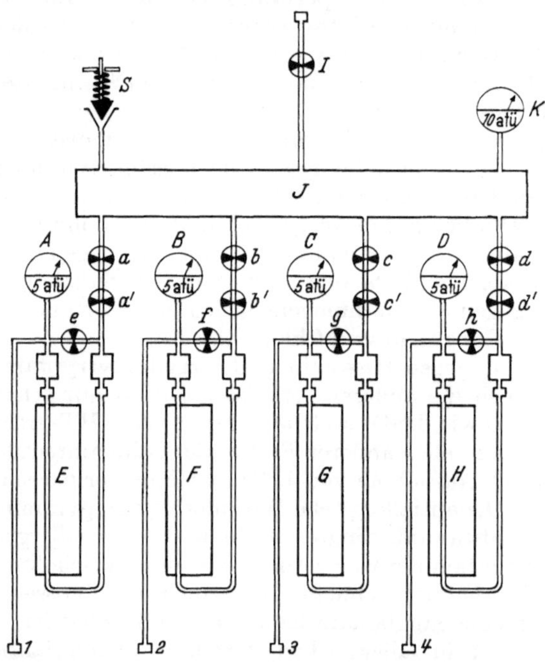

Abb. 6. Preßluftverteiler. *i* Preßluftzuführung mit Ventil, *J* zugehöriger Behälter, *S* Sicherheitsventil, *K* Manometer, *1—4* Zweigleitungen, *A—D* zugehörige Manometer, *a—d* Absperrhähne, *a'—d'* Regulierventile, *e—h* Stauventile, *E—H* zugehörige Wasserdifferentialmanometer. [Aus: H. Friebel u. A. Basold, Naunyn-Schmiedebergs Arch. exp. Path. Pharmak. **217**, 13—20 (1953)]

willkürlich im Versuch zu steuern, um am Asthma gleichbleibender Intensität quantitative Wirksamkeitsbestimmungen von Pharmaka durchzuführen. Das Prinzip der Methode beruht darauf, daß zunächst in üblicher Weise mit einem relativ konzentrierten asthmaerzeugenden Aerosol ein mittelschwerer Asthmazustand hervorgerufen wird. Durch Fortsetzung der Aerosolzufuhr, dann jedoch in geringerer Konzentration, wird das Asthma in gleichbleibender Stärke unterhalten. Die folgende Beschreibung der Versuchstechnik folgt weitgehend den Angaben von Friebel und Basold [87].

Das Verneblergerät besteht aus einer Gruppe von 4 Pari-Triplex-Zerstäubern. Die verwendeten Düsen müssen einen gleichgroßen Luftdurchtritt (etwa 6 l pro Minute bei 1,8 atü) und ein übereinstimmendes Ansaugvermögen für die zu vernebelnde Flüssigkeit haben (nefelometrisch und gravimetrisch geprüft). Die erforderliche Preßluft wird durch ein Filter geschickt und einem Preßluftverteiler zugeleitet (Abb. 6). In diesem wird die Luftzuführung in 4 Zweige gegabelt und außerdem eine Druckminderung vorgenommen. Der Druck von 4—6 atü in der Hauptleitung wird über 4 Regulierventile auf 1,8 atü im Zweig reduziert. Die laufende Kontrolle des durchfließenden Luftvolumens erfolgt an 4 Wasserdifferentialmanometern, die den Druckabfall an je einem geeichten Stauventil messen. Der Preßluftverteiler sorgt damit für einen gleichgroßen und gleichbleibenden Betriebsdruck in den nebelerzeugenden Düsen. Störungen der Luftzuführung sowie Absinken des Druckes lassen sich an den Differentialmanometern ablesen.

Die nebelabführenden Kanäle werden kurz hinter den Zerstäubern in einer Glasmischkugel zusammengefaßt. Der anschließend zum Versuchsraum führende Schenkel wird durch ein Tyndallmeter hindurchgeleitet, in dem nefelometrische Dichtebestimmungen möglich sind. Der Nebelstrom wird von einer konstanten Lichtquelle her durchleuchtet und die Intensität des in den Nebeltröpfchen abgebeugten Lichtes mit einer Sperrschichtphotozelle gemessen. Eine Verzweigung in der Nebelführung sorgt dafür, daß der in das Versuchsgefäß führende Aerosolstrom zum Teil oder auch ganz um den Versuchsraum herumgeführt werden kann.

Die Prüfung der Tröpfchengröße des Nebels wird vor dem Versuchsbeginn durchgeführt. Die in den Versuchsraum einfallenden Tröpfchen werden mit dem Ocularmikrometer unter dem Mikroskop gemessen. Hierbei dient die Thomasche Zählkammer als Absolutmaßstab. Das Gerät liefert unter den angegebenen Bedingungen Tröpfchen von 0,5—6,0 μ Durchmesser.

Der Versuchsraum (Abb. 7) besteht aus einem oben offenen Glasgefäß, in den das Meerschweinchen aufrecht hineingesetzt wird. Der Kopf des Tieres wird durch den Deckel des Glasgefäßes gesteckt. Der Luftraum des Gefäßes ist während des Versuchs geschlossen, der Deckel schließt am Rand des Gefäßes und am Hals des Tieres luftdicht ab. Verbindung nach außen hat das Gefäß durch mehrere Ansatzstutzen, von denen einer zur Entleerung von Harn und Kot dient, ein zweiter mit einer Mareyschen Kapsel in Verbindung steht, ein dritter über ein Ventil direkt in die Außenluft mündet. Über das Gefäß und den herausragenden Meerschweinchenkopf wird eine Glasglocke gestülpt, in die der Nebelstrom von oben eingeleitet und unter der er abgeführt wird. Der Rand der Glasglocke taucht zur Abdichtung in eine wassergefüllte Rinne.

Das Aerosol wird durch ein weitlumiges Rohr in die Außenluft abgeführt. Ein gasbetriebenes Verbrennungsgerät sorgt für die Vernichtung der organischen Aerosolbestandteile und für einen konstanten leichten Sog in den abführenden Wegen.

Die graphische Registrierung des Asthmas erfolgt mit Hilfe einer Mareyschen Kapsel, welche die Druckschwankungen im Innern des Versuchsgefäßes auf eine Kymographionschleife überträgt. Durch geeignete Dämpfung des Registriersystems läßt sich das ganze für den Formcharakter der Atemkurve verantwortliche Frequenzgemisch darstellen. Hierzu wird ein Teil der Druckdifferenz zwischen Versuchsgefäß und Außenluft über ein Ventil ausgeglichen. Der richtige Dämpfungsgrad läßt sich empirisch leicht finden und im Bedarfsfalle neu einregulieren. Während des Asthmaanfalles wird die Ventilöffnung so lange vergrößert und verkleinert, bis die Einstellung gefunden ist, bei der alle Feinheiten der typischen Asthmakurve am besten aufgezeichnet werden. Befriedigende Ergebnisse bekommt man, wenn die Amplitudengröße nicht weniger als 1,5 mm und nicht mehr als 5 mm von Spitze zu Spitze gemessen beträgt (Abb. 8). Ein Vergleich der aus dem Versuchsgefäß registrierten Druckschwankungen mit einer aus der Atemmaske gewonnenen Druckkurve zeigt in spiegelbildlicher Darstellung eine völlige Übereinstimmung des Kurvenverlaufes. Ebenso entsprechen sich die Volumenkurven aus dem Gefäß und aus der Maske (Abb. 9). Die Versuchsanordnung registriert demnach ausschließlich Volumenänderungen, die durch Atembewegungen des Tieres bedingt sind. Im ungedämpften System kommen ebenfalls ausschließlich Volumenschwankungen zur Darstellung, die Eigentümlichkeiten der im Asthma veränderten Atmung werden jedoch verdeckt.

Als Versuchstiere werden junge gesunde männliche oder weibliche Meerschweinchen von 250—300 g Gewicht verwendet.

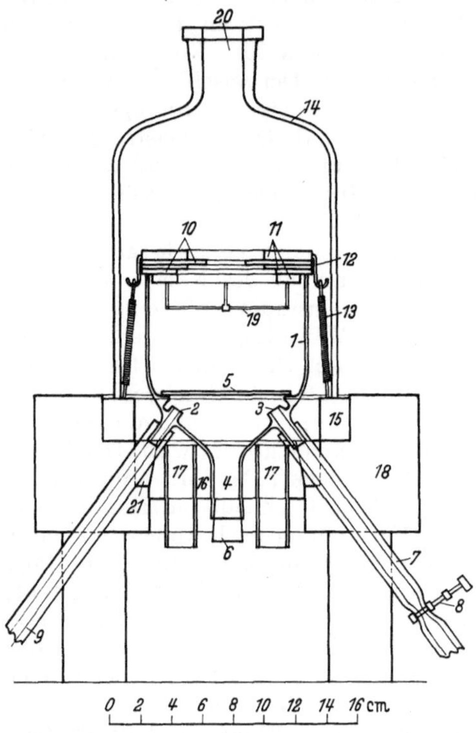

Abb. 7. *1* Glastrog zur Aufnahme des Versuchstieres. *2, 9* Ansatzstutzen und Schlauchverbindung zur Mareyschen Kapsel. *3, 7, 8* Ansatzstutzen zum Druckausgleich mit Gummirohr und Schraubklemme. *4, 6* Ansatzstutzen für Harn- und Kotentleerung mit Stopfen. *5* Einlegerost. *10—13, 19* Trogdeckel mit Gummidichtung, Spannfedern und Drahtgestell zum Aufsetzen der Vorderpfoten. *14, 20* Glashaube mit Öffnung für die Aerosolzuführung. *15, 16, 18, 21* Werkstücke für die Aufnahme des Troges und der Haube. *17* Abführende Nebelkanäle. [Aus: H. Friebel u. A. Basold, Naunyn-Schmiedebergs Arch. exp. Path. Pharmak. **217**, 13—20 (1953)]

Die Aerosolerzeugung in vier gleichartigen Zerstäubern ermöglicht eine weitgehende qualitative und quantitative Veränderung des Aerosols während des Versuchs. Die Variationsmöglichkeiten erweitern sich, wenn die Verzweigung der Nebelwege in Betrieb genommen wird. Durch die Abzweigung eines Teils des Aerosolstromes kann die dem Tier zugeführte Nebelmenge beliebig verringert werden, während das Verhältnis der einzelnen im Aerosol enthaltenen Wirkstoffe zueinander konstant bleibt. Auf diese Weise können asthmaerzeugende und -lösende Mittel einzeln oder gemeinsam gegeben werden, ihr Mengen- und Konzentrationsverhältnis kann den Versuchsbedingungen und der Reaktionsweise des Versuchstieres angepaßt werden. Die Aufzeichnung der Atemkurve ermöglicht die Auswertung von Arzneimittelwirkungen.

Friebel *et al.* [82—84, 88] untersuchten mit dieser Methode am allergischen sowie am durch Histamin und am durch Acetylcholin hervorgerufenen Asthma die Wirkungen einer Reihe von Arzneimitteln, welche entweder parenteral oder zusammen mit dem asthmaerzeugenden Aerosol zugeführt wurden.

Bei der Prüfung der Wirkung von Arzneimittelaerosolen wurde folgendermaßen vorgegangen:

Das asthmaerzeugende Aerosol wird mit einem Wasseraerosol gleichzeitig gegeben. Dieses wird 10 min nach dem Einsteuern in ein gleichbleibendes Asthma gegen das arzneimittelhaltige Aerosol ausgetauscht. Nebeldichte, Tröpfchengröße und Durchflußgeschwindigkeit müssen dabei unverändert bleiben. Die vergleichende Prüfung wird mit verschiedenen Konzentrationen des Arzneimittels in der Vernebelungsflüssigkeit vorgenommen und ein „Grenzwert" ermittelt. Dieser bezeichnet die molare Arzneimittellösung, deren Aerosol bei 4 von 5 Tieren innerhalb 40 min das Asthma gerade noch völlig aufhebt.

Bei parenteraler Zufuhr des Antagonisten wird prinzipiell in gleicher Weise vorgegangen. Die Injektion wird 10 min nach

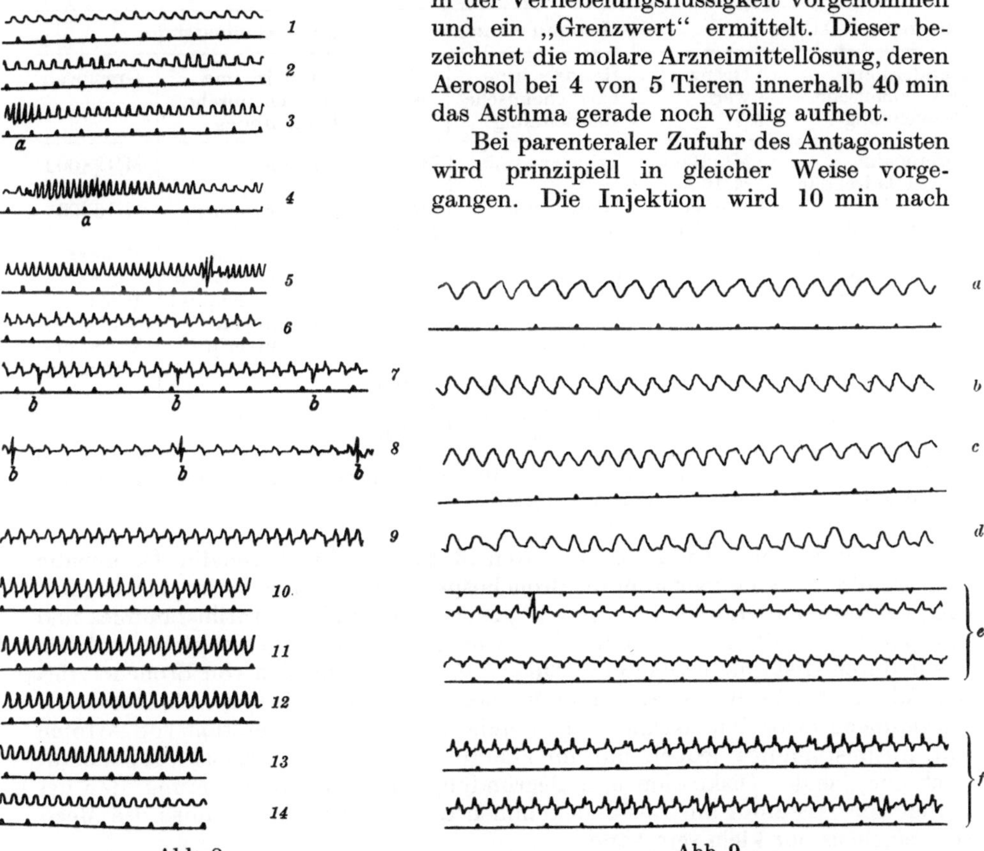

Abb. 8 Abb. 9

Abb. 8. Ausschnitte aus einer Atemkurve in verschiedenen Krankheitsstadien. *1—3* Normale Atmung. *3a* und *4a* Vorübergehende Erhöhung der Atemfrequenz aus psychischer Ursache. *5* Beginn der kontinuierlichen Tachypnoe. *6* und *7* Mittelschweres Asthma mit typischer in- und exspiratorisch veränderter Kurvenzeichnung. Bei *b* rhythmische Unterbrechungen der sonst regelmäßigen Atmung. *8* Schweres Asthma mit erheblicher Behinderung der Atemmechanik. *9—13* Rückläufige Veränderungen beim Auslaufen des Anfalls. *14* Wieder erreichte Normalatmung. [Aus: H. Friebel u. A. Basold, Naunyn-Schmiedebergs Arch. exp. Path. Pharmak. **217**, 13—20 (1953)]

Abb. 9. Vergleich der Atemvolumen- und Druckkurven bei direkter und indirekter Registrierung der Luftvolumenänderungen. *a* Normale Atemvolumenkurve aus der Atemmaske über ein kleines Spirometer geschrieben. *b* Normale Atemvolumenkurve aus dem Trog über das gleiche Meßinstrument geschrieben. *c* Atemvolumenkurve wie bei *a* im Asthmaanfall. *d* Atemvolumenkurve wie bei *b* im Asthmaanfall. *e* Asthmadruckkurve aus der Atemmaske über eine Mareysche Kapsel geschrieben. *f* Asthmadruckkurve aus dem Trog über eine Mareysche Kapsel geschrieben. [Aus: H. Friebel u. A. Basold, Naunyn-Schmiedebergs Arch. exp. Path. Pharmak. **217**, 13—20 (1953)]

Eintritt einer konstant bleibenden Asthmareaktion gegeben. Definition des „Grenzwertes" wie oben. Dosen bzw. Konzentrationen werden um den Faktor 2 gestuft.

Einige der mit dieser Methode gewonnenen Ergebnisse der Wirksamkeitsprüfung einiger Antihistaminica, von Atropin und von Bronchospasmolytica sind in Tabelle 4 angeführt. Im acetylcholinbedingten Asthma wird die Wirkung von

Tabelle 4. *Broncholytische Grenzwerte einer Reihe von Arzneimitteln, die an den jeweils geeigneten Asthmaformen ermittelt wurden*

Allergisches Asthma		Histaminasthma		Acetylcholinasthma	
Handelsname bzw. chemische Bezeichnung	Grenzwert	Handelsname bzw. chemische Bezeichnung	Grenzwert	Handelsname bzw. chemische Bezeichnung	Grenzwert
Isoprenalin	M/32000	Tripelennamin	M/8000	Atropin	M/128000
N-Äthyladrenalin	M/16000				
Adrenalin	M/4000	Mepyramin	M/8000	MTB-Brunnengräber	M/16000
Nor-Adrenalin	M/2000	*p*-Brom-Tripelennamin	M/4000		
N-Propyladrenalin	M/1000			Thiazinamium	M/4000
N-Butyladrenalin	M/1000	Clemizol	M/2000	Butylscopolamin	M/2000
N-Oktyladrenalin	M/100 unwirksam	Pheniramin	M/2000	Trihexyphenidyl	M/500
		Phenindamin	M/2000	Caramiphen	M/250
		Bamipin	M/2000	Bietamiverin	M/100 unwirksam
		Histapyrrodin	M/1000		
		Chloropyramin	M/1000		
		Antazolin	M/250		

Nach H. Friebel, Klin. Wschr. **33**, 1—4 (1955). Die in der Originalarbeit angegebenen Warenzeichen wurden durch Freinamen ersetzt.

Atropin von keiner der übrigen geprüften Stoffe erreicht. Adrenalin, Isoprenalin und weitere adrenalinverwandte Bronchospasmolytica wirken im histaminbedingten und im allergischen Asthma in gleichen Dosen. Von Antihistaminica und Atropin sind im allergischen Asthma 4—10mal höhere Dosen etwa gleich wirksam wie in durch Histamin erzeugten Asthma. Durch Kombination von Broncholytica der Adrenalinreihe mit Antihistaminica lassen sich beträchtliche Wirksamkeitssteigerungen in beiden Asthmaformen erzielen, durch Kombination von Atropin mit Antihistaminica jedoch nur im allergischen Asthma. Friebel [84] kommt nach eingehender Diskussion und Begründung zu der Schlußfolgerung, daß der Anteil von Histamin am Zustandekommen des allergischen Asthmas des Meerschweinchens nur klein sein kann.

c) Thorako-Abdomino-Motographie

Noelpp und Noelpp-Eschenhagen [147] registrierten die Atmung des nichtnarkotisierten Meerschweinchens im Asthma in folgender Weise (die Beschreibung folgt weitgehend den Angaben von Noelpp *et al.* [147, 152]).

Dem in der Inhalationskammer von etwa 1400 ml Rauminhalt frei beweglichen Tier wird ein kleiner speziell konstruierter Thorakograph aus Leichtmetall in Thoraxhöhe angelegt, von dem aus die Respirationsbewegungen mittels Luftübertragung über eine hochempfindliche Mareysche Kapsel auf ein Rußkymographion erfolgt. Die vom Thorakographen abführende Schlauchleitung wird so leicht wie möglich, aber ausreichend lang gehalten, um eine zusätzliche Belastung und Behinderung des Tieres zu vermeiden. Die Thorakographie wird durch Anlegung eines zweiten Rezeptionsapparates in Flankenhöhe („Abdominographie")

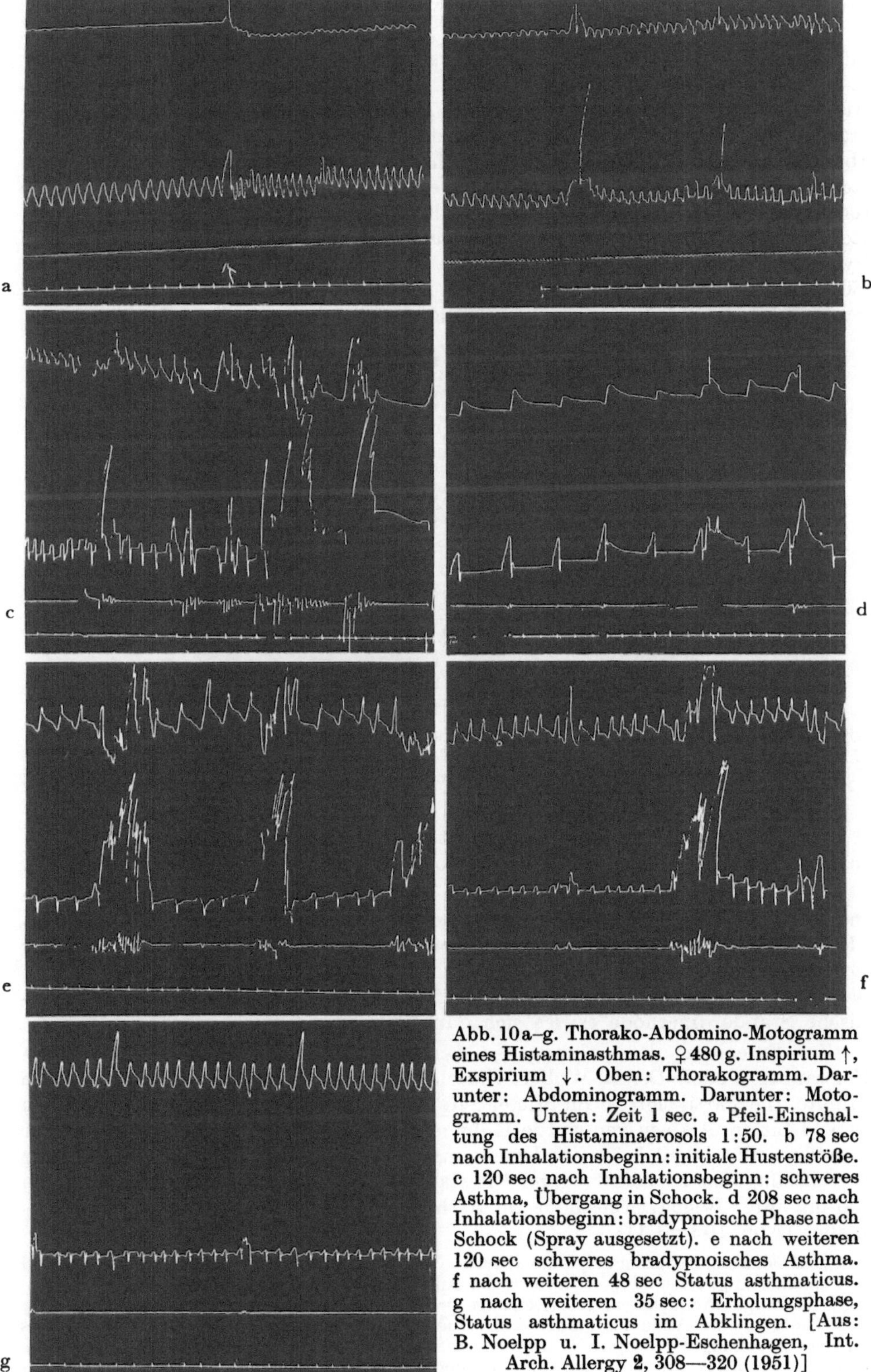

Abb. 10a–g. Thorako-Abdomino-Motogramm eines Histaminasthmas. ♀ 480 g. Inspirium ↑, Exspirium ↓. Oben: Thorakogramm. Darunter: Abdominogramm. Darunter: Motogramm. Unten: Zeit 1 sec. a Pfeil-Einschaltung des Histaminaerosols 1:50. b 78 sec nach Inhalationsbeginn: initiale Hustenstöße. c 120 sec nach Inhalationsbeginn: schweres Asthma, Übergang in Schock. d 208 sec nach Inhalationsbeginn: bradypnoische Phase nach Schock (Spray ausgesetzt). e nach weiteren 120 sec schweres bradypnoisches Asthma. f nach weiteren 48 sec Status asthmaticus. g nach weiteren 35 sec: Erholungsphase, Status asthmaticus im Abklingen. [Aus: B. Noelpp u. I. Noelpp-Eschenhagen, Int. Arch. Allergy **2**, 308—320 (1951)]

mit analogem Übertragungsmechanismus ergänzt, um durch gleichzeitige Erfassung der Abdominalatmung zu einer noch präziseren Analyse zu gelangen. Als weitere Vervollkommnung wird eine gleichfalls synchron arbeitende „Motographie" entwickelt, um im Kurvenbild die Respiration von der Gesamtmotorik abzugrenzen. Die Basisplatte der Versuchskammer wird zu einem empfindlichen Rezeptionsinstrument ausgebaut, welches jede Bewegung des Versuchstieres registriert. Mit Rücksicht auf eine möglichst synchrone Abstimmung der drei Registrierungskomponenten muß auf gute Übereinstimmung der lufthaltigen Systeme hinsichtlich Rauminhalt und Schlauchlänge geachtet werden. Die Eichung des Systems ergab, daß sich die Hebelausschläge im Bereich einer mittleren Exkursionsbreite, welche durch die Amplitude auch der asthmatiformen

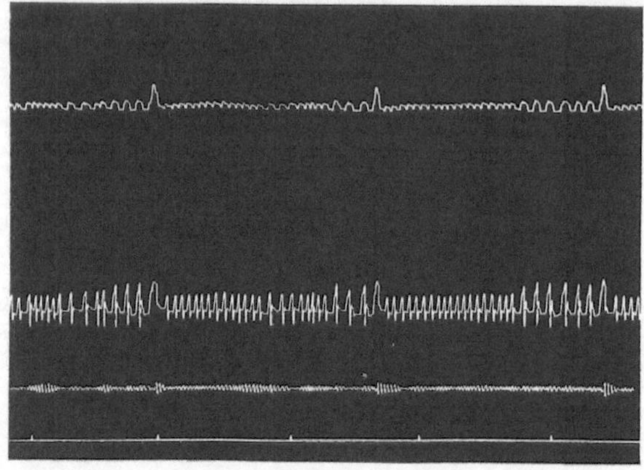

Abb. 11. Thorako-Abdomino-Motogramm: Periodische Atmung bei anaphylaktischem Asthma. ♀ 380 g. Oben: Thorakogramm. Darunter: Abdominogramm. Darunter: Motogramm. Unten: Zeit 6 sec. [Aus: B. Noelpp u. I. Noelpp-Eschenhagen, Int. Arch. Allergy **2**, 308—320 (1951)]

Atmung für gewöhnlich nicht überschritten wird, linear proportional zum Ausmaß der Bewegungen an den Registrationspunkten verhalten (Abb. 10 und 11).

Noelpp *et al.* [147, 152] überprüften die Zuverlässigkeit ihrer gewöhnlichen mechanischen Registrierung durch optische trägheitslose Verfahren (Seifenblasenmethode, Spiegelstethographie, stethographisch-optische Aufzeichnung der Exkursionen von Thorax und Abdomen, Pneumotachographie) und stellten weitgehende Übereinstimmung fest. Die für Routineversuche geeignetere mechanische Standardmethode erwies sich damit als brauchbar.

Zur Erzeugung des asthmogenen Aerosols verwendeten Noelpp *et al.* einen Zerstäuber Modell Dr. R. Wolfer, Zürich. Der Luftdurchgang betrug 13,9 l pro Minute, die Partikelgröße im Mittel 3 μ. Die Aerosolkammer hatte ein Volumen von 14 Litern. Als Antigen wurde Hühnereiweiß verwendet, Konzentration in der Zerstäuberflüssigkeit 1:50. Zur Erzeugung von histaminbedingtem Asthma wurde eine Lösung von $1—2 \times 10^{-2}$ g·ml^{-1} Histamin vernebelt. Noelpp *et al.* beschreiben die mit ihrer Registriermethode im Asthma erhaltenen Kurvenbilder folgendermaßen (Abb. 10 und 11):

„Bei normaler Atmung zeigt die Kurve einen meist ebenmäßig wellenförmigen Verlauf mit annähernd gleicher Länge des in- und exspiratorischen Anteils ohne erkennbare exspiratorische Pause (Frequenz ca. 100 Atemzüge pro min), wobei das Verhältnis der Amplituden von Thorako- und Abdominogramm individuell variabel ist. Bei Asthmaeintritt kommt es zu einer Erhöhung der Amplitude, zu einer anfänglichen Steigerung und späteren Verminderung der Frequenz sowie zu charakteristischen Veränderungen im Kurvenbilde der Einzelexkursion, wobei Thorako- und Abdominogramm gewisse typische Unterschiede aufweisen. Übereinstimmend in beiden Ableitungen registrieren wir die zeitliche Phasenverschiebung des in- und exspiratorischen Anteils mit starker Verkürzung des bei dieser Methode aufwärts gerichteten Inspiriums und Verlängerung des Exspiriums. Während aber der exspiratorische Schenkel im Thorakogramm einen zwar durch jetzt stark ausgeprägte Treppungen unterbrochenen, insgesamt jedoch kontinuierlich abfallenden Verlauf zeigt, sehen wir im Abdominogramm schwer analysierbare bizarre Deformierungen der exspiratorischen Komponente (überschießende Zackenbildungen, Arkadenformen) in Erscheinung treten. Treppenbildungen sieht man mitunter auch bei Normalatmung, selten im Thorakogramm, relativ häufig im Abdominogramm; sie erreichen jedoch bei weitem nicht den Grad und die qualitative Ausprägung wie bei der Stenoseatmung. Beide Ableitungen, synchron geschrieben, vermitteln ein gut auswertbares Bild der Kompensationsmechanismen, die das Tier zur Überwindung des endothorakalen (vorwiegend exspiratorischen) Hemmungsvorganges im Asthma einsetzt, wobei der eigenartige Verlauf des Abdominogramms durch die forcierte Aktion der abdominalen Atemmuskulatur (‚Flankenziehen') zustande kommt. Das Thorakogramm ähnelt weitgehend einer von Hofbauer im Handbuch der normalen und pathologischen Physiologie gezeigten und von Urbach und Gottlieb in ihr Lehrbuch der Allergie aufgenommenen ‚pneumographischen' Kurve des menschlichen Bronchialasthmas.

Nur bei sehr protrahierter Registration kommt es zu einer Beeinflussung des Atemtyps durch das Rezeptionsinstrument; es kann sich eine — von uns ‚Schnappatmung' genannte — Kurvenform entwickeln, bei der tiefe Inspirationen mit flacheren abwechseln, so daß ein eigentümlich unruhiges Gesamtbild entsteht. Diese Konfiguration — meist nur im Thorakogramm, seltener und weniger deutlich ausgeprägt auch im Abdominogramm erkennbar — verschwindet völlig bei Einsetzen einer Stenoseatmung."

Dieser Atemtyp wird verglichen mit Asthmareaktionen anderer Species (Hund, Ziege, Pferd) und des Menschen und auf Übereinstimmungen hingewiesen [152].

Die weiteren Untersuchungen von Noelpp und Noelpp-Eschenhagen mit dieser Methode betreffen die Rolle bedingter Reflexe in der Pathogenese des allergischen Meerschweinchenasthmas [146], die Auslösung von Asthmareaktionen nach intra- und subcutaner, intramuskulärer und nasaler sowie enteraler Zufuhr des Antigens [151]. Noelpp *et al.* [152] diskutieren ihre Ergebnisse insbesondere als weitere experimentelle Aussagen, die die Anschauung über den Modellcharakter des experimentellen Meerschweinchenasthmas stützen und bestätigen. Die Verfasser machen keine klare Trennung zwischen allergischem und durch Histamin hervorgerufenem Asthma.

II. Methoden am narkotisierten Tier

1. Registrierungsmethoden

a) Allgemeines

Operative Eingriffe am narkotisierten Tier ermöglichen eine genauere Registrierung und damit eine detailliertere experimentelle Analyse der asthmatischen Dyspnoe und verwandter Funktionsstörungen. Solche Methoden sind zunächst an größeren Versuchstieren wie Hund und Katze entwickelt worden. An diesen Tierspecies läßt sich kein allergisches Asthma erzeugen, so daß asthmaähnliche Zustände durch Pharmaka hervorgerufen werden mußten. In der Folgezeit wurden geeignete Methoden auch dem Meerschweinchen angepaßt und Untersuchungen am experimentellen allergischen Asthma durchgeführt.

Kardinalsymptome der Asthmareaktion sind die Verringerung des Atemluftvolumens und die vorwiegend exspiratorische Dyspnoe. Beim spontan atmenden Tier kommt diese Funktionsänderung in einer vor allem exspiratorischen Verringerung der Strömungsgeschwindigkeit der Atemluft in den Luftwegen zum Ausdruck. Beim künstlich beatmeten Tier steigt der Druck im Beatmungssystem, sofern die Beatmung mit konstantem Volumen erfolgt. Wird dagegen der Beatmungsdruck konstant gehalten, verringert sich das von der Lunge aufgenommene Luftvolumen.

b) Plethysmographische Methoden

Plethysmographische Methoden zur Registrierung experimenteller Asthmareaktionen am narkotisierten Tier sind frühzeitig, jedoch relativ selten verwendet worden. Dixon und Brodie [65] verwendeten Katzen. Sie schlossen entweder einen Lungenlappen oder das ganze Tier in einen luftdichten Plethysmographen ein und registrierten Druck- bzw. Volumenänderungen bei normaler und künstlicher Atmung. Sie prüften u.a. die Wirkungen von Muscarin, Pilocarpin und Physostigmin.

Hicks und Leach [107] verwendeten die Methode von Dixon und Brodie [65] am sensibilisierten Meerschweinchen. Die Beatmung wurde eingestellt auf ein Volumen von 1 ml pro 100 g Gewicht zusätzlich zum Volumen des toten Raumes

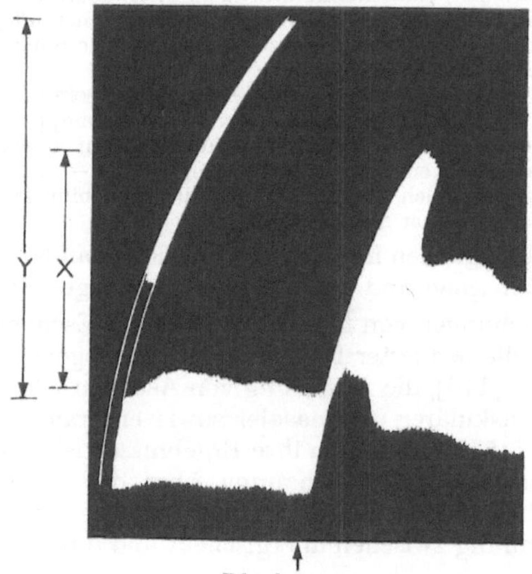

Abb. 12. Bronchoconstriction durch Antigeninjektion beim sensibilisierten Meerschweinchen (Methode Dixon u. Brodie [65]). Bestimmung der Intensität der Zunahme des Inflationswiderstandes. Bei ↑ 0,8 ml · kg^{-1} Pferdeserumantigen intravenös. X Größte Abnahme des Atemluftvolumens bei der Constriction der Bronchioli. Y Maximaler Ausschlag, hervorgerufen durch totalen Bronchialverschluß. Die Bronchoconstriction wird gemessen als prozentuale Reduktion des Atemvolumens, $100 X/Y$. [Nach R. Hicks and G. D. H. Leach, Brit. J. Pharmac. **21**, 441—449 (1963)]

des Systems, bei einer Beatmungsfrequenz von 36 pro Minute. Sie lösten Asthma durch intravenöse Injektion des Antigens aus und bestimmten den Grad der Bronchoconstriction quantitativ als prozentuale Abnahme des Beatmungsvolumens. Diese ergab sich aus dem kymographisch registrierten Verhältnis des Hebelausschlags bei der Asthmareaktion zum maximalen Ausschlag bei Abklemmen der Bifurkation (Abb. 12). Hicks *et al.* untersuchten mit dieser Methode die Beziehungen zwischen Antigendosis und Stärke der allergischen Asthmareaktion (s. S. 112).

Cloetta [44] verwendete Hunde und Katzen. Eine Thoraxwand wurde entfernt und ein Lungenlappen in den Plethysmographen eingeschlossen. Die Beatmung erfolgte durch negativen Druck. Cloetta untersuchte die Wirkung von Pilocarpin auf Druck, Volumen und Retraktionskraft der Lungen.

Jackson [109] setzte in den eröffneten Thorax dekapitierter Hunde einen starren Behälter ein, der Lungen und Herz umschloß, und beatmete durch negativen Druck. Die Registrierung der Atmung erfolgte durch eine Mareykapsel im Seitenschluß der Trachealkanüle. Mit dieser Methode untersuchte Jackson die Wirkung verschiedener Opiumalkaloide. Cameron und Tainter [35] verglichen mit gleicher Methode am decerebrierten und spinalisierten Hund die bronchodilatorischen Wirkungen verschiedener sympathomimetischer Amine am histaminbedingten Asthma.

Seibert und Handley [172] plazierten Hunde in einen Respirator vom Typ der „eisernen Lunge“. Sie untersuchten bronchodilatorische Wirkungen von N-substituierten Noradrenalinderivaten am durch Histamin erzeugten Asthma.

Yonkman *et al.* [196] untersuchten am Hund mit der Methode von Jackson [109] den Antagonismus von Histamin und Tripelennamin, Powell und Slater [161] die β-receptorblockierende Wirkung von 2-Chlorisoproterenol.

Burstein [32] verwendete Meerschweinchen in einem zylindrischen Plethysmographen. Dawes, Mott und Widdicombe [61] beschrieben einen Ganztierplethysmographen für narkotisierte Kaninchen und Katzen und registrierten die Volumenänderungen mechanisch oder oscillographisch. Die Vorrichtung erlaubte weiterhin unter anderem die Registrierung von Blutdruck und EKG. Mit dieser Methode untersuchten Kottegoda und Mott [123] die Wirkungen von 5-Hydroxytryptamin auf Kreislauf und Respiration.

Comroe, van Lingen, Stroud und Roncoroni [54] gingen in gleicher Weise vor. Sie registrierten entweder die Druckänderungen in Plethysmographen über ein Statham-Element oder die Veränderungen des Atemvolumens mittels Trachealkanüle und Spirometer elektrisch auf einem Grass-Elektroencephalographen.

c) Druckmessung bei künstlicher Beatmung

Als Kennzeichen der Asthmareaktion hervorgerufen durch elektrische Vagusreizung beim Hund registrierten Einthoven [70] und Beer [19] Druckveränderungen im Beatmungssystem in einer bestimmten Phase der künstlichen Beatmung mit konstantem Volumen. Die Druckregistrierung erfolgte mittels Manometer oder Mareykapsel. Kuschinsky [125] sowie Augstein [15] demonstrierten mit diesem Registrierverfahren an der Katze die asthmolytische Wirkung von Oxedrin (Sympatol) und einem anderen Ephedrinderivat am durch Pilocarpininjektion hervorgerufenen Bronchospasmus.

Van Arnam *et al.* [10] beatmeten das narkotisierte Meerschweinchen mit einem konstanten Volumen von 7 ml und einer Frequenz von 38 pro Minute. Eine Abzweigung der Trachealkanüle wurde mit einem Hg-Manometer verbunden und die Druckschwankungen kymographisch registriert. Histamin als intravenöse Injektion gegeben verursachte Drucksteigerung im Beatmungssystem. Van Arnam *et al.* [10] untersuchten mit dieser Methode die bronchodilatorische Wirkung von SC-10049 — L-3-{2-[2-hydroxy-2-(3,4-dihydroxyphenyl)-äthylamino]propyl}-indoltartrat.

Simke, Graeme und Sigg [174] beatmeten narkotisierte Meerschweinchen mit einem konstanten Volumen von 35 ml und einer Frequenz von 50 pro Minute. Druckänderungen im Beatmungssystem wurden über einen Nebenanschluß der Trachealkanüle auf einen Statham-Druckwandler (Bereich 0—75 mm Hg) übertragen und nach angemessener Verstärkung auf einem Offner-Dynograph registriert. Überschüssige Luft entwich durch eine weitere Abzweigung der Trachealkanüle. Simke *et al.* [174] untersuchten die bronchoconstrictorische Wirkung von Bradykinin und ihre Beeinflussung durch verschiedene Pharmaka (s. S. 121).

McCulloch, Proctor und Rand [134] registrierten ebenfalls den Ventilationsdruck mit einem Beckman-Offner-Dynograph über einen Statham-Druckwandler.

Sie untersuchten die Wirkung von Propranolol auf den histaminbedingten Bronchospasmus bei Meerschweinchen, Katzen und Hunden.

Der Haupteinwand gegen die Druckmessung im Beatmungssystem zur Kennzeichnung asthmatischer Reaktionen betrifft die Wechselwirkung von Druck und Elastizität des Lungengewebes. Durch die Rückwirkung der Drucksteigerung auf das elastische Lungengewebe und damit auf das Lungenvolumen wird die Asthmareaktion quantitativ beeinflußt und außerdem die Druckregistrierung verfälscht.

d) Atemvolumenmessung

Tiefensee [183] beatmete dekapitierte Katzen mit eröffnetem Thorax unter konstantem Druck und schaltete ein Spirometer parallel zu den Lungen. Die

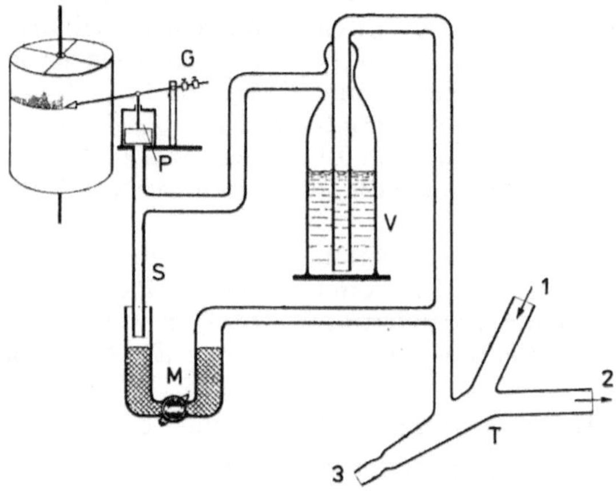

Abb. 13. Versuchsanordnung zur Registrierung des Beatmungswiderstandes nach H. Konzett u. R. Rössler, Naunyn-Schmiedebergs Arch. exp. Path. Pharmak. **195**, 71—74 (1940). Beschreibung im Text

Belastung der Spirometerglocke bestimmte den Beatmungsdruck. Veränderungen der Volumenkapazität der Lungen kamen in den Spirometerausschlägen zur Geltung. Kiese [119] untersuchte mit dieser in technischen Details von ihm vervollständigten Methode die Wirkung einiger Ephedrinabkömmlinge an Katzen. Asthmareaktionen wurden durch Arecolin, Muscarin und Pilocarpin hervorgerufen. Rietschel [165] erzeugte Bronchospasmus durch 0,05—0,1 $mg \cdot kg^{-1}$ Arecolin intravenös an der Katze und untersuchte in gleicher Versuchsanordnung die Wirkung von Ephedrin und Isalon.

Konzett und Rössler [122] vereinfachten diese Technik, indem sie das die „Überschußluft" registrierende Spirometer durch einen Pistonrekorder ersetzten. Diese ursprünglich für Anwendung an der Katze vorgesehene Versuchsanordnung ist seitdem an andere Versuchstiere angepaßt und extensiv in Untersuchungen am experimentellen Asthma angewendet worden. Die folgende Beschreibung folgt der Originalmitteilung (s. Abb. 13):

Die beiden Schenkel *1* und *2* der Trachealkanüle *T* sind mit einer Starlingschen Atmungspumpe verbunden. Zwischen den Pumpenanschlüssen der Kanüle und ihrem in die Trachea eingebundenen Ansatz *3* zweigt ein Nebenweg ab, der einerseits zu dem Hg-Manometer *M*, andererseits zu der als Wasser-Überdruckventil geschalteten Waschflasche *V* führt. Wird von der Starlingpumpe durch den Ansatz *1* Luft in die Lungen eingeblasen, so füllt sich die Lunge so lange, bis der Druck in dem System den durch die Höhe der Wassersäule in *V* eingestellten

Wert (meist 80—120 mm) erreicht hat. Die noch weiter zuströmende Luft fließt dann durch das Überdruckventil in den Pistonrekorder *P*, der den bei jeder Aufblasung verbleibenden Luftüberschuß auf einem Kymographion registriert. Um nach jeder Füllung die selbständige Entleerung des Pistonrekorders zu ermöglichen, ist das Manometer *M* als Steuerungsventil geschaltet: Die mit der Aufblasung der Lunge verbundene Drucksteigerung von 0 bis zu dem in *V* eingestellten Maximaldruck wirkt auf das Manometer, dessen Quecksilbersäule die etwa 5 mm weite Öffnung des vom Pistonrekorder kommenden Glasrohres *S* nach Beginn des Druckanstieges abschließt. Das Rohr *S*, das den Pistonrekorder mit der Außenluft verbindet, bleibt dann während der ganzen Dauer des Aufblasungsvorganges geschlossen, so daß die in *V* überfließende Luftmenge quantitativ registriert wird. Nach dem Ende der Aufblasung gibt das Ventil der Starlingpumpe den Weg nach außen frei, die Lunge entleert sich durch ihre eigene Elastizität, der Druck in der Trachea sinkt, das Manometer *M* kehrt zur Ausgangslage zurück und öffnet damit das Rohr *S*. Um den jetzt mit der Außenluft verbundenen Pistonrekorder während der Ausatmungspause wieder in seine Ausgangslage zurückzuführen, sind die Ausgleichsgewichte *G* so eingestellt, daß der Kolben mit dem Schreibhebel ein geringes Übergewicht hat und dadurch bis zum Anschlag am Boden des Zylinders absinkt.

Der Pistonrekorder muß sorgfältig gereinigt sein, um ein möglichst reibungsloses Gleiten besonders in der Abwärtsbewegung zu sichern. Das Manometer *M* soll mit Hilfe des Hahnes *H* annähernd aperiodisch gedämpft sein, da die Quecksilbersäule sonst bei der plötzlichen Druckentlastung im Beginn der Ausatmung hin und her pendelt und die Öffnung von *S* mehrmals wieder verschließt. Das Rohr *S* muß kurz und möglichst weit sein (etwa 5 mm Innendurchmesser), um den Widerstand für die Entleerung des Pistonrekorders tunlichst zu verringern. Aus diesem Grund ist auch der Innendurchmesser des Manometerrohres mit mindestens 10 mm zu bemessen.

Bei der Berechnung des Atemvolumens aus den Kurven wäre allenfalls zu berücksichtigen, daß in dem Überlaufventil *V* durch den steigenden Aufblasungsdruck zunächst das Wasser aus dem eintauchenden Rohr verdrängt wird. Dieses Wasservolumen (etwa 4—6 ml) würde vollständig mitregistriert, wenn der Nebenweg des Pistonrekorders durch *S* schon im Beginn der Ausblasung geschlossen wäre. Stellt man aber das Rohrende von *S* so ein, daß es erst kurz vor Erreichung des maximalen Aufblasungsdruckes verschlossen wird, dann kann das jetzt noch mitregistrierte Wasservolumen vernachlässigt werden.

Die Vorteile dieser Anordnung gegenüber der Registrierung mit einem Spirometer sind zunächst dadurch gegeben, daß die Einstellung des maximalen Aufblasungsdruckes mit dem Wasserventil *V* in einfachster Weise möglich ist. Die Zwischenschaltung des Wasserventils bietet aber vor allem den Vorteil, daß sich jedes volumenregistrierende Instrument verwenden läßt. Dadurch ist auch eine Anpassung der Anordnung an die Größe des Versuchstieres möglich.

Diese Methode erfaßt allerdings nicht nur den Kontraktionszustand der Bronchien, sondern den gesamten inspiratorischen Atmungswiderstand. Sie reflektiert Änderungen des Beatmungsvolumens, jedoch nicht ganz exakt quantitativ, denn die Luft wird unter positivem Druck in die Lungen befördert. Ein weiterer Fehler beruht darauf, daß während des respiratorischen Cyclus kein Gleichgewicht im Bronchialsystem erreicht wird. Die Methode ist sehr empfindlich. Änderungen der Lungengefäßfüllung infolge Änderung des pulmonalen Blutvolumens können Änderungen des Bronchialtonus vortäuschen (vgl. dazu Barer und Nusser [17], Konzett [121]). Nach Wick [192] interferiert der Kreislauf durch Veränderung der CO_2-Spannung mit der Atemluftkapazität der Lungen. Zunahme der CO_2-Spannung in der Atmungsluft bewirkt Bronchialerweiterung, Abnahme Bronchialverengerung. Wick [193] konnte zeigen, daß die Wirkung des CO_2 auf einer Veränderung der Oberflächenspannung der Alveolen beruht.

Graubner, Wick *et al.* [90, 91] wendeten die Methode von Konzett und Rössler in zahlreichen Untersuchungen am Hund an. Am Meerschweinchen wurde sie zuerst von Halpern [93] verwendet für Untersuchungen des Antihistamin-Histamin-Antagonismus. Auslösung und Registrierung reversibler allergischer Asthmaanfälle am Meerschweinchen in dieser Versuchsanordnung beschrieben Alberty [5, 6], Hicks und Leach [107], Collier *et al.* [46, 49, 50, 51] (s. S. 110).

Modifikationen

Emmelin *et al.* [71] verwendeten die Methode von Konzett und Rössler [122] zum Histaminnachweis. Sie empfehlen für Katzen und Hunde anstelle des Pistonrekorders einen Floatrekorder von 225 ml Kapazität, für Meerschweinchen einen Pistonrekorder von 31 mm Durchmesser. Weiterhin richteten sie das Steigrohr der Überdruckflasche beweglich ein, um den Beatmungsdruck variieren zu können. Sie schalten eine Auffangflasche in das Beatmungssystem ein für den Fall, daß bei spontanen Inspirationen Wasser angesaugt wird.

Halpern [93] verwendete ein Wassermanometer anstelle des Pistonrekorders. Parrot, Nicot, Laborde und Canut [153] verzichteten auf das Quecksilberventil und ersetzten den Pistonrekorder durch eine Mareykapsel.

Charlier und Vandersmissen [42] verbinden die beiden Schenkel der Trachealkanüle mit dem In- und Exspirationsanschluß der Atmungspumpe. Das im Nebenweg angeschlossene Registriersystem mit Überdruckflasche, Quecksilberventil und Pistonrekorder ersetzen sie durch eine große Mareykapsel. Nach ihrer Angabe registrieren sie auf diese Weise Volumen- und nicht Druckveränderungen im Beatmungssystem, was offensichtlich nur angenähert zutrifft. Sie beschrieben diese Technik für Anwendung am Hund.

Hansen und Zipf [94] verwenden anstelle des Pistonrekorders eine Mareykapsel, auf der sie einen Dehnungsmeßstreifen anbringen und die Überlaufluft mittels dieser Vorrichtung optisch registrieren. Sie untersuchten am Meerschweinchen die Beziehungen zwischen Bronchotonus und Lungenvagusafferenzen.

Castro de la Mata, Penna und Aviado [41] registrieren das von der Lunge nicht aufgenommene Luftvolumen quantitativ mit einer von Bellville und Seed [20] angegebenen Technik: Die Überflußluft wird durch einen Pneumotachographen geleitet und ihr Volumen mittels Transducer, Verstärker und Analog-Computer quantitativ registriert (vgl. auch S. 124). Castro de la Mata *et al.* [41] untersuchten am narkotisierten Hund die Umkehr der adrenergischen Bronchodilatation durch Dichloroisoproterenol.

Rosenthale und Dervinis [167] verbinden den Kolben des Pistonrekorders über eine Rolle mit einem Sanborn 7-DCDT-1000-Displacement-Transducer und registrieren mittels Oscillographen.

Beatmungsdruck und -frequenz

Der Beatmungsdruck richtet sich nach dem normalen Atemluftvolumen des Versuchstieres und kann zweckmäßig und leicht dem individuellen Versuchstier angepaßt werden. Konzett und Rössler [122] geben für die Katze 80—120 mm H_2O an. Sie öffnen den Thorax. Die meisten Untersucher folgen diesen Angaben. Graubner, Wick *et al.* [90, 91] beatmen Hunde mit Drucken zwischen 60 und 140 mm H_2O und einer Frequenz von $20 \cdot min^{-1}$. Die Angaben anderer Autoren entsprechen diesen Größen. Für das Meerschweinchen werden folgende Werte angegeben:

80 mm H_2O	Rosenthale *et al.* [167];
100 mm H_2O	Collier *et al.* [48, 52];
7— 15 mm Hg	Collier *et al.* [48, 52];
100—200 mm H_2O	Hansen und Zipf [94];
160—200 mm H_2O	Alberty [5, 6];
200—250 mm H_2O	Halpern [93].

Collier *et al.* [48—53] und Holgate und Warner [108] klemmen in der Erholungsphase nach einer bronchospastischen Reaktion den zum Wassermanometer führenden Schlauch kurzfristig ab, um kollabierte Lungensegmente zu eröffnen. Collier und James [49] applizieren während der Registrierung alle 30 sec automatisch für 10 sec einen Überdruck von 70—100 mm Hg. Sie stellten nicht die Frage, wie leicht und in welchem Ausmaß hierbei Alveolen zerrissen werden können. Eine forcierte Inflation kann nach D'Silva und Lewis [67] (s. auch S. 109) durchaus auch länger anhaltende Wirkung auf die Reaktivität der Bronchien haben.

Die Beatmungsfrequenzen für das Meerschweinchen werden folgendermaßen angegeben: 34—36 pro Minute (Alberty [6], Hicks *et al.* [107], 64—72 pro Minute (Rosenthale *et al.* [167], Collier *et al.* [48]). Bhoola *et al.* [25] beatmen Meerschweinchen mit 75—100 mm H_2O und einer Frequenz von 72—92 pro Minute. Bei *Ratten* verwenden sie einen Druck von 50 mm H_2O und 92 Pumpenhübe pro Minute.

e) Pneumotachographie und Bronchialwiderstand

Das wesentliche Kennzeichen der asthmatischen Dyspnoe ist eine Erhöhung des respiratorischen Widerstandes. Die bisher besprochenen Methoden messen die dadurch verursachten relativen oder absoluten Druck- und/oder Volumenveränderungen, geben aber wenig Auskunft über die dynamischen Widerstandsverhältnisse im Respirationssystem.

Detaillierte Veränderungen der Atemphasen im Asthmaanfall werden durch Pneumotachographie (Fleisch [76]), d.h. durch Registrierung der Atemströmungsgeschwindigkeit, erfaßt. Diese beruht auf dem Poiseuilleschen Gesetz, wonach das Stromvolumen bei gleitender Strömung durch ein starres Rohr proportional der Druckdifferenz an zwei Stellen dieses Rohres ist. Die pneumotachographischen Kurven zeigen direkt Atemtyp und -frequenz, Inspirations- und Exspirationsdauer und ermöglichen die Bestimmung des Atemvolumens (vgl. Anthony [9]). Die gleichzeitige Bestimmung des Pleural- bzw. Alveolardrucks ermöglicht die Berechnung des Bronchialwiderstandes (Atemströmungswiderstandes).

Die Pneumotachographie ist im Prinzip eine Druckdifferentialmessung und erfolgt durch Registrierung des Tracheal-Seitendrucks an zwei Stellen, am einfachsten unter Verwendung eines handelsüblichen Pneumotachographen nach Fleisch in geeigneter Größe. Die Registrierung kann optisch erfolgen oder über geeignete Verstärker mit Hilfe eines der modernen Direktschreiber (Grass, E. und M.-Physiograph u.a.). Die gleichzeitige Registrierung des dynamischen Pleuradrucks kann nach dem Vorgehen von Neergaard und Wirz [143, 144], die Bestimmung des Alveolardrucks nach Vuilleumier [187] erfolgen. Durch Eichung und mit Hilfe geeigneter Druckwandler und Integratoren in Verbindung mit modernen Direktschreibegeräten läßt sich das Atemvolumen ebenso wie andere gewünschte Atemgrößen direkt registrieren.

Die Beziehungen zwischen Pleuradruck bzw. Alveolardruck, Strömungswiderstand und Bronchialwiderstand R sind in vereinfachter Darstellung wie folgt:

$$\text{Bronchialwiderstand } R = k\,\frac{P}{V}.$$

Hierbei ist P die Druckdifferenz zwischen Alveolen und Außenluft = Alveolardruck und V die Atemstromstärke. Der Alveolardruck P läßt sich aus dem synchron registrierten Pleuradruck P_{pl} bestimmen. Letzterer hängt ab von den elastischen Eigenschaften der Lunge = Retraktionskraft P_{el} und dem Alveolardruck in folgender Weise:

$$P_{pl} = P_{el} \pm P.$$

Für die ausführliche Begründung und Ableitung s. Neergaard und Wirz [143, 144], Viulleumier [187], Wyss und Schmidt [195] u.a.. Das normale Pneumotachogramm wurde von Proctor und Hardy [162] experimentell analysiert. Als methodisches Beispiel, aus dem gleichzeitig die technischen Prinzipien der Methode hervorgehen, sei die Versuchsanordnung von Lopez-Botet *et al.* [129] zitiert, mit der diese Autoren Untersuchungen am experimentellen Histaminasthma des Meerschweinchens ausführten:

„Die Pneumotachographie wurde durch Registrierung des Seitendrucks der Trachea mit Hilfe einer T-förmigen eingebundenen Kanüle durchgeführt. Auf die Verwendung längerer vorgeschalteter Rohrsysteme wurde im Interesse der Herabsetzung des toten Raumes verzichtet. Der Seitendruck der Trachea wurde nicht unmittelbar, sondern nach einstufiger pneumatischer Übertragung registriert. Der Zweck dieser Übertragung bestand in erster Linie darin, die Registrierung im Interesse der Verzerrungsfreiheit möglichst wenig mit Volumverschiebung zu belasten. Gleichzeitig wurde auch eine geringfügige Verstärkung des Drucks mit der Übertragung erreicht.

Die Anordnung ist in Abb. 14 wiedergegeben und ausführlicher beschrieben.

Die wichtige Frage der Trägheit wurde durch die Bestimmung der Halbanstiegszeit geprüft.

Abb. 15 zeigt die Registrierung eines rechtwinkligen Druckanstiegs. Die Halbanstiegszeit ist mit 0,02 sec genügend kurz, um die Registrierung als ausreichend trägheitsfrei zu bezeichnen. Der Tachograph wurde mit Luftströmen bekannter Geschwindigkeit geeicht.

Die erhaltenen pneumotachographischen Kurven geben unmittelbar Aufschluß über den vorliegenden Atemtyp, die Frequenz der Atmung, das Verhältnis der Inspirationsdauer zur Exspirationsdauer und erlauben außerdem durch Planimetrie die Ermittlung des Atemvolumens und damit des Minutenvolumens.

Für die Registrierung des Pleuradrucks wurde ein dünner, mit Ringer-Lösung gefüllter Kunstgummischlauch (Durchmesser 1,5 mm), der eine seitliche Öffnung besitzt, mit Hilfe einer Nadel in den Pleuraspalt eingeführt und ebenfalls mit einer druckübertragenden Anordnung verbunden. Auch diese Registrierung wurde mit Hilfe bekannter Drucke geeicht.

Diese zweite Registrierung ergibt unmittelbar den sog. dynamischen Pleuradruck, der eine weitere für die Atmung charakteristische Größe darstellt und der außerdem nach dem Neergaardschen Vorgehen zusammen mit der Atemstromstärke zur Ermittlung des Bronchialwiderstandes (Atemströmungswiderstandes) benützt werden kann.

Das Prinzip dieses Verfahrens ist folgendes. Abb. 16 zeigt die gleichzeitige Registrierung von Strömungsgeschwindigkeit und Pleuradruck sowie die Auswertung nach Neergaard für normale Atmung und asthmatische Atmung. Die Änderungen des Pleuradruckes sind durch zwei Momente bestimmt. Einmal gehört zu jedem Lungenvolumen ein bestimmter Wert des Pleuradruckes, der gegeben ist durch den Volumwiderstand der Lunge, d.h. ihren Widerstand gegen Vergrößerung (Elastizität sowie u. U. andere Faktoren). Diese dem jeweiligen Lungenvolumen zugeordnete Druckhöhe wird als statischer Pleuradruck bezeichnet. Der Druck erfährt eine zusätzliche Änderung bei der Atmung, indem für die Exspiration der Alveolardruck erhöht, für die Inspiration herabgesetzt werden muß, was den Pleuradruck um einen entsprechenden Betrag verändert. Die resultierende Druckhöhe während der aktiven Atmung wird als der dynamische Pleuradruck bezeichnet.

Die Ermittlung des Bronchialwiderstandes aufgrund dieser Gegebenheiten erfolgt nach dem Vorgehen von Neergaard folgendermaßen: Die Registrierung ergibt zwei Werte für den statischen Pleuradruck, nämlich den Druck im Augenblick des Übergangs von der Exspirations- in die Inspirationsphase und von der Inspirations- in die Exspirationsphase. In diesen Augenblicken ist die Strömungsgeschwindigkeit null, der dynamische Druck daher mit dem statischen identisch. Nimmt man nun an, daß der statische Pleuradruck sich proportional mit dem Lungenvolumen ändert, so läßt sich die zeitliche Kurve des statischen Pleuradrucks approximativ auf folgende Weise gewinnen. Die vom Pneumotachogramm und der Nulllinie eingeschlossene Fläche wird in Fraktionen unterteilt, und die einzelnen Fraktionen werden planimetriert. Dadurch erhält man für eine Reihe von Punkten der Registrierkurve das jeweilige Lungenvolumen und damit aufgrund der genannten Voraussetzung den zugehörigen statischen Druck. Durch Vermehrung der Fraktionen läßt sich dieses Verfahren einer Integration des Tachogramms (die genau genommen nötig wäre) beliebig annähern. Die Differenz zwischen dem registrierten dynamischen und dem errechneten statischen Druck ergibt nun für jeden Augenblick den Alveolardruck und damit die treibende Kraft für die Luftströmung. Aus dieser treibenden Kraft und der im gleichen Augenblick registrierten

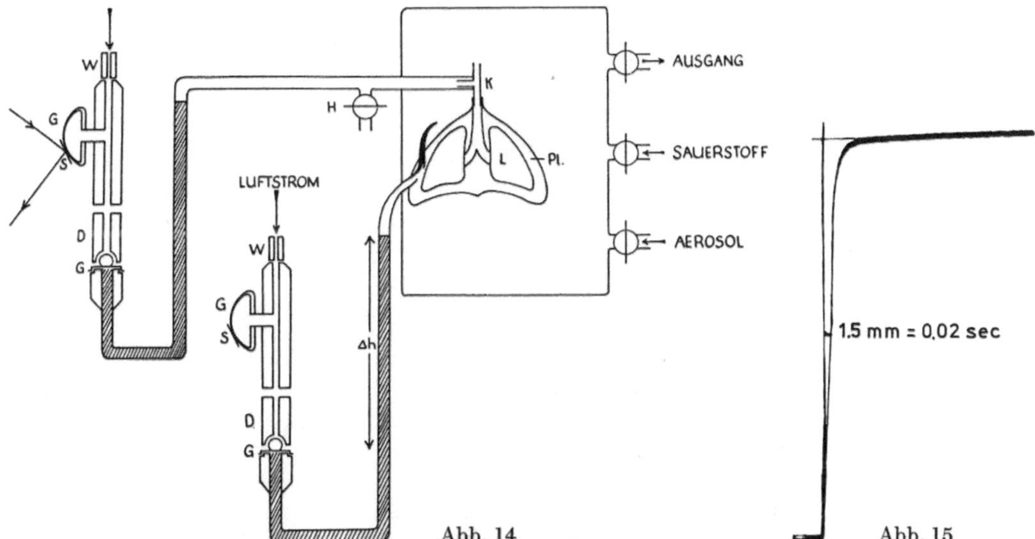

Abb. 14 Abb. 15

Abb. 14. Schema der Anordnung für die Atmungsregistrierung an Meerschweinchen. Das Tier befindet sich in einem geschlossenen Raum, der mit der Sauerstoffzufuhr bzw. der Aerosolzufuhr verbunden werden kann. Es atmet durch die Trachealkanüle *K*, deren Seitenansatz über ein teils mit Luft, teils mit Wasser gefülltes Rohrsystem mit einer Gummimembran *G* verbunden ist. Der Druck auf dieser Membran wird pneumatisch auf eine zweite mit einem Spiegel *S* versehene Gummimembran *G* übertragen und optisch registriert. Die Übertragung erfolgt mit Hilfe des durch einen Pfeil angegebenen Luftstroms, der aus einem Druckspeicher konstanten Drucks durch den hohen Widerstand *W* und die Düse *D* unter Vermittlung einer in *D* eingeschliffenen Stahlkugel auf *G* wirkt. Die in den Pleuraspalt *Pl* eingeführte Nadel trägt einen seitlich geöffneten Schlauch, der mit einem zweiten entsprechenden Druckübertragungs- und -registriersystem verbunden ist. Das erste System schreibt das Pneumotachogramm, das zweite den dynamischen Pleuradruck. [Nach E. Lopez-Botet, F. Wyss u. W. Wilbrandt, Helv. med. Acta **19**, 218—237 (1952)]

Abb. 15. Einstellkurve einer relativ trägheitsarmen Übertragung. [Nach E. Lopez-Botet, F. Wyss u. W. Wilbrandt, Helv. med. Acta **19**, 218—237 (1952)]

Strömungsgeschwindigkeit ermittelt sich nach dem Ohmschen Gesetz der Widerstand. Er wird als Atemströmungswiderstand bezeichnet.

Die Abhängigkeit des statischen Drucks vom Lungenvolumen, d.h. die für die Veränderung des Lungenvolumens um eine Volumeneinheit erforderliche Druckänderung (dP/dV) ist der ‚Volumwiderstand' der Lunge.

Abb. 16 zeigt je ein Beispiel dieser Auswertung bei normaler und asthmatischer Atmung. Von den beiden registrierten Kurven ist die obere die Kurve des Pneumotachogramms *Pt*, die untere diejenige des dynamischen Pleuradrucks PD_{dyn}. Die Punkte *A* und *B* auf der Pleuradruckkurve entsprechen der Strömungsgeschwindigkeit null und ergeben damit zwei Werte des statischen Pleuradrucks. Die geknickte Verbindungslinie PD_{stat} stellt die Kurve des statischen Pleuradruckes dar. Die Druckdifferenzen zwischen dem dynamischen Pleuradruck PD_{dyn} und dem statischen PD_{stat} entsprechen den zugehörigen Alveolardrucken P_{alv}.

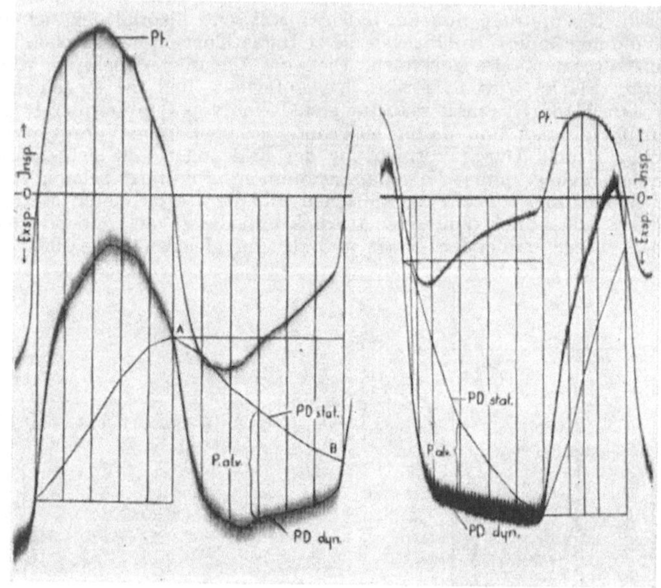

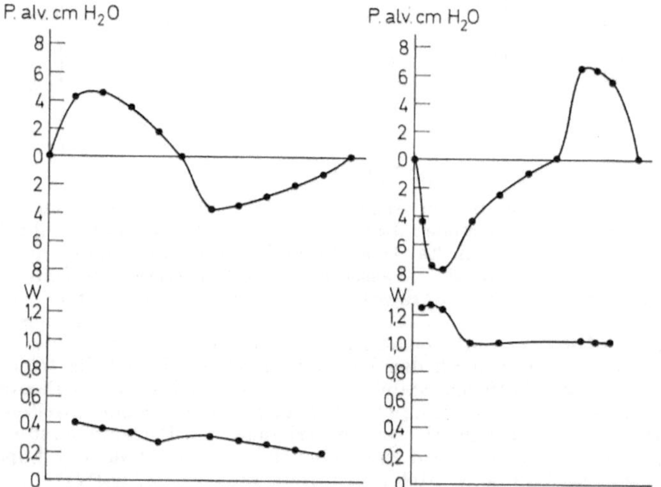

Abb. 16. Zwei Beispiele für die Registrierung des Pneumotachogramms *Pt* und des dynamischen Pleuradrucks PD_{dyn} und ihre Auswertung zur Ermittlung des statischen Pleuradrucks PD_{stat}, des Alveolardrucks P_{alv} und des Atemströmungswiderstandes *W*. [Nach E. Lopez-Botet, F. Wyss u. F. Wilbrandt, Helv. med. Acta **19**, 218—237 (1952).

Die Erzeugung des Asthmas erfolgte mit Hilfe eines Histaminaerosols. Der benützte Zerstäuber war der von Halpern [93] beschriebene Typ, die Histaminkonzentration betrug 0,5%.

Nach Ausbildung des gewünschten Grades asthmatischer Erscheinungen wurde die Respiration von aerosolhaltiger Luft auf aerosolfreien Sauerstoff umgeschaltet. Unter diesen Bedingungen erholten sich die Tiere, wenn das Aerosol nicht zu lange eingewirkt hatte, rasch.

Für die Untersuchung der mechanisch stenosierten Atmung wurden Trachealkanülen abgestufter Durchmessers verwendet. Der ‚Normaldurchmesser', der praktisch keinen Widerstand darstellt, betrug bei den üblicherweise verwendeten Kanülen 2 mm. Zur Erzeugung einer mechanischen Stenose wurden auswechselbare Ansatzstücke mit 1,5, 1,0 und 0,8 mm Durchmesser verwendet."

Mit gewissen technischen Abwandlungen sind die Prinzipien der vorstehend geschilderten Messungen für Untersuchungen mit verschiedenen Fragestellungen verwendet worden.

D'Silva und Lewis [67] bestimmten den mittleren Bronchiolardurchmesser durch Messung der elastischen Eigenschaften des Lungengewebes und des Strömungswiderstandes an Meerschweinchen, Kaninchen und Katzen. Sie erzeugten Asthma durch Histaminaerosol oder Methacholin als Aerosol oder intramuskuläre Injektion. Sie beatmeten mit konstantem Volumen bei breit eröffnetem Thorax und retrahiertem Diaphragma und registrierten das Druck-Volumendiagramm

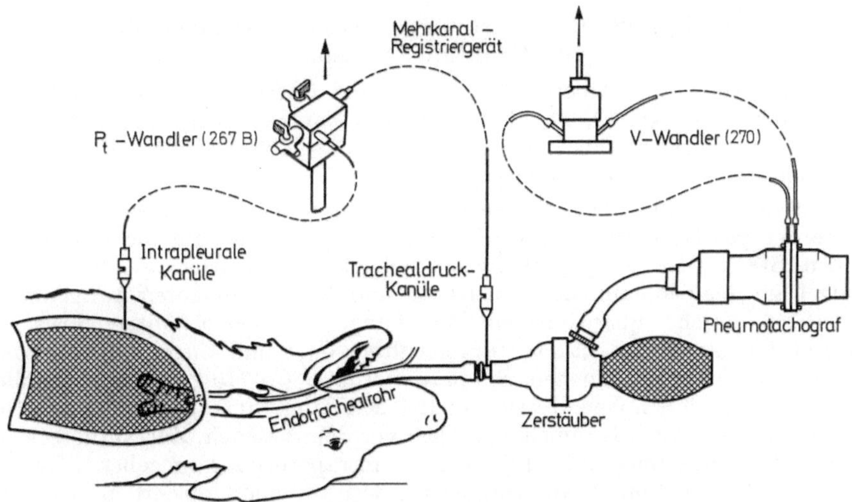

Abb. 17. Versuchsanordnung zur Messung des pulmonalen Widerstandes. [Nach L. Diamond, Arch. int. Pharmacodyn. **168**, 239—250 (1967)]

m Verlauf des Versuches. Hinsichtlich methodischer Einzelheiten und mathematischer Begründung der Berechnungen wird auf die Originalarbeit verwiesen.

Diamond [64] ermittelte den pulmonalen Widerstand durch Bestimmung von transpulmonalem Druck, Atemluftvolumen und Strömungsvolumen nach dem in Abb. 17 illustrierten Verfahren. Am narkotisierten Hund wurde Strömungsvolumen und Atemluftvolumen mittels Pneumotachograph sowie Pleural- und Trachealdruck registriert. Asthmareaktionen wurden durch Histaminaerosol hervorgerufen. Cho, Aviado und Lish [43] gingen in im wesentlichen gleicher Weise vor.

f) Aperiodische Messung der Bronchialweite

Eichler und Mügge [68] gaben eine solche Methode zur Messung der Bronchialweite am lebenden Tier (Kaninchen) an. Hierbei wird der Thorax des narkotisierten künstlich beatmeten Tieres eröffnet und eine Kanüle in einen Nebenbronchus eingebunden. Ein oder mehrere Bronchiolen werden eröffnet. Aus einem Gasometer wird kontinuierlich Luft unter konstantem Druck von 7—8 cm H_2O durchgeblasen. Im Nebenschluß liegt eine Mareykapsel, mit welcher Druckveränderungen im System kymographisch aufgezeichnet werden. Eichler und Mügge geben in ihrer Publikation die ausführliche mathematische Ableitung dieser aperiodischen Messung der Bronchialweite an einem derartigen Präparat. Dei Nachteil der Methode liegt in der nicht ganz einfachen Operation. Der Vorteil liegt in der hohen Empfindlichkeit. Außerdem kommt eine Einwirkung der Elastizität bei Atelektase nicht in Frage. Es besteht auch die Möglichkeit, durch Steuerung der Beatmung mit Hilfe des Zwerchfells das Verhalten des Atemzentrums gleichzeitig mit der Bronchialschreibung zu beobachten. Mit dieser Methode wurde beim Kaninchen die fortschreitende Tachyphylaxie der Bronchien verfolgt. Ebenso ließ sich zeigen, daß Säure bzw. CO_2 auf die Bronchien eindeutig erschlaffend wirkt.

2. Allergisches Asthma am narkotisierten Versuchstier

a) Auslösung und Beziehungen zwischen Antigendosis und Reaktionsintensität

Schaepdryver [169], Alberty [6, 7], Carr und Curry [39], Hicks und Leach [107], Collier *et al.* [46, 49, 50, 51] lösten Asthmareaktionen durch intravenöse Injektion des Antigens aus. Noelpp *et al.* [150—152], Koller [120] führten Antigen als Aerosol der Beatmungsluft zu.

Kabat und Landow [115] hatten in ihren Untersuchungen über quantitative Aspekte der passiven Anaphylaxie beim Meerschweinchen auf die Beziehungen zwischen Stärke des anaphylaktischen Schocks des ganzen Tieres oder der Schultz-Dale-Reaktion am isolierten Uterus und der verabreichten Antigenmenge hingewiesen. Solche quantitativen Beziehungen zwischen Antigendosis und Intensität von Asthmareaktionen untersuchten Carr und Curry [39] an passiv sensibilisierten Meerschweinchen. Sie präparierten 380—715 g schwere männliche Meerschweinchen mit hohen Dosen von 15—20 ml·kg^{-1} intraperitoneal von Eieralbumin-Antiserum von Kaninchen, 2 Tage vor dem Versuch. Zur Narkose wurde Paraldehyd mindestens 0,7—1,0 ml·kg^{-1} intraperitoneal gegeben. Zweimal rekristallisiertes Ovalbumin als Antigen wurde intravenös injiziert in Dosen von 0,001—100 mg·kg^{-1} in isotonischer Verdünnungsflüssigkeit. Carr und Curry registrierten das Atemluftvolumen mittels Spirometer und den intrapleuralen Druck mechanisch von einer intercostalen Kanüle über eine Mareykapsel. Sie bestimmten die Veränderungen des Verhältnisses von Ventilation und mittlerem intrapleuralem Druck (Compliance) in ml·(mm Hg)$^{-1}$. Sie untersuchten 21 mit gleicher Antiserumdosis präparierte Meerschweinchen. Je drei Tiere wurden für jede Antigendosis verwendet. Es ergab sich eine positive Korrelation zwischen Antigendosis und den prozentualen Veränderungen der Compliance.

Am aktiv sensibilisierten Tier beobachtete Alberty [6, 7] ebenfalls gleichartige Beziehungen zwischen Antigendosis und Intensität der Asthmareaktion. Im Laufe der Verabreichung steigender Antigendosen interferierte die zunehmende Desensibilisierung in bestimmter Weise. Alberty [7] erzeugte am gleichen Tier zahlreiche nicht maximale reversible Asthmareaktionen durch intravenöse Einzelinjektionen von Antigen in ansteigenden Dosen. Er ging in folgender Weise vor:

Meerschweinchen beiderlei Geschlechts zwischen 500 und 700 g Gewicht wurden verwendet. Für Versuche an allergischen Reaktionen wurden 200—300 g schwere Tiere sensibilisiert durch zwei intraperitoneale Injektionen von 0,1 ml frischem Hühnereiklar in 0,5 ml physiologischer Kochsalzlösung, verabreicht an 2 Tagen mit 1 Tag Intervall. Die Tiere wurden frühestens 6, im allgemeinen jedoch erst 8—25 Wochen danach oder später in den Versuch genommen. Zur Narkose wurde von einer 8% Urethan und 0,65% Chloralose enthaltenden Lösung

10 ml·kg^{-1} Gewicht intraperitoneal gespritzt. Bei ungenügender Narkosetiefe im Beginn oder im Verlauf des Versuches wurden weitere 1—2,5 ml·kg^{-1} intramuskulär oder intravenös gegeben. Der Blutdruck in einer Arteria carotis communis wurde mittels Quecksilber-Manometer in üblicher Weise mechanisch aufgezeichnet. Zur Verhinderung von Blutgerinnung wurde die Arterien-Glaskanüle mit Heparinlösung (5000 IE/ml) gefüllt. Änderungen der „Bronchialweite" wurden nach der von Konzett und Rössler [122] angegebenen Technik registriert.

Antigen wurde in ansteigenden Dosen intravenös injiziert. Für jeden Versuch wurde eine Verdünnungsreihe von Hühnereiklar in physiologischer Kochsalzlösung frisch hergestellt. Die Antigenkonzentration stieg stufenweise um den Faktor 2 von 2^{-22} bis 2^{-1} ml Eiklar in ml Lösung. Die Injektionsvolumina betrugen 0,25—0,5 ml pro kg. Antigeninjektionen wurden mit unterschwelligen Dosen von 2^{-22} bis 2^{-20} ml Eiklar pro kg Gewicht intravenös begonnen und in Abständen von etwa 15 min mit jeweils zwei- oder viermal höherer Dosis fortgesetzt. Um maximale Schockreaktionen zu vermeiden, wurde jede Antigendosis, die eine stärkere Reaktion ausgelöst hatte, nach deren Abklingen wiederholt. Die nächst höhere, die doppelte Antigenmenge enthaltende Stufendosis wurde erst dann gegeben, wenn die vorausgegangene Dosis nicht — oder nicht mehr — beantwortet wurde.

Auf diese Weise konnten am gleichen Tier stets mehrere bis zahlreiche in der Regel nicht maximale allergische Reaktionen ausgelöst werden. Da diese als Bruchstücke des potentiellen anaphylaktischen Schocks aufzufassen sind, wurden sie als „*Schockfragmente*" bezeichnet. Diese bestanden hier nur aus einem oder beiden objektiv registrierten Leitsymptomen — Veränderungen des Atmungsluftvolumens und/oder des Blutdrucks.

Der nach Zahl und Intensität der Schockfragmente wesentlichste Anteil des potentiellen Schocks wurde in einem relativ engen, 3 bis höchstens 5 Stufen umfassenden Bereich der Antigendosenreihe, in der Mehrzahl der Versuche mit Dosen zwischen 2^{-13} und 2^{-10} ml Eiklar-Antigen pro kg, entwickelt. In diesem bevorzugten Antigendosenbereich („*Hauptreaktivitätsbereich*") wurden mehrere aufeinanderfolgende Stufendosen, in der Regel manche von diesen mehrmals, mit einem Schockfragment beantwortet. Diese Reaktionen waren auch die intensivsten des Versuches an diesem Tier. Von der mit der niedrigsten wirksamen Antigendosis ausgelösten ersten Reaktion bis zum Beginn des Hauptreaktivitätsbereiches konnten nur vereinzelte Schockfragmente hervorgerufen werden, deren Intensität mit der Antigendosis zunahm. Nach Überschreiten des Hauptreaktivitätsbereiches wurden die Reaktionen wieder seltener und ihre Intensität zeigte abnehmende Tendenz mit Zunahme der Antigendosis. Die allergische Reaktivität brach endgültig meist relativ abrupt ab und klang in der Regel nicht mit immer schwächer werdenden Reaktionen aus. Annäherung an eine partielle Desensibilisierungsstufe kündigte sich nicht immer durch wesentliches Schwächerwerden der mit wiederholt gegebener gleicher Antigendosis ausgelösten Schockfragmente an. Nach Überschreitung der ersten reaktionsauslösenden Antigendosenschwelle kennzeichnete Unwirksamkeit oder Erlöschen der Wirksamkeit einer bestimmten Antigendosis eine Desensibilisierung nur gegenüber dieser und allen niedrigeren Antigendosen (partielle Desensibilisierung, Hyposensibilisierung). Einer größeren Antigendosis, mitunter auch bereits der nächst höheren Stufendosis der um den Faktor 2 ansteigenden Antigendosenreihe, konnte wieder eine Reaktion folgen. Zunehmende Hyposensibilisierung war also durch Ansteigen der reaktionsauslösenden Antigendosenschwelle charakterisiert. Komplette Desensibilisierung wurde in der Regel erst spät, mitunter erst auf der höchsten Dosenstufe 2^{-1} ml Antigen·kg^{-1}, erreicht.

Asthmareaktionen verliefen als „Asthmaanfälle" von verschiedener Intensität und Dauer. Ein typischer ausgeprägter Asthmaanfall ist in Abb. 18 wiedergegeben. Der Asthmaanfall begann frühestens 20—30 sec nach Antigeninjektion. Es wurden aber auch Latenzzeiten von bis zu 3 min beobachtet. Das Asthma erreichte in meist kontinuierlicher Zunahme innerhalb von etwa 1—6 min seinen Höhepunkt. Es klang dann langsamer je nach Intensität im Verlauf von 5—45 min wieder ab. Deutliche Beziehungen zwischen Latenzzeit, Geschwindigkeit des Intensitätsanstiegs, Stärke des initialen Reaktionsmaximums sowie Rückbildungsverlauf und -geschwindigkeit der Bronchostenose waren nicht erkennbar. Neben leichten kurzdauernden und schweren langdauernden Asthmaanfällen konnten auch heftige Reaktionen schnell abklingen und ein leichteres Asthma lange anhalten. Mäßige Verringerung des ursprünglichen Atmungsluftvolumens konnte auch nach leichteren, besonders langdauernden Asthmaanfällen bestehen bleiben.

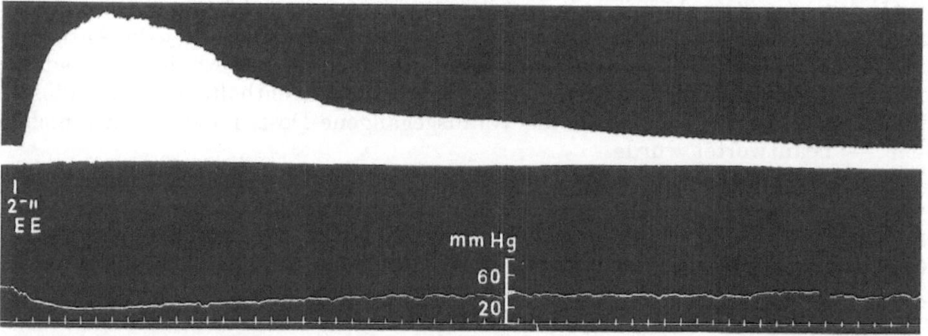

Abb. 18. Allergischer Asthmaanfall des narkotisierten Meerschweinchens, registriert nach der Methode von Konzett und Rössler [122]. [Nach J. Alberty, Int. Arch. Allergy 14, 162—204 (1959)]

Die allergische Kreislaufreaktion verhielt sich hinsichtlich Auftreten, Intensität und Dauer als vom Asthmaanfall fakultativ unabhängiges Symptom eines Schockfragments. Sie bestand in der Regel in einem mehr oder weniger schnell einsetzenden Blutdruckabfall. Nicht asphyktisch bedingte Blutdrucksteigerungen waren sehr selten. Die Latenzzeit von Antigeninjektion bis Reaktionsbeginn lag zwischen 15 und 70 sec, selten darüber bis höchstens 2 min. Sie war im Mittel kürzer als für die Asthmareaktion. Bei leichteren Reaktionen sank der Blutdruck schnell um 5—15 mm Hg und kehrte im Laufe von 2—15 min wieder zur Ausgangslage zurück. Bei stärkeren Reaktionen erfolgte im Laufe von 2—6 min ein schneller oder mehr protrahierter Abfall auf Werte von 40—30—25 mm Hg, und Atmungs- und Pulsamplitude wurden minimal. Zwischen Dauer der Latenzzeit und Reaktionsstärke war eine deutliche gesetzmäßige Verknüpfung nicht erkennbar. Leichtere und mittelschwere allergische Blutdrucksenkungen waren reversibel. Bei ausgeprägtem Kreislaufkollaps ging die Erholung meist nur sehr langsam vonstatten und der Ausgangswert wurde häufig auch nach Stunden nicht mehr erreicht. Schwere Kollapszustände konnten mit Infusion relativ großer Flüssigkeitsmengen, auch Plasmaersatzmitteln, in der Regel nur vorübergehend beeinflußt werden. Aber auch anscheinend spontane Erholung von schwerem Kreislaufkollaps wurde gelegentlich beobachtet.

Die Beziehung zwischen Antigendosis und Intensität der Kreislaufreaktionen im Versuchsverlauf zeigte im Prinzip die gleichen Merkmale wie bei den anaphylaktischen Asthmareaktionen.

Hicks und Leach [107] gingen in prinzipiell gleicher Weise wie Alberty [7] am narkotisierten Meerschweinchen vor. Sie registrierten das Asthma nach der Methode von Dixon und Brodie [65] (s. S. 100) oder nach der Methode von Konzett und Rössler [122] (s. S. 102) und bestimmten die Reaktionsintensität quantitativ als prozentuale Reduktion des Beatmungsvolumens, gemessen am Verhältnis von maximalem Schreibhebelausschlag im Asthmaanfall und maximalem Hebelausschlag bei totalem Bronchialverschluß (Abklemmen der Bifurkation bzw. Trachea, s. Abb. 12, S. 100). Nach ihren Beobachtungen entspricht die

Beziehung zwischen dem Logarithmus der Antigendosis und der Stärke des Asthmas einer normalen pharmakologischen Dosis-Wirkungsbeziehung und wird durch eine Sigmoidkurve charakterisiert. Die progressive Abnahme der Sensibilisierung bei wiederholter Gabe der gleichen Antigendosis folgt einer exponentiellen Kurve.

b) Atemmechanik

Untersuchungen der Atemmechanik im allergischen Asthma des narkotisierten Meerschweinchens führten Noelpp und Noelpp-Eschenhagen [150] sowie Noelpp, Noelpp-Eschenhagen und Lottenbach [151] durch. Sie verwendeten eine Reihe verschiedener Registriermethoden (vgl. Noelpp-Eschenhagen und Noelpp [152]. Bei der Auswertung von Pneumotachogramm, Pleuradruck- und Alveolardruckmessung fanden sie eine starke Zunahme des Volumelastizitätsmoduls und des Gewebedeformationswiderstandes und schlossen aus ihren Beobachtungen, daß die Ursache der asthmatischen Dyspnoe in einer strukturellen Veränderung des Lungengewebes selbst zu suchen sei.

Eingehende Untersuchungen über Atmungs- und Kreislaufreaktionen im allergischen Asthma des narkotisierten Meerschweinchens unternahm Koller [120]. Er sensibilisierte die Versuchstiere durch subcutane Injektionen von je 0,7 ml einer 5%igen Lösung von kristallisiertem Ovalbumin an zwei aufeinander folgenden Tagen. Nach 3 Wochen wurde eine Minimaldosis des Antigens als Aerosol der Atmungsluft zugesetzt und so ein reversibles allergisches Asthma ausgelöst. Die Auslösung des Asthmas im eigentlichen Versuch erfolgte durch Zumischung von Antigenaerosol zur Beatmungsluft an den Ansaugstutzen der Beatmungspumpe oder direkt in die Trachealkanüle. Die Aerosolzufuhr dauerte höchstens 60 sec. Koller führte Versuchsserien mit teilweise gleichzeitiger Registrierung folgender Größen durch:

1. Beatmungswiderstand nach Konzett und Rössler [122].
2. Zwerchfellaktivität mechanisch: Am breit thorakotomierten Tier wurde das Zwerchfell im Zentrum tendineum über eine Rolle mit einem isotonischen Registrierhebel verbunden.
3. Spontanatmung mittels Ganztierplethysmographie. Der Plethysmograph bestand aus einem Plexiglaszylinder von 25 cm Länge und 1000 ml Inhalt und wurde in einem Wasserbad von 28° C Temperatur untergebracht. Das Tier atmete durch eine Trachealkanüle, die in die Zylinderwand eingelassen war. Weitere Anschlüsse dienten der Registrierung des Blutdrucks mittels Hg-Manometer. Die Volumenschwankungen des Plethysmographen wurden über eine Mareykapsel kymographisch aufgezeichnet.
4. Elektromyographische Analyse der Atemreaktionen durch bipolare Ableitung der Aktivität des Zwerchfells und des M. obliquus externus.
5. Blutdruck mittels Hg-Manometer und EKG mittels Nadelelektroden.

Koller [120] beschreibt zahlreiche Beobachtungen über das Verhalten des Beatmungswiderstandes, der Spontanatmung, der Zwerchfellaktivität und des Kreislaufs bei Antigenzufuhr, über die im einzelnen in der Originalarbeit nachzulesen ist. Im Beginn des Asthmaanfalls treten inspiratorische Reaktionen auf, für die nervöse Mechanismen, später chemische Atmungsreize verantwortlich gemacht werden. Im späteren Verlauf imponieren exspiratorische Verschlüsse, die zum Teil als Folge des Kollapses der Schleimhaut der Bronchiolen und Alveolargänge angesehen werden. Diese Mechanismen komplizieren die Bronchoconstriction. Anzeichen für eine besondere Beteiligung von Zwerchfellkontraktionen am Zustandekommen der Dyspnoe werden nicht gefunden. Reversible Blutdrucksenkung und Tachykardie werden als Folgen der inspiratorischen Atmungsaktivierung gedeutet. Wesentliche Kreislaufreaktionen durch das inhalativ gegebene Antigen werden nicht beobachtet. Alberty [6, 7] beobachtete dagegen wechselnd starke, vom Asthmaanfall fakultativ unabhängige Kreislaufreaktionen als selbständige „Schockfragmente“ bei intravenöser Auslösung (s. oben).

c) Pharmakologische Aspekte des allergischen Asthmas

Pharmakologische Aspekte des allergischen Asthmas sind von mehreren Autoren am narkotisierten Tier bearbeitet worden. Zielsetzungen solcher Versuche betrafen sowohl Untersuchungen über humorale Mechanismen des allergischen Asthmas wie auch die Prüfung asthmolytischer Wirkungen von Arzneimitteln.

Carr und Curry [39] verglichen mit vorher beschriebener Methode (s. S. 110) die Wirkungen des Histaminfreisetzers 48/80, von Histamin und von Antigen beim passiv sensibilisierten Meerschweinchen. Die Wirkung von Histamin in Dosen von 0,5—1000 μg (Base) $\cdot$ kg^{-1}, im Mittel 3—30 μg $\cdot$ kg^{-1} intravenös, auf Atemvolumen und Verhalten des intrapleuralen Drucks entsprach den Veränderungen im allergischen Asthmaanfall. Von Verbindung 48/80 lösten 0,5 mg $\cdot$ kg^{-1} respiratorische Wirkungen aus. Zum Unterschied gegenüber den histaminbedingten oder allergischen Reaktionen verkleinerten sich jedoch meist die Ausschläge der intrapleuralen Druckschwankungen.

Alberty [6, 7] verglich quantitativ die asthmolytische Wirkung von unspezifischen Bronchospasmolytica, spezifischen Antihistaminica und von Atropin im allergischen und im histaminbedingten Asthma. Er registrierte das Beatmungsvolumen nach der Methode von Konzett und Rössler [122] und erzeugte reversible Asthmaanfälle in vorher beschriebener Weise durch intravenöse Antigeninjektionen (s. S. 110). Histaminbedingte Asthmareaktionen vergleichbarer Intensität wurden am gleichen Tier durch intravenöse Dauerinfusion von Histamin (als Bihydrochlorid) in einer Dosierung von 2—15 μg $\cdot$ kg^{-1} $\cdot$ min^{-1} ausgelöst. Folgende Ergebnisse werden beschrieben:

Die bronchospasmolytische Wirksamkeit von intravenös injiziertem Adrenalin, Isopropylnoradrenalin, Papaverin und Aminophyllin im allergischen Asthmaanfall entsprach ihrer Wirkung in vergleichbaren durch intravenöse Histamininfusion hervorgerufenen Asthmareaktionen. In beiden Asthmareaktionen wirkten Noradrenalin und Ephedrin nicht immer und Dihydroxypropyltheophyllin nicht asthmolytisch. Im Vergleich zu ihrer Wirksamkeit im durch Histamininfusion hervorgerufenen Asthma, wirkten die spezifischen Antihistamine Diphenhydramin und Mepyramin im anaphylaktischen Asthmaanfall nur unsicher, wesentlich geringer und nur in begrenztem Maße. Atropin wirkte dagegen in hohen, unspezifisch histamin-antagonistisch wirksamen Dosen in beiden Asthmareaktionen gleich stark asthmolytisch oder war im anaphylaktischen Asthma schwächer wirksam.

Es wurde der Schluß gezogen, daß der anaphylaktische Bronchospasmus nicht auf der Wirkung freigesetzten Acetylcholins und nur zu einem relativ geringen und begrenzten Teil auf der Wirkung freigesetzten Histamins beruht. Alberty nimmt eine Beteiligung anderer, nicht mit Histamin identischer, durch die Antigen-Antikörper-Reaktion freigesetzter Stoffe an.

Collier *et al.* [49—51] versuchten die Natur solcher am Zustandekommen des allergischen Asthmas beteiligter humoraler Faktoren weiter zu klären. Sie registrierten den Beatmungswiderstand nach Konzett und Rössler [122] mit folgendem Vorgehen: Alle 30 sec wird die Abzweigung zur Überdruckflasche und Pistonrekorder für die Dauer von 10 sec abgeklemmt („forced reinflation"), um kollabierte Lungenteile zu belüften und die Erholung zu unterstützen. Der Beatmungsdruck wird mit 7—15 mm Hg, bei der forcierten Blähung mit 70—100 mm Hg angegeben (Collier und James [49]). Die Tiere wurden sensibilisiert durch Injektionen von Ovalbumin, je 100 mg intraperitoneal und subcutan sowie 2 Wochen später Zink-Ovalbumin-Komplex 100 mg subcutan. Die Auslösung des Asthmas erfolgte durch intravenöse Injektion einer eine submaximale Reaktion erzeugenden Dosis zwischen 0,25 und 10 $mg \cdot kg^{-1}$ Ovalbumin.

Collier *et al.* [50] verglichen die Wirkung selektiver Antagonisten von Histamin, Acetylcholin, 5-Hydroxytryptamin, Bradykinin und SRS-A sowie von Catecholaminen auf das allergische Asthma (s. Tabelle 5). Der Antagonist wurde in den meisten Fällen intravenös 5 min vor Antigeninjektion gegeben. Nach einer

Tabelle 5. *Dosen verwendeter spezifischer oder selektiver Antagonisten und die Wirkungsstärken einiger von ihnen unter den Versuchsbedingungen*

Das Dosenverhältnis ist das Verhältnis äquiaktiver Dosen des Agonisten, verabreicht nach und vor der angegebenen Dosis des Antagonisten. Dosenverhältnisse wurden am Konzett-Rössler-Präparat des Meerschweinchens in vivo bestimmt, 5 und 15 min nach intravenöser Injektion des Antagonisten. Jeder Wert ist das geometrische Mittel von 5 Ergebnissen. Die Bestimmung des Dosenverhältnisses eines Antagonisten diente der Verwendung in therapeutischen Tests zur Kennzeichnung des entsprechenden Agonisten in der anaphylaktischen Bronchoconstriction. Propranolol und Pronethanol wurden intraperitoneal (i.p.) 30 min und intravenös 5 min vor dem Agonisten gegeben. Tachyphylaxie gegen Kinine wurde durch wiederholte Injektion von Bradykinin (20 µg i.v.) hervorgerufen, gegen SRS-A durch wiederholte Injektion von SRS-A (1 mg i.v.). Meclofenamat ist das Natriumsalz von N-(2,6-Dichlor-m-tolyl)-anthranilsäure. —: nicht geprüft; rep.: wiederholte Injektion. Ausgenommen wo Tachyphylaxie gegen Bradykinin oder SRS-A hervorgerufen wurde, sind die Dosen in $mg \cdot kg^{-1}$ angegeben.

Humoraler Faktor	Antagonist	Dosis	Dosenverhältnis	
			5 min	15 min
Catecholamine	Tolazolin	5 i.v.	—	—
	Propranolol	10 i.p. + 5 i.v.	—	—
	Pronethalol	10 i.p. + 5 i.v.	—	—
Acetylcholin	Atropin	1 i.v.	288	179
	Hexamethonium	5 i.v.	—	—
5-Hydroxytryptamin	Methysergid	0,1 i.v.	48	35
Histamin	Mepyramin	0,2 i.v.	642	477
Kinine	Bradykinin	20 µg i.v. rep.	—	—
	Meclofenamat	1 i.v.	92	87
SRS-A	SRS-A	1 mg i.v. rep.	—	—
	Meclofenamat	1 i.v.	20	13

Nach H. O. J. Collier, and G. W. James, Brit. J. Pharmacol. **30**, 283—301 (1967).

Testdosis des gerade in Frage stehenden Agonisten wurde eine submaximale allergische Asthmareaktion ausgelöst und 10 min lang in der oben angegebenen Weise registriert. Zum Schluß des Versuches wurde das Maximum des Beatmungsluft-Überlaufes bestimmt als Differenz zwischen dem Hebelausschlag bei Abklemmen der Trachea und der Basislinie vor Asthmaauslösung. Die Reaktionsstärke wurde in Prozent des maximalen Schreibhebel-Ausschlages als Funktion der Zeit nach Antigeninjektion bestimmt. Um die Beteiligung eines humoralen Faktors abzuleiten, wurde die Differenz der Zeit-Wirkungsmittelwert-Kurven der Gruppe vorbehandelter Tiere und der Kontrollgruppe aufgezeichnet. Die Ergebnisse wurden statistisch ausgewertet. Dosis-Wirkungskurven von Histamin und Bradykinin nach Vorbehandlung mit den gleichen Dosen der entsprechenden Antagonisten wurden an je 5 Tieren bestimmt. Sie dienten als Hinweis für die Menge dieser möglicherweise am Zustandekommen der allergischen Asthmareaktion beteiligten humoralen Faktoren.

Weitere Versuche wurden nach Dekapitierung und Zerstörung des Rückenmarks, nach Vagotomie und an adrenalektomierten Tieren durchgeführt.

Nach in einigen Details widersprüchlichen Beobachtungen kommen Collier *et al.* [46—51] zu der Schlußfolgerung, daß Kinine und SRS-A (slow-reacting substance — anaphylaxis, s. unten) neben Histamin am Zustandekommen des allergischen Bronchospasmus beim Meerschweinchen beteiligt sind. Kinine verursachen gleichzeitig Freisetzung von Catecholaminen aus den Nebennieren, wodurch die allergische Asthmareaktion modifiziert wird. Nachdem durch Meclofenamat oder Acetylsalicylsäure der durch Kinine und SRS-A verursachte Teil, durch Mepyramin der durch Histamin verursachte Teil der allergischen Asthmareaktion aufgehoben ist, bleibt ein weiterer unbekannter bronchoconstrictorischer Faktor wirksam.

Asthma durch SRS-A

Berry und Collier [21] präparierten SRS-A aus perfundierten Lungen sensibilisierter Meerschweinchen nach einem Verfahren von Brocklehurst [28, 30] und erzeugten mit dieser Asthmareaktionen an nicht sensibilisierten Meerschweinchen. Sie registrierten in der Versuchsanordnung von Konzett und Rössler [121]. SRS-A erzeugte bei intravenöser Injektion Asthma. Die Latenzzeit von Injektion

Tabelle 6. *Antagonistische Wirkung von Pharmaka gegen SRS-A und Bradykinin an der Meerschweinchenlunge in vivo*

Die minimale effektive Dosis (MED) ist definiert als die kleinste intravenöse Dosis eines Antagonisten, bei einer Dosenfolge von 1, 2, 4, 8 mg · kg⁻¹ usw., die die Reaktion auf eine Antagonistendosis, die doppelt so groß wie die vorausgegangene Dosis ist, auf weniger als die Hälfte der vorausgegangenen Reaktion reduziert, ohne die Reaktion auf Histamin zu beeinträchtigen [52, 53].

Pharmakon	MED ($mg \cdot kg^{-1}$) gegen	
	SRS-A	Bradykinin
Acetylsalicylsäure	2	2[a]
Natrium-Acetylsalicylsäure	1	2[a]
Calcium-Acetylsalicylsäure	2	2[a]
Natriumsalicylat	64	64—128[a]
Salicylamid	> 64	> 64
Natriumsalicylamid-*o*-acetat	> 64	> 64
Natriumgentisat	> 32	> 32
Natrium-4-Hydroxyisophthalat	> 32	> 64[a]
Paracetamol	64	16[a]
Cinchophen	16	32[a]
3-OH-Cinchophen	2	2
Natriumphenylbutazon	1	4[a]
Oxyphenbutazon	32	32
Amidopyrin	4	8[a]
Phenazon	16	8[a]
α-(4-Phenylphenoxy)propionsäure	4	4
Indomethacin	1	1
Ibufenac	16	16
Natriumanthranilat	> 32	> 32
Natriumflufenamat	1	1[a]
Natriummefenamat	1	1[a]
Amodiachin	>8	> 16[a]
Chlorochin	>8	> 16[a]
Amopyrochin	>8	>8
Hydrocortison	> 16	>32[a]
Dexamethason	> 16	> 16
Paramethason	> 64	> 64
Morphinsulfat	> 32	> 32[a]

[a] Collier und Shorley [52, 53].
Aus P. A. Berry, and H. O. J. Collier, Brit. J. Pharmacol. 23, 201—216 (1964).

bis Reaktionsbeginn war länger als bei Auslösung einer Asthmareaktion durch Histamin oder Bradykinin, die Zeit von Reaktionsbeginn bis Reaktionsmaximum kürzer als nach Bradykinin. Die Wirkung klang langsamer ab als die von Histamin, aber schneller als die von Bradykinin. Durch Zerstörung des Rückenmarks oder Quetschung der Vagi und der Halssympathici wurde die Reaktion auf SRS-A nicht verändert. SRS-A wirkte auch bei lokaler Applikation auf die Pleura. Mepyramin, Atropin und Brom-Lysergsäurediäthylamid beeinflußten die durch SRS-A ausgelöste Asthmareaktion nicht. SRS-A zeigte weiterhin eindeutige Unterschiede gegenüber Kininen, es verursachte keine gekreuzte Desensibilisierung mit Bradykinin. Acetylsalicylsäure und andere Substanzen der Antipyretica-Analgetica-Gruppe, einige Antimalariastoffe und Corticosteroide wirkten dagegen am durch SRS-A hervorgerufenen Asthma ebenso wie am durch Kinine, insbesondere Bradykinin erzeugten Asthma (vgl. Tabelle 6). Berry und Collier [21] fassen die Charakteristika der antagonistischen Wirkung von Substanzen der Analgetica-Antirheumatica-Gruppe gegenüber der asthmogenen Wirkung von SRS-A folgendermaßen zusammen:

1. Der Antagonismus ist peripher und lokal, denn er ist in vivo am spinalisierten Meerschweinchen, nach Vago- und Sympathicotomie sowie an der isolierten Trachea zu demonstrieren.
2. Der Antagonismus ist wahrscheinlich kompetetiv, denn er kann durch höhere Dosen Acetylsalicylsäure überwunden werden, und Acetylsalicylsäure verursacht eine Parallelverschiebung der Dosis-Wirkungskurve.
3. Die gleichen Substanzen sind unwirksam gegen SRS-A und gegen Bradykinin.
4. Die antagonistische Wirkungsstärke von SRS-A-Antagonisten ist gleich ihrer antagonistischen Wirksamkeit gegen Bradykinin.
5. Aktive Antagonisten von SRS-A und Bradykinin zeigen keine antagonistische Wirkung gegen andere Bronchoconstrictoren.

3. Durch Pharmaka erzeugtes Asthma des narkotisierten Versuchstieres

a) Allgemeines

Asthmareaktionen werden mit verschiedenen Pharmaka durch intravenöse Injektion oder Infusion, auch mit inhalativer Zufuhr als Aerosol, hervorgerufen. Eine Übersicht über verwendete Pharmaka, Zufuhrwege und Dosierung wurde bereits auf S. 81 und 82 gegeben. Histamin und Pilocarpin haben bevorzugte Anwendung gefunden. Acetylcholin bringt nach Graubner und Wick [91] ein Maximum an unerwünschten Nebenwirkungen hervor. 5-Hydroxytryptamin und Bradykinin werden als neue, möglicherweise am allergischen Asthma des Meerschweinchens beteiligte Substanzen verwendet (5-HT: Comroe *et al.* [54], Kottegoda *et al.* [123], Konzett [121], Westermann *et al.* [190], Holgate *et al.* [108]; Bradykinin: Collier *et al.* [47—53], Bhoola *et al.* [25].

Durch Pharmaka hervorgerufene Asthmareaktionen werden zur Unterscheidung vom allergischen („anaphylaktischen") Asthma von manchen Autoren bezeichnet als „experimentelles Asthma", „experimenteller Bronchospasmus", „Bronchospasmus". Ohne Zweifel ist ein Bronchospasmus einer der Hauptmechanismen der durch irgendeines der aufgeführten Pharmaka erzeugten Asthmareaktionen. Er ist aber auch für das experimentell ausgelöste allergische Asthma des Meerschweinchens in der Regel ein bestimmender Faktor. Andererseits können die beiden anderen klassischen Asthmamechanismen, Schleimhautödem und Bronchialsekret, außer im allergischen Asthma auch z.B. im durch Histamin erzeugten Asthma beträchtlichen Einfluß gewinnen, besonders wenn Histamin als Infusion gegeben wird (Alberty [6]). Das gleiche dürfte auch für durch Kinine erzeugtes Asthma gelten. Eine scharfe Trennung von allergischem Asthma gegen pharmakonbedingten Bronchospasmus ist somit oft schwer zu begründen und wird in dieser Darstellung nicht vorgenommen.

b) Atemmechanik

Untersuchungen über das Verhalten der elastischen Lungenspannung und des Gewebsdeformationswiderstandes im histaminbedingten „Modellasthma" führten Noelpp *et al.* [150—152] durch. Sie registrierten Pneumotachogramm, Alveolarseitendruck und Pleuradruck am narkotisierten Meerschweinchen und führten Histamin als Aerosol zu. In den gleichen Untersuchungen wurden jedoch auch allergische Asthmaanfälle registriert und zusammen mit den im Histaminasthma erhaltenen Ergebnissen ausgewertet. Noelpp *et al.* [150—152] deuten ihre Resultate als Zunahme des Elastizitätsmoduls und des Gewebsdeformationswiderstandes und schließen daraus, daß die Ursache der asthmatischen Dyspnoe in einer strukturellen Veränderung des Lungengewebes selbst zu suchen ist. Sie gehen nicht auf Unterschiede zwischen histaminbedingtem und allergischem Asthma ein.

Lopez-Botet, Wyss und Wilbrandt [129] gingen am experimentellen Histaminasthma des Meerschweinchens ebenfalls der Frage nach, welchen Anteil die Bronchostenose an der asthmatischen Dyspnoe hat. Sie registrierten Pneumotachogramm und Pleuradruck (s. S. 106) sowie den Volumwiderstand und führten Histamin als Aerosol zu. Ihre Ergebnisse zeigen, daß eine Reihe von Atemgrößen, die in der Form des Pneumotachogramms zum Ausdruck kommen, in der gleichen Weise verändert werden wie im allergischen Asthma des Menschen. Im Gegensatz zum letzteren finden sie beim Meerschweinchen jedoch wie Noelpp *et al.* [150] eine starke Zunahme des Deformationswiderstandes der Lunge, die sie auf totalen Verschluß einzelner Bronchialäste zurückführen. Sie deuten ihre Befunde als Anzeichen für eine wesentliche Beteiligung eines Zwerchfellkrampfes am Zustandekommen der Dyspnoe, wie sie u. a. auch von Wyss und Schmidt [195] für den Menschen postuliert wird. Diese Deutung wird von Koller [120] auf Grund seiner Untersuchungen am allergischen Asthma des Meerschweinchens abgelehnt (s. auch S. 113). Demgegenüber fand Wick [194] in Versuchen am Hund mit der Methode nach Konzett und Rössler [122] reflektorische Bronchodilatation bei Tonuszunahme des Zwerchfells.

D'Silva und Lewis [67] bestimmten an Meerschweinchen, Kaninchen und Katzen die Veränderungen der mittleren Bronchiolarweite im Asthma durch Methacholin oder Histamin (s. S. 109) und fanden, daß der Durchmesser der Bronchiolen in der Asthmareaktion einen kritischen Wert erreichen kann, bei dem es zum totalen Bronchialverschluß kommt. Hierbei kommt es zu entsprechenden Veränderungen der elastischen Eigenschaften des Lungengewebes. Beim Meerschweinchen betrug der kritische Wert 60% der normalen Weite der Bronchiolen und konnte leicht erreicht werden. Bei Kaninchen und Katze waren erheblich höhere Dosen erforderlich und der kritische Durchmesser wurde nicht erreicht, da die Wirkungen der Bronchoconstrictoren auf die Herztätigkeit interferierten. Kollabierte Alveolargebiete öffneten sich nicht spontan, sondern bedurften der Anwendung von Überdruck. Durch entsprechende Inflation geöffnete Alveolareinheiten blieben für beträchtliche Zeit auch nach Abbrechen der Druckinflation weit offen.

c) Arzneimittelwirkungen und verschiedene pharmakologische Aspekte

Für die Wirkungsprüfung unspezifischer wie auch spezifischer Bronchodilatoren ist das durch Pharmaka erzeugte Asthma ein geeignetes Versuchsobjekt.

Histamin und Cholinergica

Kuschinsky [125] und Augstein [15] untersuchten an der narkotisierten Katze mit einfacher Methode die Wirkung von Oxedrin und von 2-Amino-1-oxyhydrinden am Pilocarpinspasmus. Kiese [119] (s. S. 102) verwendete als Asthmogene Pilocarpin, Arecolin, Acetylcholin, Histamin und Fliegenpilzextrakt und prüfte die antagonistische Wirkung von Atropin, Adrenalin, Oxedrin (Sympatol), Ephedrin und anderen Ephedrinderivaten. Rietschel [165] verwendete in gleicher Versuchsanordnung Arecolin 0,05—0,1 mg als Asthmogen und fand ebenso wie Kiese, daß Ephedrin nur in gleichzeitig blutdrucksteigernden Dosen broncholytisch wirkt und auch bronchoconstrictorische Wirkungskomponenten aufweist.

Am Hund untersuchten mit plethysmographischer Methode (s. S. 100) Cameron und Tainter [35] sowie Seibert und Handley [172] die Wirkung sympathomimetischer Amine auf histaminbedingte Asthmareaktionen. Die erstgenannten Autoren verabreichten Histaminbihydrochlorid als intravenöse Injektion alle 30 min, beginnend mit 0,3 $mg \cdot kg^{-1}$ und jedesmaliger Vergrößerung der Dosis um 0,1 $mg \cdot kg^{-1}$. Sie fanden abnehmende antagonistische Wirksamkeit in folgender Ordnung: Adrenalin, Epinin, 3,4-Dihydroxyephedrin, Ethylnoradrenalin, Noradrenalin, Metaoxedrin (Neosynephrin), Corbadrin (Cobefrin), und schwache bis fehlende Wirkung von 3-Hydroxyephedrin, Ephedrin, Amphetamin, Octamylamin, Ephetonal, Propadrin, m-Hydroxynorephedrin, p-Hydroxyephedrin. Atropin wirkte prompt, aber unvollständig. Seibert und Handley [172] untersuchten verschiedene N-substutierte Derivate von Noradrenalin und fanden die N-2-[1-(4-methoxyphenyl)-propyl]-substituierte Verbindung ebenso wirksam wie Isoprenalin (= Isopropydrin). Den Antagonismus von Tripelennamin und Histamin untersuchten Yonkman *et al.* [196] am Hund mit plethysmographischer Methode.

Die Methode von Konzett und Rössler [122] wurde insbesondere von Graubner und Wick [90, 91] für die Wirkungsprüfung von Asthmolytica am Hund ausgebaut. Sie verwendeten Pilocarpin (Dosierung s. S. 82) zur Auslösung von Asthmareaktionen und prüften verschiedene Sympathomimetica, insbesondere Isoprenalin (Aludrin). Atanackovic und Schaepdryver [14] untersuchten mit gleicher Methode am Hund die broncholytische Wirkung von Procain (20 bis 50 $mg \cdot kg^{-1}$) gegen die durch Acetylcholin (10—20 $\mu g \cdot kg^{-1}$) und Eserin (0,2 $mg \cdot kg^{-1}$) hervorgerufene Asthmareaktion.

Cho, Aviado und Lish [43] bestimmten am Hund den pulmonalen Widerstand (s. S. 109) und erzeugten ein „locked-lung syndrome", d.h. Wirkungslosigkeit oder paradoxe bronchoconstrictorische Wirkung des Bronchospasmolyticums Isoprenalin. Sie erreichten dieses durch wiederholte inhalative Administration von Isoprenalin in Abständen von 1—6 min oder durch Hyperkapnie. Außerdem verwendeten sie spontan Isoprenalin-refraktäre Tiere. In allen diesen Fällen blieb der Bronchodilator MJ-1992 (Soterenol), 2-Hydroxy-5-(1-hydroxy-2-isopropylaminoäthyl)-methansulfonanilid wirksam bei intravenöser, intraduodenaler oder inhalativer Zufuhr.

Halpern [93] verwendete die Methode von Konzett und Rössler [122] am Meerschweinchen. Er prüfte die histaminantagonistische Wirkung von Phenbenzamin (2339 RP, Antergan) und anderen Antihistaminica und erzeugte Asthmareaktionen durch intravenöse Injektion von 10—25 $\mu g \cdot kg^{-1}$ Histamin und 50—100 $\mu g \cdot kg^{-1}$ Acetylcholin. Schaepdryver [169] untersuchte die antagonistische Wirkung von Caramiphen (Parpanit), Diethazin (Diparcol) und Antazolin (Antistin) an der Asthmareaktion des Meerschweinchens hervorgerufen durch Injektion von Histamin 60 $\mu g \cdot kg^{-1}$ und Acetylcholin 50 $\mu g \cdot kg^{-1}$.

Alberty [5, 6] verglich am Meerschweinchen die Wirkung unspezifischer Bronchospasmolytica sowie von Atropin und einigen Antihistaminica am durch Histamininfusion erzeugten und am allergischen Asthma (s. S. 110 und 114). Er gab Histamin als Lösung des Bihydrochlorids in physiologischer Kochsalzlösung als intravenöse Dauerinfusion in Dosen von 2 bis höchstens 15 $\mu g \cdot kg^{-1} \cdot min^{-1}$. Die Infusionsvolumina betrugen 0,02—0,15 $ml \cdot kg^{-1} \cdot min^{-1}$. Änderung der Dosierung erfolgte durch Änderung der Infusionsgeschwindigkeit, bei größeren Differenzen durch Konzentrationswechsel der Infusionslösung. Die zur Lyse des histaminbedingten Asthmas erforderlichen Dosen von Isoprenalin, Adrenalin, Aminophyllin, Papaverin entsprachen den beim Menschen antiasthmatisch wirksamen Dosen.

Eine antagonistische Wirkung von 10 $\mu g \cdot kg^{-1}$ Lysozym aus Eiweiß am histaminbedingten Asthma des Meerschweinchens beschrieben Parrot *et al.* [153].

5-Hydroxytryptamin

Die Wirkungen von 5-Hydroxytryptamin (5-HT) auf Atmung und Kreislauf untersuchten Comroe *et al.* [54] sowie Kottegoda *et al.* [123] an der narkotisierten Katze. Comroe *et al.* zeigten, daß 5-HT bei schneller intravenöser Injektion von 0,5 $\mu g \cdot kg^{-1}$ unter anderem Bronchoconstriction verursacht. Kottegoda *et al.* beschrieben Veränderungen der Entladungen der pulmonalen Dehnungsreceptoren durch 100—200 μg 5-HT intravenös als Zeichen einer direkten bronchoconstrictorischen Wirkung. Konzett [121] untersuchte in der von ihm und Rössler [122] angegebenen Versuchsanordnung die Wirkung von 5-HT an Katzen und Meerschweinchen. Er bestätigte die direkte, nichtreflektorische Wirkung von 5-HT auf die Bronchialmuskulatur. Spezifische Antagonisten dieser Wirkung sind nach den Ergebnissen von Konzett D-Lysergsäurediäthylamid sowie 1-Acetyl- und 2-Bromlysergsäurediäthylamid in Dosen von 8—32 $\mu g \cdot kg^{-1}$. Diese Stoffe hemmten nicht die durch intravenöse Gabe von Histamin, Acetylcholin oder Pilocarpin hervorgerufenen Asthmareaktionen. Partielle und weniger spezifische 5-HT-antagonistische Wirkungen zeigten Atropin in Dosen über 0,3 $mg \cdot kg^{-1}$ und Thenalidin (1-Methyl-4-amino-N'-phenyl-N'-(2'-thenyl)-piperidin, Sandosten) in Dosen von 80—150 $\mu g \cdot kg^{-1}$.

Antagonistische Wirkungen von Antihistaminica, LSD-Derivaten sowie Atropin gegen 5-hydroxytryptamin-, histamin- und acetylcholinbedingte Asthmareaktionen bestimmten auch Holgate und Warner [108] am Meerschweinchen mit gleicher Methode. Sie berechneten antagonistische Wirkungsstärken als das Verhältnis gleichwirksamer Dosen des Antagonisten während und vor der Antagonistenwirkung. Außerdem bestimmten sie das Verhältnis der per os und intravenös gleichwirksamen Antagonistendosen. Sie prüften folgende Substanzen: Chlorpheniraminmaleat, Diphenhydraminhydrochlorid (0,4 $mg \cdot kg^{-1}$), Mepyraminmaleat (0,04 $mg \cdot kg^{-1}$), Lysergsäurediäthylamintartrat (0,05 $mg \cdot kg^{-1}$), 2-Brom-LSD-tartrat, Atropinsulfat (0,1 $mg \cdot kg^{-1}$).

Westermann, Balzer und Knell [190] erzeugten am Meerschweinchen anhaltenden Bronchospasmus durch intravenöse Injektion von 2—4 mg 5-Hydroxytryptophan („5-HTP"), was offenbar auf Decarboxylation von 5-HTP zu 5-HT im Organismus zurückzuführen ist: α-Methyldopa verhinderte die Wirkung von 5-HTP, hatte aber keinen Einfluß auf die asthmaerzeugende Wirkung von 5-HT.

Peptide

Die Erzeugung von Asthmareaktionen durch Bradykinin am Meerschweinchen studierten Collier, Holgate, Schachter und Shorley [47, 48] in der Versuchsanordnung von Konzett und Rössler [122]. Bradykinin erwies sich als etwa ebenso wirksam wie Histamin (bei Dosenvergleich), zeigte aber eine erheblich stärker ausgeprägte Tachyphylaxie. Wespenkinin verhielt sich weitgehend ähnlich. Die Wirkung von Bradykinin beruht offenbar vorwiegend auf Bronchoconstriction, denn sie wird von gleichzeitig gegebenem Adrenalin (2 $\mu g \cdot kg^{-1}$) oder Isoprenalin (0,6 $\mu g \cdot kg^{-1}$) unterdrückt. Sie beruht offenbar nicht auf einer Freisetzung von Histamin oder 5-Hydroxytryptamin, denn Mepyramin oder LSD haben keinen Einfluß auf die Bradykininwirkung. Acetylsalicylsäure, Amidopyrin und Phenylbutazonnatrium erwiesen sich als starke Antagonisten. Die Autoren vermuten eine Beteiligung von Bradykinin oder eines ähnlichen Peptides beim allergischen Asthma, was sie in späteren Untersuchungen experimentell zu klären suchen (vgl. S. 114).

Aarsen [1] bestätigte die Ergebnisse von Collier *et al.* teilweise. Er beobachtete, daß die Antibradykininwirkung von Acetylsalicylsäure (als Calciumsalz) durch das Narkoticum beeinflußt wird. Sie war stärker bei Tieren in Mebumal-(Pentobarbital-)Narkose als bei Tieren in Urethannarkose. Durch Steigerung der Dosis von Acetylsalicylat von 2 auf 8 $mg \cdot kg^{-1}$ konnte er meist keine stärkere Wirkung erzielen. Vagotomie verringerte die antagonistische Wirkung. Acetylsalicylat und andere Analgetica wirkten nicht bradykininantagonistisch an der isolierten Lunge (s. S. 129 und 132). Aarsen zieht aus seinen Ergebnissen die Schlußfolgerung, daß die antagonistische Wirkung von Acetylsalicylat am bradykinininduzierten Asthma des narkotisierten Meerschweinchens indirekt, wahrscheinlich über das Zentralnervensystem zustande kommt.

Collier und Shorley [52] erweiterten die Beobachtungen von Collier *et al.* [47, 48], wonach Acetylsalicylsäure und andere antipyretische Analgetica die asthmogene Wirkung von Bradykinin antagonisieren. An der durch Bradykinin erzeugten Asthmareaktion des Meerschweinchens erwiesen sich Acetylsalicylsäure, Phenylbutazon, Amidopyrin und Phenazon als hochwirksame spezifische Antagonisten (s. Tabelle 7). Sie waren jedoch nur gering wirksam im Versuch am isolierten Meerschweinchenileum und zeigten keine antagonistische Wirkung am isolierten Duodenum der Ratte oder den Hautcapillaren des Meerschweinchens. Paracetamol, Cinchophen, Natriumsalicylat und Acetanilid waren mäßig effektive Antagonisten der Bradykinin-Asthmareaktion. Phenacetin, Salicylamid und 4-Hydroxyisophthalsäure hatten keine nennenswerte Wirkung. Cortison, Hydrocortison, Aldosteron, Amodiachin und Morphin waren unwirksam oder wirkten unspezifisch. Eine nennenswerte Wirkung des spezifischen Bradykininantagonisten Acetylsalicylsäure im allergischen Asthma konnten Collier und Shorley in dieser Untersuchung, im Gegensatz zu späteren Ergebnissen (Collier *et al.* [49—51], s. S. 114) nicht feststellen.

In einer weiteren Untersuchung demonstrierten Collier und Shorley [53] die antagonistische Wirkung von Natrium-Mefenamat und Natrium-Flufenamat (N-(2,3-xylyl)-anthranilsaures Natrium und N-(α,α,α-trifluoro-m-tolyl)-anthranilsaures Natrium) gegen Asthmareaktionen des Meerschweinchens hervorgerufen durch die Kinine Bradykinin oder Kallidin-10. Die Wirkung war spezifisch — keine acetylcholin-, histamin- oder 5-hydroxytryptaminantagonistische Wirkung — und zeigte die Kennzeichen eines kompetetiven Antagonismus. Die Wirksamkeit der genannten Antagonisten entsprach der von Acetylsalicylsäure, deren antagonistische Wirkung jedoch nur im niedrigeren Dosenbereich kompetetiven Charakter hatte.

Simke, Graeme und Sigg [174] untersuchten die Wirkung verschiedener Pharmaka auf die durch Bradykinin hervorgerufene Asthmareaktion des narkotisierten Meerschweinchens mittels Registrierung von Druckveränderungen im Beatmungssystem bei Beatmung mit konstantem Volumen. Sie beobachteten Ver-

Tabelle 7. *Wirkungsstärken verschiedener Substanzen zur Unterdrückung der Bronchoconstriction verursacht durch Bradykinin am Meerschweinchen*

Die minimal effektive Dosis (MED) ist die kleinste Dosis eines Antagonisten, welche die Reaktion auf eine intravenöse Bradykinindosis, die doppelt so groß ist wie die vorausgegangene Dosis, auf weniger als die Hälfte der vorausgegangenen Reaktion reduziert, ohne die Reaktion auf Histamin zu beeinträchtigen.

Agens	MED (mg Säure oder Base · kg^{-1})			
	intravenös	oral	intraduodenal	andere Zufuhrwege
Acetylsalicylsäure	2[a]	32	64	—
Natriumsalicylat	64	> 512	256	—
Salicylamid	—	> 256	> 512	—
4-Hydroxyisophthalsäure	> 64[b]	—	> 512	i.p. > 512
Chinchophen	32[b]	> 512	256	—
Natriumphenylbutazon	4	16	16	—
Amidopyrin	8	16	16	—
Phenazon	8	64	128	
Acetanilid	—	> 512	256	—
Phenacetin	—	> 512	512	—
Paracetamol	16	512	128	—
Amodiachinsphosphat	—	> 512	> 512	—
Cortison	—	—	—	i.m. > 25
Hydrocortison-natriumsuccinat	unspezifisch bei 100	—	—	—
D,L-Aldosteron	> 2	—	—	—
Morphinsulfat	> 32	—	—	—
1-(1-Phenylcyclohexyl)piperidinhydrochlorid	> 16	—	—	—

[a] Verabreicht als Calciumsalz.
[b] Verabreicht als Natriumsalz.
—: nicht geprüft; i.p.: intraperitoneal; i.m.: intramuskulär.
Aus H. O. J. Collier, and P. G. Shorley, Brit. J. Pharmacol. 15, 601—610 (1960).

stärkung der Bradykininwirkung durch Antiadrenergica wie Guanethidin, Reserpin und Pronethalol (Nethalide) sowie 6-Mercaptopurin und Amethopterin und verschiedenen anderen Stoffen wie ε-Aminocapronsäure, Verbindung 48/80 und Tripelennamin. Biphasische Wirkungen, in der Regel initiale Hemmung mit anschließender Verstärkung der Bradykininwirkung, verursachten Chlorochin, Atropin und Isoproterenol. Antagonistische Wirkungen zeigten Substanzen der Analgetica-Antipyretica-Gruppe sowie Phenoxybenzamin und Chlorpromazin (s. Tabelle 8).

Weitere antiinflammatorisch wirksame nichtsteroide Pharmaka sowie andere Stoffe testeten Collier, James und Piper [51] auf ihre bradykininantagonistische Wirksamkeit an der Asthmareaktion des Meerschweinchens. Das Prinzip der Auswertung und die Ergebnisse gehen aus Tabelle 9 hervor. Demnach wirken alle geprüften antiinflammatorischen Pharmaka bradykininantagonistisch mit Ausnahme von Benzydamin. Besonders starke Wirksamkeit zeigte Meclofenamat. Von andersartigen geprüften Substanzen zeigten die Monoaminooxydaseinhibitoren Phenelzin und Mebanazin eine antagonistische Wirkung. Diese wurde von Propranolol nicht aufgehoben, beruhte also nicht auf einer Potenzierung endogener Catecholamine. Im Gegensatz zu Simke *et al.* [174] fanden sie keine bradykininantagonistische Wirkung von Chlorpromazin und Phenoxybenzamin. Über den Vergleich der Wirkungen dieser Substanzen mit ihrer Wirkung am allergischen Asthma des Meerschweinchens sowie am Asthma hervorgerufen durch SRS-A (aus Lungen sensibilisierter Meerschweinchen durch Antigenapplikation freigesetzt) s. S. 116.

Tabelle 8. *Inhibitoren der Bradykinin-Bronchoconstriction beim Meerschweinchen*

Anzahl der Versuche	Agens	Dosis (mg · kg⁻¹)	Prozent Hemmung	
			26 min nach Injektion	60 min nach Injektion
	I. Intraduodenale Verabreichung			
8	CI 583[a]	0,25	85	100
5	Mefenamsäure	2,5	60	34
10	Phenylbutazon Natrium	2,5	50	56
2	Phenylbutazon	12,5	45	68
8	Oxyphenbutazon	100,0	20	80
10	Sulfinpyrazon	25,0	30	70
5	Indomethacin	2,5	40	100
4	Antipyrin	20,0	60	70
5	Phenacetin	40,0	35	30
7	Acetylsalicylsäure	40,0	30	33
3	Chlorpromazin	2,0	15	100
	II. Intravenöse Injektion			
6	Phenylbutazon Natrium	1,25	55	—
5	Aminopyrin	0,75	50	—
13	Acetylsalicylsäure	0,75	50	—
6	UML 491[b]	0,1	0	—
8	Phenoxybenzamin	1,0	55	—

[a] N-(2,6-Dichlor-m-tolyl)-anthranilsäure.
[b] Methysergid.
Aus J. Simke, M. L. Graeme, and E. B. Sigg, Arch. int. Pharmacodyn. 65, 291—301 (1967).

Über die starke bradykininantagonistische Wirkung im Asthmaversuch am Meerschweinchen von zwei neuen Antiphlogistica berichteten Jahn und Wagner-Jauregg [110]. Es handelte sich um 1,2 Pentylmalonyl-1,2-dihydro-4-phenyl-cinnolin (Scha 306) und 1,2-Propylmalonyl-3-dimethylamino-7-methyl-1,2-dihydro-1,2,4-benztriazin.

Die asthmaerzeugende Wirkung anderer Peptide außer Bradykinin untersuchten Bhoola, Collier, Schachter und Shorley [25] an Kaninchen, Meerschweinchen und Ratte. Asthmareaktionen konnten am Meerschweinchen erzeugt werden durch Kallidin-10 6—12 $\mu g \cdot kg^{-1}$, Substanz P 50—100 $E \cdot kg^{-1}$, Angiotensin 25—35 $\mu g \cdot kg^{-1}$. Lysin- oder Arginin-Vasopressin und Oxytocin waren unwirksam. Kallidin war etwa ein Drittel so wirksam wie Bradykinin. Angiotensin wirkte erheblich schwächer als die anderen Peptide und zeigte keine Dosis-Wirkungsbeziehung. Acetylsalicylsäure verminderte die Wirkung von Kallidin wie die von Bradykinin, aber nicht die Wirkung der beiden anderen Peptide. Bradykinin verringerte ebenso wie Acetylcholin und Histamin das Atemluftvolumen des Kaninchens. Die Ratte reagierte erst auf so hohe Dosen von Bradykinin oder Acetylcholin wie 450 μg, dagegen schon auf 10—100 $\mu g \cdot kg^{-1}$ 5-Hydroxytryptamin. Acetylsalicylsäure antagonisierte an Kaninchen und Ratte die Bradykininwirkung nicht.

Über die hemmende Wirkung von Chlordiazepoxid in Dosen von 0,05 bis 5,0 $mg \cdot kg^{-1}$ intravenös auf die Asthmareaktion hervorgerufen durch Histamin, Acetylcholin, 5-Hydroxytryptamin und Bradykinin am Meerschweinchen in der Versuchsanordnung nach Konzett und Rössler berichteten Kovács und Görög [124]. Nach Vorbehandlung mit Dichlorisoprenalin blieb nur die histaminantagonistische Wirkung von Chlordiazepoxid erhalten (vgl. auch S. 91 und 131).

Tabelle 9. *Minimal effektive Dosen einiger neuer antiinflammatorischer und anderer Pharmaka gegen die bradykininbedingte Bronchoconstriction beim Meerschweinchen*

Eine effektive Dosis ist die intravenöse Dosis eines Antagonisten, welche die bronchoconstrictorische Wirkung von Bradykinin nach Gabe des Antagonisten auf weniger als die Hälfte der Wirkung der gleichen Bradykinindosis vor Antagonistengabe reduziert, ohne die Reaktion auf Acetylcholin zu verringern. Eine minimal effektive Dosis (MED) ist die kleinste in einer Mehrzahl von Tests wirksame Dosis. An jedem Tier wurden bis zu zwei Dosen eines Stoffes geprüft, wobei die Dosen zwischen jedem Test um das Vierfache gesteigert wurden.

Pharmakon		Gesamt-versuchszahl	MED ($mg \cdot kg^{-1}$ i.v.)
Klasse	Stoff		
Antiinflammatorisch	Benzydamin	22	> 32
	Glafenin	25	4
	Ibufenac	26	8
	Indomethacin	29	2
	Indoxol	29	0,25
	Meclofenamat	10	0,06
	Mi 85[a]	21	1
	Scha 87/2[b]	19	0,125
	Scha 306[c]	20	0,06
Andere Klassen	γ-Aminobuttersäure	15	> 64
	Chlorpromazin	18	> 4
	2,4 Dinitrophenol	10	> 8
	Iproniazid	23	> 32
	Mebanacin	37	16
	Phenelzin	28	8
	Phenoxybenzamin	15	> 32
	Trancylpromin	17	> 16

[a] 5-(Dimethylamino)-9-methyl-1 H-pyrazolo [1,2-a][1,2,4]-benzotriazin-1,3-(2 H)dion (als Natriumsalz).
[b] 2-Butyl-1 H-pyrazolo[1,2-a]cinnolin-1,3(2 H)-dion (als Natriumsalz).
[c] 2-Pentyl-1H-pyrazolo [1,2-a]cinnolin-1,3-(2 H)-dion (als Natriumsalz).
Aus H. O. J. Collier, G. W. L. James, and P. J. Piper, Brit. J. Pharmacol. 34, 76–87 (1968).

Asthmareaktionen, asthmolytische Wirkungen und adrenergische Receptoren

Die Umkehr der bronchodilatorischen Wirkung von Isoprenalin und Adrenalin durch Dichlorisoproterenol zeigten Powell und Slater [161] sowie Castro de la Mata, Penna und Aviado [41] am Hund. Die letztgenannten Untersucher konnten die bronchoconstrictorische Wirkung von Dichlorisoproterenol durch Tolazolin aufheben. Sie schlossen daraus, daß Erregung der adrenergischen α-Receptoren der Bronchialmuskulatur Bronchoconstriction, Erregung der β-Receptoren Bronchodilatation verursacht.

Farmer und Lehrer [72] untersuchten die broncholytische Wirkung von Isoprenalin und ihre Beeinflussung durch Pronethalol (0,1—10 $\mu g \cdot kg^{-1}$) unter anderem an der durch Histamin und Acetylcholin hervorgerufenen Asthmareaktion des Meerschweinchens. Da Pronethalol die Isoprenalinwirkung in den verschiedenen Asthmareaktionen gleich stark hemmt, wird angenommen, daß nur ein gleicher Typ von β-Receptoren beteiligt ist.

James [111] untersuchte am Meerschweinchen in der Versuchsanordnung nach Konzett und Rössler die Rolle der Nebennieren und der adrenergischen α- und β-Receptoren bei der Wirkung von Asthmolytica in Asthmareaktionen verursacht durch Histamin, Acetylcholin, 5-Hydroxytryptamin und Bradykinin. Die unspezifisch bronchodilatorische Wirksamkeit nahm ab in der Reihenfolge Isoprenalin, Adrenalin, Noradrenalin, Metaoxedrin (= Penylephrin). Die gleichen Stoffe zeigten bronchoconstrictorische Wirkungseigenschaften, die in dieser

Reihenfolge zunahmen. Die bronchodilatorische Wirkung konnte durch Hemmung der adrenergischen α- oder β-Receptoren, Tolazolin oder Pronethalol aufgehoben werden. Versuche am adrenalektomierten Tier zeigten, daß die bronchodilatorische Wirkung von Aminophyllin, Papaverin, Metaoxedrin (Phenylephrin) und Noradrenalin zum Teil auf die Wirkung freigesetzter Catecholamine aus den Nebennieren zurückzuführen war.

Den Mechanismus der potenzierenden Wirkung von Propranolol (0,1 bis 3 $mg \cdot kg^{-1}$) auf den durch Histamin ausgelösten Bronchospasmus untersuchten McCulloch *et al.* [134] am Meerschweinchen. Sie vermuteten nach ihren Ergebnissen, daß die Wirkungen bronchoconstrictorischer Stoffe normalerweise modifiziert werden durch reflektorisch freigesetzte Catecholamine, deren Wirkung durch Propranolol blockiert wird (s. auch Herxheimer und Langer [105], S. **91**).

Lish *et al.* [128] untersuchten die bronchodilatorische Wirkung des α-adrenergischen Blockers Phentolamin an der durch Histaminaerosol hervorgerufenen Asthmareaktion des Meerschweinchens. Sie kamen zu der Schlußfolgerung, daß diese auf Freisetzung von Adrenalin aus den Nebennieren oder aus anderen Gewebedepots zurückzuführen ist.

Hansen und Zipf [94] untersuchten den Zusammenhang zwischen Bronchustonus, registriert nach der Methode von Konzett und Rössler, und Lungenvagusafferenzen. Die durch Histamin, Acetylcholin oder 5-Hydroxytryptamin ausgelöste Asthmareaktion war eng korreliert mit einer Vermehrung der exspiratorischen Lungenvagusafferenzen. Adrenalin, Atropin, Procain, Papaverin und Chlorphenoxamin hemmten diese Wirkung von Histamin und Acetylcholin. Adrenalin und Procain, nicht aber Chlorphenoxamin, hemmten auch die Wirkung von 5-Hydroxytryptamin. Diese Stoffe beeinflußten nicht die durch Veratridin verursachte isolierte Erregung der Lungendehnungsreceptoren, welche nicht von einem Bronchospasmus begleitet war. Die durch Histamin, Acetylcholin oder 5-Hydroxytryptamin bewirkte Erregung der Lungendehnungsreceptoren kann unabhängig vom weiterbestehenden Bronchospasmus durch Benzonatat, Dodecylnonaäthylenoxydäther, Tetracain und Lidocain vermindert werden. Es wird geschlossen, daß die Vermehrung der Lungenvagusafferenzen durch Histamin, Acetylcholin und 5-Hydroxytryptamin ursächlich mit dem Bronchospasmus zusammenhängt und daß ihre Verminderung durch die genannten Spasmolytica durch die Bronchospasmolyse bedingt ist. Daneben ist aber eine echte Endoanaesthesie der Dehnungsreceptoren unabhängig vom Bronchospasmus möglich.

III. Asthmareaktionen an der isolierten Lunge

Untersuchungen an der isolierten Lunge können über die von extrapulmonalen Einwirkungen freien Reaktionen des Organs Aufschluß geben. Dabei darf andererseits nicht übersehen werden, daß die isolierte Lunge von vornherein in einem weitgehend unphysiologischen Milieu reagiert. Dazu kommen mehr oder weniger starke Schädigungen des empfindlichen Gewebes durch die zur Isolierung notwendigen operativen Manipulationen. Für die Beurteilung und Verwertung von Versuchsergebnissen müssen dementsprechende Einschränkungen beachtet werden.

1. Versuchsanordnungen

a) Künstliche Beatmung und Perfusion des Gefäßsystems

α) Beatmung mit positivem Druck

Bei dieser Versuchsanordnung wird die Lunge von den meisten Untersuchern im breit eröffneten Thorax belassen. Die Registrierung der pulmonalen Reaktion kann in gleicher Weise erfolgen wie am narkotisierten Tier. Die Perfusion des

Gefäßsystems wird im offenen oder geschlossenen Lungenkreislauf durchgeführt. Pharmaka werden in die Perfusionsleitung unmittelbar vor deren Einmündung in die Arteria pulmonalis injiziert und als Dosen angegeben, oder der Perfusionsflüssigkeit in definierter Konzentration zugesetzt. Gleichzeitig mit Veränderungen von Beatmungsgrößen können Reaktionen des Gefäßsystems als Veränderungen der Perfusionsrate registriert werden.

Als Perfusionsflüssigkeiten dienen in der Regel Tyrode-, Ringer-, Locke- oder ähnlich zusammengesetzte Lösungen, oder defibriniertes Blut.

Meerschweinchenlunge

Baehr und Pick [16] führten wohl als erste Studien an der isolierten, überlebenden, in situ belassenen, von der Arteria pulmonalis durchströmten Meerschweinchenlunge durch. Sie bestimmten die Tropfenzahl der abfließenden Perfusionsflüssigkeit und beobachteten das Verhalten der Lunge unter der Wirkung zahlreicher Pharmaka.

Bartosch, Feldberg und Nagel [18] verwendeten sensibilisierte Meerschweinchen. Die Atemexkursionen wurden über einen Faden, der am Rande eines Lungenflügels befestigt war, auf einen Hebel übertragen und kymographisch aufgezeichnet. Nach Antigenzusatz zur Perfusionsflüssigkeit wurde die aus dem linken Herzohr abfließende „Schockflüssigkeit" in das gleichartig isolierte Lungenpräparat eines nichtsensibilisierten Meerschweinchens geleitet, wo sie eine Lungenstarre auslöste.

Daly *et al.* bestätigten und erweiterten die vorstehend genannten Untersuchungen mit gleicher Methode. Anstelle der mechanischen Aufzeichnung der Lungenbewegungen registrierten sie den Beatmungsdruck im Respirationssystem mittels Wassermanometer bei gleichbleibendem Beatmungsvolumen (Einthoven [70]) (vgl. S. 101).

Mit gleicher Technik führten Dale und Narayana [56] Untersuchungen über die Nervenversorgung der pulmonalen Blutgefäße durch. Petrovskaia [155] untersuchte die Wirkungen von Acetylcholin, Adrenalin und Ergotoxin sowie peripherer Vagus- und Sympathicusreizung. Hebb [97] beobachtete Bronchoconstriction bei Reizung des Ganglion stellatum, welche ebenso wie die durch Acetylcholin verursachte Bronchoconstriction durch Eserin potenziert und durch Adrenalin, Ergotoxin und Atropin unterdrückt wurde.

Isolierte, mit Tyrodelösung durchströmte und in der Versuchsanordnung von Konzett und Rössler beatmete Meerschweinchenlungen verwendeten Collier *et al.* [48, 52] in ihren Untersuchungen über die bronchoconstrictorische Wirkung von Bradykinin. Die wirksamen Dosen von Histamin und Bradykinin, injiziert in die Durchströmungsflüssigkeit, waren 10—20mal höher als die intravenös am ganzen Tier wirksamen Dosen. Die relativen Wirksamkeiten waren gleich. Wespengiftkinin wirkte ebenfalls bronchoconstrictorisch.

Rattenlunge

Foggie [77] untersuchte mit gleicher Methode wie Daly *et al.* [57] an der Rattenlunge die Wirkung von Adrenalin, Acetylcholin und Histamin. Als Perfusionsflüssigkeit diente glucosefreie Tyrodelösung, die Perfusionsrate wurde mittels Tropfenzähler registriert. Acetylcholin erzeugte Bronchoconstriction ohne Gefäßwirkung in Dosen von 0,2—5 μg, in zehnfach höheren Dosen auch Vasoconstriction. Histamin hatte in Dosen von 0,01—1 mg nur geringe bronchoconstrictorische Wirkung. Adrenalin 0,05 μg verursachte Vasodilatation, 0,5 μg Vasoconstriction. Adrenalininfusion verstärkte die Wirkung von Acetylcholin und Histamin.

Went und Martin [189] und Martin und Went [133] registrierten die Reaktion der durchströmten Rattenlunge onkometrisch. Sie fanden die Bronchialmuskulatur resistent gegen Histamin, Cholin und Antigen. Acetylcholin wirkte erst in einer Konzentration von 10^{-5} g·ml^{-1}.

Katzenlunge

Nisell [145] führte Untersuchungen an der künstlich beatmeten, mit Blut durchströmten Katzenlunge durch. Die Lungen wurden vollständig aus dem Organismus excidiert. Nisell registrierte den Bronchialwiderstand nach dem Verfahren von Konzett und Rössler [122] (s. S. 102), das Lungenvolumen plethysmographisch sowie den Perfusionsdruck. Die Versuchstechnik ist folgende:

Katzen zwischen 1,8 und 4,2 kg Gewicht wurden verwendet. Narkoseeinleitung mit Äther, darauf 0,05 $g \cdot kg^{-1}$ Chloralose intravenös und 10 mg Heparin intravenös. Entbluten des Tieres 1—2 Std nach Narkosebeginn. Das Blut wird in einem Gefäß mit 10 mg Heparin aufgefangen. Die Lungen werden zusammen mit Herz, Oesophagus und thorakaler Aorta excidiert, gegebenenfalls zusammen mit den nervösen Verbindungen zum Ganglion stellatum oder cervicalem Vagosympathicus. Kanülen werden durch den rechten Ventrikel in die Arteria pulmonalis sowie in das linke Herzohr und in die Trachea eingebunden. Die Lungen werden in ein dicht schließendes Glasgefäß eingebracht, aus dem die Kanülen herausführen. Dieses ist zusammen mit dem Blutreservoir und der Perfusionspumpe in einem Thermostaten von 37—38° C untergebracht. Die Lungen werden mit einer Dale-Schuster-Pumpe mit konstanter Frequenz von ca. 140/min und konstantem Fördervolumen durchströmt. In der Regel wurde 50 ml Blut des Tieres mit 20 ml Ringer-Lösung verdünnt. Der Perfusionsdruck wurde auf 20 bis 30 cm H_2O eingestellt und registriert mittels Wasser- oder Quecksilbermanometer, welches mit einem Pistonrekorder verbunden war.

Die Lungen wurden mit konstantem Druck, gewöhnlich 10 cm H_2O, beatmet. Die von den Lungen nicht aufgenommene Luft wurde mittels Spirometer gemessen. Dieses Spirometer maß Veränderungen des Bronchialwiderstandes. Ein zweites Spirometer war mit dem extrapulmonalen Raum des Glasgefäßes verbunden und zeigte Veränderungen des Beatmungsluftvolumens sowie des totalen Lungenvolumens an.

Nisell [145] untersuchte mit dieser Methode die Wirkung von Sauerstoff und CO_2 auf die Bronchiolen und Blutgefäße der Lunge. Bronchiolen, die durch Carbachol, Muscarin oder Histamin kontrahiert waren, erweiterten sich, wenn die Lungen mit CO_2-haltigem oder wenig O_2-haltigem Gas ventiliert wurden. Zwischen O_2- und CO_2-Druck der Beatmungsluft und dem Grad der Bronchoconstriction bestand eine quantitative Beziehung. Die Ergebnisse zeigten, daß der bronchiolare O_2-Druck im lebenden Organismus den Kontraktionsgrad der Lungengefäße wie auch der Bronchiolen reguliert. Es wird postuliert, daß der bronchiale O_2-Druck auch beim intakten Organismus außer der Weite der Pulmonalgefäße auch die Bronchialweite beeinflußt, so daß alveolarer O_2-Druck, Ventilation und Durchblutung in jedem Lungenbezirk in passendem Gleichgewicht sind. Die Entstehung von Bronchiektasen, Asthmaanfälle durch Hyperventilation und die Besserung asthmatischer Zustände bei Aufenthalt in Höhenlagen könnten so durch die Wirkung von Sauerstoff auf die Bronchiolen erklärt werden.

In situ perfundierte Froschlunge

Brecht [27] gab ein Vagus-Lungen-Präparat des Frosches an, bei dem die Lunge des mit Urethan narkotisierten Tieres in situ belassen und durch die Arteria pulmonalis durchströmt wird. Als Durchströmungsflüssigkeit dient Ringer-Lösung nach Barkan, Broemser und Hahn, der Perfusionsdruck beträgt 15–20 cm H_2O. Die Registrierung der ausfließenden Tropfen erfolgt mittels Zeitordinatenschreiber. Die Lunge wird etwas aufgeblasen und durch eine Trachealkanüle mit einem Wassermanometer verbunden, welches Volumen-Druck-Veränderungen registriert. Heim und Meves [98] untersuchten mit dieser Methode die Wirkungen von Histamin und Antazolin. Sie registrierten die Bewegungen des Flüssigkeitsmeniscus im Manometer photographisch als Schattenprojektion auf einem Photokymographion. Die Histamin-

Schwellenkonzentrationen lagen bei 10^{-7} bis 10^{-5} g ml^{-1}, bei empfindlichen Winterfröschen bis zu 10^{-14} g ml^{-1}. Histamin konnte an Sommerfröschen auch gefäßerweiternd und lungenerschlaffend wirken. Antazolin zeigte in Konzentrationen unter 10^{-5} g ml^{-1} histaminähnliche Wirkungen, in Konzentrationen über diesem Wert Gefäß- und Bronchialerweiterung. Unterschwellige Antazolinkonzentrationen hoben die broncho- und vasoconstrictorische Histaminwirkung auf.

β) Beatmung mit negativem Druck

Die künstliche Beatmung der isolierten Lunge durch Anwendung periodischen negativen Drucks auf die Außenfläche der Lungen entspricht eher den Verhältnissen bei der normalen Atmung als die Beatmung mittels Insufflation.

Alberty [4] beschrieb die Verwendung der isolierten Meerschweinchenlunge, die an der eingebundenen Trachealkanüle in einem luftdichten Glasgefäß suspendiert wird. Die Beatmung erfolgt mittels Beatmungspumpe, deren Ansaugstutzen an das Organgefäß angeschlossen ist, mit gleichbleibendem Hub von 30 pro Minute. Als Atmungsluft wird der Trachealkanüle Carbogen zugeführt. Der CO_2-Zusatz verhindert frühzeitigen Bronchospasmus des Präparates. Gleichzeitig wird das Gefäßsystem durch eine in die Arterie pulmonalis eingebundene Kanüle mit Tyrodelösung konstanter Temperatur durchströmt. Pharmaka werden in der Perfusionsflüssigkeit gelöst. Wechsel des zugeführten Pharmakons oder dessen Konzentration erfolgt durch Wechsel der Perfusionsflüssigkeit. Veränderungen des Atemluftvolumens werden durch die Luftbewegungen in der Trachea reflektiert, die am einfachsten durch eine Mareykapsel im Nebenschluß registriert werden können. Quantitative Registrierung kann z. B. durch einen Pneumotachographen erfolgen. Die Registrierung der Druckschwankungen im Organgefäß während der Beatmung gibt Aufschluß über Elastizitätsveränderungen der Lunge während des Versuches. Alberty [4] führte mit dieser Methode quantitative Untersuchungen über die histaminantagonistische (und acetylcholinantagonistische) Wirksamkeit von Tripelennamin, Antazolin und Atropin durch und fand geringere Wirkungsstärke der Antihistamine als im Versuch am isolierten Meerschweinchendarm, aber Übereinstimmung mit der Wirkungsstärke am ganzen Tier.

Jenden und Tureman [114] beschrieben eine mit der vorstehenden praktisch identische Versuchsanordnung. Modifikationen, Erweiterungen und Verbesserungen der von Alberty [4] angegebenen Methode wurden beschrieben von Bhattacharya, Delaunois, King, Dautrebande und Heymans [24, 58, 63], Bianchi [26], Giertz *et al.* [89] sowie Greeff und Moog [92].

Bhattacharya und Delaunois [24] sowie Delaunois und King [63] ergänzten die vorstehend beschriebene Methode in technischen Details wie Einbau des Organgefäßes in einen Thermostaten und eine Anordnung zur Messung der Perfusion mittels Tropfenzähler. Sie injizierten Pharmaka in die Perfusionsleitung. Dautrebande, Delaunois und Heymans [58, 59] beschrieben zu dieser Versuchsanordnung eine Technik zur Applikation von Stoffen in Form mikromicellarer Aerosole von Flüssigkeits- oder Staubpartikeln $\leqq 1\ \mu$ Durchmesser (s. Abb. 19).

Um die Volumenveränderungen der Lungen unter Einwirkung von Pharmaka zu demonstrieren, installierten Dautrebande und Heymans [59] eine Kamera, die im Versuchsverlauf in verschiedenen Atmungsphasen das Präparat photographiert. Die Aufnahmen werden dann planimetrisch ausgewertet. Für Einzelheiten und technische Angaben wird auf die Originalarbeit verwiesen.

Bianchi *et al.* [26] beschrieben ein Vagus-Lungen-Präparat in dieser Versuchsanordnung. Sie isolierten beide cervicalen Vagi und untersuchten die Wirkung der Vagusreizung und ihre Beeinflussung durch verschiedene Antagonisten und Bronchodilatoren.

Weitere Untersuchungen mit den vorstehend angegebenen Methoden betreffen die bronchospastische Wirkung von 5-Hydroxytryptamin und die antagonistische Wirkung von Lysergsäurediäthylamid, Dihydroergotamin, Antihistaminica, Antiadrenergica, Atropin und Adrenalin (Bhattacharya [22]) sowie die antagonistische Wirkung von Procain gegen u. a. Acetylcholin, Pilocarpin, Histamin und 5-Hydroxytryptamin (Bhattacharya und Atanackovic [23]).

Dautrebande *et al.* [58, 59] führten Untersuchungen über die Wirkungen und Wechselwirkungen von Aerosolstaubpartikeln, Sympathomimeticaaerosolen und Bronchoconstrictoren aus. Sie postulieren aufgrund ihrer Ergebnisse, daß die Wirkung ihrer Mikroaerosole sich hauptsächlich in der Alveolarregion der Lunge lokalisiert.

Nagasaka *et al.* [140, 141] untersuchten den Antagonismus von Pronethalol auf Wirkungen verschiedener Adrenergica und schlossen aus ihren Ergebnissen auf nur spärliches Vorkommen von α-Receptoren in der Lunge.

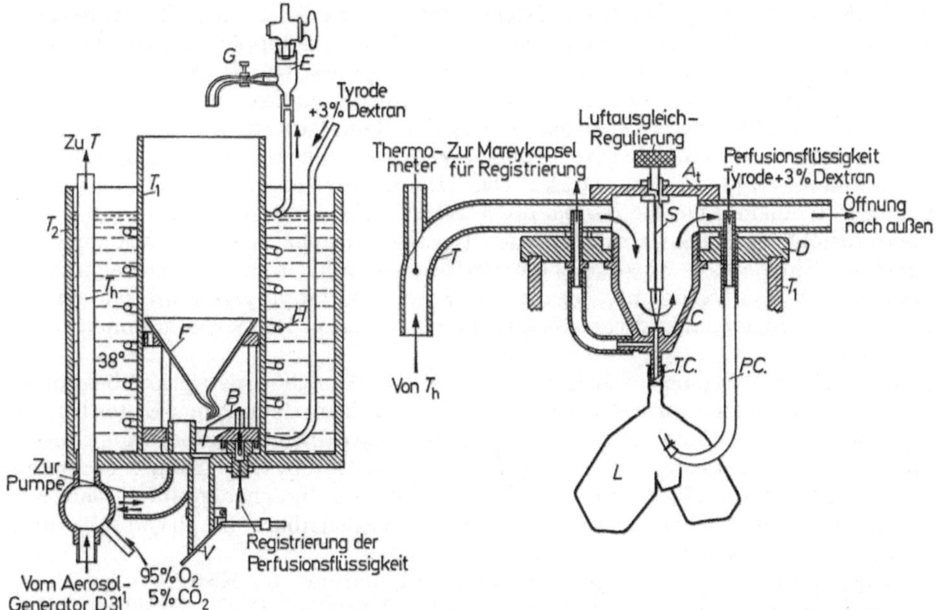

Abb. 19. **Versuchsapparatur für Versuche an der isolierten Lunge nach A. L. Delaunois u. T. O. King [63] sowie für Aerosolapplikation in dieser Versuchsanordnung nach L. Dautrebande, A. L. Delaunois u. C. Heymans. Links: Künstlicher Thorax und Wasserbad. T_1 Inneres Gefäß; T_2 Wand des äußeres Gefäßes; *F* Trichter; *B* Elektroden zur Perfusionsregistrierung; *H* Spiralrohr zur Erwärmung der Perfusionsflüssigkeit; *E* Luftblasenfalle; *G* Klemme zur Regulierung der Perfusionsrate. *Th* Kupferschlange zum Erwärmen der Beatmungsgase; *V* Einwegventil. Rechts: Oberteil des künstlichen Thorax. *D* Deckplatte aus Perspex; A_t Perspexbefestigung; *C* Konusförmige Befestigung aus Messing; *T.C.* Trachealkanüle; *P.C.* Perfusionskanüle; *S* Inneres Netz; *T* Zuleitungsrohr für Beatmungsgase und Aerosol; *L* Lunge. [Aus: J. Physiol. (Lond.) 135, 14P—15P (1956)]**

Stormorken [178] verwendete Lungen sensibilisierter Meerschweinchen in der von Bhattacharya *et al.* [24, 63] angegebenen Versuchsanordnung. Er injizierte große Antigendosen in die Perfusionsflüssigkeit (10^{-2} g Ovalbumin in 1 ml) und berichtet über uneinheitliche Reaktionen. Das Antihistaminicum Thenalidin (Sandosten) verhinderte die allergische Asthmareaktion. Ein Mischpräparat enthaltend Isoprenalin, Cyclopentylamin, Atropin und Procain hemmte die Asthmareaktion bei Verabreichung sowohl vor als auch nach Antigeninjektion.

Aarsen [1] untersuchte die Wirkung von Bradykinin außer am narkotisierten Tier (s. S. 121) und an der durch das Bronchialsystem perfundierten Lunge (s. S. 132) auch in der vorstehend beschriebenen Versuchsanordnung. Bradykinin erzeugte in Dosen von 2—6 μg, in die Perfusionsflüssigkeit injiziert, Bronchoconstriction mit gleichzeitiger starker Vasoconstriction. Im Gegensatz zu ihrer antagonistischen Wirkung am ganzen Tier beeinflußten Acetylsalicylat, 40 $\mu g \cdot ml^{-1}$, Natriumsalicylat, Natriumphenylbutazon und Phenazon in gleicher Dosierung die Bradykininwirkung nicht, und 20 $\mu g \cdot ml^{-1}$ Amidopyrin wirkte nur in 1 von 3 Versuchen antagonistisch.

Giertz, Hahn, Opferkuch und Schmutzler [89] führten an der isolierten Lunge vergleichende Untersuchungen über allergische sowie über durch Anaphylatoxin und durch Histamin verursachte Asthmareaktionen durch. Sie modifizierten die von Alberty [4] angegebene und von Bhattacharya *et al.* [24, 63] abgewandelte Methode folgendermaßen:

Der doppelwandige Mantel des Organgefäßes wurde von einem Thermostaten mit Wasser von 37° C durchströmt. Durch einen Lauf der doppelläufigen Trachealkanüle wurde Carbogen in konstantem Strom zugeführt. Durch den anderen Lauf wurde die Atemluft über ein Ventil abgeleitet. Mit diesem konnte der auf Trachea und Mareykapsel lastende Gasdruck, der in der Regel auf 15 mm H_2O eingestellt wurde, variiert werden. Die Atempumpe erlaubte willkürliche Veränderung des Hubvolumens während des Laufs. Die Druckverhältnisse im Kammerinnern wurden mit einem Quecksilbermanometer fortlaufend registriert und auf einen „Pleuradruck" zwischen 0 und 12 mm Hg (Exspirations- — Inspirationsphase) eingestellt. Substanzen wurden in die Perfusionsleitung injiziert. Als Perfusionsflüssigkeit wurde Tyrode mit Zusatz von 3,5% Polyvinylpyrrolidon verwendet. Bei einem Perfusionsdruck von 5—20 mm H_2O betrug das Stromvolumen 6 bis 10 $ml \cdot min^{-1}$.

Bei Asthmareaktionen wurde die Stärke der Bronchoconstriction bestimmt durch Messung des zu ihrer Überwindung notwendigen Beatmungs-Unterdrucks. Hierzu wurde 15 min nach Auslösung einer Asthmareaktion der Beatmungsunterdruck stufenweise gesteigert bis zum Wiederauftreten der Atemexkursionen (registriert durch die Mareykapsel im Nebenschluß der Trachealkanüle). Dadurch konnten dem allergischen Asthma quantitativ vergleichbare anaphylatoxin- und histaminbedingte Asthmareaktionen erzielt werden.

Anaphylatoxin wurde hergestellt durch Inkubation von Ratten- oder Meerschweinchenserum mit 5 $mg \cdot ml^{-1}$ Dextran für 1 Std bei 37° C. Mit allergischen Reaktionen vergleichbares Asthma wurde erzeugt durch Injektion von 5—10 $ml \cdot kg^{-1}$ Anaphylatoxin oder 0,6 $mg \cdot kg^{-1}$ Histaminbihydrochlorid (die in die Perfusionsflüssigkeit der isolierten Lunge injizierten Dosen sind hier auf das Körpergewicht des ganzen Tieres bezogen). Als spezifische Antagonisten wurden Mepyramin, Lysergsäurediäthylamid und Atropin verwendet.

Giertz *et al.* [89] kommen u. a. zu dem Ergebnis, daß das durch Anaphylatoxin erzeugte Asthma ausschließlich auf Histaminfreisetzung beruht. Das allergische Asthma am isolierten Organ kann jedoch nur zum Teil auf Histaminfreisetzung zurückgeführt werden. Hiermit kommen diese Autoren in ihren Versuchen an isolierten Lungen zu den gleichen Schlußfolgerungen wie seinerzeit Friebel [84, 85] und Alberty [6] am ganzen Tier. Giertz *et al.* [89] fanden keinen überzeugenden Hinweis für eine Beteiligung von 5-Hydroxytryptamin oder Bradykinin an dieser allergischen Reaktion und konnten die Bildung von SRS in der allergischen Reaktion in dieser Versuchsanordnung nicht aufzeigen.

Greef und Moog [92] verglichen die broncho- und vasoconstrictorischen Wirkungen der Polypeptide Bradykinin, Kallidin, Eledoisin und Hypertensin mit der Wirkung von Histamin, Acetylcholin und 5-Hydroxytryptamin an der isolierten Lunge von Ratten, Meerschweinchen und Katzen. Sie verwendeten die vorstehend beschriebene Versuchsanordnung mit einigen Modifikationen: Der

Perfusionsdruck wurde auf -2 bis 0 cm H_2O eingestellt, so daß Perfusionsflüssigkeit bei der Inspiration angesaugt wurde. Der Unterdruck bei der Inspirationsphase betrug 8—10 mm Hg. Die Perfusionsrate ebenso wie die Druckschwankungen in der Trachea wurden über Stathamelemente auf Direktschreiber registriert. In die Trachea war ein Polyäthylenkatheter von 1 mm Innendurchmesser eingeführt, durch den während der Inspiration Carbogen angesaugt wurde. Eine entsprechende Menge Atemluft konnte während der „Exspiration“ durch den gleichen Katheter entweichen. Dadurch wurde ein vollständiges Kollabieren der Lunge verhindert und eine gleichmäßigere Belüftung erreicht. Greef *et al.* [92] erhielten folgende Ergebnisse:

An der isolierten Meerschweinchenlunge verursachten Bradykinin, Kallidin und Eledoisin Bronchoconstriction und starke Vasoconstriction. Eledoisin war an der Bronchialmuskulatur etwa zweimal stärker als Bradykinin, Kallidin war etwa fünfmal schwächer wirksam als Bradykinin. Hypertensin hatte, verglichen mit seiner vasoconstrictorischen, nur eine schwache bronchoconstrictorische Wirkung. Acetylcholin und 5-Hydroxytryptamin verursachten dagegen starke Bronchoconstriction. Histamin wirkte etwa gleich stark broncho- und vasoconstrictorisch und war etwa 5—10mal schwächer als Bradykinin. Phenylbutazon und Acetylsalicylsäure verminderten die broncho- und vasoconstrictorischen Wirkungen von Bradykinin, die durch Histamin oder 5-Hydroxytryptamin verursachte Bronchoconstriction wurde dagegen nicht beeinflußt. Katzen- und Rattenlungen waren gegen alle untersuchten Stoffe weniger empfindlich. Bradykinin hatte auch in 100fach höherer Dosierung keine sichere bronchoconstrictorische Wirkung. An der Katzenlunge wirkte 5-Hydroxytryptamin stärker bronchoconstrictorisch als Histamin. Beide Amine wirkten vorwiegend vasoconstrictorisch an der Rattenlunge.

Kovács und Görög [124] verwendeten die gleiche Versuchsanordnung. Sie beobachteten, daß vorausgegangene Injektion von 100 μg Chlordiazepoxid die Bronchoconstriction durch Histamin, Bradykinin, Adenosintriphosphat und Hypertensin verhindert. Die allergische Asthmareaktion an der isolierten Meerschweinchenlunge wurde durch vorausgegangene Injektion von 0,5 mg Chlordiazepoxid verhindert. Die Wirkung von Acetylcholin wurde dagegen nur geringfügig und die von 5-Hydroxytryptamin nicht beeinflußt. Chlordiazepoxid verhinderte nur die durch Histamin gleichzeitig verursachte Vasoconstriction (vgl. auch S. 91 und S. 123).

b) Perfusion des Bronchialsystems

α) *Perfusion mit Flüssigkeit*

Sollmann und Oettingen [177] durchströmten die isolierte Lunge von der Trachea aus mit Lockes Lösung unter konstantem Druck. Die Perfusionsflüssigkeit fließt durch die Lungenoberfläche ab. Pharmaka werden in die Perfusionsleitung injiziert. Als Maß der Bronchoconstriction dient die Perfusionsgeschwindigkeit, gemessen durch Tropfenzählung oder Registrierung der Luftblasen, die in die Mariottsche Flasche konform mit dem Auslaufen der Perfusionsflüssigkeit eintreten.

Warnant [188] verwendete diese Methode am Meerschweinchen und brachte an der Lungenoberfläche mit einer feinen Nadel eine Serie von Löchern an, um das Abfließen zu erleichtern. Er durchströmte mit Ringer-Lösung. Das Präparat blieb empfindlich für etwa 60 min. Er beobachtete Bronchoconstriction durch K- und Ca-Ionen, Pilocarpin, Ergotamin und Antigen, Bronchodilatation durch Mg-Ionen, Coffein und Adrenalin. Adrenalin wirkte spasmolytisch gegen alle bronchospastisch wirkenden Agentien, Ephedrin gegen histaminbedingten und durch Antigen ausgelösten Bronchospasmus.

Swanson und Webster [180] verwendeten Lungen von Kaninchen, Katzen und Hunden in dieser Versuchsanordnung. Sie prüften die Wirkung von Ephedrin, Pseudoephedrin und Adrenalin am Bronchospasmus, hervorgerufen durch Pilocarpin, Physostigmin, Arecolin, Histamin, Morphin und Diäthylmorphin.

McDowall und Thornton [135] erweiterten die Methode von Sollmann und Oettingen durch gleichzeitige separate Perfusion des Gefäßsystems von der Arteria pulmonalis. Als Perfusionsflüssigkeit verwendeten sie van Dyke & Hastings-Lösung. Der Bronchialwiderstand wurde als Perfusionswiderstand mittels Manometer registriert. Histamin 0,01 mg injiziert in die Zuleitung zur Gefäßperfusion verursachte einen Druckanstieg im Bronchialperfusionssystem von mindestens 30—40 mm H_2O.

Thornton [182] demonstrierte mit dieser Methode Bronchoconstriction durch Histamin, Pilocarpin und Alkaliionen innerhalb physiologischer Bereiche sowie Bronchodilatation durch Adrenalin, durch Atropin bei pilocarpinbedingtem Bronchospasmus, und durch Säureionen. Das Präparat des sensibilisierten Tieres zeigte bei Antigenzusatz allergische Kontraktion mit nachfolgender Desensibilisierung.

Tainter, Pedden und James [181] verglichen in dieser Versuchsanordnung die bronchodilatorischen Wirkungen von 13 sympathomimetischen Aminen an der Meerschweinchenlunge. Sie scarifizierten die Lungenoberfläche. Bronchoconstriction wurde erzeugt durch Injektion von Pilocarpin, Histamin oder $BaCl_2$, die Bronchodilatoren wurden gleichzeitig injiziert. Mit gleicher Methode untersuchten Lands *et al.* [126, 127] und Siegmund *et al.* [173] die Wirkungen von Isoprenalin, sek-Butyl-Noradrenalin und Ethylnoradrenalin sowie von 1-(3′,4′-Dihydroxyphenyl)-2-aminoäthan an der Meerschweinchenlunge. Siegmund *et al.* [173] erzeugten Kontraktion der Tracheobronchialmuskulatur durch Perfusion der Lungen sensibilisierter Tiere mit antigenhaltiger Flüssigkeit und erhielten auch hierbei die stärkste bronchialerweiternde Wirkung mit Isoprenalin.

Yonkman, Oppenheimer, Rennick und Pellet [196] verwendeten Lungen von mit Pferdeserum sensibilisierten Meerschweinchen. Injektion von Tripelennamin oder Phenbenzamin (25—50 μg) hemmten den histaminbedingten Bronchospasmus, beeinflußten dagegen die allergische Reaktion, ausgelöst durch Antigeninjektion, nur geringfügig oder gar nicht.

Schaepdryver [168] registrierte die Perfusionsrate durch Tropfenzähler am Abfluß. Er untersuchte die Wirkung einer Reihe von Substanzen an Lungen normaler und sensibilisierter Meerschweinchen. Die verwendeten Injektionsdosen waren relativ hoch. Bronchoconstrictorische Wirkungen wurden erhalten durch Injektionen von Acetylcholin, Pilocarpin, Pituitrin, Histamin und Ovalbuminantigen. Caramiphen 0,5—2 mg wirkte bronchodilatorisch gegen alle erwähnten Agonisten und gegen den allergischen Spasmus. Antazolin 20 mg (!) wirkte selbst bronchodilatorisch und unterdrückte den allergischen und den durch Histamin, Acetylcholin und Pilocarpin verursachten Spasmus. Dibenamin 0,25 mg wirkte bronchoconstrictorisch und hemmte die bronchialerweiternde Wirkung von Adrenalin am Bronchospasmus hervorgerufen durch Pilocarpin, Pituitrin und Antigen.

Freyburger *et al.* [81] beobachteten nur geringe vorübergehende bronchoconstrictorische Wirkung von 5-Hydroxytryptamin an der Kaninchenlunge in dieser Versuchsanordnung.

Bhoola *et al.* [25] erzielten Bronchoconstriction durch Injektion von Bradykinin in die Bronchialperfusion. Aarsen [1] benötigte z. T. erheblich höhere Dosen und konnte in dieser Versuchsanordnung keine bradykininantagonistische Wirkung von Acetylsalicylat oder Phenylbutazon (bis 80 $\mu g \cdot ml^{-1}$) erzielen. Phenazon 40 $\mu g \cdot ml^{-1}$ wirkte dagegen hemmend, die Wirkung von Amidopyrin war wechselnd (vgl. S. 129).

β) Perfusion mit Luft

Arunlakshana und Schild [12, 13] durchströmten die isolierte Meerschweinchenlunge mit Luft in der in Abb. 20 dargestellten Weise (vgl. dazu die Methode

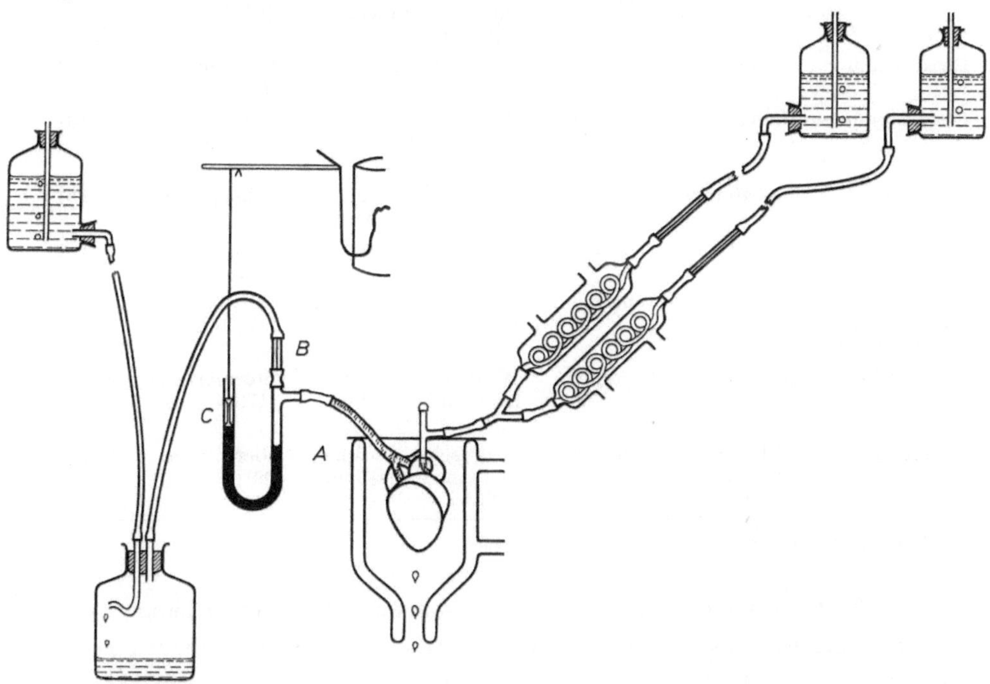

Abb. 20. Versuchsanordnung zur Perfusion der iolierten Meerschweinchenlunge mit Luft. Die Trachea ist mit der Abzweigung *A* des Quecksilbermanometers verbunden. Unter gleichbleibendem Druck strömt Luft durch den Capillarwiderstand *B* und entweicht aus Scarifikationen der Lungenoberfläche. *C* balancierter Ebonitschwimmer, mit einem Stirnschreiber verbunden. In die Pulmonalarterie wird vorgewärmte Tyrodelösung eingeleitet. [Nach O. Arunlakshana and H. O. Schild, J. Physiol. (Lond.) **14**, 48—58 (1959)]

von Eichler und Mügge [68] am ganzen Tier, s. S. 109). Luftdruckveränderungen infolge Änderungen der Bronchialweite wurden mittels Quecksilbermanometer registriert, dessen Bewegungen über einen vergrößernden Schreibhebel kymographisch aufgezeichnet wurden. Der Luftdurchfluß betrug etwa 1 $ml \cdot min^{-1}$. Gleichzeitig wurde die Lunge durch die Arteria pulmonalis mit Tyrodelösung von 37° Temperatur durchströmt. Pharmaka waren der Perfusionsflüssigkeit zugesetzt oder wurden in diese injiziert. Histamin wirkte in Dosen von 2,5—10 μg. Arunlakshana *et al.* untersuchten in dieser Versuchsanordnung quantitative Aspekte des Antagonismus Acetylcholin-Atropin, Histamin-Antihistamin und Acetylcholin-Cinchonidin und fanden nahe quantitative Übereinstimmungen mit gleichartigen Untersuchungen an anderen Organen.

2. Allergisches Asthma an der isolierten Lunge

Eine Übersicht über die verwendeten Methoden gibt Tabelle 10.

Tabelle 10. *Allergisches Asthma an der isolierten Lunge des Meerschweinchens*

Antigen	Dosierung	Zufuhrweg	Fragestellung der Untersuchung	Autoren	Kapitel im Text
Ovalbumin	5—10 mg	bronchial	allgemeine Reaktivität, Adrenergica, Atropin u. a.	Warnant [188]	S. 131
Ovalbumin	10 mg	a. pulmon.	allgemeine Reaktivität, Adrenergica, Atropin u. a.	Thornton [182]	S. 131
Pferdeserum	5 mg	a. pulmon.	Wirkung von Adrenalinderivaten	Siegmund *et al.* [173]	S. 131
Pferdeserum	10 mg	bronchial	Wirkung von Tripelennamin und Phenbenzamin	Yonkman *et al.* [196]	S. 131
Ovalbumin	5—40 mg	bronchial	Wirkung von verschiedenen Substanzen	Schaepdryver [168]	S. 131
Ovalbumin	10—15 mg	a. pulmon.	Wirkung von Schockflüssigkeit	Bartosch *et al.* [18]	S. 125
Ovalbumin Pferdeserum Hammelserum	1—15 mg 0,01 ml	a. pulmon.	Wirkung von Schockflüssigkeit	Daly *et al.* [57]	S. 125
Ovalbumin	10 mg	a. pulmon.	Wirkung von Antihistaminica und Cortison	Stormorken [178]	S. 128
Ovalbumin	0,1—10 $mg \cdot kg^{-1}$ [a]	a. pulmon.	allergisches Asthma und Anaphylatoxinasthma	Giertz *et al.* [89]	S. 128

[a] Bezogen auf das Gewicht des ganzen Tieres.

3. Durch Pharmaka verursachtes Asthma an der isolierten Lunge

Eine Übersicht über die verwendeten Methoden geben die Tabellen 11—13.

Tabelle 11. *Erzeugung von Asthmareaktionen an der isolierten Lunge durch Histamin (Dosierungsbeispiele)*

Tierart	Dosierung (Inj. a. pulmon. oder i. v. bzw. Konz. in Perf.flüss.)	Fragestellung	Autoren
		Künstliche Beatmung und Perfusion des Gefäßsystems	
		Beatmung mit positivem Druck	
Meerschweinchen	10^{-5} $g \cdot ml^{-1}$	pharmakologische Studien	Baehr *et al.* [16]
Meerschweinchen	0,2—0,5 μg	Vergleich mit allergischen Reaktionen	Daly *et al.* [57]
Meerschweinchen	20 μg	Wirkung von Bradykinin	Collier *et al.* [48]
Katze	10—20 μg	Wirkung von O_2 und CO_2	Nisell [145]
Ratte	10—1000 μg	Wirkung Histamin, Acetylchl. u. a. Substanzen	Foggie [77]
Frosch	(10^{-14}) 10^{-7} bis 10^{-5} $g \cdot ml^{-1}$	Wirkung von Antazolin	Heim *et al.* [98]

Tabelle 11 (Fortsetzung)

Tierart	Dosierung (Inj. a. pulmon. oder i.v. bzw. Konz. in Perf.flüss.)	Fragestellung	Autoren
		Beatmung durch negativen Druck	
Meerschweinchen	0,2 μg	Wirkung von Chlordiazepoxid	Kovács [124]
Meerschweinchen	1—6 μg	Methode	Jenden *et al.* [114]
		Wirkung von Procain u.a.	Bhattacharya *et al.* [23, 24],
		Methodik u.a. Fragen	Dautrebande *et al.* [58, 59]
		Analgetica und Bradykinin	Aarsen [1]
	2—5 × 10^{-7} g · ml^{-1}, Perfusion	Wirkung von Antihistaminica und Atropin	Alberty [4]
	10^{-2} g · ml^{-1} Aerosol	Meth. Aerosoladministration	Delaunois *et al.* [59, 62]
Katze	1—5 μg	Bradykinin, Histamin und 5-Hydroxytryptamin	Greeff et al. [92]
Ratte	10—50 μg	Bradykinin, Histamin und 5-Hydroxytryptamin	Greeff *et al.* [92]
		Perfusion des Bronchialsystems mit Flüssigkeit	
Nicht angegeben	20—1000 μg	Methode. Wirkung verschiedener Pharmaka	Sollman *et al.* [177]
Katze, Kaninchen, Hund	1,5—3,0 mg	Wirkung von Adren., Ephedr. und -deriv., Morphin	Swansson *et al.* [180]
Ratte, Meerschweinchen, Kaninchen, Katze	10 μg (auch Inj. a. pulmon.)	allgemeine pharmakologische Reaktivität	Thornton [182]
Meerschweinchen	25—100 μg	Wirkung von 17 adrenergischen Aminen	Tainter *et al.* [181]
	50 μg	Antihistaminica	Yonkman *et al.* [196]
Meerschweinchen	40—400 μg	pharmakologische Wirkungen, allergische Reaktion	Schaepdryver [168]
	8—320 μg 0,1—1,0 μ (auch Inj. a. pulmon.)	Analgetica und Bradykinin Wirkung von Peptiden	Aarsen [1] Bhoola *et al.* [25]
		Perfusion des Bronchialsystems mit Luft	
Meerschweinchen	2,5—10,5 μg, Inj. a. pulmon.	Antagonismus von Pharmaka quantitativ	Arunlakshana *et al.* [13]

Tabelle 12. *Erzeugung von Asthmareaktionen an der isolierten Lunge durch cholinergische Pharmaka (Dosierungsbeispiele)*

Tierart	Dosierung (Inj. a. pulmon. oder i.v. bzw. Konz. in Perf.flüss.)	Fragestellung	Autoren
	Künstliche Beatmung und Perfusion des Gefäßsystems		
	Beatmung mit positivem Druck		
	Acetylcholin		
Meerschweinchen	0,2—0,5 μg	s. Tabelle 11	Daly *et al.* [57]
Meerschweinchen	5—20 μg	Nervenversorgung der Pulmonalgefäße	Dale *et al.* [56]
Meerschweinchen	1—1000 μg	Stimul. Ggl. stellat.	Hebb [97]
Ratte	0,2—0,5 μg	s. Tabelle 11	Foggie [77]
Ratte	0,001 μg	Sensibilisierung und Emplichkeit gegen Acetylcholin, Histam. u.a.	Martin *et al.* [133] Went *et al.* [189]
	Carbacholin		
Katze	2,5—25 μg	s. Tabelle 11	Nisell [145]
	Pilocarpin		
Meerschweinchen	10^{-5}—10^{-4} g · ml^{-1}	s. Tabelle 11	Baehr *et al.* [16]
	Beatmung durch negativen Druck		
	Acetylcholin		
Meerschweinchen	0,25—5 μg	s. Tabelle 11	Bhattacharya *et al.* [23], Greeff *et al.* [92], Jenden *et al.* [114], Kovács [124]
Meerschweinchen	4—20 × 10^{-9} g · ml^{-1}	s. Tabelle 11	Alberty [4]
	Carbacholin		
Meerschweinchen	5 × 10^{-3} g · ml^{-1} (Aerosol)	Methode	Delaunois *et al.* [62]
Meerschweinchen	2 × 10^{-2} g · ml^{-1} (Aerosol)	Methode	Dautrebande *et al.* [59]
	Pilocarpin		
Meerschweinchen	50 μg	s. Tabelle 11	Bhattacharya *et al.* [23]
	Vagusreizung		
Meerschweinchen	10 Hz, 5 msec, 2—25 V	Methode und Wirkung von Pharmaka	Bianchi *et al.* [25, 26]
	Perfusion des Bronchialsystems mit Flüssigkeit		
	Acetylcholin		
Meerschweinchen	1000 μg	s. Tabelle 11	Schaepdryver [168]
Meerschweinchen	0,05—0,2, auch Inj. a. pulmon.	Wirkung von Peptiden	Bhoola [24]
	Pilocarpin		
Katze, Kaninchen, Hund	1—3 mg	s. Tabelle 11	Swansson *et al.* [180]
Ratte, Meerschweinchen, Kaninchen Katze	2 mg	s. Tabelle 11	Thornton [182]

Tabelle 12 (Fortsetzung)

Tierart	Dosierung (Inj. a pulmon. oder i.v. bzw. Konz. in Perf.flüss.)	Fragestellung	Autoren
Meerschweinchen	0,05—0,25—2,0 mg	s. Tabelle 11	Tainter *et al.* [181], Schaepdryver [168]
	Arecolin		
Kaninchen, Katze, Hund	0,8—3 mg	s. Tabelle 11	Swansson *et al.* [180]
	Diisopropylfluorophosphat		
Meerschweinchen	1—4 mg	s. Tabelle 11	Schaepdryver [168]
	Perfusion des Bronchialsystems mit Luft		
	Acetylcholin		
Meerschweinchen		s. Tabelle 11	Arunlakshana *et al.* [12]

Tabelle 13. *Erzeugung von Asthmareaktionen an der isolierten Lunge durch verschiedene Pharmaka (Dosierungsbeispiele)*

Tierart	Dosis, Zufuhr	Versuchsmethode	Autoren (Nr. des Literaturverzeichnisses)
	5-Hydroxytryptamin		
Meerschweinchen	0,5—2,0 μg a. pulmon.	Beatm. neg. Druck	[92, 124]
Meerschweinchen	10—25 μg a. pulmon.	Beatm. neg. Druck	[23, 24]
Ratte	10—100 μg a. pulmon.	Beatm. neg. Druck	[92]
Kaninchen	bronchial	bronch. Perfus.	[81]
Katze	5—20 μg a. pulmon.	Beatm. neg. Druck	[92]
	Bariumchlorid		
Meerschweinchen	1 mg bronchial	bronch. Perfus.	[177]
Meerschweinchen	5—25 mg bronchial	bronch. Perfus.	[181]
	Bradykinin		
Meerschweinchen	0,005—0,05 μg a. pulmon.	Beatm. neg. Druck	[92, 124]
Meerschweinchen	2—6 μg a. pulmon.	Beatm. neg. Druck	[1]
Meerschweinchen	0,5—5,0—16,8 μg bronchial	bronch. Perfus.	[1, 24]
Meerschweinchen	100 μg a. pulmon.	Konzett-Rössler	[48]
	Kallidin		
Meerschweinchen	0,1—0,2 μg	Beatm. neg. Druck	[92]
	Eledoisin		
Meerschweinchen	0,02—0,05 μg	Beatm. neg. Druck	[92]
	Hypertensin		
Meerschweinchen	0,5—1,0 μg	Beatm. neg. Druck	[92]
	Hypophysenhinterlappenextrakt		
Meerschweinchen	1—2 E bronchial	bronch. Perfus.	[168, 188]
	Anaphylatoxin		
Meerschweinchen	5—10 ml·kg^{-1} [a]	Beatm. neg. Druck	[89]
	Titanstaub, kolloid. Silica		
Meerschweinchen	als Aerosol	Beatm. neg. Druck	[59, 62]

[a] Bezogen auf das Gewicht des ganzen Tieres.

IV. Spasmus der isolierten Bronchial- oder Trachealmuskulatur

1. Versuchsanordnungen

Der Bronchialmuskelspasmus ist einer der Mechanismen, wenn auch in der Regel einer der wichtigsten, der am Zustandekommen des allergischen unkomplizierten Asthma bronchiale beteiligt ist. Asthmareaktionen können auch allein durch einen Bronchialmuskelspasmus hervorgerufen werden. Experimentelle Untersuchungen an der isolierten Bronchialmuskulatur betreffen somit eine der Komponenten des Asthma bronchiale und müssen deshalb in dieser Darstellung berücksichtigt werden.

Unter diesem Gesichtspunkt wäre die Muskulatur der Bronchiolen das eigentliche Versuchsobjekt. Ihre Isolierung und experimentelle Verwendung mit herkömmlichen Methoden ist aber technisch nur in besonderen Fällen und nicht allgemein zu verwirklichen. Auch Versuche an isolierter Bronchialmuskulatur setzen bereits die Verwendung größerer Tierspecies voraus. Von den meist üblichen kleineren und mittelgroßen Versuchstierspecies sind nur Muskelpräparate aus Bronchien 1. Ordnung und Trachea zu erhalten. Die meisten Untersuchungen sind deshalb auch an isolierten Trachealmuskelpräparaten durchgeführt worden. Die Bedeutung der an solchen Präparaten erhaltenen Befunde unterliegt Beschränkungen nicht nur solcher Art, wie sie für die Ergebnisse von Versuchen an isolierten Organen im allgemeinen angeführt werden können. Die Muskulatur von Trachea und Bronchien braucht sich durchaus nicht in gleicher Weise zu verhalten wie die Muskulatur der Bronchioli (vgl. Brocklehurst [29], Siro-Brigiani [175]). Rückschlüsse von Versuchsergebnissen an diesen Versuchsobjekten auf das Asthma bronchiale bedürfen daher starker Zurückhaltung. Andererseits geben diese relativ einfachen Präparate wertvolle Möglichkeiten zum Studium grundsätzlicher Fragen der experimentellen Asthmaforschung wie auch anderer pharmakologischer Probleme.

a) Isolierte Bronchioli

Wegen ihrer Kleinheit lassen sich Bronchioli nicht als isolierte Muskelpräparate herstellen und in der üblichen Weise für quantitative Untersuchungen montieren. Für qualitative Untersuchungen finden sich zwei Verfahren: Die mikroskopische Beobachtung von überlebenden Gewebsschnitten und Bronchographie.

Sollmann und Gilbert [176] stellten manuell dünne Schnitte von frischen Lungen in folgender Weise her (die Beschreibung folgt weitgehend den Originalangaben).

Das Tier wird durch Genickschlag (Kaninchen) oder durch Stickoxydul getötet. Die Lungen werden excidiert und in warme Ringer-Lösung gelegt. Eine Kanüle wird in die Trachea (bei größeren Tieren in einen Bronchus) eingebunden. Man läßt warme Ringer-Lösung mit 10% Gelatine in die Lungen fließen, bis diese ungefähr ihre normale Größe im Thorax erreicht haben (etwa 20 ml der Lösung für ein 1,5 kg schweres Kaninchen). Die Trachea wird dann abgebunden und die Lungen werden unverzüglich in eiskalte Ringer-Lösung gelegt und im Eisschrank für 1 Std aufbewahrt, bis die Gelatine hart geworden ist. Das Gewebe kann auch später verwendet werden. Der Bronchialmuskel reagiert recht gut innerhalb etwa 48 Std. Ein Lungenlappen wird dann von Hand mit einem scharfen Rasiermesser in dünne Scheiben von etwa 0,1—0,3 mm Dicke geschnitten, wobei die Lunge auf einem Paraffinblock liegt. Das Schneiden wird erleichtert durch Befeuchten des Messers mit Ringer-Lösung. Die Schnitte werden in eine flache Schale getan, welche luftdurchperlte Ringer-Lösung von Zimmertemperatur enthält. Jeder Schnitt wird auf einem Korkring in einer 9 cm-Petri-Schale befestigt, welche

50 ml Ringer-Lösung enthält. Für diesen Zweck wird ein flaches Stück Kork von etwa 3 mm Dicke und 15 mm Durchmesser mit einem Bohrloch von 3—5 mm Durchmesser versehen und mittels Bienenwachs im Zentrum der Petri-Schale befestigt. Die Petri-Schale wird auf den Objekttisch eines Mikroskops gestellt und die Lösung auf 37° erwärmt. Nach etwa einer halben Stunde hat sich das Präparat gewöhnlich von dem Trauma und dem Abkühlen erholt und reagiert auf Pharmaka. Luftzufuhr ist nicht erforderlich, da es sich nur um eine kleine Menge Gewebe in Flüssigkeit handelt, deren große Oberfläche der Luft ausgesetzt ist. Vergrößerungen von 40—100 sind am zweckmäßigsten. Es ist empfehlenswert, die Veränderungen von Lumen und Wand der Bronchioli durch Camera lucida-Zeichnungen festzuhalten (heutzutage würde Mikrophotographie oder -kinematographie als elegantestes Verfahren zu empfehlen sein). Bestimmung der Flächeninhalte und ihrer Veränderungen ermöglichen quantitative Angaben. Beobachtung der Cilienbewegungen sind in weniger als 8 Std alten Schnitten von Lungen möglich. Nach dieser Zeit läßt die Aktivität der Cilien gewöhnlich nach oder hört ganz auf. Durch Aufbringung von Rußteilchen auf längsgeschnittene Bronchien kann man die Richtung der Cilienbewegungen von den kleineren zu größeren Bronchien beobachten.

Sollman und Gilbert [176] verwendeten Lungen von Ratten, Meerschweinchen, Kaninchen, Katzen, Hunden und Menschen und prüften die Wirkung von Methacholin, Physostigmin, Pilocarpin, Histamin, $BaCl_2$, Amphetamin (Benzedrin), Nicotin, NaCN und spezifischem Antigen als Constrictoren sowie von Atropin und Adrenalin als Dilatoren. Antigenzusatz verursachte Kontraktion der Bronchioli sensibilisierter Kaninchen. Die Bronchioli von Hund und Katze reagierten auf Parasympathomimetica und andere glatte Muskulatur kontrahierende Substanzen. Menschliches Lungengewebe reagierte im wesentlichen in gleicher Weise. Die Bronchiolen der Ratte reagierten nicht auf Histamin, die des Kaninchens nur schwach auf Adrenalin. Meerschweinchenlungen erwiesen sich als ungeeignet, die Bronchioli kontrahierten sich beim Schmelzen der Gelatine irreversibel.

Kallós und Kallós-Deffner [116, 117] beobachteten mit gleicher Technik auch an Schnitten von Meerschweinchenlungen bronchiolare Reaktionen. Sie erhielten Kontraktion durch Histamin und Ziegenserum sowie in Schnitten sensibilisierter Tiere durch Antigen. Theophyllin-monoäthylamin hemmte die Kontraktion bzw. erschlaffte die kontrahierten Bronchiolen.

Jänkälä und Virtanen [113] demonstrierten eine selektive kontrahierende Wirkung von Bradykinin auf die Sphincter der respiratorischen Bronchioli am Meerschweinchen bronchographisch. Nach intravenöser Injektion von Bradykinin (1—600 $\mu g \cdot kg^{-1}$) wurde Propyliodon in 50%iger wäßriger Lösung (Dionosil aqu.) tropfenweise in die Trachea injiziert bei aktiver Inspiration. Nach Füllung von Bronchialsystem und Trachea wurden Trachea und Lungen excidiert und röntgenphotographiert mit einer Siemens-Feinstruktur-Röntgenröhre Ab 30 mit Kupferanode und Berylliumfenster, 30 kV, Focus-Film-Abstand 30 cm.

b) Isoliertes Trachealrohr

Fink und Akiyama [75] suspendierten die Trachea des Meerschweinchens in van Dyke-Hastings-Lösung, die mit Carbogen durchperlt wurde. Ihre Versuchstechnik geht aus Abb. 21 hervor. Sie fanden in dieser Versuchsanordnung, daß 0,5—2,0 mM Morphin allein geringe Kontraktion verursachte und in Konzentrationen von 0,1—1,5 mM die Wirkung von Acetylcholin signifikant verstärkte. Pethidin (Meperidin) 0,001—1,0 mM hatte dagegen keine Wirkung auf den normalen Trachealmuskel und blockierte in Konzentrationen von 0,1—1,0 mM die Acetylcholinwirkung vollständig.

Die von Jamieson [112] publizierte Versuchsanordnung entspricht im Prinzip der von Fink und Akiyama [75] beschriebenen Technik. Sie verwendete ein Capillarmanometer, deren Spiegel vor und nach Applikation von Pharmaka abgelesen wurde. Jamieson verglich die Wirkungsstärken verschiedener Pharmaka am Trachealpräparat von Meerschweinchen und Ratte. Ihre Ergebnisse gehen aus Tabelle 14 hervor

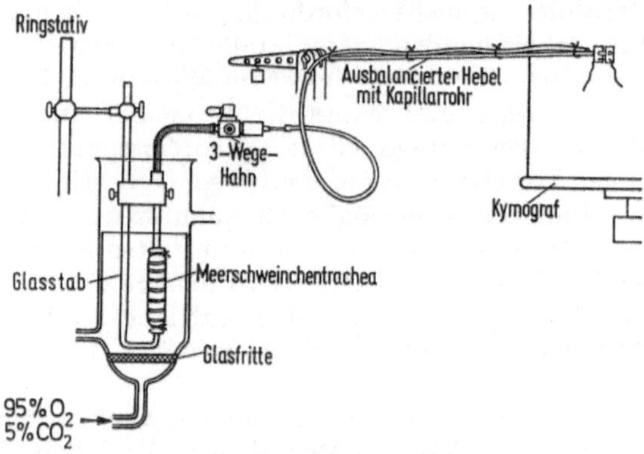

Abb. 21. Versuchsanordnung zur Registrierung von Volumänderungen der isolierten Trachea des Meerschweinchens. [Nach L. D. Fink and J. Akiyama, Arch. int. Pharmacodyn. **91**, 322—329 (1952)]

Tabelle 14. *Minimale Konzentrationen von Substanzen (g · ml⁻¹), die eine Reaktion des Tracheapräparates verursachen*

Verbindung	Meerschweinchen-trachea	Rattentrachea
Acetylcholin	2×10^{-8}	10^{-8}
5-Hydroxytryptamin	5×10^{-8}	$2{,}5 \times 10^{-8}$
Histamin	4×10^{-8}	$> 10^{-3}$
Adrenalin	10^{-9}	$> 10^{-3}$
Aminophyllin	10^{-5}	$> 10^{-3}$

Aus D. Jamieson, Brit. J. Pharmacol. **19**, 286—294 (1962).

Elektrische Reizung der Trachea

Foster [79] beschrieb eine Versuchsanordnung für transmurale elektrische Reizung der intakten isolierten Trachea des Meerschweinchens. Die Versuchsanordnung geht aus Abb. 22 hervor. Stimulation erfolgte alle 10 min mittels Rechteckimpulsen von 0,1 msec, gewöhnlich 3 Hz, und 60 V, für 30 sec. Ablesungen des Manometermeniscus wurden alle 2 min vorgenommen. Stimulation verursachte eine biphasische Reaktion: Initiale Kontraktion gefolgt von Erschlaffung. Die initiale Kontraktion wurde durch Atropin blockiert. Die Relaxation wurde aufgehoben durch Dichlorisoprenalin oder Dichlornoradrenalin, Procain und Cocain in höheren Konzentrationen. Sie trat nicht auf nach Vorbehandlung des Versuchstieres mit Reserpin oder Vorbehandlung des isolierten Präparates mit Bretylium oder Guanethidin. Hexamethonium hatte keinen Einfluß auf die Erschlaffung durch elektrische Reizung. Nach diesen Ergebnissen führt Foster [80] die Wirkung elektrischer Reizung auf Erregung postganglionärer adrenergischer Nerven zurück, welche β-Receptoren innervieren.

Carlyle [37] erweiterte diese Untersuchungen mit gleicher Methode und untersuchte insbesondere den Mechanismus der initialen Kontraktion. Diese trat am besten bei Reizung mit hohen Frequenzen (bis 50 Hz) auf. Sie wurde durch Atropin aufgehoben, durch den Cholinesteraseinhibitor Fluor-N,N-diisopropylphosphodiamid (Mipafox) dagegen verstärkt. Der Nachweis einer Acetylcholinfreisetzung durch elektrische Reizung in Gegenwart von Mipafox konnte an der Trachealkette des Kaninchens erbracht werden. Dieses Präparat reagiert auf Acetylcholin in Größenordnungen von ng·ml^{-1} und ist unempfindlich gegen Histamin und 5-Hydroxytryptamin. An der Trachealkette des Meerschweinchens (s. S. 145) zeigte Carlyle [36], daß die durch Physostigmin und Neostigmin hervorgerufene Kontraktion eher durch Acetylcholinfreisetzung als durch Cholinesterasehemmung zustandekommt.

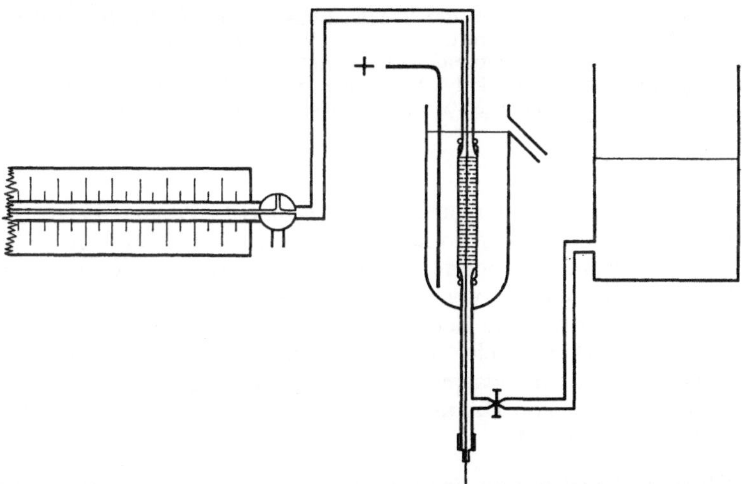

Abb. 22. Versuchsanordnung zur transmuralen elektrischen Reizung der isolierten Trachea des Meerschweinchens. Die Vorrichtungen zur Erwärmung des Organbads, Wechsel sowie Carbogendurchlüftung der Badflüssigkeit und zur elektrischen Reizung sind nicht abgebildet. Die Perfusion des Trachealllumens und die Einstellung des Ausgangspunktes des Meniscus wird gehandhabt durch die Höheneinstellung des Vorratsgefäßes, die Klemme am Einlaß in das Organgefäß und den 3-Wegehahn. [Nach R. W. Foster, J. Pharm. Pharmacol. **16**, 125—128 (1964)]

c) In verschiedener Weise geschnittene isolierte Muskelpräparate aus Bronchien oder Trachea

Muskelstreifen, Bronchialringe

Die Reaktion der bronchialen oder trachealen Muskulatur kann als Volumenänderung des beiderseits verschlossenen Rohres registriert werden, wie aus dem vorausgegangenen Abschnitt hervorgeht. Um Längenänderungen der Ringmuskulatur von Bronchus oder Trachea als solche direkt zu registrieren, muß das röhrenförmige Organ zerschnitten werden. Verwendet werden Ringmuskelstreifen, spiralig oder in anderer Weise geschnittene Präparate oder die „Kette" aus zusammenhängenden bzw. -gebundenen Bronchial- oder Trachealringen in mannigfachen Variationen.

Die Verwendung isolierter Bronchialmuskulatur zu pharmakologischen Untersuchungen geht auf P. Trendelenburg [185] zurück. Er präparierte Muskelstreifen aus Rinderbronchien, suspendierte sie in Ringerlösung und registrierte die Muskelbewegungen kymographisch. Trendelenburg beschrieb u. a. die bronchialmuskelkontrahierende Wirkung von parasympathomimetischen Alkaloiden wie Muscarin, Pilocarpin, Arecolin, die antagonistische Wirkung von Atropin, und die bronchialmuskulaturerschlaffende Wirkung von Adrenalin, Cocain, Coffein, Chinin, Morphin, Emetin und anderen Stoffen. Auf Pepton und Histamin reagierte der Bronchialmuskel des Rindes nicht.

Macht und Ting [131] verwendeten Bronchialmuskulatur des Schweines in der Versuchsanordnung von Trendelenburg [185]. Sie beobachteten Kontraktion durch Fliegenpilzextrakt, Pilocarpin und $BaCl_2$ und Relaxation durch Adrenalin, Papaverin, Narcotin, Narcein, Cocain, Phenacain und andere Lokalanaesthetica. Morphin, Codein, Thebain und Heroin wirkten nicht oder verursachten nur schwache Kontraktion. Nicotin, Lobelin und Gelsemin verursachten langsame Relaxation.

Wick [191] untersuchte am Trachealmuskelpräparat des Hundes in gleicher Versuchsanordnung die Wirkung von Kohlendioxyd. Das durch 10^{-7} g · ml^{-1} Pilocarpin oder 10^{-6} g · ml^{-1} Acetylcholin zu Eigenrhythmen angeregte Präparat reagierte auf schwache CO_2-Konzentrationen mit einer geringen Kontraktion, auf stärkere CO_2-Konzentrationen mit ausgiebiger Erschlaffung. Nach 2×10^{-6} g · ml^{-1} Atropin kam es zu einer Umkehr der CO_2-Wirkung. Unter der Wirkung von CO_2 kommt es zu einer Verringerung der Empfindlichkeit für Acetylcholin. Diese ist reversibel.

Mohme-Lundholm [139] fand an der Trachealmuskulatur des Rindes in der Versuchsanordnung von Trendelenburg quantitative Parallelen zwischen dem Grad der erschlaffenden Wirkung von Adrenalin, Noradrenalin, Isoprenalin und Ephedrin und dem Milchsäuregehalt des Muskelpräparates. Glykolysehemmung durch Ammoniumkarbonat, Cu-Ionen, NaF, Monojodacetat, Natriumacid, Natriumarsenat sowie $CaCl_2$ verhinderten die relaxierende Wirkung.

„Trachealkette"

Castillo und de Beer [40] beschrieben die isolierte „Trachealkette" des Meerschweinchens: Die Trachea wird excidiert und in etwa 12 Ringe geschnitten, die zu einer Kette zusammen gebunden werden. Das Präparat wird in van Dyke-Hastings-Lösung suspendiert, der 0,05% Glucose zugesetzt ist und die mit Carbogen durchperlt wird. Die Belastung des Schreibhebels ist gering und entspricht etwa dem Eigengewicht des Präparates. Castillo und de Beer untersuchten die Wirkungen von Spasmolytica und spezifischen Antagonisten auf die kontrahierende Wirkung von Histamin, Acetylcholin und $BaCl_2$. Die Ergebnisse sind in Tabelle 15 aufgeführt.

Tabelle 15. *Maximale Verdünnungen (in g · ml^{-1}) der Spasmolytica, die unter den hier beschriebenen Bedingungen (I) eine Dilatation der normalen oder unbehandelten Trachea entsprechend einer Senkung der registrierten Kurve von etwa 1 cm verursachten, und (II) eine definitive Erschlaffung (75-100%) der durch Histamin, Acetylcholin oder Bariumchlorid hervorgerufenen Kontraktion verursachten*

	Normaler Muskel	Histamin phosphat 2×10^{-6}	Acetylcholin-bromide 10^{-6}	Barium-chlorid 2×10^{-4}
Adrenalin	10^{-8}	5×10^{-8}	5×10^{-8}	$1{,}25 \times 10^{-8}$
Aminophyllin	5×10^{-6}	4×10^{-5}	2×10^{-4}	5×10^{-5}
Papaverin	5×10^{-7}	2×10^{-6}	$2{,}5 \times 10^{-5}$	2×10^{-6}
Atropinsulfat	keine Werte	2×10^{-5}	2×10^{-8}	keine Werte
Novatropin	keine Werte	keine Werte	5×10^{-8}	keine Werte
Syntropan	keine Werte	keine Werte	5×10^{-6}	keine Werte
Trasentin	keine Werte	keine Werte	8×10^{-6}	keine Werte
Diphenhydramin	keine Werte	$6{,}1 \times 10^{-8}$	4×10^{-6}	keine Werte

Nach J. C. Castillo, and E. J. De Beer, J. Pharmacol. exp. Ther. **90**, **104—109** (1947).

Lu und Allmark [130] verwendeten diese Versuchsanordnung zum Vergleich der bronchodilatorischen Wirkung von Adrenalin und Noradrenalin und als Versuchspräparat zur biologischen Gehaltsbestimmung von Adrenalin in Lösungen, welche gleichzeitig Noradrenalin enthalten.

Van Arman *et al.* [10] demonstrierten an der Trachealkette die erschlaffende Wirkung von SC-10049 = L-3-{2-[2-hydroxy-2-(3,4-dihydroxyphenyl)-äthylamino]-propyl}-indoltartrat (vgl. auch S. 101), welches in dieser Versuchsanordnung etwa zehnmal wirksamer als Isoprenalin war.

Rosa und McDowall [166] fanden die Kette aus Bronchialringen des Menschen geeigneter als ein spiralig geschnittenes Präparat (s. später). Sie reagierte in gleicher Weise wie die Trachealkette des Meerschweinchens auf Histamin und Acetylcholin mit Kontraktion und auf Adrenalin mit Erschlaffung. Bei der Präparation wurde, ebenso wie bei Antigenzusatz zur Suspensionsflüssigkeit des Präparates eines Allergikers, eine histaminähnliche Substanz freigesetzt.

Hawkins und Schild [96] fanden ebenfalls die isolierte Bronchialkette aus menschlichen Lungen geeignet. Sie verwendeten 3—4 zusammengebundene Ringe aus Bronchien 2.—5. Ordnung von Operationspräparaten, in Ringer-Lösung durchlüftet mit Carbogen, und untersuchten an diesen die Wirkung von Cholinergica quantitativ. Die Größenordnung von Konzentrationen, die abstufbare bronchoconstrictorische Wirkungen hervorriefen, war für Acetylcholin 10^{-6}, für Pilocarpin und Histamin 4—5×10^{-7} g·ml^{-1}. Carbachol wirkte stärker als Acetylcolin, Eserin 10^{-7} g·ml^{-1} potenzierte die Acetylcholinwirkung. Mepyramin antagonisierte die Histaminwirkung in Konzentrationen von 10^{-9} g·ml^{-1}, was der am isolierten Meerschweinchendarm wirksamen Konzentration entspricht. Die Größenordnungen für bronchodilatorische Wirkungen betrugen für Isoprenalin und Adrenalin 10^{-8}, Noradrenalin 10^{-6} und Ephedrin sowie Aminophyllin 10^{-5} g·ml^{-1}. Gleich wirksame Dosen der untersuchten Substanzen waren bezogen auf DL-Adrenalin = 1 für Isoprenalin 0,19, DL-Noradrenalin 23, L-Ephedrin 710 und Aminophyllin 1900.

Schild, Hawkins, Mongar und Herxheimer [171] untersuchten mit gleicher Methode die Reaktionen isolierter Bronchialringpräparate von Lungen von Asthmatikern auf Zusatz des spezifischen Antigens (s. S. 147).

Die Wirkung von 5-Hydroxytryptamin auf die isolierte Trachealkette des Meerschweinchens in der Versuchsanordnung nach Castillo und de Beer untersuchten Freyburger *et al.* [81]. Sie beobachteten Kontraktion durch Konzentrationen von 4×10^{-6} des Kreatininsulfates.

Powell und Slater [161] demonstrierten an der Trachealkette des Meerschweinchens die Hemmung der erschlaffenden Adrenalinwirkung durch 1-(3′,4′-Dichlorophenyl)-2-isopropylaminoäthanol.

Hawkins und Paton [95] untersuchten die Wirkung ganglionaktiver Pharmaka, Adrenergica, Antiadrenergica und Antihistaminica vergleichend an Bronchialringpräparaten von Meerschweinchen, Katze und Mensch in der Versuchsanordnung von Castillo und de Beer. Suspensionsflüssigkeit war Krebs-Henseleit-Lösung, die mit Carbogen durchlüftet wurde. Die Trachealkette des Meerschweinchens wurde durch Nicotin erschlafft. Diese Wirkung blieb aus nach Vorbehandlung mit Nicotin selbst, Hexamethonium, Lobelin, Coniin, Cytysin, Spartein, Anagyrin oder Cocain. Sie wurde vermindert durch Ergotoxin, Ergotamin oder Dihydroergotamin in annähernd gleicher Stärke wie die Wirkung von Adrenalin oder Isoprenalin. Beträchtlich größere Konzentrationen waren zur Aufhebung der Wirkung von Noradrenalin nötig. Atropin oder Mepyramin in acetylcholinantagonistisch bzw. histaminantagonistisch wirkenden Konzentrationen hemmten die relaxierende Nicotinwirkung nicht. Es wird angenommen, daß Nicotin adrenergische Ganglienzellen erregt, welche einen Transmitter freisetzen, welcher eher Adrenalin oder Isoprenalin gleicht als Noradrenalin. Wenn der Tonus der Trachealkette reduziert ist, oder nach Vorbehandlung mit Physostigmin, verursacht Nicotin Kontraktion, die durch Ganglienblocker oder Atropin aufgehoben wird. Diese Wirkung von Nicotin wird als Erregung cholinergischer Ganglienzellen gedeutet.

Primäre Bronchien des Meerschweinchens zeigten außer den vorstehend beschriebenen Reaktionen eine dritte Komponente der Nicotinwirkung, eine langsam einsetzende und lang anhaltende Tonussteigerung. Diese konnte durch Hexamethonium oder Cocain aufgehoben werden, war aber nicht beeinflußbar durch Mepyramin, B_1-Pyrimidin, Physostigmin oder Atropin in spezifisch wirksamen Konzentrationen. Diese Wirkung wurde als eine ganglionäre Reaktion gedeutet, welche nicht durch Acetylcholin oder Histamin vermittelt wird, dagegen möglicherweise durch eine „slow reacting substance".

Isolierte Trachealringe von Katzen zeigten keinen Ruhetonus. Nicotin (20 bis 400 $\mu g \cdot ml^{-1}$) verursachte geringe flüchtige Kontraktionen. Physostigmin potenzierte, Hexamethonium, Cocain oder Atropin hemmten diese Reaktion. Nicotin (20—50 $\mu g \cdot ml^{-1}$) erschlaffte die durch Pilocarpin tonisierte Trachea. Diese Reaktion wurde durch Nicotin oder Hexamethonium blockiert. Die Reaktionen auch dieses Präparates werden auf Stimulierung adrenergischer und cholinergischer Ganglien zurückgeführt.

Carminati und Cattorini [38] verglichen an der Trachealkette des Meerschweinchens nach Castillo und de Beer [40] die Wirksamkeit von Adrenergica, Anticholinergica und muskulotropen Spasmolytica untereinander sowie mit ihrer Wirkung am isolierten Darmpräparat. Nur Isoprenalin und Adrenalin zeigen eine wirklich spezifische antispasmodische Wirkung an der isolierten Meerschweinchentrachea.

Offene Trachealkette

Akçasu [2] modifizierte das von Castillo und de Beer [40] angegebene Versuchspräparat, indem er jeden Trachealring im Knorpelteil öffnete. Nach seinen Angaben wird durch diese Maßnahme eine bis zu dreifache Vergrößerung der Reaktion erreicht.

Akçasu [3] verglich die pharmakologische Reaktivität von in dieser Weise modifizierten Präparaten von Meerschweinchen, Ratte, Kaninchen, Katze, Hund und Mensch. Er fand die Präparate von Katze, Kaninchen und Ratte unempfindlich gegen Histamin, die von Mensch, Hund und Meerschweinchen in dieser Reihenfolge zunehmend empfindlich: die wirksamen Konzentrationsbereiche waren in gleicher Folge 10^{-5}, 10^{-6} und 10^{-7} $g \cdot ml^{-1}$. Alle Präparate reagierten auf Acetylcholin mit Kontraktion, am empfindlichsten die Muskulatur des Hundes (10^{-9} $g \cdot ml^{-1}$), am wenigsten empfindlich menschliche Bronchialmuskulatur (10^{-5} $g \cdot ml^{-1}$). Kein Präparat reagierte auf Nicotin. Kaliumionen verursachten Kontraktion, die nicht durch Curare oder Atropin beeinflußt wurde. Magnesiumionen hatten keine direkte Wirkung, hemmten aber die Wirkung von Acetylcholin und Kalium. Calcium blockierte die stimulierende Kaliumwirkung und verstärkte die Wirkung von Acetylcholin.

Türker und Kiran [186] untersuchten in dieser Versuchsanordnung das Verhalten der isolierten Trachealmuskulatur der Katze. Abweichend von Befunden am Meerschweinchen wirkte Noradrenalin stärker relaxierend als Adrenalin. Die Wirkung von Isoprenalin, Noradrenalin und Adrenalin wurde durch Pronethalol 1—10 $\mu g \cdot ml^{-1}$ blockiert, aber durch Phenoxybenzamin potenziert. Der letztgenannte Effekt wird als Erregung unspezifischer Receptoren gedeutet und gefolgert, daß die relaxierende Wirkung von Catecholaminen ausschließlich durch adrenergische β-Rezeptoren vermittelt wird.

Farmer und Lehrer [72] fanden in der gleichen Versuchsanordnung am Präparat des Meerschweinchens, daß Isoprenalin wie auch Adrenalin und Noradrenalin ebenso wie am ganzen Tier die bronchospastische Wirkung von Histamin stärker als die von Acetylcholin hemmt. Pronethalol hemmt jedoch die äquieffektiven Dosen von Isoprenalin gleich stark, so daß die Isoprenalinwirkung sich ausschließlich an β-adrenergischen Receptoren abspielen dürfte, ohne direkte Beteiligung des Acetylcholin- oder Histaminreceptors.

Paarige Trachealkette

Foster [78] verwendete die Tracheen zweier Meerschweinchen von 600—800 g Gewicht. Von diesen werden jeweils 6—8 Ringe geschnitten und von den fortlaufend numerierten Ringen die geraden der einen Trachea mit den ungeraden der anderen Trachea zu einer Kette verbunden. Die Ringe werden nach dem vorstehend geschilderten Vorgehen von Akçasu im knorpeligen Teil durchschnitten. Die auf diese Weise erhaltenen Präparate werden in Krebs-Henseleit-Lösung von 38° suspendiert. Die Badflüssigkeit wird mit Carbogen durchlüftet. Belastung 240 mg, diese wird während des Wechsels der Badflüssigkeit entfernt und jeweils 5 min vor Zugabe eines Pharmakons angebracht. Die beiden Präparate sind praktisch identisch und verhalten sich in ihrer pharmakologischen Reaktivität dementsprechend gleich. So kann das eine als Kontrolle von Pharmakonwirkungen am anderen dienen. Da die Reaktionen beider Präparate direkt miteinander vergleichbar sind, wird dementsprechend Zeit eingespart.

Foster [80] untersuchte in dieser Versuchsanordnung die Natur der adrenergischen Receptoren der Meerschweinchentrachea. Er bestimmte quantitativ die Wirkungsstärken der Catecholamine Isoprenalin, Adrenalin und Noradrenalin sowie die Wirkungen der Antagonisten Piperoxan, Thymoxamin, Hydergin, Phentolamin und Phenoxybenzamin als α-Antiadrenergica sowie Dichlorisoprenalin, Dichlornoradrenalin, Propranolol und Pronethalol als β-Antiadrenergica. Die Ergebnisse begründen die Annahme, daß die isolierte Meerschweinchentrachea β-Receptoren enthält. Für die Anwesenheit von adrenergischen α-Receptoren fand sich dagegen kein Anhalt.

In einer weiteren Untersuchung bestimmte Foster [80] die Beziehungen zwischen Konzentrationslogarithmus und Potenzierung der Noradrenalin- und Isoprenalinwirkung von Abkühlung sowie von folgenden Substanzen: Desipramin, Cocain, Phentolamin, Phenoxybenzamin, Guanethidin und Metanephrin.

Carlyle [36] untersuchte mit gleicher Methode an der Trachealmuskulatur des Meerschweinchens den Wirkungsmechanismus von Neostigmin und Physostigmin. Er führte die kontrahierende Wirkung dieser Pharmaka auf die Freisetzung von Acetylcholin von postganglionären parasympathischen Nervenendigungen zurück.

Zusammenhängend geschnittene Trachealpräparate

Nach dem Vorschlag von Timmermann und Scheffer [184] wird die Trachealkette des Meerschweinchens alternierend von den Seiten her eingeschnitten, so daß eine zusammenhängende Kette entsteht und das zeitraubende Zusammenbinden der einzelnen Ringe entfällt.

Patterson [154] fand größere Empfindlichkeit der spiralig aufgeschnittenen Trachea des Meerschweinchens. Diese Möglichkeit wurde vorher von Rosa und McDowall [166] angegeben, die jedoch die Kette aus Bronchialringen, jedenfalls für Untersuchungen an menschlicher Bronchialmuskulatur, geeigneter fanden. Die von Constantine [55] veröffentlichte Präparation ist identisch mit der Trachealspirale von Patterson [154].

Bhoola *et al.* [25] spalten die Trachea auf der Dorsalseite longitudinal und schneiden zwischen den Ringen von jeder Seite alternierend horizontal ein, so daß ein Z-förmig zusammenhängendes Präparat entsteht. Dieses wird in üblicher Weise in Krebs-Henseleit-Lösung suspendiert. Bhoola *et al.* untersuchten u. a. (s. S. 123 und 132) auch in dieser Versuchsanordnung die Wirkung von Peptiden am isolierten Trachealpräparat von Meerschweinchen, Kaninchen und Hund. Bradykinin 0,4—2,1 $\mu g \cdot ml^{-1}$ kontrahierte das Trachealpräparat des Meerschweinchens. Phenylbutazon und Amidopyrin wirkten stärker antagonistisch als gegen histaminbedingte Kontraktionen. Am isolierten Bronchialpräparat des Hundes hatte Bradykinin bis 15 $\mu g \cdot ml^{-1}$ und auf die menschliche Bronchialmuskulatur bis 667 $\mu g \cdot ml^{-1}$ keine Wirkung.

Am Trachealpräparat der Katze in der Präparationstechnik nach Akçasu [2] erhielten Türker *et al.* [186] dagegen relaxierende Wirkung von Bradykinin, welche durch Pronethalol nicht blockiert wurde. Eledoisin wirkte an diesem Präparat nicht.

Eine vergleichende Untersuchung der Wirkungen von bronchoconstrictorischen und -dilatorischen Pharmaka in verschiedenen der vorstehend beschriebenen Versuchstechniken an Präparaten von Maus, Ratte, Meerschweinchen, Kaninchen, Katze, Schaf, Hund, Pferd, Rind und Mensch publizierte Siro-Brigiani [175].

2. Allergischer Spasmus der isolierten Tracheo-Bronchialmuskulatur

Im folgenden werden Versuche am allergischen Spasmus isolierter Bronchial- bzw. Trachealmuskelpräparate kurz im Zusammenhang besprochen. Für Einzelheiten wird auf die vorausgegangene methodische Darstellung verwiesen.

Kaninchen

Eine Bronchialmuskelkontraktion ist nicht die typische allergische Reaktion dieser Species. Sollman und Gilbert [176] beobachteten dennoch Kontraktion der Bronchiolen in überlebenden Lungenschnitten.

Meerschweinchen

An Lungenschnitten sensibilisierter Meerschweinchen in der Versuchsanordnung nach Sollman und Gilbert beobachteten Kallós und Kallós-Deffner [116, 117] Kontraktion der Bronchiolen auf Antigenzusatz. Diese wurde durch Theophyllinmonoäthylamin gehemmt.

Hawkins und Paton [95] verwendeten das Bronchial- bzw. Trachealringpräparat nach Castillo und de Beer [40]. Meerschweinchen wurden sensibilisiert durch je eine Injektion von 100 mg Ovalbumin intraperitoneal und subcutan 4 Wochen vor dem Versuch. Hexamethonium 2—$20 \times 10^{-5}\, g \cdot ml^{-1}$ hatte keinen Einfluß auf die allergische Kontraktion ausgelöst durch Zusatz von $10^{-4}\, g \cdot ml^{-1}$ des Antigens zur Badflüssigkeit.

Patterson [154] sensibilisierte Meerschweinchen mit dreimaliger intraperitonealer Injektion von je 4 mg kristallisierten Ovalbumins in physiologischer Salzlösung. Er suspendierte die spiralig aufgeschnittene Trachea in Ringer-Locke-Lösung. Zusatz von Antigen verursachte Kontraktion, die durch Diphenylhydramin $3 \times 10^{-5}\, g \cdot ml^{-1}$ oder Adrenalin $3 \times 10^{-6}\, g \cdot ml^{-1}$ aufgehoben wurde. Zusatz von Hydrocortison hemisuccinat $3 \times 10^{-5}\, g \cdot ml^{-1}$ zur Badflüssigkeit oder Inkubation des Präparates in der gleichen Konzentration für 45 min vor Antigenzugabe beeinflußte die allergische Kontraktion nicht. Histamin verursachte weitere Kontraktion des durch Antigenzugabe maximal kontrahierten Präparates.

Hawkins und Schild [96] fanden keinen Einfluß von Hexamethonium 2×10^{-5} bis $2 \times 10^{-4}\, g \cdot ml^{-1}$ auf die allergische Kontraktion der isolierten Trachealkette des Meerschweinchens in der Versuchsanordnung nach Castillo und de Beer.

Alberty und Huurrekorpi [7] verwendeten gleichfalls die Trachealkette nach Castillo und de Beer. Sie sensibilisierten mit frischem Hühnereiklar 0,1 ml in 0,5 ml physiologischer Kochsalzlösung intraperitoneal, verabreicht an 2 Tagen mit einem Tag Intervall. Allergische Kontraktionen wurden ausgelöst durch Zugabe von 2×10^{-6} bis 10^{-3}, in der Regel mit 5×10^{-4} ml Antigen pro ml Badflüssigkeit. Am gleichen Präparat konnten mit steigenden Antigendosen häufig mehrere allergische Kontraktionen ausgelöst werden. Alberty *et al.* setzten der Badflüssigkeit den Histaminaseinhibitor B_1-Pyrimidin zu und prüften nach Auslösung der allergischen Kontraktion die Aktivität der Badflüssigkeit an der isolierten Trachealkette oder am isolierten Darm eines nichtsensibilisierten Meerschweinchens. Die durch diese „Schockflüssigkeit" hervorgerufenen Kontraktionen waren langsamer und wesentlich geringer als die allergische Kontraktion, gemessen an der Wirkung zugegebenen Histamins. Dieses wurde als Beteiligung nicht mit Histamin identischer, die glatte Muskulatur kontrahierender „H-Substanzen" an der allergischen Bronchialmuskelkontraktion gedeutet.

Berry und Collier [21] präparierten solche „H-Substanz" als partiell gereinigte histaminfreie „SRS-A" (slow reacting substance — anaphylaxis) aus dem Lungenperfusat sensibilisierter Meerschweinchen nach Antigenzusatz und prüften deren Wirkung unter anderen an der isolierten Trachealkette des Meerschweinchens und Kaninchens (über die Versuche am Präparat nach Konzett und Rössler und an der isolierten Lunge s. S. 114 bzw. 126). Sie erhielten langsame Kontraktion an Trachealpräparaten von Meerschweinchen. Die Substanz verursachte nur in 8 von 14 Fällen Kontraktion von Kaninchentrachea-Präparaten, welche alle auf Acetylcholin und 5-Hydroxytryptamin, aber nicht auf Histamin oder Bradykinin reagierten. Am Trachealpräparat des Meerschweinchens antagonisierte 10^{-4} g·ml^{-1} Acetylsalicylsäure die Wirkung von SRS-A in einigen Versuchen, ohne die Acetylcholinwirkung zu beeinflussen.

Mensch

Rosa und McDowall [166] verwendeten kleine Bronchien aus Operationspräparaten und suspendierten sie als Spirale oder als Kette. Letzteres Verfahren fanden sie geeigneter. Sie beobachteten Kontraktion durch Zusatz spezifischen Antigens (Fußbodenstaubextrakt) zur Badflüssigkeit von Präparaten sensibilisierter Individuen. Dabei konnten sie die Freisetzung einer histaminähnlichen Substanz demonstrieren. Chlorcyclizin hemmte die allergische Kontraktion.

Schild, Hawkins, Mongar und Herxheimer [171] studierten diese Beobachtung ausführlicher und mit dem Ziel quantitativer Aussagen. Sie verwendeten ebenfalls die Bronchialkette nach der Technik von Castillo und de Beer [40]. Die Bronchien stammten aus operativ gewonnenem Lungengewebe von Asthmatikern. Auf Zufügung des spezifischen Antigens erfolgte Kontraktion und spezifische Desensibilisierung. Das gleiche Präparat reagierte auf Zusatz eines anderen Antigens, gegen das der Patient ebenfalls sensibilisiert war. Mepyramin und Promethazin hemmten die allergische Kontraktion nur unvollständig und erst in Konzentrationen, die um mehrere Zehnerpotenzen höher waren (8×10^{-6} bis 8×10^{-5} g·ml^{-1}) als histaminantagonistische Konzentrationen (8×10^{-10} g·ml^{-1}). In weiteren Versuchen bestimmten Schild *et al.* die Freisetzung von Histamin durch spezifisches Antigen aus Lungengewebe und Bronchien des Menschen. Diese war von derselben Größenordnung wie die Freisetzung aus entsprechenden Geweben des Meerschweinchens, etwa 2—3 µg/g Gewebe entsprechend 10—16% des Gesamtgehaltes.

3. Durch Pharmaka hervorgerufener Spasmus der isolierten Tracheo-Bronchialmuskulatur

Die folgende Zusammensetzung gibt eine Übersicht über die Größenordnungen wirksamer Konzentrationen derjenigen Pharmaka, die meist zur Auslösung von Kontraktionen isolierter Bronchial- bzw. Trachealmuskulatur in verschiedenen Versuchsanordnungen angewendet werden: Tabelle 16.

Tabelle 16. *Spasmus der isolierten Bronchial- oder Trachealmuskulatur. (Konzentrationsangaben in g · ml^{-1}, sofern nicht anders angegeben.) (Konzentrationsbeispiele; vgl. auch die Angaben von Siro-Brigiani [175])*

Species	Versuchsanordnung	Acetylcholin	Andere Cholinergica	Histamin	5-Hydroxy-tryptamin	Andere Pharmaka oder Maßnahmen	Literatur (Nr. im Literatur-verzeichnis)
Rind, Schwein, Hund	Ringmuskelstreifen	 10^{-6}	Pilocarpin 10^{-6} Pilocarpin 4×10^{-5} Pilocarpin 10^{-7}	Ø Wirkung		Arecolin, Muscarin Muscarin	[139, 185] [131] [191]
Ratte Meerschweinchen	Intakte Trachea („Trachealrohr")	10^{-8} 2×10^{-8}		$> 10^{-3}$ 4×10^{-8}	2 ,5 $\times 10^{-8}$ 5×10^{-8}	 Elektrische Reizung	[112] [112, 37, 79]
Meerschweinchen	Trachealkette (geschlossen)	5×10^{-7} bis 2×10^{-6}	Pilocarpin 10^{-5}	5×10^{-7} bis 5×10^{-6}	4×10^{-6}	$BaCl_2$ 2×10^{-4}	[7, 38, 40, 81, 161]
Mensch	Bronchialkette (geschlossen)	2×10^{-7} bis 5×10^{-6}		2×10^{-7} bis 2×10^{-6}			[96, 166, 171]
Meerschweinchen Hund Mensch	Trachealkette (offen)	10^{-9}—10^{-6}		10^{-7}—10^{-5}		K, Mg, Ca	[2, 3]
Ratte Kaninchen Katze	Trachealkette (offen)	10^{-9}—10^{-6}		—	(Katze) 10^{-8} bis 5×10^{-7}	Bradykinin: 1—5 $\times 10^{-6}$	[186]
Meerschweinchen	Trachealspirale	10^{-8}—10^{-6}		10^{-7} bis $2{,}5 \times 10^{-6}$	10^{-8}—10^{-6}		[55, 154]
Meerschweinchen	Z-förmig geschnittene Trachea oder Bronchus	$2{,}5 \times 10^{-7}$ bis 10^{-6}		5×10^{-7} bis 2×10^{-6}		Bradykinin: $2{,}5 \times 10^{-6}$—10^{-5}	[24]
Kaninchen		6×10^{-8} bis 5×10^{-7}		$> 6{,}25 \times 10^{-4}$		$6{,}25 \times 10^{-4}$ (Ø Wirkung)	[24]
Hund						$6{,}25 \times 10^{-4}$ (Ø Wirkung)	[24]
Mensch		2—7 $\times 10^{-7}$		7×10^{-8} bis 7×10^{-7}		$6{,}25 \times 10^{-4}$ (Ø Wirkung)	[24]

Literatur

1. Aarsen, P. N.: The influence of analgesic antipyretic drugs on the response of guinea pig lungs to bradykinin. Brit. J. Pharmacol. **27**, 196—204 (1966).
2. Akçasu, A.: The action of drugs on the isolated trachea. J. Pharm. Pharmacol. **4**, 671 (1952).
3. — The physiologic and pharmacologic characteristics of the tracheal muscle. Arch. int. Pharmacodyn. **122**, 201—207 (1959).
4. Alberty, J.: Untersuchungen über die histaminantagonistische Wirksamkeit einiger Antihistaminica und von Atropin. 2. Mitt. Antagonismus an der isolierten Meerschweinchenlunge. Arch. int. Pharmacodyn. **95**, 408—427 (1953).
5. — Experimentelle Untersuchungen am Asthma bronchiale. Acta physiol. scand. **31**, Suppl. 114, 3 (1954).
6. — Versuche über den Anteil von Histamin am anaphylaktischen Asthma sowie Beobachtungen über Auslösung und Verhalten der Asthma- und Kreislaufsymptome anaphylaktischer Schockfragmente des Meerschweinchens. Int. Arch. Allergy **14**, 162—204 (1959).
7. —, u. L. Huurrekorpi: H-Substanz-Freisetzung und anaphylaktische Reaktion der isolierten Trachealkette des Meerschweinchens. Acta allerg. (Kbh.) **14**, 386—396 (1959).
8. Alexander, H. L., W. G. Becke, and J. A. Holmes: Reactions of sensitized guinea pigs to inhaled antigens. J. Immunol. **11**, 175—189 (1926).
9. Anthony, A. J.: Methodisches zur Registrierung der Atmung. Naunyn-Schmiedebergs Arch. exp. Path. Pharmak. **169**, 498—502 (1933).
10. Arman, C. G. van, L. M. Miller, and M. P. O'Malley: SC-10049: A catecholamine bronchodilator and hyperglycemic agent. J. Pharmacol. exp. Ther. **133**, 90—97 (1961).
11. Armitage, P., H. Herxheimer, and L. Rosa: The protective action of antihistamines in the anaphylactic microshock of the guinea pig. Brit. J. Pharmacol. **7**, 625—636 (1952).
12. Arunlakshana, O., and H. O. Schild: The air-perfused bronchial tree. J. Physiol. (Lond.) **111**, 48 P (1950).
13. — — Some quantitative uses of drug antagonists. Brit. J. Pharmacol. **14**, 48—58 (1959).
14. Atanackovic, A., et A. de Schaepdryver: Actions pharmacologiques sur les bronches du chien. Arch. int. Pharmacodyn. **85**, 209—216 (1951).
15. Augstein, W.: Über (2)-Amino-(1)-Oxyhydrinden, eine ephedrinartige Substanz. Naunyn-Schmiedebergs Arch. exp. Path. Pharmak. **169**, 114—118 (1933).
16. Baehr, G., u. E. P. Pick: Pharmakologische Studien an der Bronchialmuskulatur der überlebenden Meerschweinchenlunge. Naunyn-Schmiedebergs Arch. exp. Path. Pharmak. **74**, 41—64 (1913).
17. Barer, G. R., and E. Nusser: The part played by bronchial muscles in pulmonary reflexes. Brit. J. Pharmacol. **8**, 315—320 (1953).
18. Bartosch, R., W. Feldberg u. E. Nagel: Das Freiwerden eines histaminähnlichen Stoffes bei der Anaphylaxie des Meerschweinchens. Pflügers Arch. ges. Physiol. **230**, 129—153 (1932).

— — — Die Übertragung der anaphylaktischen Lungenstarre auf die Lunge normaler Meerschweinchen. Pflügers Arch. ges. Physiol. **230**, 674—679 (1932).

19. Beer, Th.: Über den Einfluß der peripheren Vagusreizung auf die Lunge. Arch. Anat. Physiol., Suppl. Physiol. Abt. 101—216 (1892).
20. Bellville, J. W., and J. C. Seed: Respiratory carbon dioxide response curve computer. Science **130**, 1079—1083 (1959).
21. Berry, P. A., and H. O. J. Collier: Bronchoconstrictor action and antagonism of a slow reacting substance from anaphylaxis of guinea pig isolated lung. Brit. J. Pharmacol. **23**, 201—216 (1964).
22. Bhattacharya, B. K.: A pharmacological study on the effect of 5-hydroxytryptamine and its antagonists on the bronchial musculature. Arch. int. Pharmacodyn. **103**, 357—369 (1955).
23. —, and D. Atanackovic: On the pharmacology of procaine and its antagonists on the bronchial musculature. Arch. int. Pharmacodyn. **104**, 275—284 (1956).
24. —, and A. L. Delaunois: An improved method for the perfusion of isolated lung of guinea pig. Arch. int. Pharmacodyn. **101**, 495—501 (1955).
25. Bhoola, K. D., H. O. J. Collier, M. Schachter, and P. G. Shorley: Actions of some peptides on bronchial muscle. Brit. J. Pharmacol. **19**, 190—197 (1962).
26. Bianchi, A., and R. G. de Vleeschhouwer: Effects of vagal stimulation on the isolated guinea pig's lungs. Arch. int. Pharmacodyn. **125**, 248—249 (1960).

— — Effects of various pharmacological compounds on the vagal induced lung constriction. Arch. int. Pharmacodyn. **135**, 472—480 (1962).

27. Brecht, K.: Über die Wirkung elektrischer Reizung des Vagosympathicus auf die glatte Muskulatur der Froschlunge und ihre Beeinflussung durch Ionen bei künstlicher Durchströmung. Pflügers Arch. ges. Physiol. **249**, 94—111 (1947).
28. Brocklehurst, W. E.: Occurrence of an unidentified substance during anaphylactic shock in cavy lung. J. Physiol. (Lond.) **120**, 16P—17P (1953).
29. — The action of 5-hydroxytryptamine on smooth muscle. 5-Hydroxytryptamine (G. P. Lewis, ed.), p. 172—176. London: Pergamon Press 1958.
30. — The release of histamine and formation of a slow-reacting substance (SRS-A) during anaphylactic shock. J. Physiol. (Lond.) **151**, 416—435 (1960).
31. Bucher, K.: Zum Wirkungsmechanismus der Antihistaminica. Arch. int. Pharmacodyn. **79**, 336—342 (1949).
32. Burstein, M.: Recherches sur les circulations sanguine et aérienne dans les poumons du cobaye. J. Physiol. Path. gén. **36**, 62—71 (1938).
33. Busson, B.: Über Eiweißanaphylaxie von den Luftwegen aus. Wien. klin. Wschr. **1911**, 1492—1497.
34. —, u. N. Ogata: Gibt es Beziehungen zwischen den menschlichen Idiosynkrasien und der tierexperimentellen Anaphylaxie? Wien. klin. Wschr. **1924**, 820—823.
35. Cameron, W. M., and M. L. Tainter: Comparative actions of sympathomimetic compounds: Bronchodilator actions in bronchial spasm induced by histamine. J. Pharmacol. exp. Ther. **57**, 152—169 (1936).
36. Carlyle, R. F.: The mode of action of neostigmine and physostigmine on the guinea-pig trachealis muscle. Brit. J. Pharmacol. **21**, 137—149 (1963).
37. — The responses of the guinea-pig isolated intact trachea to transmural stimulation and the release of an acetylcholine-like substance under conditions of rest and stimulation. Brit. J. Pharmacol. **22**, 126—136 (1964).
38. Carminati, G. M., e M. Cattorini: L'attivitá broncodilatatoria in vitro sugli anelli tracheali de cavia. Arch. int. Pharmacodyn. **163**, 186—198 (1966).
39. Carr, E. A. Jr., and Ch. F. Curry: Comparative effects of compound 48/80, histamine and antigen, and the relation between challenging dose of antigen and anaphylactic response in guinea pigs sensitized to egg albumin. Int. Arch. Allergy **8**, 271—283 (1956).
40. Castillo, J. C., and E. J. de Beer: The tracheal chain. I. A preparation for the study of antispasmodics with particular reference to bronchodilator drugs. J. Pharmacol. exp. Ther. **90**, 104—109 (1947).
41. Castro de la Mata, R., M. Penna, and D. M. Aviado: Reversal of sympathomimetic bronchodilation by dichloroisoproterenol. J. Pharmacol. exp. Ther. **135**, 197—203 (1962).
42. Charlier, R., et L. Vandersmissen: Une méthode simple d'enregistrement des modifications du volume pulmonaire chez le chien anesthésié. Arch. int. Physiol. **4**, 433—444 (1954).
43. Cho, W. Y., D. M. Aviado, and P. M. Lish: Efficacy of a new bronchodilator, soterenol, on experimental locked-lung syndrome in dogs. J. Allergy **42**, 36—48 (1968).
44. Cloetta, M.: Zur experimentellen Pathologie und Therapie des Asthma bronchiale. Naunyn-Schmiedebergs Arch. exp. Path. Pharmak. **73**, 233—250 (1913).
45. Colldahl, H.: Gaswechsel und Gewebsatmung beim experimentellen Asthma des Meerschweinchens. Acta physiol. scand. **6**, Suppl. 13, 1—171 (1943).
46. Collier, H. O. J., A. R. Hammond and B. Whiteley: Anti-anaphylactic action of acetylsalicylate in guinea pig lung. Nature 1963, **200**, 176—178.
47. — J. A. Holgate, M. Schachter, and P. G. Shorley: An apparent bronchoconstrictor action of bradykinin and its suppression by some anti-inflammatory agents. J. Physiol. (Lond.) **149**, 54P—55P (1959).
48. — — — — The bronchoconstrictor action of bradykinin in the guinea-pig. Brit. J. Pharmacol. **15**, 290—297 (1960).
49. —, and G. W. L. James: Bradykinin and slow-reacting substance in anaphylactic bronchoconstriction of the guinea-pig in vivo. J. Physiol. (Lond.) **185**, 71P—72P (1966).
50. — — Humoral factors affecting pulmonary inflation during acute anaphylaxis in the guinea-pig in vivo. Brit. J. Pharmacol. **30**, 283—301 (1967).
51. — —, and P. J. Piper: Antagonism by fenamates and like-acting drugs of bronchoconstriction induced by bradykinin or antigen in the guinea-pig. Brit. J. Pharmacol. **34**, 76—87 (1968).
52. —, and P. G. Shorley: Analgesic antipyretic drugs as antagonists of bradykinin. Brit. J. Pharmacol. **15**, 601—610 (1960).
53. — — Antagonism of mefenamic and flufenamic acids of the bronchostrictor action of kinins in the guinea pig. Brit. J. Pharmacol. **20**, 345—351 (1963).

54. Comroe, J. H., B. van Lingen, R. C. Stroud, and A. Roncoroni: Reflex and direct cardiopulmonary effects of 5-OH-tryptamine (serotonin). Amer. J. Physiol. **173**, 379—383 (1953).
55. Constantine, J. W.: The spirally cut tracheal strip preparation. J. Pharm. Pharmacol. **17**, 384—385 (1965).
56. Dale, A. S., and B. Narayana: Observations on the perfused lungs of the guinea pigs. Quart. J. exp. Physiol. **25**, 85—97 (1935).
57. Daly, I. de Burgh, S. Peat, and H. Schild: The release of a histamine-like substance from the lungs of guinea-pigs during anaphylactic shock. Quart J. exp. Physiol. **25**, 33—59 (1935).
58. Dautrebande, L., A. L. Delaunois, and C. Heymans: Method for administering micromicellar aerosols to guinea-pig isolated lungs. J. Physiol. (Lond.) **135**, 14P—15P (1956).
59. —, and C. Heymans: Studies on aerosols. VIII. A method for recording changes in volume of guinea pigs excised lungs after breathing constricting of dilating aerosols. Arch. int. Pharmacodyn. **122**, 448—462 (1959).
60. — E. Philippot, F. Nogarède et R. Charlier: Aérosols médicamenteux. I. Pénétration dans l'organisme et action à distance de substances médicamenteuses introduites par voie transpulmonaire. Arch. int. Pharmacodyn. **66**, 138—167 (1941).
61. Dawes, G. S., J. C. Mott, and J. G. Widdicombe: Respiratory and cardiovascular reflexes from the heart and lungs. J. Physiol. (Lond.) **115**, 258—291 (1951).
62. Delaunois, A. L., L. Dautrebande, and C. Heymans: Method for administering micromicellar aerosols to guinea-pig isolated lungs. Arch. int. Pharmacodyn. **108**, 238—251 (1956).
63. —, and T. O. King: Improvements in an isolated perfused lung technique. Arch. int. Pharmacodyn. **108**, 90—92 (1956).
64. Diamond, L.: Utilization of changes in pulmonary resistance for the evaluation of bronchodilator drugs. Arch. int. Pharmacodyn. **168**, 239—250 (1967).
65. Dixon, W. E., and T. G. Brodie: Contribution to the physiology of the lungs part. I. The bronchial muscles, their innervation, and the action of drugs upon them. J. Physiol. (Lond.) **29**, 97—173 (1903).
66. Doerr, R.: Die Immunitätsforschung, Bd. 8: Allergie. Wien: Springer 1951.
67. D'Silva, J. L., and A. F. Lewis: The measurement of bronchoconstriction in vivo. J. Physiol. (Lond.) **157**, 611—622 (1961).
68. Eichler, O., u. H. Mügge: Zur Methodik der Messung der Bronchialweite am lebenden Tier. Arch. exp. Path. Pharmak. **159**, 613—632 (1931).
— — Mechanismus der Histaminwirkung am Kaninchen. Arch. exp. Path. Pharmak. **159**, 633—656 (1931).
69. — M. Höbel, D. Meroske, K. Wegener u. H. T. Lauer. Quantitative Bestimmung der Aufnahme von Kobalt nach Verabreichung in Aerosolform. I. Beschreibung der Methode und ihrer Anwendung bei Toxizitätsbestimmungen. Aerosolforschung **13**, 526—534 (1967).
70. Einthoven, W.: Über die Wirkung der Bronchialmuskeln, nach einer neuen Methode untersucht, und über Asthma nervosum. Pflügers Arch. ges. Physiol. **51**, 367—445 (1892).
71. Emmelin, N., G. Kahlson, and F. Wicksell: Histamine in plasma and methods of its estimation. Acta physiol. scand. **2**, 123 (1941).
72. Farmer, J. B., and D. N. Lehrer: The effect of isoprenaline in the contraction of smooth muscle produced by histamine, acetylcholine or other agents. J. Pharmacol. **18**, 649—656 (1966).
73. Feinberg, S. M., and S. Malkiel: Protective effect of cortisone on induced asthma in the guinea pig. Proc. Soc. exp. Biol. (N.Y.) **81**, 104—105 (1952).
— —, and F. C. McIntire: The effect of stress factors on asthma induced in guinea pigs by aerolized antigens. J. Allergy **24**, 302—308 (1953).
74. Findeisen, W.: Über das Absetzen kleiner, in der Luft suspendierter Teilchen in der menschlichen Lunge bei der Atmung. Pflügers Arch. ges. Physiol. **236**, 367—379 (1935).
75. Fink, L. D., and J. Akiyama: Response of the excised guinea pig tracheal muscle to morphine and meperidine. Arch. int. Pharmacodyn. **91**, 322—329 (1952).
76. Fleisch, A.: Der Pneumotachograph; ein Apparat zur Geschwindigkeitsregistrierung der Atemluft. Pflügers Arch. ges. Physiol. **209**, 712—722 (1925).
77. Foggie, P.: The action of adrenaline, acetylcholine, and histamine on the lungs of the rat. Quart. J. exp. Physiol. **26**, 225—233 (1937).
78. Foster, R. W.: The paired tracheal chain preparation. J. Pharm. Pharmacol. **12**, 189—191 (1960).

79. Foster, R. W.: A note on the electrically transmurally stimulated isolated trachea of the guinea pig. J. Pharm. Pharmacol. **16**, 125—128 (1964).
80. — The nature of the adrenergic receptors of the trachea of the guinea pig. J. Pharm. Pharmacol. **18**, 1—12 (1966).
— The potentiation of the response to noradrenaline and isoprenaline of the guinea pig isolated tracheal chain preparation by desipramine, cocaine, phentolamine, phenoxybenzamine, guanethidine, metanephrine and cooling. Brit. J. Pharmacol. **31**, 466—482 (1967).
81. Freyburger, W. A., B. E. Graham, M. M. Rapport, P. H. Seay, W. M. Govier, O. F. Swoap, and M. J. Vander Brook: The pharmacology of 5-hydroxytryptamine (serotonin). J. Pharmacol. exp. Ther. **105**, 80—86 (1952).
82. Friebel, H.: Studien am langdauernden Asthma des Meerschweinchens. Naunyn-Schmiedebergs Arch. exp. Path. Pharmak. **217**, 21—34 (1953).
83. — Über die Prüfung von Antihistaminkörpern am tierexperimentellen Asthma. Naunyn-Schmiedebergs Arch. exp. Path. Pharmak. **217**, 35—42 (1953).
84. — Histamin und anaphylaktischer Schock. Z. Aerosolforsch. Beih. 1 (1953).
85. — Über das experimentelle allergische Asthma der Meerschweinchen und seine Beziehungen zum Asthma des Menschen. 1. u. 2. Mitt. Int. Arch. Allergy **5**, 377—395 (1954).
86. — Tierexperimentelle Untersuchungen im Rahmen der Asthmaforschung. Klin. Wschr. **33**, 1—4 (1955).
87. —, u. A. Basold: Über das steuerbare Meerschweinchenasthma. Naunyn-Schmiedebergs Arch. exp. Path. Pharmak. **217**, 13—20 (1953).
88. —, und H. Flick: Über das steuerbare Meerschweinchenasthma. II. Mitt. Versuche mit Acetylcholin. Naunyn-Schmiedebergs Arch. exp. Path. Pharmak. **221**, 258—266 (1954).
89. Giertz, H., F. Hahn, W. Opferkuch u. W. Schmutzler: Vergleichende Untersuchungen über den anaphylaktischen Schock und den Anaphylatoxinschock an der isolierten Meerschweinchenlunge. Naunyn-Schmiedebergs Arch. exp. Path. Pharmak. **242**, 42—64 (1961).
90. Graubner, W., G. Peters u. H. Wick: Gleichzeitige Anwendung zweier Methoden zur Untersuchung der Bronchialweite und zur Prüfung bronchoaktiver Substanzen. Wien. klin. Wschr. **64**, 635—638 (1952).
91. —, u. H. Wick: Der Bronchialmuskelkrampf des Hundes und seine Beziehung zur medikamentösen Asthmatherapie. Arch. int. Pharmacodyn. **84**, 337—347 (1950).
92. Greeff, K., u. E. Moog: Vergleichende Untersuchungen über die bronchoconstrictorische und gefäßconstrictorische Wirkung des Bradykinins, Histamins und Serotonins an isolierten Lungenpräparaten. Naunyn-Schmiedebergs Arch. exp. Path. Pharmak. **248**, 204—215 (1964).
93. Halpern, B. N.: Les antihistaminiques de synthèse. Essais de chimiothérapie des états allergiques. Arch. int. Pharmacodyn. **68**, 339—408 (1942).
94. Hansen, K., u. H. F. Zipf: Beziehungen zwischen Bronchotonus und Lungen-Vagusafferenzen und ihre pharmakologische Beeinflussung. Naunyn-Schmiedebergs Arch. exp. Path. Pharmak. **240**, 253—274 (1960).
95. Hawkins, D. F., and W. D. M. Paton: Responses of isolated bronchial muscle to ganglionically active drugs. J. Physiol. (Lond.) **144**, 193—219 (1958).
96. —, and H. O. Schild: The action of drugs on isolated human bronchial chains. Brit. J. Pharmacol. **6**, 682—690 (1951).
97. Hebb, C. O.: Bronchomotor responses to stimulation of the stellate ganglia and to injection of acetylcholine in isolated perfused guinea pig lungs. J. Physiol. (Lond.) **99**, 57—75 (1940).
98. Heim, F., u. H. Meves: Die Wirkungen von Histamin und Antistin an der in situ durchströmten Froschlunge. Naunyn-Schmiedebergs Arch. exp. Path. Pharmak. **211**, 462—467 (1950).
99. Herxheimer, H.: Repeatable "microshocks" of constant strength in guinea-pig anaphylaxis. J. Physiol. (Lond.) **117**, 251—255 (1952).
100. — The bronchial reaction of guinea pigs to 5-hydroxytryptamine. J. Physiol. (Lond.) **120**, 65P (1953).
101. — Protection against anaphylactic shock by various substances. Brit. J. Pharmacol. **10**, 160—162 (1955).
102. — The 5-hydroxytryptamine shock in the guinea-pig. J. Physiol. (Lond. **128**, 435—445 (1955).
103. — Bronchoconstrictor agents and their antagonists in the intact guinea-pig. Arch. int. Pharmacodyn. **106**, 371—380 (1956).

104. Herxheimer, H.: The bronchoconstrictor action of propranolol aerosol in the guinea pig. J. Physiol. (Lond.) **190**, 41 P (1967).
105. —, u. J. Langer: Untersuchungen über die bronchoconstrictorische Wirkung des β-Receptorblockers Propranolol bei Meerschweinchen und Patienten mit Asthma bronchiale. Klin. Wschr. **45**, 1149—1153 (1967).
106. Heubner, W.: Über Inhalation zerstäubter Flüssigkeiten. Z. ges. exp. Med. **10**, 269—332 (1920).
107. Hicks, R., and G. D. H. Leach: Quantitative evaluation of guinea-pig anaphylaxis in vivo. Brit. J. Pharmacol. **21**, 441—449 (1963).
108. Holgate, J. A., and B. T. Warner: Evaluation of antagonists of histamine, 5-hydroxytryptamine, and acetylcholine in the guinea-pig. Brit. J. Pharmacol. **15**, 561—566 (1960).
109. Jackson, D. E.: A note on the pharmacological action of opium alcaloids. J. Pharmacol. exp. Ther. **6**, 57—72 (1914).
110. Jahn, U., u. Th. Wagner-Jauregg: Vergleich von zwei neuen Klassen antiphlogistischer Substanzen im Collier-Test. Arzneimittelforsch. **18**, 120—121 (1968).
111. James, G. W. L.: The role of the adrenal glands and of α- and β-adrenergic receptors in bronchodilation of guinea-pig lungs in vivo. J. Pharm. Pharmacol. **19**, 797—802 (1967).
112. Jamieson, D.: A method for the quantitative estimation of drugs on the isolated intact trachea. Brit. J. Pharmacol. **19**, 286—294 (1962).
113. Jänkälä, E. O., and P. Virtanen: Bronchographic demonstration of the bronchoconstrictor effect of bradykinin in the guinea-pig. Ann. Med. exp. Fenn. **41**, 436—440 (1963).
114. Jenden, D. J., and J. R. Tureman: New technique for study of drug actions on bronchial resistance in isolated lungs. Proc. Soc. exp. Biol. (N.Y.) **91**, 275—279 (1956).
115. Kabat, E. A., and H. Landow: A quantitative study of passive anaphylaxis in the guinea pig. J. Immunol. **44**, 69—74 (1942).
116. Kallós, P., u. L. Kallós-Deffner: Modellversuche zum Verständnis des allergischen Bronchialasthmas. Acta med. scand. **116**, 409—440 (1944).
117. — — Über die Beeinflußbarkeit des experimentellen Asthmas durch ein Adrenalinpräparat mit Depotwirkung. Acta med. scand. **116**, 441—446 (1944).
118. —, u. W. Pagel: Experimentelle Untersuchungen über Asthma bronchiale. Acta med. scand. **91**, 292—305 (1937).
119. Kiese, M.: Pharmakologische Untersuchungen an der glatten Muskulatur der Lunge (insbesondere mit einigen ephedrinartigen Substanzen). Naunyn-Schmiedebergs Arch. exp. Path. Pharmak. **178**, 342—366 (1935).
120. Koller, E. A.: Atmung und Kreislauf im anaphylaktischen Asthma bronchiale des Meerschweinchens. I. Atmungs- und Kreislaufreaktionen des „Normaltieres". Helv. physiol. pharmacol. Acta **25**, 287—308 (1967).
121. Konzett, H.: The effects of 5-hydroxytryptamine and its antagonists on tidal air. Brit. J. Pharmacol. **11**, 289—294 (1956).
122. —, u. R. Rössler: Versuchsanordnung zu Untersuchungen an der Bronchialmuskulatur. Naunyn-Schmiedebergs Arch. exp. Path. Pharmak. **195**, 71—74 (1940).
123. Kottegoda, S. R., and J. C. Mott: Cardiovascular and respiratory actions of 5-hydroxytryptamine in the cat. Brit. J. Pharmacol. **10**, 66—72 (1955).
124. Kovács, I. B., and P. Görög: Effect of chlordiazepoxide on bronchoconstriction. Arch. int. Pharmacodyn. **173**, 27—33 (1968).
125. Kuschinsky, G.: Untersuchungen über Sympatol, einen adrenalinähnlichen Körper. Naunyn-Schmiedebergs Arch. exp. Path. Pharmak. **156**, 290—308 (1930).
126. Lands, A. M., F. P. Luduena, J. I. Grant, and E. Ananenko: The pharmacologic action of some analogs of 1-(3,4-dihydroxyphenyl)-2-amino-1-butanol (ethylnorepinephrine). J. Pharmacol. exp. Ther. **99**, 45—56 (1950).
127. — V. L. Nash, H. M. McCarthy, H. R. Granger, and B. L. Dertinger: The pharmacology of N-alkyl homologues of epinephrine. J. Pharmacol. exp. Ther. **90**, 110—119 (1947).
128. Lish, P. M., S. I. Robbins and K. W. Dungan: Mode of the bronchodilator action of phentolamine. J. Pharmacol. exper. Ther. **163**, 11—16 (1968).
129. Lopez-Botet, E., F. Wyss u. W. Wilbrandt: Untersuchungen über das experimentelle Histaminasthma beim Meerschweinchen. Helv. med. Acta **19**, 218—237 (1952).
130. Lu, F. C., and M. G. Allmark: A comparison of the bronchodilator activities of adrenaline and noradrenaline: A proposed procedure for the biological assay of adrenaline solutions containing noradrenaline. J. Pharm. Pharmacol. **6**, 513—521 (1954).
131. Macht, D. J., and G. C. Ting: Response to drugs of excised bronchi from normal and diseased animals. J. Pharmacol. exp. Ther. **18**, 111—119 (1921).
— — A study of antispasmodic drugs on the bronchus. J. Pharmacol. exp. Ther. **18**, 373—398 (1921).

132. Manteufel, P., u. R. Preuner: Experimentelle Untersuchungen über den anaphylaktischen Schock als Modellversuch für allergische Krankheiten. Z. Immun.-Forsch. **80**, 65—74 (1933).
133. Martin, J., u. S. Went: Einfluß der Sensibilisierung auf die Histamin-, Cholin- und Acetylcholinempfindlichkeit von Meerschweinchen und Ratten. Naunyn-Schmiedebergs Arch. exp. Path. Pharmak. **193**, 308—311 (1939).
134. McCulloch, M. W., C. Proctor, and M. J. Rand: The enhancement of histamine bronchospasm after blockade of pulmonary sympathetic function. J. Physiol. (Lond.) **191**, 130P—131P (1967).
135. McDowall, R. J. S., and J. W. Thornton: A method of recording the movements of isolated bronchi. J. Physiol. (Lond.) **70**, 44 (1930).
136. Meltzer, S. J.: Bronchial asthma as a phenomenon of anaphylaxis. J. Amer. med. Ass. **55**, 1021—1024 (1910).
137. Mendes, E.: Action of prednisone on experimental asthma of the guinea pig. Acta allerg. (Kbh.) **11**, 181—187 (1957).
138. — Experimental asthma in the guinea pig provoked by anaphylatoxin. Acta allerg. (Kbh.) **13**, 8—18 (1959).
139. Mohme-Lundholm, E.: Effect of adrenaline, noradrenaline, isopropylnoradrenaline and ephedrine on tone and lactic acid formation in bovine tracheal muscle. Acta physiol. scand. **37**, 1—4 (1956).
— Effect of calcium ions upon the relaxing and lactic acid forming action of adrenaline on smooth muscle. Acta physiol. scand. **37**, 5—7 (1956).
140. Nagasaka, M., J. Bouckaert, A. F. de Schaepdryver, and C. Heymans: Adrenergic constriction in isolated guinea-pig lung revealed by nethalide. Arch. int. Pharmacodyn. **149**, 237—242 (1964).
141. — A. F. de Schaepdryver, and C. Heymans: The antiadrenergic property of nethalide on the isolated guinea-pig lung. Arch. int. Pharmacodyn. **149**, 232—236 (1964).
142. Neely, F. L.: Experimental asthma: Treatment with histaminase. J. Lab. clin. Med. **27**, 319—328 (1941).
143. Neergaard, K. v., u. K. Wirz: Über eine Methode zur Messung der Lungenelastizität am lebenden Menschen, insbesondere beim Emphysem. Z. klin. Med. **105**, 35—50 (1927).
144. — — Die Messung der Strömungswiderstände in den Atemwegen des Menschen, insbesondere bei Asthma und Emphysem. Z. klin. Med. **105**, 51—82 (1927).
145. Nisell, O. I.: The action of oxygen and carbon dioxide on the bronchioles and vessels of the isolated perfused lungs. Acta physiol. scand. **21**, Suppl. 73 (1950).
146. Noelpp, B., u. I. Noelpp-Eschenhagen: Die Rolle bedingter Reflexe beim Asthma bronchiale. Helv. med. Acta **18**, 142—158 (1951).
147. — — Das experimentelle Asthma bronchiale des Meerschweinchens. I. Mitt.: Methoden zur objektiven Erfassung (Registrierung) des Asthmaanfalles. Int. Arch. Allergy **2**, 308—320 (1951).
148. — — Das experimentelle Asthma bronchiale des Meerschweinchens. III. Mitt.: Studien zur Bedeutung bedingter Reflexe, Bahnungsbereitschaft und Haftfähigkeit unter „Stress". Int. Arch. Allergy **3**, 108—136 (1952).
149. — — Das experimentelle Asthma bronchiale des Meerschweinchens. IV. Mitt.: Zum Modellcharakter des experimentellen Meerschweinchenasthmas. Int. Arch. Allergy **3**, 207—217 (1952).
150. — — Das experimentelle Asthma bronchiale des Meerschweinchens. V. Mitt.: Experimentelle pathophysiologische Untersuchungen. Int. Arch. Allergy **3**, 302—323 (1952).
151. — — u. K. Lottenbach: Das Verhalten der elastischen Lungenspannung und des Gewebs-Deformationswiderstandes bei der experimentellen asthmatiformen Dyspnoe. Int. Arch. Allergy **5**, 245—260 (1954).
152. Noelpp-Eschenhagen, I., and B. Noelpp: New contributions to experimental asthma. Progr. Allergy **4**, 361—456 (1954).
153. Parrot, J. L., G. Nicot, C. Laborde et P. Canut: Inhibition de diverses actions biologiques de l'histamine par le lysozyme. J. Physiol. (Paris) **54**, 739—748 (1962).
154. Patterson, R.: The tracheal strip: Observations on the response of tracheal muscle. J. Allergy **29**, 165—172 (1958).
155. Petrovskaia, B.: Broncho- and vaso-motor responses of guinea-pig lungs. Quart. J. exp. Physiol. **29**, 121—137 (1939).
156. Preuner, R.: Allergiestudien. I. Die Wirkung der Witterung auf das experimentelle Asthma bronchiale. Z. Hyg. **121**, 559—568 (1939).
157. — Allergiestudien. II. Die Beziehungen zwischen experimentellem Asthma bronchiale und Witterung. Z. Hyg. Infekt.-Kr. **122**, 320—352 (1940).

158. Preuner, R.: Die Prüfung histaminantagonistischer und antiallergischer Eigenschaften des 1-Dimethylphenyliminothiazolidins am allergischen Inhalationsasthma des Meerschweinchens. Ärztl. Forsch. **5**, 64—71 (1951).
159. — Untersuchungen über ein neues Asthmatherapeuticum. Med. Klin. **46**, 1273—1274 (1951).
160. — J. von Prittwitz und Gaffron u. W. Brehmer: Experimentelle Untersuchungen zur Therapie des Asthma bronchiale. Arzneimittel-Forsch. **3**, 337—341 (1953).
161. Powell, C. E., and I. H. Slater: Blocking of inhibitory receptors by a dichloro analog of isoproterenol. J. Pharmacol. exp. Ther. **122**, 480—488 (1958).
162. Proctor, D. F., and J. B. Hardy: Studies on respiratory air flow. 1. Significance of the normal pneumotachogram. Bull. Johns Hopk. Hosp. **85**, 253—289 (1949).
163. Ratner, B.: Experimental asthma. Critical analysis of the literature. Ann. Allergy **9**, 677—694 (1951).
164. Reichel, F.: Diss. Göttingen 1942 (zit. R. Preuner [158]).
165. Rietschel, H.: Zur Pharmakologie von Ephedrin und Isalon. Klin. Wschr. **14**, 1649 (1935).
166. Rosa, L. M., and R. J. S. McDowall: The action of the local hormones on the isolated human bronchus. Acta allerg. (Kbh.) **4**, 293—304 (1951).
167. Rosenthale, M. E., and A. Dervinis: Improved apparatus for measurement of guinea pig lung-overflow. Arch. int. Pharmacodyn. **172**, 91—94 (1968).
168. Schaepdryver, A. de: Actions pharmacologiques sur le muscle bronchique des poumons isolés du cobaye normal et anaphylactisé. Arch. int. Pharmacodyn. **79**, 231—256 (1949).
169. — Actions pharmacologiques sur les bronches du cobaye. Arch. int. Pharmacodyn. **82**, 207—219 (1950).
170. Schaumann, O.: Über eine neue Klasse von Verbindungen mit spasmolytischer und zentralanalgetischer Wirksamkeit unter besonderer Berücksichtigung des 1-Methyl-4-phenyl-piperidin-4-carbonsäure-äthylesters (Dolantin). Naunyn-Schmiedebergs Arch. exp. Path. Pharmak. **196**, 109—136 (1940).
171. Schild, H. O., D. F. Hawkins, J. L. Mongar, and H. Herxheimer: Reaction of isolated human asthmatic lung and bronchial tissue to a specific antigen. Histamine release and muscular contraction. Lancet **71**, 376—382 (1951).
172. Seibert, R. A., and C. A. Handley: The evaluation of some N-substituted arterenol derivatives as bronchodilators. J. Pharmacol. exp. Ther. **110**, 304—308 (1954).
173. Siegmund, O. H., H. R. Granger, and A. M. Lands: The bronchodilator action of compounds structurally related to epinephrine. J. Pharmacol. exp. Ther. **90**, 254—259 (1947).
174. Simke, J., M. L. Graeme, and E. B. Sigg: Bradykinin induced bronchoconstriction in guinea pigs and its modification by various agents. Arch. int. Pharmacodyn. **165**, 291—301 (1967).
175. Siro-Brigiani, S.: Reattività farmacologica dei muscoli tracheo-bronchiali di dieci specie animali. Arch. Ital. Sci. farmacol. **15**, 214—231 (1965).
176. Sollmann, T., and A. J. Gilbert: Microscopic observations of bronchiolar reactions. J. Pharmacol. exp. Ther. **61**, 272—285 (1937).
177. —, and W. F. von Oettingen: Bronchial perfusion of isolated lung as a method for studying pharmacologic reactions of bronchiolar muscle. Proc. Soc. exp. Biol. (N.Y.) **25**, 692—695 (1927).
178. Stormorken, H.: On the pharmacology of the isolated sensitized guinea pig lung. Arch. int. pharmacodyn. **119**, 238—244 (1959).
179. Stresemann, E.: Desensitization in the guinea-pig by anaphylactic microshock repeated at different intervals. J. Physiol. (Lond). **159**, 384—390 (1961).
180. Swanson, E. E., and R. K. Webster: The action of ephedrine, pseudoephedrine and epinephrine on the bronchiolar muscle of the isolated lung. J. Pharmacol. exp. Ther. **38**, 327—342 (1930).
181. Tainter, M. L., J. R. Pedden, and M. James: Comparative actions of sympathomimetic compounds: Bronchodilator actions in perfused guinea pig lungs. J. Pharmacol. exp. Ther. **51**, 371—386 (1934).
182. Thornton, J. W.: Reactions of isolated bronchi. Quart. J. exp. Physiol. **21**, 305—314 (1932).
183. Tiefensee, K.: Pharmakologische Studien an der Bronchialmuskulatur. I. Mitt.: Methodik. Naunyn-Schmiedebergs Arch. exp. Path. Pharmak. **139**, 129—138 (1929).
— Pharmakologische Studien an der Bronchialmuskulatur. II. Mitt: Über die Bedeutung der Blutbeschaffenheit für den Tonus der Bronchialmuskulatur und ihr Ansprechen auf Gifte. Naunyn-Schmiedebergs Arch. exp. Path. Pharmak. **139**, 139—153 (1929).

184. Timmermann, H., and N. G. Scheffer: A new tracheal strip preparation for the evaluation of β-adrenergic activity. J. Pharm. Pharmacol. **20**, 78—79 (1968).
185. Trendelenburg, P.: Physiologische und pharmakologische Untersuchungen an der isolierten Bronchialmuskulatur. Naunyn-Schmiedebergs Arch. exp. Path. Pharmak. **69**, 79—107 (1912).
186. Türker, K., and B. K. Kiran: Adrenergic mechanisms in the isolated cat tracheal muscle and effect of some polypeptides. Arch. int. Pharmacodyn. **158**, 286—291 (1965).
187. Vuilleumier, P.: Über eine Methode zur Messung des intraalveolären Druckes und der Strömungswiderstände in den Atemwegen des Menschen. Z. klin. Med. **143**, 698—717 (1944).
188. Warnant, H.: Recherches pharmacologiques sur le muscle bronchique des poumons isolés du cobaye normal et sensibilisé. Arch. int. Pharmacodyn. **37**, 61—86 (1930).
189. Went, St., u. J. Martin: Über die Schockresistenz der weißen Ratte. Naunyn-Schmiedebergs Arch. exp. Path. Pharmak. **191**, 545—552 (1939).
190. Westerman, E., H. Balzer u. J. Knell: Hemmung der Serotoninbildung durch α-Methyl-Dopa. Naunyn-Schmiedebergs Arch. exp. Path. Pharmak. **234**, 194—205 (1958).
191. Wick, H.: Über die Wirkung der Kohlensäure auf das Trachealpräparat des Hundes. Arch. int. Pharmacodyn. **88**, 450—457 (1952).
192. — Die Beeinflussung der Tracheobronchial- und Alveolarweite durch lokale Einwirkung des Kohlendioxyds. Arch. int. Pharmacodyn. **88**, 461—472 (1952).
193. — Über die Änderung der Lungenelastizität durch Kohlensäure. Arch. int. Pharmacodyn. **89**, 21—27 (1952).
194. — Zwerchfellspannung und Bronchialweite. Naunyn-Schmiedebergs Arch. exp. Path. Pharmak. **215**, 52—57 (1952).
195. Wyss, F., u. F. Schmid: Beruht die bronchialasthmatische Dyspnoe auf einer Bronchialstenose? Schweiz. med. Wschr. **81**, 916—920 (1951).
196. Yonkman, F. F., E. Oppenheimer, B. Rennick, and E. Pellet: Pharmacodynamic studies of a new antihistaminic agent, pyribenzamine [N,N-dimethyl-N′-benzyl-N′-(α-pyridyl)-ethylene diamine hydrochloride]. II. Effects on smooth muscle of the guinea pig and dog lung. J. Pharmacol. exp. Ther. **89**, 31—41 (1947).

Das experimentelle Lungenödem

K. Karzel

Mit 17 Abbildungen

Definition und Abgrenzung des Begriffes Lungenödem

Als Lungenödem wird eine abnorme Ansammlung seröser Flüssigkeit bezeichnet, die aus den Lungencapillaren stammt und intracellulär, interstitiell und/oder intraalveolär im Lungengewebe deponiert ist (s. z.B. Cameron, 1948; Hegglin, 1956; Luisada und Cardi, 1956; Visscher *et al.*, 1956). Die Ödemflüssigkeit ist demnach ein Plasmafiltrat mit einem mehr oder weniger hohen Eiweißgehalt. Einige Autoren schließen auch Blutextravasate (primär hämorrhagisches, toxisches Ödem) in die Definition Lungenödem mit ein (Assmann, 1949; Grosse-Brockhoff, 1951; Halmágyi, 1957), andere (Visscher *et al.*, 1956) sehen Hämorrhagien nur als gelegentliche Komplikationen des Lungenödems an und grenzen sie von diesem scharf ab. Nicht immer wird man die Herkunft von Blutzellen in der Ödemflüssigkeit aufklären können. Sie können nicht nur als unmittelbare Folge ödemerzeugender Schädigungen, sondern auch sekundär bei der Tötung der Versuchstiere infolge intrapulmonaler Gefäßruptur oder Blutaspiration in die Alveolen gelangt sein (Lauche, 1958).

Weitere Schwierigkeiten bietet die Unterscheidung zwischen experimentellem Lungenödem und pneumonischer Exsudation (Luisada und Cardi, 1956; Reichsman, 1946; Robin und Thomas, 1954). Letztere ist zwar im allgemeinen durch ihren Fibrin- und Blutzellengehalt charakterisiert; in den Anfangsstadien der Lobärpneumonie (Büchner, 1955), bei hypostatischer (Giese, 1960) und Viruspneumonie (Harford und Hara, 1950) kann das Exsudat in den Alveolen aber auch weitgehend zellfrei sein (s. auch Spencer, 1962). Außerdem ist die für die Pneumonie charakteristische Blutanschoppung in den Alveolarcapillaren ein häufiges Vor- oder Begleitsymptom des Lungenödems. Schließlich kann eine experimentelle Schädigung der Lunge (z.B. durch Phosgen) zunächst zu rein ödematösen Erscheinungen führen, im Lauf der weiteren Entwicklung aber auch zu entzündlichen Veränderungen mit Zellaustritten aus den Gefäßen (Laqueur und Magnus, 1921a), die möglicherweise durch Sekundärinfektionen verursacht oder kompliziert sind (Heitzmann, 1921; Moon und Morgan, 1936). Eiweißreiche Ödemflüssigkeit in den Alveolen bietet einen guten Nährboden für Erreger (Harford und Hara, 1950). Andererseits erleichtert die Kenntnis der experimentellen Bedingungen und des Versuchsablaufs die Abgrenzung von Lungenödem und pneumonischer Herdbildung, selbst wenn gelegentlich beide gleichzeitig auftreten, wie es z.B. nach Vagotomie der Fall sein kann (Farber, 1937a; Rusznyák *et al.*, 1957).

Pathologische Zustände, bei denen es ausschließlich oder bevorzugt zur Flüssigkeitssekretion in die Bronchien oder Bronchioli kommt, müssen vom Lungenödem abgegrenzt werden (Grosse-Brockhoff, 1957; Schoedel und Grosse-Brockhoff, 1961). Auch hier gelingt die Unterscheidung nicht immer, weil einerseits zum Bild mancher Formen des Lungenödems vermehrte Sekretion der Bronchialschleimhaut zu gehören scheint (Kisch, 1958) und andererseits exzessive Vermehrung der

Speichel- oder Bronchialsekretion ein Lungenödem vortäuschen kann, besonders dann, wenn die Sekrete aspiriert werden (Aviado und Schmidt, 1959; Hahn, 1948; Heinz, 1906; Surtshin *et al.*, 1948). Die chemische Analyse der Trachealflüssigkeit kann die Diagnose erleichtern. Einige Autoren benutzen den Ausdruck Lungenödem ohne Rücksicht darauf, ob die Ödemflüssigkeit aus den Capillaren stammt oder in die Luftwege injiziert wurde (Harford und Hara, 1950; Laqueur und Magnus, 1921a). Klinisch werden akutes, subakutes und chronisches Lungenödem unterschieden. Beim experimentellen Lungenödem wird fast ausschließlich die akute Form erzeugt. Andere Einteilungsprinzipien werden von Halmágyi (1957), Hegglin (1956), Rusznyák *et al.* (1957) vorgeschlagen.

Anatomische und physiologische Vorbemerkungen

1. Alveolar- und Capillarwand

Die Alveolen der menschlichen Lunge sind nach elektronenmikroskopischen Befunden mit einer lückenlosen Cytoplasmaschicht ausgekleidet, die von den Alveolarepithelien ausgeht (v. Hayek, 1957; Schulz, 1959, dort weitere Lit.). Soweit untersucht, gilt das auch für die Laboratoriumstiere der Säugerklasse (Kisch, 1958; Lauche, 1958; Schlipköter, 1958; Schulz, 1959). Die Cytoplasmaschicht bedeckt in einer Stärke von 40—300 mμ etwa 90% der Alveolarwand (Giese, 1960). Sie ist wahrscheinlich an Änderungen der Alveolar- oder Capillargröße anpassungsfähig. Im Kernbereich nimmt die Wandstärke auf 5—15 μ zu. Die Alveolarepithelzellen haben neben ihrer Beteiligung am Gasaustausch vermutlich sekretorische (v.Hayek, 1952, 1953, 1957, dort weitere Lit.) und resorptive (Cameron und Courtice, 1946; Courtice und Phipps, 1946) Funktionen. Sie sondern ein mucopolysaccharidhaltiges Sekret (Clemens, 1956; Macklin, 1954) ab, das nach Macklin einen benetzenden Überzug der Alveolaroberfläche bildet, der etwa 0,2 μ dick ist (Stary, 1959) und dem Teilchentransport aus den Alveolen zu den Luftwegen dient (Friedberg, 1960; Gross, 1953). Ihm wird außerdem ein Einfluß auf die Oberflächenspannung bzw. die Alveolarweite, den Gasaustausch sowie eine Schutzfunktion gegen Austrocknung und gegen das Eindringen von Mikroorganismen zugeschrieben. Die Resorption intratracheal injizierter kolloidaler Teilchen (von der Größe der Plasmaeiweißmoleküle) ist elektronenmikroskopisch nachgewiesen worden (Gieseking, 1959). Glatte Muskelfasern, die von den Bronchiolen ausgehen, erstrecken sich bis in die Alveolargänge (Sturm, 1948; v.Hayek, 1953) und sind wahrscheinlich an der Regulation der Alveolarbelüftung beteiligt.

Die Plasmaschicht der Alveolarepithelien liegt auf der etwa 150 mμ breiten, homogenen Basalmembran. Diese wird damit einerseits von der basalen Zellmembran der Alveolarepithelzellen, andererseits von den Capillarendothelzellen begrenzt. Das Capillarendothel ist im Kernbereich 3—5 μ, in den übrigen Anteilen etwa 200 mμ dick. Der gesamte Luft-Blut-Weg beträgt nach Schulz (1959) 285—640 mμ. Ähnliche Werte werden von Giese (1960), Thews (1961) und von v.Hayek (1957) angegeben. Die 150—500 mμ dicke alveolocapilläre Membran nimmt nach der Schätzung von Giese etwa 80% der Alveolarwandfläche ein.

2. Capillarnetz und Pulmonalkreislauf

Das Capillarnetz um die Alveolen ist engmaschig. Die Räume zwischen den Capillaren sind oft schmaler als die Capillardurchmesser (v.Hayek, 1953). Das Capillarvolumen der Lungencapillaren beträgt nach Piiper (1960) 38% des gesamten Lungengefäßvolumens. Giese (1960) unterscheidet zwischen den an der Basis der Alveolen gelegenen 20—40 μ weiten Strom- oder Ruhecapillaren und den fakultativ durchströmten 6—11 μ weiten Netz- oder Arbeitscapillaren. Die Stromcapillaren, deren Gefäßwandstärke derjenigen der feineren Capillaren entspricht, durchlaufen streckenweise die Alveolarwand und sind dem Gasaustausch dienstbar. In Körperruhe sollen nur 6—10% aller Alveolarcapillaren durchströmt sein (v.Euler, 1951). Die Durchblutung der Alveolarcapillaren wird wahrscheinlich durch Sphincter an den Arteriolen bzw. Sphincterzellen an den Capillaren — wie sie in anderen Organen nachgewiesen wurden (Illig, 1956, 1957) — gesteuert. Die Capillaren erhalten ihren Zufluß aus muskelfreien Präcapillaren, die direkt oder über Arteriolen aus den kleinen Arterien hervorgehen. Der Abfluß des Capillarblutes erfolgt über Postcapillaren und Venolen in die Venen. Die Lobulusarterien sind Endarterien, die keine Verbindung zu Nachbararterien haben; dasselbe gilt für die Venen. Die Pulmonalarterien sind besser dehnbar als die Arterien des großen Kreislaufs und bieten daher einen geringeren Widerstand.

Wieweit arteriovenöse Anastomosen in der Lunge existieren und für die wechselnde Durchblutung der Lunge von Bedeutung sind, ist umstritten. v. Hayek (1953) ist der Meinung, daß bis zu 20% der Gesamtblutmenge des Lungenkreislaufs durch arteriovenöse Kurzschlußwege (Stromcapillaren ausgeschlossen) strömt, ohne mit der Alveolarluft in Berührung zu kommen. Dagegen kommen Bostroem und Piiper (1955) aufgrund eigener Untersuchungen zu dem Ergebnis, daß arteriovenöse Anastomosen bei der Durchblutung der Lunge keine wesentliche Rolle spielen. Mehrere Autoren (Bartels und Rodewald, 1953; Lochner, 1957; Piiper, 1961) geben für die Kurzschlußdurchblutung des gesunden Menschen einen Wert von 2% des Herzminutenvolumens an. Giese (1957) konnte mit einer verfeinerten Arteriographiemethode im Läppchenbereich keine arteriovenösen Anastomosen nachweisen. Demgegenüber scheint das Vorhandensein arterioarterieller und venovenöser Anastomosen zwischen Bronchial- und Pulmonalgefäßen gesichert zu sein (Giese, 1957; v.Hayek, 1953; Heimburg *et al.*, 1961; Mürtz, 1961; Schoedel, 1956; Schoedel *et al.*, 1961).

3. Lymphgefäße der Lunge

In den Alveolarsepten der menschlichen Lunge befinden sich keine Lymphgefäße, sondern nur intercelluläre Spalten (v.Hayek, 1953; Schulz, 1959). Den Alveolarsepten der Rattenlungen scheinen dagegen nicht nur Lymphgefäße, sondern auch diese Spalten zu fehlen (Meessen und Schulz, 1957). Die Gewebsflüssigkeit wird im Bereich der Präcapillaren in die Lymphgefäße überführt. Die Lymphgefäße besitzen im Unterschied zu den Gewebsspalten eine Endothelauskleidung und Klappen. Sie begleiten zunächst die kleinen Arterien und gehen schließlich in die peribronchialen Lymphgefäße oder die der größeren Arterien über. An der Lungenoberfläche breiten sich subpleurale Lymphgefäße aus, die sich im Hilusbereich mit den tiefen Lymphgefäßen vereinigen. Die Lymphgefäße durchsetzen die an der Bronchialwand und der Lungenwurzel bzw. im hinteren Mediastinum gelegenen Lymphknoten und münden im Ductus thoracicus, am Angulus venosus und im Truncus bronchomediastinalis dexter. Ausführliche Beschreibung bei Rusznyák u. Mitarb. (1957) und Drinker (1950).

4. Die Innervation der Lunge

Darstellungen der Lungeninnervation geben Aviado (1961), Daly (1960), Halmágyi (1957, 1959), v. Hayek (1953), Sturm (1948) und Visscher u. Mitarb. (1956). Hier bestehen noch erhebliche Wissenslücken. Die Blutgefäße der Lungen einschließlich der Alveolarcapillaren werden von sympathischen und parasympathischen Fasern versorgt. Neuere Untersuchungsbefunde machen wahrscheinlich, daß die arteriellen, capillären und venösen Anteile des Lungengefäßsystems unabhängig voneinander durch zentrale Impulse beeinflußt werden können und daß zentral ausgelöste Kaliberänderungen der Gefäße als ödemgenetischer Faktor in Betracht gezogen werden müssen (Aravanis *et al.*, 1957). Auch in der Wand der Lungenlymphgefäße sind vegetative Nervenfasern nachgewiesen worden.

5. Vergleichende Morphologie

Der anatomische und histologische Aufbau der Nagetierlunge scheint nicht wesentlich von dem der menschlichen Lunge abzuweichen. Nach Lauche (1958), der die Differenzen ausführlicher darstellt, unterscheidet sich die Rattenlunge am wenigsten von der menschlichen Lunge. Nach Schulz, der — wie mehrere andere (Lit. bei Schulz, 1959) — den submikroskopischen Bau der Lungen einiger Säugetierarten studierte, ähnelt die Hundelunge der menschlichen Lunge am meisten.

6. Der Gasaustausch in der Lunge

Der Gasaustausch in der Lunge erfolgt wahrscheinlich durch Diffusion (Lit. s. Giese, 1961). Er wird daher vom Partialdruck des betreffenden Gases in der Alveolarluft, von der Kontaktzeit zwischen Alveolarluft und Capillarblut (Bartels und Rodewald, 1953), von der Kontaktfläche und den physikochemischen Eigenschaften des Luftblutweges sowie der weiteren Diffusionswege (Plasma, Erythrocyt) abhängen. Über die theoretischen Voraussetzungen für die Sauerstoffdiffusion in der Lunge haben Kreuzer (1953) und Thews (1961) zusammenfassend berichtet; die O_2-Leitfähigkeit eines Mediums ist nach Kreuzer vor allem von seinem Eiweißgehalt abhängig. Die O_2-Sättigung des Blutes hängt außerdem von der Belüftung der Alveolen, der Durchblutung der Capillaren und dem Verhältnis beider Größen zueinander im Bereich der einzelnen Alveole ab (Piiper, 1961).

Beim Lungenödem bildet sich je nach dem Schweregrad ein mehr oder weniger eiweißreiches Exsudat (s. S. 164f.) und der Luftblutweg wird auf das 4—5fache der Norm verlängert (Meessen und Schulz, 1957). Veränderungen der Belüftung und Durchblutung kommen hinzu, lassen sich aber weniger genau erfassen. Alle diese Faktoren bewirken eine — gegebenenfalls hochgradige — Gasaustauschstörung. Rossier u. Mitarb. (1958) fanden bei akutem Lungenödem trotz O_2-Atmung ein Absinken der arteriellen O_2-Sättigung auf 40—70%.

7. Die Permeabilität der Lungencapillaren

Die Capillarpermeabilität wurde kürzlich in einer Übersichtsarbeit von Renkin und Pappenheimer (1957) ausführlich behandelt (s. auch Bennhold und Ott, 1961). Nach Renkin und Pappenheimer sind Muskelcapillaren von Poren mit einem Radius von etwa 31 Å durchsetzt, die den Durchtritt von Wasser und wasserlöslichen Substanzen gestatten. Die Porenzahl pro cm^2 Membranoberfläche wird für Skeletmuskelcapillaren mit $1—2 \cdot 10^9$ angegeben. Als Porenradius von Glomeruluscapillaren wurden 38 Å errechnet; er überschreitet also den Radius der Muskelcapillarporen nicht sehr, doch ist die Zahl der Poren pro Flächeneinheit hier wesentlich höher. Werte für Lungencapillaren sind nicht bekannt, man kann nur vermuten, daß sie in einer ähnlichen Größenordnung liegen oder etwas kleiner sind (Halmágyi, 1957; Hughes *et al.*, 1958a).

Die Austauschvorgänge durch die Capillarwand können auf Filtration und Reabsorption oder Diffusion beruhen. Filtrations- und Reabsorptionsvorgänge hängen — zumindest partiell — vom hydrostatischen und kolloidosmotischen

Druck des Blutes bzw. der extracellulären Flüssigkeit im betreffenden Capillarabschnitt ab. Die Diffusionsrate zwischen Blut und extracellulärer Flüssigkeit wird durch den Konzentrationsgradienten, die Molekülgröße und die zur Verfügung stehende Porenfläche begrenzt.

Kleinere Moleküle werden vor allem durch Diffusion ausgetauscht, Filtration und Absorption haben einen relativ geringen Anteil. Mit zunehmender Molekülgröße wird die Diffusionsrate kleiner. Große, lipoidunlösliche Moleküle (Eiweiß) verlassen das Capillarlumen vorwiegend durch Filtration. In Abhängigkeit von der Capillarpermeabilität und Filtrationsrate können im Verlauf von Stunden erhebliche Eiweißmengen aus den Capillaren auswandern. Sie werden mit der Lymphflüssigkeit dem Blut wieder zugeführt. Da die Capillarpermeabilität von Kaliberänderungen der Gefäße beeinflußt wird (Aviado und Schmidt, 1959; Hughes *et al.*, 1958a; Mack, 1952) und diese der nervösen und humoralen Steuerung unterliegen, können Änderungen der Capillarpermeabilität indirekt — vielleicht auch direkt — über beide Mechanismen induziert werden. Direkte nervöse Einwirkungen auf die Capillarpermeabilität sind häufig diskutiert (Bickel und Dieckhoff, 1954; Driesen und Rummel, 1949; Halmágyi, 1957; Weiser und Rienmüller, 1933), aber experimentell nicht eindeutig nachgewiesen worden (Sarnoff und Sarnoff, 1952a). Einige ödemerzeugende Faktoren wirken vorwiegend durch Steigerung der Capillarpermeabilität. Ob Sauerstoffmangel die Permeabilität der Lungencapillaren erhöht (Drinker, 1950) ist zweifelhaft (Aviado und Schmidt, 1959; Courtice und Korner, 1952; Visscher *et al.*, 1956). Ammoniak, 2-Naphthylthioharnstoff, Phosgen, Ozon und andere reizende Gase und Dämpfe, Virus- und Bakteriengifte, Röntgenstrahlen sollen permeabilitätssteigernde Wirkungen ausüben (Spencer, 1962). In einer Übersichtsarbeit hat Spector (1958) kürzlich über Substanzen, die die Capillarpermeabilität beeinflussen, berichtet.

Beim Austritt von Ödemflüssigkeit aus den Capillaren wirkt nach elektronenoptischen Befunden (s. S. **166** f.) außer Filtration und Diffusion offensichtlich noch ein besonderer pathogenetischer Mechanismus mit. Im Endothelcytoplasma bilden sich Vacuolen, deren Inhalt unter Zerreißung der Vacuolenaußenwand in den pericapillären Spalt abfließt.

Kleine lipoidlösliche Moleküle und Atemgase durchdringen die Capillarwand, ohne Poren in Anspruch zu nehmen. Größere lipoidlösliche Moleküle (Phosphatide, Cholesterol), die in der Regel an Eiweißmoleküle gebunden sind, passieren die Capillarwand mit ihren Trägermolekülen durch die Poren. Blutzellen können nur dann aus Capillaren austreten, wenn die Kittsubstanz zwischen den Capillarwandzellen oder die Zellen selbst fermentativ (Hyaluronidase) oder auf andere Art aufgelöst worden sind (Bennhold und Ott, 1961). Ob und wieweit aktiver Transport bei Austauschvorgängen durch die Capillarwand eine Rolle spielt, ist noch nicht entschieden.

8. Lungenblutvolumen und hydrostatischer Gefäßdruck

Da das gesamte Herzzeitvolumen, das bei der Arbeit das 6fache des Ruhewertes erreichen kann, den Lungenkreislauf durchströmt, muß sich dieser an die großen Schwankungen dieser Zirkulationsgröße anpassen können. Die Strombahn kann durch Einbeziehung neuer Gefäßbezirke (Reservecapillaren) erheblich erweitert werden. Weiterhin setzen die Lungengefäße aufgrund ihres anatomischen Baues einer gesteigerten Blutzufuhr weniger Widerstand entgegen als die Arterien in den übrigen Teilen des Gefäßsystems; wieweit Druckänderungen in den Pulmonalgefäßen bei der Erhöhung des Herzzeitvolumens auftreten, kann noch nicht abschließend beurteilt werden (Cournand, 1950; Lochner, 1957). Die normalen Druckwerte (Methoden s. Lagerlöf, 1955) im Lungenkreislauf sind wesentlich niedriger als die vergleichbaren Werte im großen Kreislauf.

Der hydrostatische Druck in den Lungencapillaren beträgt 5—7 mm Hg. In den übrigen Abschnitten des kleinen Kreislaufs des Menschen wurden in Ruhe gemessen: In der Pulmonalarterie 8—12 mm Hg diastolisch und 20—25 mm Hg systolisch, in den Venen etwa 5 mm Hg und im linken Vorhof 4 mm Hg (s. z.B. Campbell *et al.*, 1951; Cournand, 1950; Grosse-Brockhoff, 1951; Rossier *et al.*, 1958). Für verschiedene Säugetierarten werden Werte in der gleichen Größenordnung angegeben, z. B. für den Hund: arterieller Mitteldruck 20 mm Hg; Druck im linken Vorhof 7 mm Hg (Rusznyák *et al.*, 1957; Sarnoff und Berglund, 1952), für das Meerschweinchen und Kaninchen ein Pulmonalvenendruck von 3,4 bzw. 3,8 mm Hg (Drenckhahn, 1958). Eine Erhöhung des Alveolarcapillardruckes über ein Niveau von 30—35 mm Hg verursacht in der Regel Lungenödem (s. z.B. Drenckhahn, 1958; Hayward, 1955; Hughes *et al.*, 1958a). Die Zirkulationsgrößen des Lungenkreislaufs können durch physikalische und chemische Faktoren beeinflußt werden. In einer Übersichtsarbeit hat Aviado (1960) die Wirkung derartiger Faktoren besprochen.

9. Der kolloid-osmotische Druck

a) Intravasal

Der kolloidosmotische Druck des Plasmas von Säugetieren liegt in einem Bereich von 20—30 mm Hg (Spector, 1956); er ist nicht nur von der absoluten Eiweißkonzentration des Plasmas, sondern auch vom prozentualen Anteil der einzelnen Eiweißfraktionen und vom pH-Wert abhängig (Scatchard *et al.*, 1944). Normalerweise ist der kolloidosmotische Plasmadruck entlang des ganzen Verlaufes der Alveolarcapillaren höher als der hydrostatische Druck in diesen (z. B. Cournand, 1950). Eine alleinige Verminderung des kolloidosmotischen Druckes des Blutes wird für die Ausbildung eines Lungenödems daher weniger bedeutungsvoll sein als für ödematöse Prozesse in anderen Körperteilen. Der *effektive* kolloidosmotische Druck des Plasmas kann allerdings wesentlich geringer als 20—30 mm Hg sein, wenn der kolloidosmotische Druck der extracellulären Flüssigkeit infolge extravasaler Eiweißanreicherung erhöht ist (Hughes *et al.*, 1958). Der kolloidosmotische Plasmadruck wird gelegentlich artifiziell durch i.v. Infusionen verändert. Wenn dieser Faktor und die damit verbundene Hypervolämie zu schon bestehenden Schäden (z. B. infolge von Blutverlusten, chronischen Herz- oder Nierenkrankheiten) hinzukommt, kann Lungenödem provoziert werden (Eaton, 1950; Spencer, 1962).

b) Im Extracellulärraum

Der kolloidosmotische Druck im Bindegewebsraum ist im allgemeinen um etwa 40% niedriger als der des Blutplasmas (Ehrich, 1956). Es ist fraglich, wieweit das auch für das Lungengewebe gilt. Es wird vermutet, daß der kolloidosmotische Druck des Lungengewebes aufgrund eines höheren Eiweißgehaltes der extracellulären Flüssigkeit verhältnismäßig groß ist (Rusznyák *et al.*, 1957; Hughes *et al.*, 1958a).

10. Der mechanische Gewebsdruck

Einen gewissen Einfluß auf die Entwicklung des Lungenödems hat der mechanische Gewebsdruck. Das geht z. B. daraus hervor, daß das intraepitheliale Ödem im Bereich der Capillarvorwölbungen beginnt, wo der Widerstand des Gewebes am schwächsten ist (Schulz, 1959).

Der mechanische Druck des Lungengewebes ist auch von den Druckverhältnissen in der Alveolarlichtung abhängig. Wahrscheinlich ist er im Gegensatz zu den Verhältnissen in anderen Körpergeweben negativ (Rusznyák *et al.*, 1957; Drinker, 1950) und somit ein filtrationsfördernder Faktor. Drinker schätzt diese Sogwirkung auf 5—10 mm Hg bei normaler Atmung.

11. Lymphbildung, -zusammensetzung und -transport

Die Problematik der Lymphbildung und des Lymphtransportes in der Lunge wird ausführlich von Rusznyák u. Mitarb. (1957) diskutiert. Es ist ungeklärt, ob trotz des niedrigen hydrostatischen Druckes im Pulmonalsystem unter normalen Verhältnissen Filtration aus den Alveolarcapillaren erfolgt. Rusznyák u. Mitarb. kommen aufgrund ihrer Untersuchungen zu einer bejahenden Antwort. Der Abstrom der Lymphe aus den Lympgefäßen wird vor allem durch aktive oder passive Bewegungen — hier also der Atembewegungen — gewährleistet; dazu kommen die atmungsbedingten Druckschwankungen, der Einfluß der arteriellen Pulsation und evtl. rhythmische Kontraktionen der Lymphgefäße selbst (Smith, 1949), denn in ihrer Wand sind glatte Muskelfasern sowie sympathische bzw. parasympathische Nervenfasern nachgewiesen worden; Kaliberänderungen bis zum Verschluß von Lymphgefäßen sind möglich (Rusznyák *et al.*, 1957). Es wäre denkbar, daß bestimmte Substanzen durch Einwirkungen auf die Lymphgefäße bzw. den Lymphtransport einen ödemfördernden oder -hemmenden Effekt haben. Adrenalin und Pituitrin z.B. können einen Lymphangiospasmus hervorrufen, Procain verursacht eine Abnahme der Kontraktilität bei gleichzeitiger Erweiterung der Lymphgefäße (Smith, 1949). Der Druck in den Lymphcapillaren beträgt unter normalen Verhältnissen nur 1—2 cm H_2O, er ist in größeren Lymphgefäßen starken Schwankungen unterworfen (Rusznyák *et al.*, 1957; Hansen, 1958) und überschreitet im Ductus thoracicus in der Regel den Venendruck (Paine *et al.*, 1950). Eine Erhöhung des Venendrucks im großen Kreislauf kann den Lymphabfluß beeinträchtigen (Altschule, 1956; Paine *et al.*, 1950; Rusznyák *et al.*, 1957).

Die normale Transportkapazität der Lungenlymphgefäße kann um etwa das 3fache überschritten werden (Rusznyák *et al.*, 1957; Spencer, 1962). Reicht diese Kapazität für die Abfuhr von Flüssigkeit aus der Lunge nicht aus, entsteht Lungenödem.

Der Eiweißgehalt der Lungenlymphe (gewonnen aus dem Truncus lymph. dexter) des Hundes wird mit 3,6% angegeben (Cameron und Courtice, 1946; Rusznyák *et al.*, 1957; Warren und Drinker, 1942), der Eiweißgehalt des Plasmas dieser Hunde mit 5,2% (Cameron und Courtice) bzw. 6,6% (Rusznyák *et al.*).

Die Rückführung eiweißhaltiger Flüssigkeit aus den Alveolen in den Kreislauf wird über das Lymphgefäßsystem vollzogen. Wasser und Elektrolyte können auch unmittelbar in den Blutkreislauf aufgenommen werden. Eiweißmoleküle werden vielleicht auch an Ort und Stelle enzymatisch gespalten. Die N-haltigen Spaltprodukte könnten dann durch die Blutcapillaren abtransportiert werden (Drinker, 1950). Eine aktive Beteiligung der Alveolarepithelien an der Rückresorption von Flüssigkeit aus der Alveolarlichtung konnte bisher nicht nachgewiesen werden, doch ist aus elektronenmikroskopischen Untersuchungen bekannt, daß Partikel in der Größe von Eiweißmolekülen die Alveolardeckzellen auch vom Lumen zum Interstitium hin durchdringen können (Gieseking, 1959).

12. Flüssigkeitsresorption aus der Lunge

Die Resorption intratracheal injizierter Flüssigkeit kann rasch erfolgen. Diesbezügliche ältere Literatur hat Heubner (1925) besprochen. Courtice und Phipps

(1946) und Courtice und Simmonds (1949a) verfolgten an Kaninchen und Hunden die Resorption von Wasser, physiologischer NaCl-Lösung und Serum, die in die Trachea instilliert wurden. 80% des injizierten Wassers war nach 1 Std, eine annähernd gleiche Menge NaCl-Lösung nach 24 Std aus der Lunge verschwunden. Die Resorption der entsprechenden Serummenge dauerte länger als 4 Tage. Mit der Isotopentechnik konnten Qualls *et al.* (1953) den Ablauf der Resorption am intakten Hund verfolgen; sie erzielten ähnliche Ergebnisse wie frühere Untersucher. Auch bei ödemkranken Tieren wurden prinzipiell gleichwertige Befunde erhoben. Auf dem Höhepunkt des α-Naphthylthioharnstofflödems in die Trachea von Ratten injiziertes Wasser oder NaCl-Lösung wurden schnell resorbiert, während heparinisiertes Blut lange in der Lunge festgehalten wurde (Starzecki und Halmágyi, 1961).

13. Zusammensetzung der Ödemflüssigkeit

Über die Zusammensetzung der Ödemflüssigkeit können keine allgemeingültigen Angaben gemacht werden. Bis heute besitzen wir keine Methode, die ihre Gewinnung direkt aus den Alveolen ermöglicht. Sie wird üblicherweise von narkotisierten Tieren gewonnen, denen eine Trachealkanüle eingebunden worden ist (z.B. nach der Methode von Boyd, s. S. 168f.). Bei diesem Verfahren wird von gesunden Tieren Bronchialsekret geliefert (ausführliche Besprechung unter: „Experimentelle Untersuchung der Bronchialsekretion“), von ödemkranken Tieren ein Gemisch von Bronchialsekreten und Ödemflüssigkeit, wobei zu berücksichtigen ist, daß bei Lungenödem auch die Sekretion von Bronchialschleim erheblich gesteigert sein kann (Kisch, 1958). Eine Beimengung von Bronchialsekret ist auch dann möglich, wenn die Flüssigkeit aus den Atemwegen unmittelbar nach Eintritt des Todes gewonnen wird, z.B. durch Ausfließenlassen aus der Nase nach Druck auf den Thorax (Poulsen, 1954a; Flury, 1925) oder bei Hängelage des Tieres (Cameron und Courtice, 1946). Hierbei muß außerdem an die Beimischung von Speichel, Nasensekret, Blut aus dem Nasen-Rachen-Raum (Luisada und Sarnoff, 1946a) und evtl. Mageninhalt gedacht werden.

Die Zusammensetzung der „Ödemflüssigkeit“ ist von der Ödemursache und dem Ödemstadium abhängig. Sie wird ferner von Rückresorptionsvorgängen in den Atemwegen beeinflußt; Elektrolyte und ihr Lösungswasser werden schneller rückresorbiert als Eiweiß (Hughes *et al.*, 1958a; s. auch S. 163f.).

Die Veränderungen, die in der über die Trachealkanüle gewonnenen Expektorationsflüssigkeit im Verlaufe einer Phosgenschädigung auftreten, sind von Boyd und Perry (1960) an Kaninchen studiert worden. Das Volumen und die Zusammensetzung (abgesehen von der Elektrolytkonzentration) blieben in den Anfangsstadien des Phosgenödems unverändert. Erst kurz vor Eintritt des Todes stieg das Flüssigkeitsvolumen stark an und der Gehalt an Elektrolyten und Lipoiden näherte sich in dieser Phase ungefähr dem Plasmagehalt dieser Substanzen. Da Plasmalipoide an Eiweißmoleküle gebunden sind, erlauben die Ergebnisse einen indirekten Schluß auf die Eiweißkonzentration in der expektorierten Flüssigkeit. Koenig u. Mitarb. (1952) fanden beim alkalotisch bedingten Ödem von Katzen mit ähnlicher Methodik einen Eiweißgehalt von 0,8—1,4%. Bei zusätzlich mit Dibenamin behandelten Tieren wurden 4,6—4,9 g-% Eiweiß gemessen. Im Anfangsstadium des Ammoniumchloridödems war die Ödemflüssigkeit von Katzen und Meerschweinchen z.T. eiweißfrei (Koenig und Koenig, 1949b). Beim α-Naphthylthioharnstoff-Ödem von Hunden bewegte sich der Eiweißgehalt der aus der Trachea entnommenen Flüssigkeit zwischen 0,21 und 3,34 g-% (Halmágyi *et al.*, 1955) bzw. 4 und 4,5 g-% (Williams, 1953). Bei einem spontan auftretenden

Lungenödem betrug er 1 g-% (Halmágyi *et al.*, 1955). Ödemflüssigkeit lobektomierter Katzen enthielt 5,7 g-%, ihr Plasma 7,0 g-% Proteine (Gibbon und Gibbon, 1942). Poulsen (1954a) bestimmte den mittleren Wassergehalt der Ödemflüssigkeit von Mäusen (CO_2-Ödem) mit 94,9%, woraus auf einen Eiweißgehalt von 4—5% geschlossen werden kann. Cheng (1948) ermittelte den Eiweißgehalt der Ödemflüssigkeit bei verschiedenen Formen des experimentellen Lungenödems. Die Ergebnisse seiner Versuche gibt Tabelle 1 wieder.

Tabelle 1. *Eiweißgehalt der Ödemflüssigkeit bei experimentellem Lungenödem nach* CHENG *(1948)*

Ödemprovokation durch	Tierart	Eiweißgehalt der Ödemflüssigkeit in g-%
Methylsalicylat i. v.	Kaninchen	7,62
Adrenalin i. v.	Ratte	5,20
O_2-Vergiftung für 5 Tage	Meerschweinchen	4,25
Intracisternale Fibrininjektion	Kaninchen	5,50
Intracisternale Fibrininjektion	Ratte	4,68
NaCl-Infusion in die Art. carotis	Kaninchen	1,25
Ligatur der Aorta	Kaninchen	5,30

Cameron und Courtice (1946) fanden bei voll entwickeltem Phosgenödem im Plasma bzw. in der nach dem Tod gewonnenen Ödemflüssigkeit folgende Eiweißkonzentrationen (Tabelle 2):

Tabelle 2. *Eiweißgehalt des Plasmas und der Ödemflüssigkeit bei Phosgenödem*

	Eiweißgehalt des Plasmas in g/100 ml $\pm \sigma_M$		Eiweißgehalt der Ödemflüssigkeit in g/100 ml $\pm \sigma_M$
	vor Phosgenschädigung	nach Phosgenschädigung	
Kaninchen	$5{,}57 \pm 0{,}12$	$4{,}37 \pm 0{,}18$	$4{,}79 \pm 0{,}24$
Hunde	$5{,}74 \pm 0{,}17$	$4{,}51 \pm 0{,}19$	$5{,}15 \pm 0{,}38$
Ziegen	$7{,}38 \pm 0{,}32$	$5{,}27 \pm 0{,}41$	$5{,}04 \pm 0{,}39$

Ähnliche Werte geben Laqueur und Magnus (1921a) für die Ödemflüssigkeit des Phosgenödems beim Menschen (6,4—7,8% Eiweiß) und bei der Katze (5,9—7,7% Eiweiß) an. Bei klinischen Fällen von akutem Lungenödem wurden 2,5—3,5 g-% Eiweiß in der expektorierten Flüssigkeit gefunden (Hayward, 1955). Ödemflüssigkeit aus perfundierten Kaninchenlungen enthielt 4,7 g Eiweiß pro 100 ml; das Perfusionsblut 6,6 g/100 ml (Hughes *et al.*, 1958a).

14. Blut- und Lymphzusammensetzung bei Lungenödem

Die Blutzusammensetzung von Versuchstieren kann sich während der Entwicklung von Lungenödemen erheblich ändern. Richter (1952) zeigte, daß bei der α-Naphthylthioharnstoff-Vergiftung von Ratten eine Verminderung der durch Entbluten gewonnenen Blutmenge von 3,6 auf 1% des Körpergewichtes eintrat. Spezifisches Gewicht, Eiweiß- sowie Kalium- und Natriumgehalt des Serums bzw. des Plasmas waren dabei kaum verändert. Der Hämatokrit stieg jedoch von etwa 50% bis auf Werte von 80% an. Da der Wassergehalt des Vollblutes (ca. 78%) wesentlich geringer als der des Serums (ca. 92%) ist, muß mit diesem Anstieg des Hämatokrits eine Abnahme des Wassergehaltes einhergehen. Laqueur und Magnus (1921a) berichten über beträchtliche Bluteindickung (Anstieg der Hämoglobinwerte auf das Doppelte) beim Phosgenödem des Menschen und der Katze. Der Wassergehalt des Serums (92%) und der Erythrocyten (66%) phosgenvergifteter Katzen entsprach dabei der Norm, während der Wassergehalt des Gesamtblutes von etwa 82% (Kontrollen) auf 77% (Ödemtiere) absank. Boyd und Perry (1960) konnten dagegen beim Phosgenödem des Kaninchens nur geringe Anstiege des Hämatokrits nachweisen. Auch Cameron und Courtice (1946) fanden beim Phosgenödem des Kaninchens keine eindeutige Veränderung des Hämoglobingehaltes des Blutes und der Erythrocytenzahl, während der Plasma-Eiweiß-Gehalt abnahm. Wurden die Tiere jedoch einige Tage vor dem Versuch auf Trockendiät gesetzt, so stieg nach der Phosgeneinwirkung der Hämoglobingehalt als Ausdruck einer Konzentrationszunahme des Blutes erheblich an. Beim Phosgenödem von Hunden wurden Anstieg des Hämoglobingehaltes, der Erythrocytenzahl und des Hämatokrits sowie der Abfall des Plasmavolumens und des Eiweißgehaltes des Plasmas auch bei normaler Diät beobachtet. Ziegen verhielten sich ähnlich wie Hunde (Cameron und Courtice, 1946). Ähnliche Ergebnisse erzielten Winternitz und Lambert (1919) beim Phosgen- und Chlorpikrinödem von Hunden; der Eindickung des Blutes ging eine Konzentrationsabnahme voraus. Bluteindickung trat auch beim osmotischen Ödem (Injektion hypertonischer Glucoselösung in die Trachea) auf (Laqueur, 1920). Der durch die Bluteindickung bedingte relative Anstieg der Erythrocytenzahl bewirkt eine Zunahme der Blutviscosität. Sie kann erhebliche Grade erreichen und den Kreislauf stark beeinträchtigen (Laqueur und Magnus, 1921a).

Der Eiweißgehalt der Lungenlymphe (gewonnen aus dem Truncus lymphaceus dexter) verändert sich bei Lungenödem nur geringfügig. Bei Phosgenödem von Hunden fiel er von 4,0 auf 3,3%, als Folge eines von 5,2 auf 4,1% verminderten Eiweißgehaltes des Blutes (Cameron und Courtice, 1946).

15. Die pathogenetischen Faktoren und ihre Beziehungen zum mikroskopischen und submikroskopischen Bild

Die Pathogenese des Lungenödems ist in den letzten Jahren zusammenfassend von Altschule (1954, 1956), Aviado und Schmidt (1959), Halmágyi (1957), Hayward (1955), Hilden (1949), Rusznyák u. Mitarb. (1957), Spencer (1962), Visscher u. Mitarb. (1956) diskutiert worden. Die Bedeutung einzelner pathogenetischer Faktoren wurde in zahlreichen Arbeiten untersucht (s. hierzu: Abschnitt III, Erzeugung von Lungenödem). In Abhängigkeit von den Versuchsbedingungen (insbesondere von der ödemauslösenden Noxe) gewinnen sie von Fall zu Fall eine unterschiedliche Bedeutung. In der Regel werden mehrere Faktoren beteiligt sein. Als direkte Determinanten kommen in Frage: 1. Erhöhung des hydrostatischen Drucks in den Alveolarcapillaren; 2. Vergrößerung der Filtrationsfläche; 3. Steigerung der Capillarpermeabilität; 4. Verminderung des kolloidosmotischen Druckes des Plasmas; 5. Zunahme des kolloidosmotischen Drucks im extracellulären Raum; 6. Insuffizienz des Lymphtransportsystems; 7. Änderungen des mechanischen Gewebedrucks.

Der morphologische Aspekt derartiger Faktoren ist lichtmikroskopisch untersucht worden (Ceelen, 1931; Giese, 1960; v. Hayek, 1943; Spencer, 1962). Einzelne Ödemformen z.B. durch Phosgen haben eine besonders intensive Bearbeitung erfahren (Heitzmann, 1921; Laqueur und Magnus, 1921a). Tiefere Einblicke in die pathophysiologischen Vorgänge brachten erst elektronenoptische Untersuchungen. Elektronenmikroskopische Befunde beim Adrenalinlungenödem (Kisch, 1958; Gieseking, 1959), beim Histamin- (Gieseking, 1959), beim α-Naphthylthioharnstoff-, beim Thiosemicarbazid- (Meessen und Schulz, 1957; Schulz, 1959), beim

CO_2-Lungenödem (Meessen und Schulz, 1957) haben gezeigt, daß diese experimentellen Ödemformen mit einer Schwellung und Vacuolisierung der Capillarendothelien beginnen. Die Vacuolen vergrößern sich, bis ihre Außenwand zerreißt und der Vacuoleninhalt in das Interstitium der Alveolarsepten abfließt (Gieseking, 1959). Der Austritt von Flüssigkeit aus der Capillare erfolgt also, ohne daß die Kontinuität der Endothelzellage gegenüber dem Gefäßvolumen unterbrochen wird. Kisch (1958) hat aber auch — gleichfalls beim Adrenalinlungenödem — vereinzelte Capillarrupturen mit Blutaustritten in das Interstitium und die Alveolen beobachtet. Die aus den Capillaren in das Interstitium übergetretene Flüssigkeit breitet sich dort aus und diffundiert in die Alveolarepithelien. Gleichzeitig kommt es zur Schwellung der Basalmembran, zu schleusenartigen Öffnungen in den basalen Zellmembranen der Alveolarepithelzellen (Schulz, 1959) und zur Schwellung der Alveolarepithelien. Diese runden sich ab und zerreißen auf der der Alveole zugekehrten Seite. Außer diesem Mechanismus der intraalveolären Ödementstehung (Schulz, 1959) ist die Transsudation eiweißarmer Flüssigkeit aus den Capillaren in die Alveolen auch bei morphologisch intakten Membranen möglich (Schulz, 1959). Im Falle des Adrenalinlungenödems trägt die stark vermehrte Bronchialsekretion zur Bildung der Ödemflüssigkeit bei (Kisch, 1958). Ob alle Formen experimentellen Lungenödems von gleichartigen morphologischen Veränderungen begleitet werden, kann noch nicht entschieden werden (Giese, 1961).

Die Diagnose des Lungenödems

A. Erkennung und quantitative Bewertung des Lungenödems beim lebenden Versuchstier

1. Symptomatik

Veränderungen des Atemmodus — insbesondere Dyspnoe — können bei Lungenödem vorhanden sein, sind aber kein selektives Anzeichen für diesen Krankheitszustand; auch müssen Flüssigkeitsanreicherung der Lunge und Stärke der Dyspnoe nicht parallel verlaufen (Luisada u. Sarnoff, 1944, 1946a; Winternitz u. Lambert, 1919). So erzeugt z.B. Hypervolämie durch Infusion von Blut schweres Lungenödem mit nur mäßiger Dyspnoe, während nach Infusion eines gleich großen Volumens NaCl-Lösung nur leichtes Lungenödem, aber schwere Dyspnoe auftritt (Luisada u. Sarnoff, 1946a). Aus der Beobachtung der Versuchstiere allein können daher in der Regel noch keine eindeutigen Schlüsse auf ein bestehendes Lungenödem gezogen werden. Erst Austritt von schaumiger Flüssigkeit aus Mund und Nase ist im allgemeinen für Lungenödem beweisend. Dieses Symptom wird aber erst bei schwersten Krankheitszuständen sichtbar (Boyd u. Perry, 1960) und ausnahmsweise können auch starke Hypersekretion der Bronchien und Bronchiolen (Aviado u. Schmidt, 1959; Heinz, 1906), vermehrte Salivation (Hahn, 1948; Surtshin *et al.*, 1948) sowie Blutungen aus Mund- oder Nasenschleimhaut (Luisada u. Sarnoff, 1946a) ein ähnliches Syndrom erzeugen und ein Lungenödem vortäuschen.

2. Der Röntgenbefund

Die Röntgenuntersuchung ist zur Erkennung experimentellen Lungenödems nur selten herangezogen worden (z.B. Laqueur u. Magnus, 1921a; Luisada u. Sarnoff, 1944, 1946). Eine Verschattung im Röntgenbild wird häufig erst sichtbar, wenn das Lungenödem tödliche Grade erreicht. So konnten Visscher u. Mitarb. (1956) an Schafen und Ziegen, bei denen mit anderen Methoden ein massives Lungenödem nachweisbar war, keine Verschattungen in der Lunge finden. Laqueur u. Magnus (1921a) beobachteten bei Ödem durch Phosgeneinwirkung oder nach

Flüssigkeitsinstillation in die Trachea von Katzen bzw. Kaninchen eine Verbreiterung des Thorax sowie Trübung und fleckige Beschaffenheit der Lungenfelder; doch handelte es sich auch hier um die Ansammlung großer Flüssigkeitsmengen (Laqueur u. de Vries Reilingh, 1920b). Ähnliche Befunde erhoben Luisada und Sarnoff (1946) beim hochgradigen Lungenödem des Hundes durch intravenöse Infusion großer Flüssigkeitsmengen.

Zu einer günstigeren Beurteilung der Röntgendiagnostik kommen Kimmerle und Diller (1969) aufgrund neuer Untersuchungen. Bei Beaglehunden, die in einer Inhalationskammer 10 min lang Phosgenkonzentrationen zwischen 115 und 430 mg/m³ ausgesetzt wurden, erhoben sie vor und in bestimmten Intervallen nach der Exposition den Thorax-Röntgenbefund (Aufnahmen in p.a.-Richtung) und ermittelten in Parallele dazu den Hämoglobingehalt und den Hämatocrit des Ohrvenenblutes als weitere Kriterien zur Ödemdiagnose. Aufnahmen in p.a.-Richtung erbrachten unter den gewählten Versuchsbedingungen (die Tiere waren frei beweglich) bessere Resultate als solche bei seitlichem Strahlengang. Als röntgenologische Frühzeichen des Lungenödems nennen die Autoren: Flaue streifige bis milchglasartige Trübungen, die sich zunächst meist perihilär-zentral finden, im weiteren Verlauf an Intensität und Ausdehnung zur Peripherie hin zunehmen und bald inhomogen-fleckig werden. Es zeigte sich, daß die ersten röntgenologisch erfaßbaren Lungenveränderungen stets frühzeitiger nachweisbar waren als die ersten Blutveränderungen. Die „röntgenologische Latenzzeit" war um 4—20 Std (in Abhängigkeit von der angewandten Phosgenkonzentration) kürzer als die „hämatologische Latenzzeit".

Das durch intratracheale Flüssigkeitsinstillation erzeugte Ödem läßt sich auch bei geringer Intensität röntgenologisch gut darstellen, wenn der Flüssigkeit ein Kontrastmittel, z.B. ein Wismutsalz, zugesetzt wird (Laqueur u. Magnus, 1921a).

3. Der Auskultationsbefund

Bei der Auskultation ödemkranker Versuchstiere werden in einigen Fällen verschärftes Atemgeräusch sowie Knister- und Rasselgeräusche gehört (z.B. Brunn, 1933; Farber, 1937a; Fineberg, 1954; Jarisch u. Mitarb., 1939; Luisada u. Sarnoff, 1946), in anderen Fällen sind sie nicht nachweisbar. So konnten Harrison u. Liebow (1952) bei Hunden, bei denen post mortem ein starkes Ödem festgestellt wurde, keine auskultatorischen Symptome wahrnehmen. Laqueur u. de Vries Reilingh (1920a, b) hörten beim osmotischen Lungenödem des Kaninchens (Injektion von hypertonischer Glucoselösung in die Trachea) nur vorübergehend Rasselgeräusche und nur bei einem Teil der Tiere verschärfte Atemgeräusche; aber schon nach kurzer Zeit war oft kein auskultatorischer Befund mehr zu erheben, obwohl bei der anschließenden Obduktion das Lungenödem noch vorlag. Auch beim Menschen besteht offenbar keine Korrelation zwischen der Ausbreitung von Rasselgeräuschen über kleinere oder größere Partien der Lunge und der arteriellen Sauerstoffsättigung (Vitale *et al.*, 1954). Auskultation ermöglicht für sich allein angewendet keine sichere Diagnose.

4. Gewinnung von Ödem- bzw. Expektorationsflüssigkeit

Die physikalisch-chemische Untersuchung der Expektorationsflüssigkeit erfolgt an Proben, die nach Perry u. Boyd (1941) von narkotisierten Hunden, Katzen, Kaninchen, Meerschweinchen oder Ratten gewonnen werden. Den mit Urethan narkotisierten Versuchstieren wird dicht unterhalb des Kehlkopfes eine Kanüle in die Trachea eingebunden, die einerseits der Atmung, andererseits der Ableitung der aus den tieferen Lungenteilen in die Trachea gelangenden Flüssigkeit dient. Die Flüssigkeit stammt aus mehreren Quellen; in jedem Fall aus den Bronchialdrüsen und Becherzellen, evtl. aus den Schleimhautgefäßen, im Falle von Lungenödem auch aus den Alveolarcapillaren. Angaben über Volumen und Zusammensetzung der von verschiedenen Tierarten gelieferten Flüssigkeiten findet man bei Boyd (1954).

Unter dem Einfluß ödemerzeugender Maßnahmen bleibt das Volumen der aus der Trachea gewonnenen Flüssigkeit zunächst unverändert. Erst unmittelbar vor dem Tod, wenn das Lungenödem seinen höchsten Grad erreicht hat, nimmt das Volumen zu (Boyd u. Perry, 1960). Konzentrationsänderungen der Bestandteile (Vermehrung des Na^{+}- und Cl^{-}-Gehaltes) werden im Fall des Phosgenödems schon früher erkennbar (Boyd u. Perry, 1960). Ob allerdings Veränderungen des Ionengehaltes auch bei anderer Ödemgenese nachweisbar sind, bleibt zu prüfen. Sie können sowohl durch eine Störung der Sekretion oder Transsudation der Bronchialschleimhaut als auch durch eine Beimengung von Alveolarflüssigkeit verursacht sein. Bei hochgradigem spontanem (Boyd *et al.*, 1944) oder künstlich ausgelöstem Lungenödem (Boyd u. Lapp, 1946; Boyd u. Perry, 1960) mit starker Zunahme der expektorierten Flüssigkeit wird diese in ihrer Zusammensetzung der des Blutplasmas der betreffenden Tierart (Boyd, 1954) ähnlicher.

Ein wesentlicher Faktor für das späte Auftreten ödembedingter Veränderungen in expektorierter Flüssigkeit mag das Fehlen eines geeigneten Transportsystems sein. Das physiologische Transportmittel für die Bronchialsekrete sind die flimmernden Cilien des Bronchial- und Bronchiolenepithels. Im Bereich der Bronchioli terminales und in den Alveolen fehlt das Flimmerepithel; das Alveolarepithel kann keine aktive Rolle als Transporteur spielen. Ein von Atembewegungen geförderter Flüssigkeitstransport aus den Alveolen wird diskutiert (Boyd, 1954; Gordonoff, 1938).

Ein anderer Faktor mag das Rückresorptionsvermögen der Lunge sein. Solange sich nach der Entstehung eines Lungenödems Flüssigkeitsabsonderung und -rückresorption im Alveolarbereich — selbst unter dem Einfluß ödemprovozierender Gifte — ausgleichen, kann keine Flüssigkeit aufsteigen.

Zusätzliche Schwierigkeiten ergeben sich aus den Rückwirkungen von ödemerzeugenden Mitteln auf den Transportmechanismus; Reizgase hemmen die Ciliartätigkeit (Dalhamn, 1956). Auch Narkosemittel (häufig Urethan) (Boyd u. Perry, 1944, 1960) und Operationsschädigung (s. S. 174) verändern die Ödembereitschaft, die Bronchialsekretion und den Transportmechanismus. Die meisten Narkotica und stark wirkende Analgetica, z.B. Morphin hemmen schon nach kurzer Einwirkungszeit die Ciliartätigkeit (Ernst, 1938; Dongen u. Leusink, 1953). Die Erkennung und Bewertung von Lungenödem wird demnach auch durch die quantitative und qualitative Analyse der Expektorationsflüssigkeit nicht wesentlich erleichtert.

5. Messung des Lungenlymphflusses

Die Zunahme des Lymphabflusses aus den Lungen ist von Cameron u. Courtice (1946), Paine u. Mitarb. (1949a, b), Warren u. Drinker (1942) sowie Drinker (1950) als ödemanzeigendes Merkmal verwendet worden. Die Autoren messen die aus dem Truncus lymphaceus dexter narkotisierter Hunde ausströmende Lymphe.

Paine u. Mitarb. verwenden Hunde in Nembutalnarkose, denen sie zur Markierung der Lymphgefäße 10 ml einer 1%igen Evans-Blau-Lösung in den unteren Teil der Trachea instillieren. 10 min nach der Injektion wird ein Längsschnitt entlang der rechten Vena jugularis externa bis zur ersten Rippe geführt. Die Vena jugularis wird bis zur Einmündungsstelle der Vena axillaris und der rechten Vena subclavia freipräpariert. Das an dieser Stelle mündende Lymphgefäß wird mit einer feinen Schere eröffnet, so daß die Lymphe frei abfließen kann. Bei sorgfältiger Präparation ist der Lymphfluß die einzige Flüssigkeitsquelle. Die austretende Lymphe wird von kleinen, saugfähigen Baumwollstreifen (im Gewicht von 10—20 mg) aufgenommen; die Gewichtszunahme des Baumwollstückchens pro Zeiteinheit wird registriert. — Cameron u. Courtice (1946), Warren und Drinker (1942) sowie Drinker (1950) binden eine Kanüle in das Lymphgefäß ein und wiegen die in der Zeiteinheit abfließende Lymphe. Diese Arbeitsweise ist jedoch technisch schwieriger und führt nur bei einzelnen Versuchstieren zum Erfolg. Nach Drinker wird ein Schnitt entlang der rechten Vena jugularis externa bis in den 3. Intercostalraum geführt. Die Vena jugularis wird bis zum Zusammenfluß mit der Vena subclavia freipräpariert, die abzweigenden kleinen Gefäße werden unterbunden. Die Vena jugularis wird dann nach außen gezogen. Das darunter zum Vorschein kommende Halslymphgefäß wird mit einer Ligatur versehen. Folgt man diesem Lymphgefäß entlang der Vena subclavia ins Körperinnere, so gelangt man zur Einmündung des Truncus lymphaceus dexter in die Vene. In den Truncus lymphaceus dexter wird eine Glaskanüle mit einem Außendurchmesser von maximal 1 mm eingebunden. Die Lymphe beginnt sofort auszufließen. Sie muß klar sein. Erscheint sie milchig-trüb, so sind ihr Bestandteile aus Abdominallymphgefäßen beigemischt. Auch eine Steigerung der Lymphabflußrate beim Druck auf das Abdomen ist für die Beimischung von Lymphe aus dem Bauchraum beweisend.

Bei der Beurteilung der mit dieser Methode gewonnenen Ergebnisse muß beachtet werden, daß die im Normalfall aus dem Truncus lymphaceus dexter austretende Lymphmenge bei narkotisierten Hunden stark schwankt: z. B. zwischen 4—50 mg/min (Paine *et al.*, 1949b), 3,7—59,4 mg/min (Warren u. Drinker, 1942) bzw. 0,1—8,2 ml/h (etwa 1,5—130 mg/min) (Cameron u. Courtice, 1946). Obwohl eine ödemprovozierende Reizung den Lymphfluß in der Regel verstärkt (z. B. Paine *et al.*, 1949a), kann doch angesichts so starker Spontanabweichungen vermehrter Lymphfluß nicht ohne weiteres als eindeutiger Hinweis auf ein Lungenödem angesehen werden. Die normale, durchschnittlich abfließende Lymphmenge muß um das 3—4fache überschritten sein, bevor sie für Lungenödem beweisend ist (Rusznyák *et al.*, 1957). Selbst signifikant vermehrter Lymphfluß zeigt zunächst Licht mehr als gesteigerte Filtration aus Capillaren an. Diese kann im Bereich der nunge, aber auch in der Pleura, im Herzmuskel, im Perikard, im rechten Arm und/oder der Peritonealhöhle stattfinden; denn der Truncus lymphaceus dexter führt auch Lymphe aus all diesen Körperbereichen (Drinker, 1950; Rusznyák *et al.*, 1957).

Die Lymphstrommessung muß daher in der Regel durch andere diagnostische Methoden ergänzt werden. Sie eignet sich weniger zu Routineuntersuchungen als zur Klärung spezieller Fragen der Pathogenese des Lungenödems.

6. Veränderungen der Blutkonzentration

Der quantitative Nachweis von Bluteindickung eignet sich ebenfalls nur bedingt zur Diagnose von Lungenödem. Derartige Veränderungen können aufgrund von Hämatocrit- oder Hämoglobinbestimmungen erfaßt werden. Winternitz und Lambert (1919) haben jedoch bereits darauf hingewiesen, daß das Ausmaß der bei manchen Formen von Lungenödem auftretenden Bluteindickung der Flüssigkeitsansammlung in der Lunge durchaus nicht proportional zu sein braucht. Auch in neueren Veröffentlichungen wird der Wert dieses Verfahrens trotz Anwendung verbesserter Nachweismethoden (z. B. Hämoglobinbestimmung mit der

Cyanhämintechnik) skeptisch beurteilt. So konnten Kimmerle und Diller (1969) phosgenbedingtes Lungenödem bei Hunden nur in einem Teil der Fälle aufgrund von Blutveränderungen erfassen, während gleichzeitig durchgeführte Röntgenuntersuchungen des Thorax eindeutigere diagnostische Schlüsse zuließen. Aber auch bei Tieren mit einem positiven Blutbefund waren röntgenologisch nachweisbare Lungenveränderungen stets mehrere Stunden vor dem Auftreten der Blutveränderungen erkennbar.

7. Messung des Blut- und Plasmagehaltes der Lunge

Die Anwendung radioaktiver Isotope zur Ödemdiagnose haben Aviado (1953) bzw. Aviado u. Schmidt (1952, 1957) vorgeschlagen. Bei narkotisierten Hunden, deren Blut entweder ^{32}P-markierte Erythrocyten oder ^{131}J-markiertes Albumin enthielt, wurde die Radioaktivität der Lunge mit einem Geigerzähler registriert. Der Zähler wurde der Lungenoberfläche in einem luftdichten Rohr aufgesetzt und die Brustwand um das Rohr wieder geschlossen. Veränderungen des Blutvolumens wurden aus der Zahl der ^{32}P-Impulse, Veränderungen des Plasmagehaltes bzw. Ansammlung von Ödemflüssigkeit aufgrund der ^{131}J-Impulse geschätzt. Die ^{131}J-Impulse waren lange vor dem Austritt von Schaum aus der Trachea vermehrt. Die Isotopenmethode läßt demnach ödembedingte Eiweißanreicherungen in der Lunge in vivo frühzeitiger erkennen als die anderen beschriebenen Verfahren. Sie gestattet ferner eine Kontrolle des Wirkungsablaufes therapeutischer Maßnahmen. Enthält die Ödemflüssigkeit aber wenig Eiweiß, so kann mit dieser Technik nicht mehr als die Hyperämie erkannt werden, das Ödem wird nicht angezeigt. Diese Fehlerquelle und der große Aufwand engen die Anwendung der Methode auf die Untersuchung spezieller Probleme ein.

8. Die elektrische Leitfähigkeit des Lungenparenchyms

Änderungen der elektrischen Leitfähigkeit des Lungenparenchyms sind von Lambert u. Gremels (1926) zur Überwachung der Ödementwicklung bei narkotisierten Katzen verwendet worden. Der elektrische Widerstand wurde über eine Wheatstone'sche Brückenschaltung gemessen. Eine Nadelelektrode wurde in der Trachealwand und eine Plattenelektrode zwischen Brustwand und Lungenoberfläche fixiert. Es war Vorsorge getroffen, daß das Trachealgewebe im Bereich der Nadelelektrode nicht austrocknete und die Plattenelektrode vollständig von Lungengewebe bedeckt war. Die künstliche Beatmung wurde auf konstantem Niveau gehalten. Da sich die Widerstandswerte zwischen Inspiration und Exspiration änderten, wurde immer während ein und derselben Atmungsphase gemessen. Eine Blutansammlung in der Pleurahöhle, die die Leitfähigkeit verändert hätte, wurde verhindert. Die Untersuchungsergebnisse zeigen, daß mit zunehmender Ausbildung von Lungenödem durch i.v. Infusion von NaCl-Lösung eine Abnahme des elektrischen Widerstandes des Gewebes eintritt. Die Widerstandsänderungen der Lunge wurden mit dem histologischen Bild und dem Wassergehalt des Gewebes (Entnahme kleiner Proben nach jeder Widerstandsmessung) verglichen. Zunahme des Wassergehaltes und Abnahme des elektrischen Widerstandes waren miteinander vergesellschaftet (s. Abb. 1). Zunahme der Blutdurchströmung der Lunge hingegen hatte keinen Einfluß auf ihre elektrische Leitfähigkeit.

Aviado und Schmidt (1952) versuchten die Methode der Widerstandsmessung dadurch zu verbessern, daß sie anstelle des Gleichstromwiderstandes den Wechselstromwiderstand registrierten und anstelle von Kupferelektroden Platinelektroden verwendeten. Fehler, die durch Polarisation der Elektroden zustande kommen, sollten auf diese Weise ausgeschaltet werden. Als Wechselstromquelle wurde der Oszillator Hewlett-Packard 200 C, zur Impedanzangleichung die Wechselstrombrücke General Radio Typ 650 A, als Nullpunktanzeiger das Oszilloskop Dumont Typ 304 verwendet. Der Widerstand war von der Distanz zwischen den beiden Elektroden und innerhalb eines bestimmten Bereiches von der Frequenz abhängig, oberhalb von 20000 Hz für die gewählte Distanz jedoch konstant. Für die Messungen wurde diese Frequenz gewählt. Zur Untersuchung am intakten Tier wurde der Thorax geöffnet und nach Einstich der Elektrodenspitzen an zwei Stellen eines Lappens wieder geschlossen; die Atembewegungen kamen auf dem Oszilloskop zur Darstellung. Bei normalen Tieren lag der Widerstand, abhängig von der Elektrodendistanz, zwischen 0,167 und 1,17 Ω. Registriert wurden die

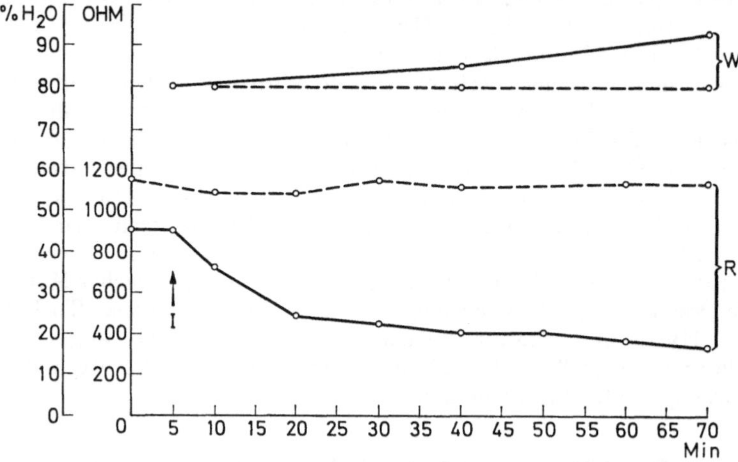

Abb. 1. Wassergehalt (W) und elektrischer Gewebswiderstand (R) der Lungen intakter Katzen bei Ödem durch Infusion von NaCl-Lösung (ausgezogene Linien) und bei Kontrolltieren (punktierte Linien). (Aus: Lambert u. Gremels, 1926)

prozentualen Änderungen des Widerstandes. Wiederholte Kontrollmessungen variierten um 3% oder weniger. Die Einführung der Elektroden durch die geschlossene Thoraxwand ist mit Hilfe von Kanülen möglich. Eine Elektrode kann auch in einem Pulmonalarterienkatheter so weit wie möglich in eine Lobararterie vorgeschoben werden, während die Gegenelektrode an der benachbarten Brustwand befestigt wird.

Ödemprovozierende Maßnahmen (Alloxaninjektion, Dampfinhalation) bewirkten Abnahmen, Blutverluste, Zunahmen des Widerstandes. Wie Messungen an der isolierten Hundelunge zeigten, registriert die Methode jedoch lediglich Änderungen des Gesamtflüssigkeitsgehaltes der Lunge; sie läßt keine Unterscheidung zwischen Ansammlung von Ödemflüssigkeit und Zunahme des Blutvolumens zu.

9. Die mechanischen Eigenschaften der Lunge

Gelegentlich ist versucht worden, Veränderungen der mechanischen Eigenschaften der Lunge für die Ödemerkennung zu verwerten. So haben Laqueur u. Magnus (1921a) Veränderungen des Dondersschen Druckes zur Beurteilung der Lungenelastizität verwendet. Unmittelbar nach Eintritt des Todes (vor Ausbildung der Totenstarre) wurde eine Kanüle, die mit einem Wassermanometer verbunden war, endständig in der Trachea des Tieres fixiert. Dann wurden beide Pleurahöhlen geöffnet, so daß die Lunge sich entsprechend ihrer Elastizität zusammenziehen konnte und der Manometerstand anstieg. Bei gesunden Katzen mit relativen Lungengewichten von 8—10 g/kg wurde ein Donderscher Druck von durchschnittlich 36 mm H_2O, bei ödemkranken Tieren mit Lungengewichten von 20—40 g/kg ein Druck von 26 mm H_2O (72% der Norm) gemessen.

In jüngeren Beiträgen (Hughes *et al.*, 1958b; Moore u. Sexter, 1956) ist die „compliance" (Dehnbarkeit der Lunge) — der reziproke Wert des elastischen Lungenwiderstandes — zur Beurteilung des Lungenödems in vivo und am perfundierten Organ herangezogen worden. Die Compliance ist definiert als das Verhältnis von Volumenänderung der Lunge zu intrathorakaler Druckänderung. Sie wird in l/cm H_2O gemessen. Diskussion der Problematik und Literaturangaben bei Borst *et al.* (1957), Lottenbach *et al.* (1956), Rossier *et al.* (1958). Verschiedene pathophysiologische Zustände der Lunge (Emphysem, Stauung, pulmonale Hypertension) verändern die Compliance im gleichen Sinne wie Lungenödem (Bondurant *et al.*, 1957; Borst *et al.*, 1957). Aus diesem Grund wird man von diesem Verfahren dort keine eindeutigen diagnostischen Hinweise erwarten können, wo der Pathomechanismus von Compliance-Änderungen nicht bekannt ist.

Hughes u. Mitarb. (1958b) bestimmten die Compliance narkotisierter Katzen (Pentobarbital i.p.). Der intrapleurale Druck wurde über einen intrapleuralen Katheter manometrisch registriert, Lungenvolumenänderungen wurden mit Hilfe eines Pneumotachographen aufgezeichnet. Die Compliance wurde aus dem intrapleuralen Druck und dem korrespondierenden Lungenvolumen im Augenblick der Atemruhelage bestimmt. Da die Druckmessung bei hoher Atemfrequenz schwierig war, wurde notfalls mit einer Injektionsspritze unter positivem Druck Luft in die Lunge geblasen, der transpulmonale Druck bei verschiedenen Füllungsvolumina gemessen und der Berechnung der Compliance zugrunde gelegt. Bei ödematösen Lungen war eine Verdoppelung des Lungengewichtes von einer Abnahme der Compliance um 30% begleitet. Gleichgroße Reduktionen der Compliance können aber auch die Folge pulmonaler Hyperämie sein. Kreislaufaktive Substanzen (wie z.B. Adrenalin, Histamin) verändern die Compliance schon nach Gaben, die zur Auslösung eines Lungenödems offensichtlich nicht ausreichen (Bucher, 1960; Meier, 1960). Werden zur Ödemprovokation Substanzen angewandt, die einen Einfluß auf die Bronchialweite ausüben (wie z.B. Histamin) oder die Bronchialsekretion anregen, muß mit einer Verfälschung des Ergebnisses gerechnet werden (Radford u. Lefcoe, 1955; Bucher, 1957, 1960).

10. Die Diffusionskapazität der Lunge

Ein von Henschler (1964) angegebenes Verfahren, das sich zur Erkennung auch geringgradiger Lungenfunktionsstörungen eignet, zieht die Diffusionskapazität der Lunge für Kohlenoxyd als diagnostisches Kriterium heran. Die zu beurteilenden Versuchstiere (verwendet wurden Mäuse oder Ratten) werden in einem geschlossenen System einer CO-Konzentration von 200 ppm ausgesetzt. Kohlendioxyd und Wasserdampf werden über eine Membranpumpe in Patronen absorbiert, während der verbrauchte Sauerstoff aus einem Spirometer nachströmt. Die CO-Konzentration wird mit Hilfe eines Infrarotanalysators bestimmt; die Abatmungsgeschwindigkeit dient als Maß der Diffusionskapazität. Die Prüfung wird am wachen, ungezwungenen Tier durchgeführt, erstreckt sich über 15 min und kann beliebig oft wiederholt werden. Zur Beurteilung der Lungenfunktionsstörung werden die vor und nach Einwirkung der Ödemnoxe ermittelten Werte für die Abatmungsgeschwindigkeit zueinander in Beziehung gesetzt.

11. Diskussion der Methoden

Keine der genannten Methoden ermöglicht in idealer Weise ein frühzeitiger und quantitatives Erkennen von Lungenödem, ja mit Ausnahme der Durchleuchtung und der Auskultation komplizieren die diagnostischen Maßnahmen die pathophysiologische Situation, denn einige können den Reizeffekt verstärken, andere abschwächen oder qualitativ verändern.

Narkotica beeinflussen die Entwicklung von Lungenödem in unterschiedliches Weise (Luisada, 1928; Luisada u. Sarnoff, 1944). Äthernarkose z.B. vermindert die Ödembereitschaft beim Ammoniumchloridödem (Cameron u. Sheikh, 1951; MacKay *et al.*, 1949), Thiosemicarbazidödem (Tennekoon, 1954), Adrenalinödem (Luisada, 1950a; Poulsen, 1954d) und CO_2-Ödem (Poulsen, 1954d); Phenobarbital verstärkt adrenalinbedingtes (Stone u. Loew, 1949) und hemmt durch Hypervolämie ausgelöstes Lungenödem (Luisada u. Sarnoff, 1946b); Pentobarbital hemmt das Thiosemicarbazidödem (Tennekoon, 1954); Aprobarbital (Allylpropymal), in narkotischer Dosis angewandt, verhindert die Ausbildung des CO_2-Ödems völlig (Poulsen, 1954c); Chloralhydrat und Urethan hemmen das Veratrinlungenödem bei Kaninchen und Meerschweinchen, bei Ratten jedoch nicht; dagegen gelingt es bei Kaninchen in Chloralosenarkose durch Veratrin Lungenödem zu erzeugen (Jarisch *et al.*, 1939). Dasselbe Narkosemittel verhindert das Ammoniumchloridödem (Cameron u. Sheikh, 1951). Äther- und in stärkerem Maße Urethannarkose hemmen vagotomiebedingtes Lungenödem (Reichsman, 1946); Barbituratnarkose oder Lokalanaesthesie sind in dieser Hinsicht anscheinend wirkungslos (Farber, 1937a, b; Lorber, 1939a, b). Das O_2-Ödem wird durch Urethan gedämpft (Gottsegen *et al.*, 1957). Der Lymphfluß von Hunden wird durch Ätherinhalation gesteigert, Lokalanaesthesie bedingt keine Zunahme, unter Pentobarbital-Na und Cyclopropan ist er vermindert (Beecher *et al.*, 1948; Flinker u. McCarrell, 1949; Hungerford u. Reinhardt, 1950). Auf Katzen wirkten Äther- und Barbituratnarkose in gleicher Weise lymphflußsteigernd (Flinker u. McCarrell, 1949). Die Narkosefolgen werden durch das Alter der Versuchstiere modifiziert. Bei 60 Tage alten Ratten waren keine durch Narkosehilfsmittel bedingte Differenzen nachweisbar, 40 Tage alte Tiere reagierten auf Äther- und Barbituratnarkose unterschiedlich (Hungerford u. Reinhardt, 1950).

Operative Eingriffe verschiedener Art können die Ödembereitschaft verändern. Abdominaloperationen wirken ödemhemmend. Polli und Luisada (1957) führen diesen Effekt auf die Auslösung einer unspezifischen Stressreaktion zurück. Tracheotomie kann bei langdauernden Versuchen von sich aus ödemprovozierend wirken, wenn durch die Ausschaltung des Kehlkopfes und das Hindernis der Trachealkanüle der normale Transport von Sekreten unterbrochen wird. Nicht selten sammeln sich vor der Kanüle Sekrete an, die die Gaspassage erschweren, Asphyxie hervorrufen und Lungenödem bewirken (Short, 1944). Künstliche Beatmung mit Atempumpen kann die Sekretion, Transsudation und Drainage von Flüssigkeit aus der Lunge und den Atemwegen in unphysiologischer Weise beeinflussen (Drinker, 1950; Lorber, 1939a). Bei Hunden hemmte Beatmung unter erhöhtem Druck (18 cm H_2O) die durch intraarterielle Flüssigkeitsinfusion provozierte Ödementstehung und förderte sie unter vermindertem Druck (Luisada u. Sarnoff, 1946a). Bei narkotisierten, im übrigen aber unbehandelten Meerschweinchen wirkte künstliche Beatmung unter hohem Druck (20 mm Hg) ödemprovozierend, während Beatmung unter geringerem Druck (6 mm Hg) auch bei langer Dauer (bis zu 25 Std) keine nachteiligen Folgen hatte (Sussman *et al.*, 1948).

Abnorme Körperlage, die narkotisierten Tieren während des Versuches nicht selten aufgezwungen wird, kann morphologische Veränderungen der Lunge zur

Folge haben und den Verlauf der Ödemkrankheit beeinflussen. Die abhängigen Partien der Lunge neigen zuerst zu vermehrter Blutfüllung (Luisada u. Sarnoff, 1946a). Drinker (1950) zeigte, daß bei narkotisierten Hunden, die in Rückenlage fixiert sind, schon nach $2^1/_2$ Std schwere Blutstauung, Atelektasen und Ödem in den Lungen, besonders in ihren abhängigen Partien nachweisbar sind. Visscher u. Mitarb. (1956) sahen bei Schafen und Ziegen, die in Rückenlage gehalten wurden, Lungenödem entstehen. Für ödematöse Kaninchen erwies sich die Rückenlage als schädlich, Kopftieflagerung als günstig (Laqueur u. de Vries Reilingh, 1920b).

B. Postmortale Erkennung und Bewertung des Lungenödems

Die diagnostischen Schwierigkeiten und Unsicherheiten, mit denen der Experimentator bei lebenden Tieren zu kämpfen hat, sind der wichtigste Grund, Versuchstiere zur Feststellung und Bewertung ihres Ödems zu opfern. Man tötet sie zu bestimmten Phasen des Versuchs, oder wartet den spontanen Eintritt des Todes ab.

1. Die Überlebenszeit

Wiederholt ist der Versuch gemacht worden, die Wirkung ödemerzeugender oder -hemmender Faktoren an der Überlebenszeit zu messen (z.B. Dieke u. Richter, 1946; Luisada, 1950a; MacKenzie u. MacKenzie, 1943). Dabei ist jedoch zu berücksichtigen, daß die Überlebenszeit nur ein sekundäres Merkmal für die Bewertung des experimentellen Lungenödems ist. Der Spontantod ist nicht immer ausschließlich ödembedingt. Er kann ganz oder zum Teil durch eine Schädigung anderer Organe verursacht sein. So sterben bei Ammoniumchloridvergiftung die Tiere nicht an dem entstehenden Lungenödem, sondern an einer Schädigung des Zentralnervensystems (Halmágyi *et al.*, 1956; MacKay *et al.*, 1949). Beugt man der zentralnervösen Schädigung durch therapeutische Maßnahmen vor, so kommt es prämortal zu einer stärkeren Ausbildung des Lungenödems (Halmágyi *et al.*, 1956). Umgekehrt kann durch Gynergen- oder Hyderginbehandlung das durch Veratrin auslösbare Lungenödem, nicht aber der Tod der Tiere verhindert werden (Horst *et al.*, 1950; Riechert, 1950).

Auch unter Bedingungen, unter denen der Tod der Tiere ausschließlich die Folge der Flüssigkeitsanfüllung der Lunge ist, gibt die Überlebenszeit kein zuverlässiges Maß für die Stärke des Ödems; denn der Grad der tolerierten Flüssigkeitsanschoppung wird von der Geschwindigkeit, mit der die Lunge sich füllt, mitbestimmt. Bei langsamer Entwicklung erreicht das Lungenödem bis zum Eintritt des Todes häufig einen höheren Grad als bei rascher Entstehung (Winternitz u. Lambert, 1919). Kommt es allerdings zur Schaumbildung, so muß mit frühzeitiger Erstickung bei verhältnismäßig geringer Flüssigkeitsansammlung gerechnet werden (Laqueur u. de Vries Reilingh, 1920b). Schaumbildung ist kein Maß für die Ausdehnung des Ödems. Schaum in den Luftwegen kann bei motorischer Aktivität eines Tieres schon bei verhältnismäßig geringgradigem Ödem auftreten, während ruhende Tiere mit schwererem Ödem schaumfrei bleiben (Laqueur u. de Vries Reilingh, 1920b).

2. Der makroskopische Obduktionsbefund

Die makroskopische Inspektion der freigelegten Atmungsorgane erlaubt eine Orientierung über größere Abweichungen von der Norm. Im Vergleich zu gesunden Organen werden Größe, Gewicht, Konsistenz, Farbe, Oberflächenbeschaffenheit der exstirpierten Lunge, das Vorhandensein schaumiger Flüssigkeit in den

Luftwegen und der Austritt von Flüssigkeit aus Schnittflächen, evtl. nach Druck auf das Gewebe, beurteilt. Die makroskopische Bewertung des Lungenbefundes ist subjektiven Einflüssen unterworfen (Harrison u. Liebow, 1952) und erfordert Blindversuchsbedingungen. An der Gestaltung der pathologischen Veränderungen wirken neben der ödemerzeugenden Noxe die Entwicklungsgeschwindigkeit und Dauer des Ödems mit (Giese, 1960). Einige Autoren (Courtice u. Korner, 1952; Haddy *et al.*, 1950; Jordan u. DeLaney, 1951; MacKay, 1950; Sussman *et al.*, 1948) versuchen anhand des makroskopischen Befundes nicht nur die Diagnose Lungenödem zu stellen, sondern auch eine quantitative Beurteilung vorzunehmen. Als Beispiel für dieses Vorgehen sei das Schema von Jordan und DeLaney (1951), das 6 Grade des Lungenbefundes unterscheidet, angeführt: Grad 0: Blutstauung oder freie Flüssigkeit in den Lufträumen nicht erkennbar; C (Congestion): Stauung, erkennbar an einer Farbänderung der Lunge von rosarot bis rot. In diesen Fällen ist in den normalerweise lufthaltigen Teilen des Gewebes keine Flüssigkeit nachweisbar. Grad 1: keine freie Flüssigkeit in den Bronchien, aber Flüssigkeitsaustritt von der Schnittfläche nach leichtem Druck; Grad 2: Flüssigkeit in den Bronchioli. 2. Ordnung und Flüssigkeitsaustritt von der Schnittfläche auf Druck; Grad 3: Schaumige Flüssigkeit fließt ohne Anwendung von Druck aus dem Lappenhauptbronchus; Grad 4: Schaumige Flüssigkeit ist auch in der Trachea enthalten. — Da die Ödementwicklung in den einzelnen Lappen verschiedene Grade erreichen kann, wird jeder Lappen für sich beurteilt. Beim Hund ergab sich eine gute Übereinstimmung von makroskopischem Befund und Wassergehalt des Lungengewebes.

3. Der mikroskopische Lungenbefund

Die mikroskopische Untersuchung fixierter und gefärbter Lungengewebsschnitte wird von einigen Autoren nicht nur für die qualitative, sondern auch für eine quantitative Ödembewertung herangezogen. Da aber von jedem Organ gewöhnlich nur wenige Schnitte durchgemustert werden, können in der Regel nur Stichprobenergebnisse erhalten werden.

Für den Erfolg der histologischen Untersuchung ist eine sachgemäße Fixation von entscheidender Bedeutung. Warme (52° C), heiße oder kochende Formalinlösung wird empfohlen, um die Ödemflüssigkeit möglichst rasch zur Gerinnung zu bringen (Farber, 1937a; Rusznyák *et al.*, 1957; Giese, 1960). Einige Autoren fixieren anstelle kleiner Gewebsproben die Lungen in toto (Farber, 1937a) oder vollständige, abgebundene Lungenlappen. Koenig u. Koenig (1949a) erzielten unter verschiedenen Methoden die besten Ergebnisse, wenn abgebundene Lungenlappen in einer Schüttelapparatur 24—48 Std lang der Einwirkung einer 10%igen Lösung von Formalin in isotonischer Kochsalzlösung ausgesetzt wurden. Altschul u. Laskin (1946) instillierten in situ in die Trachea Formalinlösung oder Heidenhain-Susa-Lösung.

Zur Einbettung wird in der Regel Paraffin, zur Färbung Hämotoxylin-Eosin (H.E.) verwendet (Altschul u. Laskin, 1946; Cameron u. De, 1949; Harford u. Hara, 1950; Henschler *et al.*, 1960; Koenig u. Koenig, 1949a; Koenig *et al.*, 1952; Meessen u. Schulz, 1957; Rusznyák *et al.*, 1957; Short, 1944; Tennekoon, 1954), gelegentlich werden andere Färbungen z. B. van Gieson, Cameron u. De, 1949; Flinker u. McCarrell, 1949; Short, 1944), Elasticafärbung (Hemingway u. Williams, 1952; Meessen u. Schulz, 1957; Short, 1944), Anilinblau und Chromotrop (zur Darstellung der Erythrocyten (Hemingway u. Williams, 1952), die Färbungen nach Mallory (Altschul u. Laskin, 1946; Rusznyák *et al.*, 1957), nach Masson (Plester u. Rummel, 1951) herangezogen. Nach Harford und Hara (1950) kann Ödemflüssigkeit mit Eisen-Hämatoxylin oder Phloxin und Methylenblau besser als mit H.E. sichtbar gemacht werden.

Da die Ödemflüssigkeit in den Anfangsstadien nur wenig Eiweiß enthält (Boyd u. Perry, 1960; Halmágyi *et al.*, 1955; Koenig *et al.*, 1952; s. auch S. 164f.) und ihre Zusammensetzung häufig erst prämortal der des Plasmas ähnelt (Boyd u. Perry, 1960) wird in histologischen Präparaten von Lungen mit akutem Ödem gelegentlich kein färbbares Material in den Alveolen angetroffen (Harrison u. Liebow, 1952; Reichsman, 1946; Visscher *et al.*, 1956), denn eiweißfreie Flüssigkeit wird bei den üblichen histologischen Färbungen nicht sichtbar. Das einzige Ödemzeichen ist in solchen Fällen die Verdickung des interstitiellen Gewebes (Visscher *et al.*, 1956).

Gottsegen u. Mitarb. (1957) unterscheiden nach der Ausdehnung der histologischen Veränderungen über die ganze Lunge, über einzelne Lappen oder verstreute Partien 3 Schweregrade; sie erheben den mikroskopischen Befund im Blindversuch (d.h. ohne Kenntnis der experimentellen Daten). Rusznyák u. Mitarb. (1957) ordnen einer Gruppe 0 die ödemfreien Tiere zu, der Gruppe I Fälle mit Ödem in verstreuten, voneinander entfernt liegenden Alveolengruppen von 15—20 Alveolen, der Gruppe II Tiere mit Flüssigkeitsansammlung in Alveolengruppen von 30—50 Alveolen, die an einzelnen Stellen konfluieren, der Gruppe III alle Fälle mit makroskopisch erkennbarem konfluierendem Ödem.

Wie Boyd und Perry (1960) am Beispiel der Phosgenvergiftung gezeigt haben, differieren die histologischen Veränderungen bei den verschiedenen Schweregraden des Ödems jedoch nicht nur hinsichtlich ihrer Ausdehnung. Bei Tieren, die durch Phosgen nur wenig geschädigt worden waren, bestand ein leichtes Ödem der Trachea, der Bronchien und des Alveolargewebes, leichtes Emphysem, sowie Stauung und Arterienkontraktionen im Alveolarbereich. Bei stärkerer Schädigung war in der Trachea und den Bronchien kein Ödem nachweisbar; dafür war es im Alveolarbereich stärker ausgeprägt. Das Emphysem war deutlicher geworden. Hämorrhagien waren aufgetreten. Bei den schwerstgeschädigten Tieren wurde maximaler Flüssigkeitsaustritt in die Alveolen gefunden; Kontraktionen der Arterien, Stauungen, Hämorrhagien und Emphysem fehlten.

4. Das Lungengewicht

Unter den diagnostischen Verfahren wird die Bestimmung des Lungengewichtes im Verhältnis zum Körpergewicht, zum Gewicht anderer Körperorgane oder zum Lungengewicht vergleichbarer (d.h. vor allem gleich schwerer) Kontrolltiere am häufigsten zur Feststellung bzw. Bewertung des Lungenödems angewendet. Gelegentlich ist auch das Lungenvolumen bestimmt und zum Körpergewicht in Beziehung gesetzt worden. Ältere Arbeiten, die sich derartiger Verfahren bedienten, sind von Laqueur u. Magnus (1921a), Flury (1925) und Winternitz und Lambert (1919) besprochen worden.

Das Lungengewicht kann bis zum 5—6fachen der Norm anwachsen. Laqueur u. Magnus (1921a) beobachteten bei der Phosgenvergiftung von Katzen eine Zunahme des Lungengewichtes von 7,5 g/kg auf durchschnittlich 30 g/kg, in Einzelfällen bis auf 54 g/kg. Auch beim Menschen ist ein Anstieg des Lungengewichtes auf das 3—5fache beobachtet worden.

Zur Isolierung der Lungen wird die Trachea abgeklemmt und der Thorax seitlich weit eröffnet. Die Lungen werden möglichst rasch freipräpariert, Herz, Oesophagus und mediastinales Fettgewebe werden entfernt, Blutreste mit angefeuchtetem Filterpapier beseitigt (Courtice u. Korner, 1952; Durlacher *et al.*, 1950; Harrison u. Liebow, 1952; Hemingway, 1950; Henschler *et al.*, 1960; Luisada u. Sarnoff, 1946a; Poulsen, 1954a; Richter, 1952; Tennekoon, 1954). Das Gewicht wird in g/kg Körpergewicht oder in % des Körpergewichtes angegeben. Der Lungen-Körpergewichtsindex ödematöser Tiere wird mit demjenigen gesunder Kontrolltiere oder einem theoretischen Wert verglichen, der Ödemgrad aus dem Verhältnis der Indices errechnet. Bei gesunden Kaninchen und Ratten fanden Testelli u. Mitarb. (1960) z.B. einen Index von 0,5%; ein Prozentsatz von 0,75 gilt als Zeichen von Stauung oder mäßigem Lungenödem, ein Wert von 1,0% oder mehr als Zeichen von schwerem Lungenödem. Harrison u. Liebow (1952) geben für gesunde Hunde im Gewicht von 7—20 kg ein relatives Lungengewicht von 0,80—1,20% an. Eine Erhöhung auf 1,21—1,40 wird als fraglicher Effekt, Steigerung auf 1,41—1,60% als leichtes, auf 1,61—2,00% als mäßiges und auf mehr als 2,01% als schweres Ödem gewertet.

Als normaler Lungen-Körpergewichtsindex (= relatives Lungengewicht) werden sehr unterschiedliche Werte angegeben (Tabelle 3). Die Variabilität der Werte dürfte art-, alters-, gewichts- (Poulsen, 1954a; Richter, 1952), jahreszeitlich

Tabelle 3. *Lungen-Körpergewichts-Index (relatives Lungengewicht) gesunder Versuchstiere*

Tierart	Lungengewicht in g/kg Körpergewicht	Lungengewicht in % des Körpergewichtes	Mittleres Körpergewicht in g bzw. kg	Bemerkungen	Literatur
Maus	5,71	0,57	25—33		Poulsen (1954b)
	9,1	0,91 (±0,062)	18,6	Decapitation nach 1 h Laufen	Sjöstrand (1935)
	14,3	1,43 (±0,056)	18,8		Sjöstrand (1935)
Ratte	3,57	0,36			Durlacher *et al.* (1950)
	4,9 (±0,34)	0,49	180—340		Courtice *et al.* (1954)
	5,0	0,50			Testelli *et al.* (1960)
	5,6	0,56 (±0,09)	325—375		Skillen *et al.* (1961)
	6,2	0,62 (±0,09)	210		Mac Kay (1950)
	8,1	0,81	180,3		Riechert (1951)
	8,2	0,82 (±0,037	174,7	Decapitation nach 1 h Laufen	Sjöstrand (1935)
	8,5 (±0,071)	0,85	150—250		Halmágyi (1956)
	8,6	0,86 (±0,024)	115—220		Koch (1956)
	9,2 (±0,05)	0,92	120—160		Henschler u. Reich (1959)
	11,0	1,10			Riechert (1941)
	13,0	1,30 (±0,16)	180,8		Sjöstrand (1935)
	13,3	1,33	80—90		Eichholtz u. Hoppe (1933)
	8,0		197		Rothlin (1940)
	7,7	0,77	212		Winter (1949)
	5,2	0,52 (±0,01)			Maire u. Patton (1954)
	5,3	0,53			Starzecki u. Halmágyi (1961)
	4,4	0,44 (±0,007)	345		Gamble u. Patton (1953)
	5,1	0,51 (±0,01)			Maire u. Patton (1956a)
	6,3	0,63 (±0,13)	200—300		Johnson u. Bean (1957)

Tabelle 3 (Fortsetzung)

Tierart	Lungengewicht in g/kg Körpergewicht	Lungengewicht in % des Körpergewichtes	Mittleres Körpergewicht in g bzw. kg	Bemerkungen	Literatur
Meerschweinchen	5,5	0,55 (±0,09)	540		Mac Kay u. Pecka (1949)
	6,9	0,69 (±0,11)	740		Mac Kay *et al.* (1949)
	7,15	0,72			Hemingway u. Williams (1952)
	7,2	0,72	310		Haddy *et al.* (1949)
	8,9 (±0,062)	0,89	400—700		Halmágyi *et al.* (1956)
	9,1	0,91			Luisada (1950)
	6,8	0,68	450		Winter (1949)
	6,2	0,62			Prasad (1958)
	7,8	0,78 (±0,07)			Schmitt u. Meyers (1957)
Kaninchen	4,07	0,41	2,59		Stone u. Loew (1949)
	4—5	0,4—0,5			Laqueur u. Magnus (1921)
	4,5	0,45 (±0,021)	1,5—2,5		Luisada (1950)
	4,6	0,46			Rosenbluth *et al.* (1952)
	4,9	0,49			
	5,0	0,50	2,0		Testelli u. Musiker (1960)
	5,0	0,50	2,0		Testelli *et al.* (1960)
Katzen	7,5	0,75			Laqueur u. Magnus (1921a)
	7,0	0,70			
	7,0—9,0				Wirth (1936)
Hund	7,0—8,0	0,7—0,8	14—18		Testelli u. Musiker (1960)
	7,0—8,0	0,7—0,8			Testelli *et al.* (1960)
	8,0	0,8	15		Wood u. Moe (1942)
	8,0	0,8			Luisada (1950)
	8,0—9,0	0,8—0,9	20—24		Aravanis *et al.* (1957)
	8,6	0,86	5—20	Winter-Frühjahr	Luisada u. Sarnoff (1946)
	13,3	1,33	5—20	Sommer	Luisada u. Sarnoff (1946)

(Harrison u. Liebow, 1952; Luisada u. Sarnoff, 1946a) und methodisch bedingt sein. Poulsen (1954a) fand bei Mäusen im Gewicht von 16—37 g, daß sich das Lungengewicht mit zunehmendem Körpergewicht von 105 auf 225 mg erhöht. Wurde jedoch das Lungengewicht in % des Körpergewichtes ausgedrückt, so nahm der Wert mit steigendem Körpergewicht von etwa 0,72 auf 0,48% ab. Zu einem ähnlichen Resultat kam Richter (1952) bei Ratten. Das relative Lungengewicht verminderte sich von 1,01% für Tiere von weniger als 50 g Gewicht bis auf 0,46% für die Gewichtsklasse von 300—350 g. Bei der Feststellung der Gewichte muß auf die Dauer des Wiegevorgangs geachtet werden (Poulsen, 1954a). Innerhalb von 1—2 min kann infolge Wasserverdunstung eine deutliche Gewichtsminderung eintreten. Jahreszeitliche Schwankungen der Indices sind möglicherweise temperaturbedingt. Luisada und Sarnoff (1946) fanden bei Hunden einen durchschnittlichen normalen Lungen-Körpergewichtsindex von 0,86 im Winter und beginnenden Frühjahr und von 1,33 im Sommer.

Eine relative Zunahme des Lungengewichtes kann nicht nur ödembedingt sein, sondern auch die Folge von Entzündung oder vermehrter Blutansammlung in den Lungengefäßen (Stauung) (Korner, 1953). Weitere zusätzliche Faktoren (Tötungsart, prämortales Verhalten des Tieres) werden am Schluß des Kapitels besprochen. Es ist daher ratsam, der Gewichtsbestimmung andere Bewertungsmethoden zur Seite zu stellen.

Mehrfach ist das „relative" Lungengewicht mit dem histologischen Befund verglichen worden. Gottsegen u. Mitarb. (1957) sowie Courtice u. Mitarb. (1954) fanden eine gute Übereinstimmung zwischen dem relativen Gewicht und der im histologischen Bild beobachteten Ausdehnung ödematöser Veränderungen. Nach Erfahrungen von Korner (1953) verlaufen beide nicht immer völlig parallel. Bei Lungen von Kaninchen, die i.v. Infusionen von Ringer-Locke-Lösung bzw. von Ringer-Locke-Lösung mit Zusatz von Noradrenalin erhalten hatten, war der Anstieg des relativen Lungengewichtes der mit Noradrenalin behandelten Tiere nicht in demselben Maße von Ödembildung begleitet wie bei den Tieren der Vergleichsgruppe; die Gewichtszunahme beruhte bei den Noradrenalintieren teilweise auf vermehrter Blutfüllung der Lungengefäße (Tabelle 4).

Tabelle 4. *Beziehung zwischen relativem Gewicht und mikroskopischem Befund ödematöser Kaninchenlungen.* (Nach Korner, 1953)

Rel. Lungengewicht in g/kg	Lungenödem provoziert durch	
	i.v. Infusion von Ringer-Locke-Lösung	i.v. Infusion von Ringer-Locke-Lösung mit Zusatz von Noradrenalin
	Lungenbefund	
5—6	leichte Lungenstauung, gelegentliche größere Ödemherde	beträchtliche Lungenstauung
6—7	Lungenstauung und weiter ausgebreitetes Lungenödem	schwere Lungenstauung mit wenigen verstreuten Ödemherden
7—8	schweres Lungenödem mit schaumiger Flüssigkeit in der Trachea	schwere Lungenstauung mit größeren Ödemherden
8—9	schweres Lungenödem und viel schaumige Flüssigkeit in der Trachea	Lungenstauung mit mäßig schwerem Lungenödem und schaumiger Flüssigkeit in der Trachea
9—10		schweres Lungenödem mit viel schaumiger Trachealflüssigkeit

Ein Vergleich des relativen Lungengewichtes mit dem makroskopischen Obduktionsbefund ist von Courtice und Korner (1952) bei Kaninchen vorgenommen worden, wobei die Bewertung des Ödems nach einer Gradeinteilung erfolgte (0: ödemfreie Tiere; 1: Stauung; 2: mäßiges, makroskopisch gleichförmiges Ödem; 3: ausgeprägtes Ödem mit Schaum in der Trachea). Das errechnete mittlere relative Lungengewicht der den einzelnen Gruppen zugeordneten Tiere war von

Grad zu Grad signifikant verschieden (Abb. 2). Ein ähnlicher Vergleich wurde von Luisada und Sarnoff (1946a) publiziert; sie unterteilten das Lungenödem von Hunden aufgrund des relativen Lungengewichtes und des bei makroskopischer Inspektion gefundenen Schaumgehaltes des Organs in 4 Grade (s. Tabelle 5).

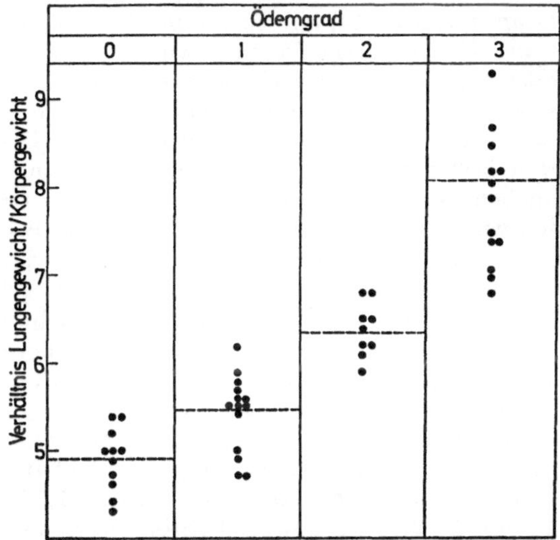

Abb. 2. Beziehung zwischen relativem Lungengewicht (g/kg) und Ödemgrad, beurteilt nach dem makroskopischen Obduktionsbefund. (Aus: Courtice u. Korner, 1952)

Tabelle 5. *Gradeinteilung des Lungenödems nach Luisada u. Sarnoff (1946)*

Lungen-Körpergewichts-Index	Schaum	Ödemgrad
1,20—1,60	kein	—
1,40—2,00	wenig	+
1,40—2,00	reichlich	++
1,60—2,75	mäßig viel	++
1,60—2,75	reichlich	+++
2,75—5,00 und mehr	reichlich	++++

Haddy u. Mitarb. (1949, 1950) und Drenckhahn (1958) bestimmten neben dem Lungen-Körpergewichtsindex den Lungen-Ventrikelgewichtsindex. Bei Meerschweinchen mit einem Durchschnittsgewicht von 310 g betrug der Lungen-Ventrikelgewichtsindex 2,4, der Lungen-Körpergewichtsindex 0,0072, d.h. 0,72%. Das Ventrikelgewicht ist keine unveränderliche Bezugsgröße; es birgt als Fehlerquelle die Neigung des Ventrikels zur Hypertrophie in sich (Haddy *et al.*, 1950); unter Umständen können auch die ödemprovozierenden Maßnahmen das Ventrikelgewicht ändern; Drenckhahn (1958) fand nach der Verabreichung von Adrenalin Blutungen im Herzmuskel, die eine Zunahme des Ventrikelgewichtes verursachten.

Das Verhältnis von Lungen- zu Herzgewicht ist von Winternitz u. Lambert (1919), Cameron u. Courtice (1946), Cameron u. De (1949); Hughes, May u. Widdicombe (1958a) sowie Tennekoon (1954) verwendet worden. Bei diesem Vorgehen müssen die für die Verwendung des Ventrikelgewichtes genannten Kriterien beachtet werden. Zusätzlich ist die schematische Einhaltung einer stets gleichen

Exstirpations- und Wägetechnik Voraussetzung für Vergleichbarkeit der Ergebnisse. Cameron u. De (1949) exstirpierten bei Ratten und Kaninchen nach Unterbindung der Trachea Herz und Lungen, trennten das Herz ab, öffneten Kammern u. Vorhöfe, spülten das Blut heraus, trockneten mit Filterpapier und wogen beide Organe. Als normales Lungen-Herzgewichtsverhältnis nehmen sie einen Wert von 2,4:1 an. Short (1944) unterband die Trachea, öffnete den Thorax und entfernte Herz und Lungen. Das Perikard wurde aufgeschnitten, das Herz herausgelöst, die großen Gefäße an ihrem Ursprungsort durchtrennt und das Blut aus den Kammern ausgespült. Beide Hauptbronchi wurden am Hilus abgebunden und die Lungen von allem anhaftenden Gewebe freipräpariert. Die Feuchtgewichte beider Organe wurden bestimmt. Das durchschnittliche Lungen-Herzgewichts-Verhältnis des Kaninchens war 2,0, die unteren und oberen Grenzen 1,65 bzw. 2,61. Bei Windhunden wurde ein mittlerer Wert von 1,3, bei Bastardhunden von 1,0, bei Kaninchen von 1,76 (Courtice u. Phipps, 1946) bzw. 1,53 ($\sigma = \pm 0{,}11$) (Hughes *et al.*, 1958a), bei Ratten von 1,5 (Tennekoon, 1954) gefunden.

Eyster (1919) und Piiper (1960) haben das Verhältnis Feucht-:Trockengewicht ödematöser Lungen auf den entsprechenden Wert von Kontrollorganen bezogen.— Einige Autoren vergleichen das Lungengewicht gleich schwerer Kontrolltiere (Cassen *et al.*, 1956; Eichholtz u. Hoppe, 1933; Horst *et al.*, 1950; Lagrange u. Promel, 1949; Sjöstrand, 1935). Bei gesunden Kaninchen mit einem mittleren Körpergewicht von 2,59 kg (n = 12) betrug das Lungengewicht 10,58 g ($S = \pm 1{,}41$); nach Adrenalin bzw. Phenobarbital und Adrenalin wurden 21,77 g ± 7,19 (2,32 kg, n = 18) bzw. 34,95 g ± 14,49 (2,60 kg) gewogen (Stone u. Loew, 1949). Als mittleres Lungengewicht gesunder Mäuse wurden 150—160 g ermittelt, bei Tieren mit schwerem Lungenödem fand man 255 bzw. 370 mg (Lagrange u. Promel, 1949; Cassen u. Kistler, 1954). Für ödemfreie Ratten mit einem mittleren Gewicht von 350 g wird ein mittleres Lungengewicht von 1,83 g angegeben, nach Adrenalininjektion stieg es auf 5,45 g (Cassen *et al.*, 1956).

Alle Methoden, die sich auf Gewichtsbestimmungen als Grundlage für die Ödembewertung stützen, setzen die Verwendung eines recht homogenen Tiermaterials voraus, eine Forderung, die z. B. bei Untersuchungen an Hunden nur schwer zu erfüllen ist.

5. Der Wassergehalt der Lunge

Einige Autoren messen ödembedingte Veränderungen am Wassergehalt der Lungen. Die Wassergehaltsbestimmung ist der einfachen Lungengewichtsbestimmung überlegen, denn der Wassergehalt ist vom Körpergewicht unabhängig. Nach Ansicht mehrerer Autoren informiert die Bestimmung des Wassergehaltes zuverlässiger über den Ödemgrad als andere Methoden (Henschler *et al.*, 1960; Joffe, 1954; Jordan u. DeLaney, 1951; Poulsen, 1954a; Wohlzogen *et al.*, 1956). Für die Bewertung des Wassergehaltes ist die Kenntnis altersbedingter Unterschiede des Wassergehaltes normaler Lungen erforderlich (Wohlzogen *et al.*, 1956).

Der Wassergehalt von Lungen oder Gewebsproben des Organs wird durch Vergleich von Feucht- und Trockengewicht bestimmt. Bei der Arbeitsweise von Joffe (1954) sowie Wohlzogen u. Mitarb. (1956) werden Meerschweinchenlungen nach der Isolierung gewogen, aufgeblasen, in diesem Zustand getrocknet und erneut gewogen. Reichsman (1946) trocknete Rattenlungen bei 100—110° C bis zur Gewichtskonstanz. Er registrierte an ödematösen Lungen eine enge Korrelation von Wassergehalt des Gewebes und makroskopischem Obduktionsbefund. Lambert und Gremels (1926) bestimmten den Wassergehalt kleiner Proben von Hundelungen (Trocknung bis zur Gewichtskonstanz bei 110° C). Mit zunehmender Ödementwicklung stieg der Wassergehalt vom Ausgangswert von 80% auf 92—93% an. Jordan und DeLaney (1951) fanden (ebenfalls an der Hundelunge) einen mittleren normalen Wassergehalt von 79% ; er stieg bei Lungenödem bis auf 87% an. Eaton (1950) trocknete etwa 15 g schwere Proben von Hundelungen 48 Std lang in einem Trockenofen bei 60° C und 24 weitere Stunden lang im Exsiccator über wasserfreiem $CaCl_2$. Aus dem Feucht- und Trockengewicht wurde ein mittlerer normaler Wassergehalt von 79,3% errechnet. Poulsen (1954a) empfiehlt die Einwirkung von Wärme auf das Gewebe zu vermeiden. Bei seinem Verfahren werden die exstirpierten Lungen nach dem Wiegen für etwa 30—40 min in einem Kühlschrank bei —20° C hängend aufbewahrt und anschließend in einem evakuierten Exsiccator bei Raumtemperatur über Silicagel getrocknet. Nach 2 Tagen ist in der Regel Gewichtskonstanz erreicht. Die auf diese Weise getrockneten Lungen sind hygroskopisch; sie müssen nach Entnahme aus dem Exsiccator rasch gewogen werden. Der Autor sieht den Vorteil der Gefriertrocknung darin, daß sich das Lungenvolumen nicht verändert und es infolgedessen nicht zum Einschluß von Wasser im Gewebe, auch nicht in den zentralen Teilen des Organs kommt.

Der Wassergehalt der Lungen gesunder Mäuse betrug im Mittel 77,11%; $\sigma = \pm 0{,}982$ (Poulsen, 1954b) bzw. 78,4%; $\sigma = \pm 1{,}02$ (Matzen, 1957b). Die Grenzen für eine statistische Sicherheit von 99% ($\pm 2{,}75\,\sigma$) errechnen sich zu 74,6—79,6% bzw. 76,6—80,8%. Darüberliegende Werte sprechen für Lungenödem. Vergleich mit dem makroskopischen Obduktionsbefund zeigte, daß dem stärksten Ödemgrad ein Wassergehalt von 84—90% entsprach. Bei einem Wassergehalt zwischen 82 und 84% war das Ödem mit bloßem Auge noch erkennbar, bei Werten unter 82% nicht mehr. Bei anderen Lungenaffektionen hatte das Organ gewöhnlich einen niedrigeren Wassergehalt als erwartet (Poulsen, 1954b). Der Wassergehalt des Blutes der Versuchstiere betrug im Mittel 78,5% (Poulsen) oder 77,8% (Matzen); er entsprach also annähernd dem Wassergehalt des Lungenparenchyms. Flüssigkeit, die aus ödematösen Lungen (nach Einwirkung von 30% CO_2 für 15 min) ausgepreßt werden konnte, enthielt im Mittel 94,9% Wasser.

Aus der Ähnlichkeit des Wassergehaltes der Lunge und des Blutes resultiert, daß Blutstauung im Pulmonalkreislauf, die eine relative Gewichtszunahme hervorruft, den Wassergehalt der Lunge nicht wesentlich verändert, während eine ödembedingte Gewichtszunahme mit einem deutlichen Anstieg des Wassergehaltes der Lunge einhergeht. In der Abb. 3 ist der Wassergehalt von ödematösen Mäuselungen gegen ihr relatives Gewicht abgetragen. Das durchgezogene Rechteck umgrenzt den 2 σ-Bereich für die Normalwerte der verwendeten Gewichtsklasse von 25—33 g. Die ausgezogenen Kurven sind Standardkurven für den Wassergehalt der Lunge bei einer Gewichtszunahme infolge Ödem (obere Kurve) oder Blutansammlung (untere Kurve). Sie ermöglichen ein Abschätzen der anteilmäßigen Beteiligung von Ödemflüssigkeit und Blut an der Gewichtszunahme ödematöser Lungen.

Zur Differenzierung zwischen Ödemflüssigkeit und Blutvolumen der Lunge werden einige weitere Verfahren vorgeschlagen. Aviado und Schmidt (1952) berechnen den Ödemanteil (einschließlich des normalen Wassergehaltes des Gewebes) aus der Differenz zwischen Gesamtwassergehalt und Blutwassergehalt excidierter Lungen unter Verwendung des Feuchtgewichts der ganzen Lunge (L_T), einer Lungengewebsprobe (L_W) (im Homogenisator 10 min lang zermahlen) und einer genau abgemessenen Blutmenge aus dem Herzen (B_W) sowie des Trockengewichts der Blut- und Gewebsproben, die 24 Std lang in einem Ofen bei 150° C getrocknet wurden (Trockengewichte L_D bzw. B_D). Der Hämoglobingehalt einer Blutprobe (H_B) und einer zerkleinerten Lungengewebsprobe (H_L) wurde colorimetrisch nach Evelyn und Malloy (1938) bzw. Greenberg und Erickson (1944) gemessen. Aus den gefundenen Parametern wurden folgende Werte errechnet: a) der Wassergehalt der ganzen Lunge $= \frac{L_W \cdot L_D}{L_W} \cdot 100$ (in %); b) das Blutvolumen der Lunge $\frac{H_L}{H_B} \cdot 100$ (in ml Blut pro 100 g Lunge); c) der Wassergehalt des Lungenblutes $= \frac{B_W - B_D \cdot \text{Blutvolumen der Lunge}}{100}$ (in g/100 g Lunge); d) die Ödemflüssigkeit in der Lunge = Wassergehalt der Lunge — Wassergehalt des Lungenblutes (in g/100 g Lunge).

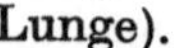

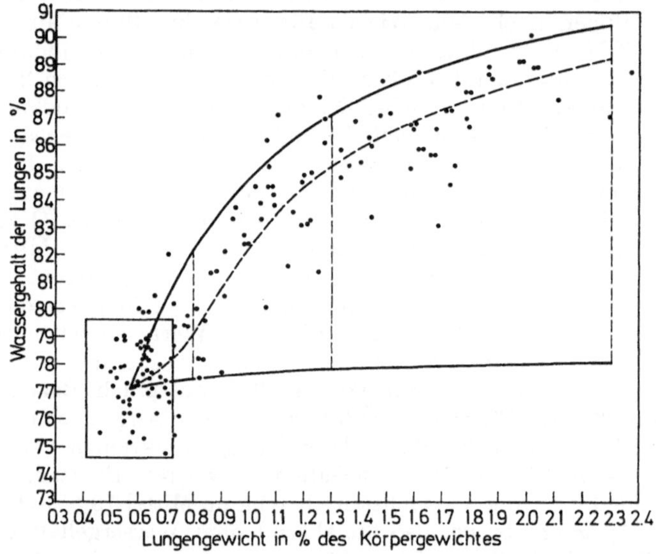

Abb. 3. Wassergehalt (Ordinate) und relatives Gewicht (Abszisse) ödematöser Mäuselungen. Punkte = Einzelwerte. Gestrichelte Linie = Mittelwertskurve. Ausgezogene Kurven: Standardkurven für Gewichtssteigerungen, die durch Ödemflüssigkeit (oben) bzw. vermehrte Blutfüllung (unten) bedingt sind. Das ausgezogene Rechteck (links unten) schließt 99% der Normalwerte für Tiere im Gewicht von 25—33 g ein. (Aus: Poulsen, 1954a)

Als Gesamtwassergehalt normaler Hundelungen wurden etwa 79%, als Blutvolumen etwa 24 ml pro 100 g Lunge und als Anteil des Gewebswassers etwa 57% ermittelt; die entsprechenden Werte ödematöser Lungen (Dampfinhalation) betrugen 84%, 16 ml pro 100 g Lunge und 71%. — Einige Untersucher bestimmten den Wasser- und Eisengehalt des Lungengewebes, um zwischen Ödem und veränderter Blutfüllung unterscheiden zu können (Boyd und Perry, 1960; Harrison und Liebow, 1952; Hughes *et al.*, 1958a). Im Anfangsstadium der Phosgenvergiftung von Kaninchen stieg der Wassergehalt der Lunge von 78,8 auf 82,4% an; gleichzeitig stieg der Eisengehalt von 420 auf 502 μg/g Trockengewicht; im Endstadium betrug der Wassergehalt 84,6%, der Eisengehalt nur 280 μg/g Trockengewicht (Boyd und Perry, 1960). Diese Ergebnisse entsprachen nicht in allen Fällen dem histologischen Befund, was verständlich erscheint, wenn man berücksichtigt, daß sich der Erythrocytenanteil des Blutes während der Ödementstehung ändern kann (s. S. 165f.), besonders dann, wenn sich neben dem Lungenödem ein Pleuraexsudat entwickelt. Beim Thioharnstoffödem der Ratte wurden z. B. Erhöhungen der Hämatokritwertebis auf 80% gefunden (Richter, 1952); damit dürfte eine erhebliche Reduzierung des Wassergehaltes des Blutes verbunden sein. Es ist zweckmäßig, die Bestimmungen des Gewebeeisens durch gleichzeitige Bestimmungen der Blutzusammensetzung zu ergänzen.

Die Verfahren zur Differenzierung von Ödem- und Blutfüllung der Lunge erfordern einen höheren Arbeitsaufwand als die Gewichtsbestimmung und sind nicht frei von Fehlerquellen. Zu den schon genannten kommt hinzu, daß die Ödemflüssigkeit nicht bei allen Ödemformen und in allen Ödemstadien dieselbe Zusammensetzung hat. Unterschiedliche Elektrolytkonzentrationen der Ödemflüssigkeit werden nur geringe Rückwirkungen auf ihren Wasseranteil haben. Hingegen kann ihr Eiweißgehalt in einem Fall unter 0,5% liegen, in einem anderen dem des Plasmas nahekommen. Ferner kann die Ödemflüssigkeit durch die Beimischung von Blutzellen oder vermehrt abgesondertem Bronchialsekret modifiziert werden.

Wird daher der Wassergehalt der Lunge zur Beurteilung von Lungenödem verwendet, ist es zweckmäßig andere Bewertungsmethoden mit heranzuziehen (Aviado u. Schmidt, 1952; Boyd u. Perry, 1960; Jordan u. DeLaney, 1951; Lambert u. Gremels, 1926; Poulsen, 1954a; Reichsman, 1946).

6. Lungenvolumen und spezifisches Gewicht

Rothlin (1940, 1941), Riechert (1941, 1950) und Hemingway (1950) haben neben anderen Größen das Lungenvolumen gemessen und auf das Körpergewicht bezogen sowie das spezifische Gewicht der Lunge errechnet. Auch Plester und Rummel (1951) legten der Ödembewertung das spezifische Gewicht zugrunde. Rothlin (1940) mißt die Flüssigkeitsmenge, die von der untergetauchten Lunge verdrängt wird. Bei Ratten im Gewicht von etwa 200 g betrug das mittlere Lungenvolumen bei ödemkranken Tieren etwa 3,0 cm^3/100 g Körpergewicht. Vergrößerungen des Lungenvolumens sind nicht immer ödembedingt, sondern können durch andere Erkrankungen, z.B. ein Emphysem, verursacht sein. Eine von Hemingway (1950) angegebene Apparatur zur Bestimmung von Lungengewicht und Lungenvolumen ist in Abb. 4 wiedergegeben. Sie besteht aus einem weithalsigen Wägegefäß, das an einem Draht aufgehängt ist. Der Hals des Gefäßes ist durch einen Schliffstopfen verschlossen, in den zentral eine kurze Capillare, die sich nach oben erweitert, eingelassen ist. An der engsten Stelle der Capillare ist eine Strichmarke angebracht. Der untere Teil des Gefäßes ist mit einer Schliffverbindung in einen Dreiwegehahn eingepaßt. Vom Dreiwegehahn führt ein Schlauch zu einer 10 ml-Bürette, die aus einem Vorratsgefäß mit 1% NaCl-Lösung gefüllt werden kann. Das Volumen des Wägegefäßes wird durch Füllung mit dem Büretteninhalt bestimmt und derselbe Vorgang nach Einbringen einer Lunge in das Gefäß wiederholt. Die Differenz der gemessenen Werte ergibt das Lungenvolumen. Aus dem Lungenvolumen und dem zuvor ermittelten Lungengewicht wird das spezifische Gewicht errechnet.

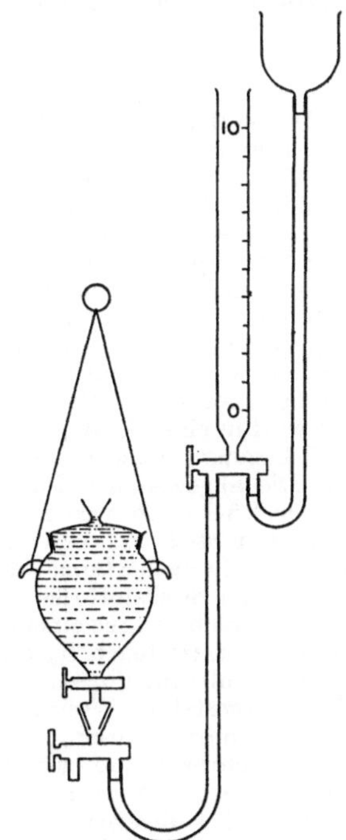

Abb. 4. „Densitometer“ zur Bestimmung von Lungengewicht und Lungenvolumen. (Nach Hemingway, 1950)

7. Pleuraexsudat

Die Volumenbestimmung von Exsudat in der Pleurahöhle ist gelegentlich zur Bewertung spezieller Ödemformen herangezogen worden (z.B. MacKenzie u.

MacKenzie, 1943). Die Anwendbarkeit dieser Methode ist begrenzt, denn Pleuraexsudate entstehen nur bei einzelnen Ödemformen, z. B. bei der Thioharnstoffvergiftung. Wird diese Substanz bei der Ratte angewendet, so bildet sich ein Pleuraexsudat nur bei den Tieren aus, die so schwer erkranken, daß sie im Verlauf von 48 Std sterben; Tiere, die diese Zeitspanne überleben und dann geopfert werden, haben kein Exsudat, wohl aber nach dem Lungen-Körpergewichtsindex ein zweifelsfreies, wenn auch nicht hochgradiges Lungenödem (Koch, 1956). Die Diskrepanz zwischen Exsudatvolumen und Ödemgrad wurde unter dem Einfluß von Therapiemaßnahmen noch deutlicher, im Extremfall hatten überlebende, exsudatfreie Tiere ein schwereres Lungenödem als gestorbene Tiere mit Pleuraexsudat (Koch, 1956).

Untersuchungen von Courtice und Simmonds (1949b) machen derartige Befunde verständlich: Generell wird eiweißhaltige Flüssigkeit aus der Pleurahöhle schneller eliminiert als aus den Alveolen. Damit ist der Exsudatbildung besser vorgebeugt als der Ödembildung. Wird die pleurale Absorptionsrate aber durch Narkoticawirkung oder infolge prämortal reduzierter Thoraxexkursionen verkleinert (Courtice u. Morris, 1953), so kann es doch zur Ansammlung von Exsudat kommen, das dann — wie Richter (1952) an thioharnstoffvergifteten Ratten bestätigte — keine zeitliche Korrelation zur Exsudatentwicklung erkennen läßt. In der Regel setzt die Ödementwicklung schneller ein und erreicht ihren Gipfel früher als die Exsudatbildung.

8. Der Eiweißgehalt der Lunge

Das Verhältnis von unlöslichem zu löslichem Lungenprotein kann nach Hemingway (1950) bzw. Hemingway und Campbell (1951) zur Ermittlung des Ödemgrades verwendet werden. Der Gehalt an unlöslichem Parenchymeiweiß bleibt bei der Ödementstehung unverändert. Die ödembedingte Gewichtszunahme der Lunge wird nur von einer Vermehrung des löslichen Eiweißes der Plasmaproteine begleitet. Die Lungen von Meerschweinchen werden unmittelbar nach der Tötung herausgenommen und von anhängendem Gewebe befreit, wobei große Gefäße dicht an der Lungenoberfläche abgeschnitten werden. Lungengewicht und -volumen werden bestimmt, wie auf S. 185 beschrieben. Die Lunge wird nach Abgießen der NaCl-Lösung aus dem Wägegefäß genommen und in einem Mörser in 8—9 g stickstofffreiem Sand zu Brei zerrieben. Der Brei wird zusammen mit der aus dem Wägegefäß abgegossenen NaCl-Lösung in ein starkwandiges Zentrifugenglas (Volumen 40 ml) gefüllt und zentrifugiert. Die überstehende Flüssigkeit wird in einen Meßzylinder abgegossen, der Rückstand wiederholt im Zentrifugenglas mit NaCl-Lösung gewaschen und erneut zentrifugiert, bis er jede Spur von roter Färbung verloren hat. Die abgegossenen Lösungen werden gesammelt und ihr Volumen bestimmt. Der unlösliche Rückstand wird zusammen mit dem Sand nach Kjeldahl auf Stickstoffgehalt untersucht. Der Stickstoff dieser Fraktion (IPN = insoluble protein nitrogen) stammt aus dem unlöslichen Eiweiß der Lunge, dem Bindegewebs-, Blutgefäß- und Parenchymeiweiß. Der Extrakt enthält den Stickstoff des löslichen Proteins (SPN = soluble protein nitrogen) einschließlich des Hämoglobins. Aus einem Teil des Extraktes wird das Eiweiß mit Wolframsäure ausgefällt und quantitativ (nach Kjeldahl) bestimmt. Zu diesem Zweck werden 10 ml des Extraktes in einem 50 ml-Zentrifugenglas, das gleichzeitig als Mikro-Kjeldahl-Röhrchen dient, mit 5 ml frisch hergestellter Wolframsäure versetzt. (Herstellung der Wolframsäure: zu 20 ml 10% Natriumwolframatlösung werden 15 ml 2/3 N H_2SO_4 und dann aus einer Bürette sowiel weitere Schwefelsäure zugefügt, bis der Farbumschlag von Kongorot erfolgt). Nach 15minütigem Stehen wird zentrifugiert; die überstehende Flüssigkeit, die den Nichteiweiß-Stickstoff enthält, wird abgegossen. Der eiweißhaltige Niederschlag und die abgegossene Flüssigkeit werden getrennt nach Kjeldahl auf Stickstoffgehalt untersucht. Aus dem Stickstoffwert des Eiweißniederschlages wird der Gehalt der Lunge an löslichem Eiweiß (Hämoglobin- und Plasmaeiweiß) errechnet.

Zur Hämoglobinbestimmung werden zwei Proben des Extraktes von je 10 ml in Bechergläsern in einem Vakuumexsiccator getrocknet. Zum Trockenrückstand werden jeweils 20 ml Äther-Alkohol-Säure-Reagens (5,7 ml Eisessig, 8,6 ml 37%ige Salzsäure, 800 ml Äthyläther und 200 ml Äthylalkohol) zugefügt. Der Rückstand wird von den Wänden und dem Boden des Glases mit einem Glasstab abgelöst, in einem Homogenisator zerkleinert, in graduierte Zentrifugenröhrchen gegossen und mit dem Lösungsmittel auf etwa 20 ml aufgefüllt. Nach 15minütigem Stehen wird mit hoher Umdrehungszahl zentrifugiert. Die überstehende rosa Flüssigkeit, die saures Hämatin in klarer Lösung enthält, wird in einen 100 ml-Meßkolben abgegossen. Der Rückstand wird wiederholt mit dem Lösungsmittel gemischt und zentrifugiert, bis er farblos geworden ist. Die abgegossenen Flüssigkeitsproben müssen klar sein; andernfalls muß länger zentrifugiert werden. Die Meßkolben werden mit dem Lösungsmittel auf 100 ml aufgefüllt. Die Farbintensität der Lösungen wird spektrophotometrisch bei einer Wellenlänge von 390 $m\mu$ gemessen. Eichwerte erhält man mit Hilfe gleichartig behandelter Blutproben (0,1 und 0,2 ml) mit bekanntem Hämoglobingehalt. Analysenwerte normaler Meerschweinchenlungen gibt Hemingway (1950) an. Zwischen dem Lungengewicht und dem Stickstoffwert des unlöslichen Lungeneiweißes (IPN) besteht bei gesunden Tieren eine enge Korrelation. Man kann den Stickstoffwert zur Schätzung der Lungengröße verwenden. Da der IPN-Wert durch ein Lungenödem nicht verändert wird, orientiert das Verhältnis Lungengewicht:IPN über die Schwere des Ödems. Weiterhin nimmt bei Ödem der Gehalt der Lunge an löslichem und Hb-Eiweiß zu, bei der Vermehrung des Lungengewichtes infolge Blutanschoppung verschiebt sich vor allem der Index Hb/IPN, bei einer Plasmaansammlung kommt es zur Vergrößerung des Index SPN/IPN. Dementsprechend fanden Hemingway u. Williams (1952) z.B. bei einer O_2-Vergiftung von Meerschweinchen einen mit der Dauer der Einwirkung fortschreitenden Anstieg der Indexzahlen für das Verhältnis von Lungengewicht zu Körpergewicht, von Lungengewicht zu IPN und von SPN zu IPN; das Verhältnis Hb zu IPN ließ dagegen in diesen Versuchen keine signifikante Abweichung vom Normalwert erkennen. Histologisch waren zwar Erythrocyten in den Alveolen und interstitiellen Räumen nachweisbar, doch war dieser Befund auf umschriebene Gebiete beschränkt.

Die Methode nach Hemingway verlangt einen großen Arbeitsaufwand. Sie wird nur dann zuverlässige Resultate liefern, wenn außer dem relativen Lungengewicht und den Werten der Gewebsanalyse auch die Blutzusammensetzung des Tieres zum Zeitpunkt seines Todes berücksichtigt wird.

Skillen *et al.* (1961a) bestimmten den Gesamteiweißgehalt der Rattenlunge und bezogen ihn auf das Körpergewicht. Beim Ozonödem nahm er von 0,09 g Eiweiß/100 g Gewicht (Kontrolltiere) auf 0,19 g/100 g zu. Das relative Lungengewicht stieg bei denselben Tieren auf das 3fache.

9. Bemerkungen zur postmortalen Ödemdiagnose

Bei der postmortalen Bewertung von Lungenödem müssen neben der ödemerzeugenden Behandlung auch die allgemeinen Lebensbedingungen der Versuchstiere, die Tötungsart und das Intervall zwischen Eintritt des Todes und Auswertung berücksichtigt werden.

Motorische Hyperaktivität schafft eine erhöhte Anfälligkeit gegen ödemerzeugende Noxen (Stokinger, 1957) und bewirkt bei Tieren mit Lungenödem möglicherweise eine vermehrte Flüssigkeitsausscheidung in die Lunge (Laqueur u. de Vries Reilingh, 1920b), während bei gesunden Tieren starke prämortale Erregung oder erzwungenes Laufen das Lungengewicht vermindern (Sjöstrand, 1935).

Die *Tötungsart* kann das Aussehen der Lungen, ihr Gewicht und das histologische Bild beeinflussen (Durlacher *et al.*, 1950; Lauche, 1958; Poulsen, 1954a; Richter, 1952; Sjöstrand, 1935). Gewaltsames Töten, z.B. Abtrennen des Kopfes mit einer großen Schere (Poulsen, 1954a), Schädelschuß (Maréchaux, 1943) oder Nackenschlag (Lauche, 1958) können profuse Blutaustritte in die Lunge, evtl. auch Blutaspiration bis in die Alveolen verursachen (Lauche, 1958; Richter, 1952). CO-Gas (Lauche) und gealterter Narkoseäther (Friedberg, 1960) können ebenfalls Blutungen verursachen. Quetschung des Cervicalmarks mit der Pinzette beeinflußt das Lungengewicht in wechselndem Maße, da Krämpfe unterschiedlicher Stärke und Dauer auftreten, wobei mehr oder weniger Blut in die Lungen gepreßt wird (Richter, 1952). Tötung durch Verletzung der Medulla oblongata (Zug am Schwanz bei fixiertem Kopf) wirkt sich auf das Lungengewicht weniger stark aus. Intraperitoneale Injektion von Kaliumcyanidlösung (25%ig, 0,1 ml pro Maus) verändert den Lungenbefund kaum. Lebensnahe Verhältnisse bestehen anscheinend nach rasch ablaufender Entblutung (Drenckhahn, 1958; Durlacher *et al.*, 1950; Richter, 1952; Sussman *et al.*, 1948). Richter (1952) öffnet die Bauchhöhle der mit Äther narkotisierten Tiere unter Schonung der Brusthöhle. Die Eingeweide werden zur Seite gelagert und der Gefäßstamm freipräpariert. Die Vena cava wird nach Injektion von 0,1 ml einer 1%igen Heparinlösung pro 100 g Körpergewicht aufgeschnitten und das austretende Blut von Wattetupfern aufgefangen. Wenn die Blutung aus der Vena cava nachzulassen beginnt, wird die Bauchaorta durchtrennt. Nach dem Ausbluten wird die Brusthöhle geöffnet und die Thoraxorgane werden entnommen. Sussman *et al.* (1948) töteten Meerschweinchen durch Entbluten aus der Art. carotis bei hochgelagertem Unterleib. Die Lungen wurden unmittelbar nach Sistieren der Blutung exstirpiert.

Harrison und Liebow (1952) obduzierten ihre Tiere unmittelbar nach dem spontanen Eintritt des Todes, öffneten das Herz und saugten das Blut mit einer Saugflasche möglichst schnell ab.

Mit zunehmendem Zeitintervall zwischen Tod und Untersuchung steigt die Wahrscheinlichkeit der postmortalen Flüssigkeitsansammlung in der Lunge (Durlacher *et al.*, 1950; Richter, 1952). Durlacher u. Mitarb. fanden bei Kaninchen, die durch Luftembolie, Barbiturat-, Äther- oder Magnesiumsulfat-Verabreichung, durch Nackenschlag oder Elektroschock getötet worden waren, bereits 3 Std nach Eintritt des Todes eine Zunahme des Lungengewichtes. Histologisch sind Blutstauung und Ödem nachweisbar; Entblutung beugt diesen Veränderungen vor.

C. Erkennung und Bewertung des Lungenödems am perfundierten Organ

1. Gewichtsänderungen

Der Ablauf der Ödementwicklung in isolierten, perfundierten Lungen wird von Born (1954) an Gewichtsveränderungen verfolgt. Narkotisierten (Urethan bzw. Äther und Chloralose) und heparinisierten Kaninchen oder Katzen wird eine ver-

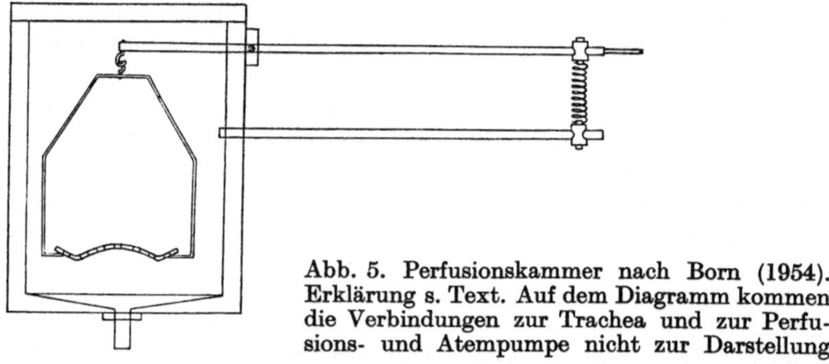

Abb. 5. Perfusionskammer nach Born (1954). Erklärung s. Text. Auf dem Diagramm kommen die Verbindungen zur Trachea und zur Perfusions- und Atempumpe nicht zur Darstellung

schließbare Kanüle in die Trachea eingebunden. Man läßt die Tiere ausbluten (Aorta), verschließt die Trachealkanüle, um ein Kollabieren der Lunge zu verhüten, und öffnet den Thorax. Lungen und Mediastinum werden herausgenommen und gewogen. Dann wird durch den geöffneten rechten Ventrikel eine gefüllte Perfusionskanüle in die Pulmonalarterie geschoben und mit einer zuvor gelegten Ligatur festgebunden. Das Präparat wird dann in eine Atmungskammer (s. Abb. 5) aus Plexiglas (Innenmaße 12,5 × 12,5 × 17,5 cm) gebracht, deren Temperatur mit Hilfe eines Wasserbades (37° C) konstant gehalten wird. Die Kammer hat Verbindungen zu einer Atempumpe und einem Wassermanometer. Durch ihre Wand können Verbindungen zwischen der Perfusionskanüle und der Perfusionspumpe sowie zwischen der Trachealkanüle und der Außenluft hergestellt werden. Im Innern der Kammer ist an einem Schreibhebel eine perforierte Plexiglasplatte zur Aufnahme der Lunge aufgehängt. Der Hebel (Innenlänge 8 cm, Außenlänge 22 cm) führt durch eine Öffnung, die Drehbewegungen in der Vertikalebene (Drehpunkt an der Kammeraußenwand) zuläßt, nach außen; die Öffnung ist durch eine Gummimembran luftdicht verschlossen. Der Hebel wird durch eine Spiralfeder an seinem äußeren Ende im Gleichgewicht gehalten. Er überträgt Gewichtsänderungen der Lunge kontinuierlich auf ein Rußkymographion. Die Lunge wird in der Kammer auf die Plexiglasplatte gelegt und die Trachealkanüle mit der Durchlaßöffnung verbunden. Zum Gewichtsausgleich können Plastilinkügelchen auf dem Schreibhebel angebracht werden, bis die Spiralfeder leicht gestreckt ist. Das System muß am Ende jeden Versuches geeicht werden. Die Trachealkanüle wird nun geöffnet, der gefettete Kammerdeckel geschlossen und die Atem- und Perfusionspumpe werden in Gang gesetzt. Die Starling-Atempumpe wird so eingestellt, daß der Druck in der Kammer 30mal pro Minute von —1 bis auf —8 cm Wassersäule vermindert wird. Als Perfusionsflüssigkeit dient Tyrodelösung (NaCl 0,8, KCL 0,02, $CaCl_2$ 0,02, $MgCl_2$ 0,01, NaH_2PO_4 0,005, $NaHCO_3$ 0,1, Glucose 0,1; alle Angaben in g/100 ml), die 25% steriles Pferdeserum enthält. Sie wird mit einer Dale-Schuster-Pumpe aus Mariotteschen Flaschen über eine Wärmespirale in die Perfusionskanüle gepumpt; die Messung des Perfusionsdruckes erfolgt über ein Bromoformmanometer. Die aus dem eröffneten linken Vorhof ausfließende Perfusionsflüssigkeit gelangt durch ein Loch im Kammerboden über ein Ventil in ein Ausflußmeßgerät (z. B. nach Stephenson, 1949). Ödemerzeugende Substanzen werden den Vorratsflaschen für Perfusionslösung zugesetzt oder in den Perfusionsschlauch gespritzt.

Am Ende des Experimentes werden das Präparat sowie die davon abgetrennten Mediastinalorgane erneut gewogen. Die Differenzen aus den Anfangs- und den Endgewichten ermöglichen die Berechnung des initialen und terminalen Lungengewichtes.

Born (1954) wertet in seinen Versuchen jeden Flüssigkeitseintritt in die Lufträume, der signifikant schneller entsteht als es gelegentlich bei Kontrolltieren der Fall ist, als Ödem. Man wird eine genügende Zahl von Kontrollversuchen durchführen müssen, da sowohl das Herz als auch die Lunge im Herz-Lungenpräparat zur spontanen Entstehung von Ödem neigen (Wood u. Moe, 1942).

2. Chemische Analyse

Daly u. Mitarb. (1946) schlossen aus Konzentrationsänderungen des Perfusionsblutes auf die Entstehung von Lungenödem. Hughes, May u. Widdicombe (1958a) versuchten zwischen Ödem und Hyperämie perfundierter Kaninchenlungen zu differenzieren, indem sie neben dem Lungenventrikelgewichtsindex den Eisengehalt des Organs bestimmten. Sie ermittelten nach der Methode von Ponder (1942) spektrophotometrisch den Eisengehalt der ödematösen Lunge, des Perfusionsblutes und der blutfrei gespülten Lunge und schlossen aus den Ergebnissen auf das Blutvolumen der Ödemlunge. In ihren Versuchen gingen bis zu 25% der Gewichtszunahme ödematöser Lungen zu Lasten einer vermehrten Blutfüllung des Organs.

3. Messung des Blut- und Plasmagehaltes

Veränderungen des Blut- oder Plasmagehaltes der perfundierten Lunge wurden von Aviado u. Schmidt (1952) mit der Isotopentechnik nach dem gleichen Prinzip wie am intakten Tier gemessen. Das Schema ihrer Versuchsanordnung ist in Abb. 6 wiedergegeben. Weitere Einzelheiten zur Technik s. S. 171.

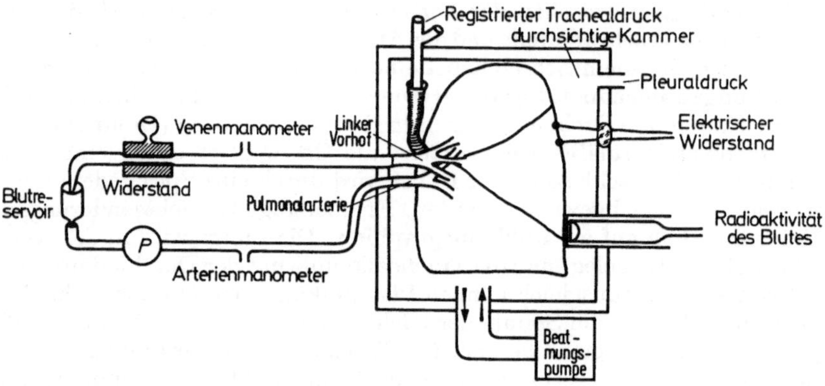

Abb. 6. Versuchsanordnung nach Aviado und Schmidt (1952) zur Ödemdiagnose am perfundierten Lungenflügel des Hundes. Radioaktiv markiertes Blut (Erythrocyten oder Plasma) wird aus einem Reservoir durch eine Dale-Schuster-Pumpe zur Pulmonalarterie befördert und gelangt vom linken Vorhof zum Reservoir zurück. Registrierung der radioaktiven Impulse über der Lungenoberfläche mit einem Geigerzähler. Beatmung durch intermittierenden Druckwechsel in der Atemkammer

4. Lymphflußrate

Paine *et al.* (1949a) verfolgten die Entstehung des Ödems im Herz-Lungenpräparat anhand der Lymphabflußrate und histologischer Schnitte (wiederholte Probeexcisionen während des Versuchs). Technik der Lymphstrommessung wie beim intakten Tier (s. S. 169f.).

5. Elektrische Leitfähigkeit des Lungengewebes

Die auf S. 171f. beschriebenen Verfahren zur Messung des elektrischen Parenchymwiderstandes können ohne methodische Abänderungen am perfundierten Organ angewandt werden. Lambert u. Gremels (1926) maßen den Gewebewiderstand an Herz-Lungenpräparaten von Hunden, die unter Kontrolle des Blutdruckes in der Pulmonalarterie und den Vorhöfen mit defibriniertem Blut durchströmt wurden. Vermehrung des Wassergehaltes der Lunge verminderte den Parenchymwiderstand, gesteigerte Blutdurchströmung war wirkungslos. Das modifizierte Verfahren von Aviado u. Schmidt (1952) läßt eine solche Unterscheidung nicht zu. Die von diesen Autoren benutzten isolierten Hundelungen beantworteten intraarterielle Injektionen von 5 ml Flüssigkeit oder intratracheale Zufuhr von 10 ml Luft mit Widerstandsänderungen.

6. Die mechanischen Eigenschaften der Lunge

Hughes u. Mitarb. (1958b) bestimmten die Dehnbarkeit (Compliance, s. S. 173) an geschädigten perfundierten Kaninchenlungen und setzten diesen Wert zum Ödemgrad in Beziehung. Die Kaninchen wurden vorausgehend durch 32—40 mg/kg Nembutal (Pentobarbital-Na) i.v. narkotisiert und erhielten 10 mg/kg Heparin. Ihre Lungen wurden in situ mit dem Blut eines Spendertieres perfundiert. Der mittlere Perfusionsdruck (Mittelwert aus arteriellem und venösem Druck), der dem Capillardruck entsprechen dürfte, betrug 10 mm Hg und konnte nach Bedarf verändert werden. Die Beatmung erfolgte mit Luft unter konstantem positivem Druck, die Exspiration gegen einen Widerstand von 2 mm Hg. Die Compliance wurde mit der Methode von Konzett u. Rössler (1940) gemessen. Dieses Verfahren zeigt bei konstantem Beatmungsdruck Änderungen des Respirationsluftvolumens an und soll damit ein Maß für die „dynamische Compliance" geben. Der Grad des Lungenödems wurde geschätzt, wobei Veränderungen des Blutvolumens in den Perfusionsgefäßen bei unverändertem Perfusionsdruck über das Ausmaß orientierten. Nach Beendigung der Versuche wurde das Ödem anhand des Verhältnisses von Lungengewicht/Herzgewicht genauer bewertet. Normalwert: 1,53 (Standardabweichung: $\pm 0{,}11$).

D. Zusammenfassende Diskussion

Es ist verhältnismäßig einfach, ein massives Lungenödem aufgrund des Obduktionsbefundes zu diagnostizieren. Schwieriger ist die Erkennung leichter Ödemformen und die quantitative Bestimmung des Ödemgrades, vor allem wenn die Diagnose in vivo gestellt werden soll. Für die ödembedingte Gaswechselstörung bzw. die diagnostische Bewertung des Lungenödems sind verschiedene Kriterien maßgebend. Neben der Flüssigkeitsansammlung in Alveolen und Interstitium sowie der Ausdehnung der ödematösen Veränderungen über die Lunge spielt der Eiweißgehalt der Ödemflüssigkeit und die Verlegung der zuführenden Luftwege durch schaumige Ödemflüssigkeit eine Rolle. Mit steigendem Eiweißgehalt wird der Gasdiffusion zunehmender Widerstand entgegengesetzt, die Rückresorption der Ödemflüssigkeit beeinträchtigt und die Schaumbildung in den Atemwegen gefördert. Der Organismus toleriert die Anwesenheit relativ großer Flüssigkeitsmengen im Lungengewebe und in den Atemwegen, solange sich kein Schaum bildet (Luisada, 1950a, b). Werden aber kleine Bronchien durch Schaum verlegt und die zugehörigen Alveolarbezirke von der Gaszufuhr abgeschnitten, so erreicht die Hypoxie leicht einen bedrohlichen Grad und bewirkt ihrerseits vermehrte Transsudation aus den Capillaren. Ödembedingte Dyspnoe bzw. Gaswechselstörung können dementsprechend bei einem gewissen Grad von Flüssigkeitsakkumulation in dem einen Fall fehlen, in einem anderen sehr deutlich sein (Laqueur u. Magnus, 1921a; Luisada u. Sarnoff, 1946a; Vitale *et al.*, 1954; Winternitz u. Lambert, 1919). Die Flüssigkeitsmenge, die sich bis zum Eintritt des Todes in der Lunge ansammelt, ist von der Entstehungsgeschwindigkeit des Lungenödems abhängig (Winternitz u. Lambert, 1919). Bei langsamer Ödementwicklung kann die Lunge mehr Flüssigkeit aufnehmen, weil die Lebensdauer durch Kompensationsvorgänge verlängert wird.

Neben den vorgenannten primären Determinanten wird der Krankheitszustand durch sekundäre Faktoren bestimmt, die einerseits Folge der ödematösen Lungenveränderungen sein, andererseits aus einer direkten Einwirkung der Ödemnoxe auf andere Organe oder Organsysteme resultieren können. In Frage kommen in erster Linie Störungen der Zirkulation infolge Bluteindickung mit Zunahme der Blutviscosität, Erhöhung des Kreislaufwiderstandes in der Lunge, Hyperämie und Hämorrhagien der Lunge sowie eine Behinderung der Gaspassage im Tracheobronchialsystem infolge Bronchoconstriction, gesteigerter Bronchialsekretion, Schleimhautschwellung oder -desquamation, Glottisödem oder -constriction. Ferner kann das — evtl. unter dem Einfluß der Ödemnoxe veränderte — Verhalten des Tieres eine Rolle spielen. Eine latente Gaswechselstörung kann unter dem Einfluß gesteigerter Muskelaktivität manifest werden; Bewegung soll zudem der Schaumbildung in den Bronchien Vorschub leisten (Laqueur u. de Vries Reilingh, 1920a, b).

Die Vielzahl der potentiellen Faktoren erklärt, daß die lebensbedrohende Hypoxämie häufig nicht in Korrelation zu einzelnen klinischen Symptomen steht. So war beim Menschen z.B. keine Beziehung zwischen der Ausdehnung von

Rasselgeräuschen über kleinere oder größere Teile der Lunge und der arteriellen Sauerstoffsättigung nachzuweisen (Vitale *et al.*, 1954) und beim Versuchstier muß die vor dem Tod beobachtete Dyspnoe nicht mit dem bei der Obduktion diagnostizierten Schweregrad des Ödems übereinstimmen (Luisada u. Sarnoff, 1944, 1946a, b; Winternitz u. Lambert, 1929).

Daher ist es auch verständlich, daß es trotz vielfältiger Bemühungen bisher nicht gelungen ist, ein Verfahren zu entwickeln, das ein frühzeitiges oder quantitatives Erkennen von Lungenödem beim lebenden Versuchstier ermöglicht. Alle Techniken (Beobachtung, Durchleuchtung oder Auskultation), die auf operative Eingriffe verzichten, liefern unzuverlässige Resultate oder zeigen erst bei hochgradigem Ödem kurz vor Eintritt des Todes einen positiven Befund. Die übrigen in vivo anwendbaren diagnostischen Methoden können von sich aus aufgrund der damit verbundenen Maßnahmen (Narkose, Operation) einen ödemfördernden oder -hemmenden Einfluß ausüben (vgl. S. 28ff.). Sie verlangen zudem einen vergleichsweise großen technischen Aufwand. Aus diesen Gründen erscheint die Mehrzahl der verfügbaren in vivo-Verfahren weniger für eine quantitative Diagnosestellung als vielmehr für die Lösung spezieller pathophysiologischer Probleme geeignet.

Sehr viel häufiger wird die Diagnose bzw. die quantitative Bewertung des Krankheitszustandes daher post mortem entweder nach Eintritt des Spontantodes oder nach Opferung des Tieres vorgenommen. Besten Aufschluß über den Schweregrad eines Ödems wird man durch Methoden erhalten, die nebeneinander mehrere Parameter wie relatives Lungengewicht, Wassergehalt des Lungengewebes, chemische Analysenwerte (vor allem Eiweißgehalt der Lunge bzw. der Ödemflüssigkeit) und histologische Daten erfassen; um das zu erreichen müssen gegebenenfalls mehrere diagnostische Maßnahmen kombiniert werden. Ein solches Vorgehen empfiehlt sich besonders dann, wenn differentialdiagnostische Erwägungen zu treffen sind. Ein spezielles Problem stellt in dieser Hinsicht die Unterscheidung zwischen Ödem und Hyperämie der Lungen dar.

Der makroskopische Obduktionsbefund erfordert zwar wenig technischen Aufwand, besitzt aber nur beschränkte Aussagekraft und muß daher mit weiteren diagnostischen Resultaten verglichen werden. Die mikroskopische Untersuchung der Lunge läßt quantitative Schlüsse ebenfalls nur bedingt zu, ermöglicht jedoch häufig erst eine Abgrenzung zwischen Ödem und anderen pathologischen Zuständen, die makroskopisch nicht erkennbar sind. Allerdings ist die Methode mit einem verhältnismäßig großen Arbeitsaufwand verbunden, der insbesondere dann ins Gewicht fällt, wenn bei Serienversuchen auf diese Weise eine quantitative Beurteilung erfolgen soll. Der histologische Befund wird deshalb in der Regel nur als Ergänzung zu anderen Daten erhoben. Das relative Lungengewicht und ähnliche Meßgrößen geben verhältnismäßig zuverlässige quantitative Hinweise bei einem auch für Serienversuche vertretbaren Arbeitsaufwand. Aufgrund derartiger Werte ist jedoch keine Unterscheidung zwischen Ödem und anderen Störungen der Lunge, die gleichfalls mit einer Gewichtszunahme des Organs einhergehen, möglich. Prinzipiell dasselbe gilt für die Bestimmung des Wassergehaltes der Lunge, wenn diese Technik auch Vorteile vor der Wägung besitzt. Werden dagegen relatives Gewicht und Wassergehalt der Lunge zueinander in Beziehung gesetzt (Poulsen, 1954a), so läßt sich — zwar auch nur unter Einschränkungen — zwischen ödembedingter und stauungsbedingter Gewichtssteigerung differenzieren. Dieses Vorgehen dürfte den im Vergleich zum Aufwand größten Informationswert besitzen und sich für die Beurteilung therapeutischer Maßnahmen am besten eignen. Die Bestimmung des Eiweißgehaltes der Lunge bzw. der Ödemflüssigkeit kann zur weiteren Klärung der Situation beitragen, wird im allgemeinen aber nur als zusätzliches Verfahren in Frage kommen; da die experimentellen Anforderungen erheblich sind, hat diese Methode bisher keine weite Verbreitung gefunden.

Die diagnostische Beurteilung pathophysiologischer Prozesse der isolierten Lunge erfolgt mittels ähnlicher Methoden, wie sie in vivo oder post mortem angewandt werden. Ein gewisser Vorteil ergibt sich aus der Möglichkeit bestimmte Vorgänge, z.B. Gewichtsveränderungen der Lunge, kontinuierlich zu registrieren. Andererseits hat die Technik insgesamt recht enge Grenzen, die ihren Einsatz auf die Untersuchung umschriebener Probleme, vor allem auf die Analyse lokal wirksamer ödemgenetischer bzw. therapeutischer Faktoren, beschränkt.

Die Erzeugung von Lungenödem im Tierversuch

Lungenödem wird von Rusznyák *et al.* (1957) als „einer der wichtigsten und häufigsten pathologischen Zustände" bezeichnet. Es tritt bei zahlreichen Krankheiten, vor allem bei Herz-, Kreislauf-, Lungen- und Nierenkrankheiten, bei Erkrankungen oder Verletzungen des zentralen Nervensystems, bei Vergiftungen und multiplen Frakturen auf (s. z.B. Cameron, 1948; Hayward, 1955; Halmágyi, 1957; Luisada u. Cardi, 1956). Vielfältig sind die pathologischen Mechanismen, die zum Lungenödem führen. Vielfältig sind auch die Möglichkeiten im Tierexperiment Lungenödem hervorzurufen. Versuche, beim Tier Lungenödem zu erzeugen, dienen entweder der Aufklärung der Ödempathogenese und des Pathomechanismus, oder der Erforschung prophylaktischer und therapeutischer Maßnahmen. Da es in der Regel klinische, werksärztliche, kurz, aus der Pathophysiologie des Menschen stammende Probleme sind, zu deren Aufklärung Laboratoriumstiere eingesetzt werden, bemühen sich viele Autoren, Ödemformen im Modellversuch herzustellen, die klinischen Ödemformen nahestehen. Bei der Bearbeitung von Problemen der Ödemprophylaxe und -therapie haben sich auch Methoden als brauchbar oder nützlich erwiesen, die in ihrer Genese kaum Beziehungen zu klinisch bekannten Ödemformen erkennen lassen, den Krankheitszustand jedoch in einfacher, leicht reproduzierbarer Weise hervorrufen.

A. Allgemeines zur Technik der Ödemprovokation

Experimentelles Lungenödem kann bei zahlreichen Tierarten erzeugt werden. Verwendet wurden Frösche (Heim u. Meves, 1950), Mäuse (Harford u. Hara, 1950; Henschler *et al.*, 1960; Poulsen, 1954a), Ratten (Dieke u. Richter, 1946; Henschler *et al.*, 1960; Koenig u. Koenig, 1949; MacKenzie, 1943), Hamster (Stokinger, 1957), Meerschweinchen (Drenckhahn, 1958; Koenig u. Koenig, 1949; Moon u. Morgan, 1936; Plester u. Rummel, 1951; Wohlzogen *et al.*, 1956), Kaninchen (Boyd u. Perry, 1960, Cameron u. Courtice, 1946; Kisch, 1958; Koenig u. Koenig, 1949; MacKay *et al.*, 1949; Sarnoff u. Sarnoff, 1952b), Katzen (Koenig u. Koenig, 1949; Koenig *et al.*, 1952; Mendenhall u. Stokinger, 1959; Wirth, 1936), Hunde (Harrison u. Liebow, 1952; Moon u. Morgan, 1936; Rusznyák *et al.*, 1957; Sarnoff u. Sarnoff, 1952b), Schafe (Visscher *et al.*, 1956), Ziegen (Cameron u. Courtice, 1946; Visscher *et al.*, 1956; Winternitz u. Lambert, 1919), Affen (Dieke u. Richter, 1946; Winternitz u. Lambert, 1919); weitere Literaturangaben s. Tabelle 4. Spontan tritt es auch bei anderen Tierarten, z.B. Pferden auf (Laqueur u. Magnus, 1921). Es kann beim intakten, wachen oder narkotisierten Tier, an der in situ perfundierten Lunge oder am isolierten Organ hervorgerufen werden.

Ein und dieselbe Noxe erzeugt nicht bei allen Versuchstierarten in gleicher Weise Ödem. Auch Rassen-, Geschlechts- und Altersunterschiede beeinflussen die Reaktivität. So ruft die i.p. Injektion von α-Naphthylthioharnstoff bei Mäusen, braunen norwegischen Wildratten, Katzen und Hunden Lungenödem hervor, bleibt aber bei Ratten eines anderen Stammes, bei Meerschweinchen, Kaninchen und Affen selbst bei vielfach höherer Dosierung wirkungslos (Dieke u. Richter, 1946). Junge Ratten im Gewicht bis zu 100 g sind wesentlich unempfindlicher gegen diese Verbindung als Tiere, die über 200 g wiegen. Erst oberhalb von 200 g bleibt das Verhältnis von wirksamer Dosis/kg Körpergewicht annähernd konstant (Dieke u. Richter, 1945; MacKenzie u. MacKenzie, 1943). Männliche und weibliche Tiere reagierten bei diesen Versuchen gleichartig. Ein anderes Thioharnstoffderivat, Thiosemicarbazid, löste nur bei Ratten Lungenödem aus (Dieke, 1949), obwohl es für artverschiedene Tiere im gleichen Dosenbereich tödlich war. Mit Ammoniumchlorid kann man bei Ratten und Meerschweinchen Lungenödem erzeugen, weniger gut bei Katzen; Kaninchen entwickeln selbst nach letalen Dosen kein Lungenödem (Koenig u. Koenig, 1949). Auch hier gibt es altersbedingte Empfindlichkeitsunterschiede; junge Ratten im Alter bis zu 2 Wochen sind resistent, bei einem Körpergewicht von 50 g reagieren sie mit leichtem, bei mehr als 100 g Gewicht mit schwerem Lungenödem (Jaques, 1954). Für ozonbedingtes Lungenödem sind junge Mäuse mit einem mittleren Gewicht von 19 g viel empfänglicher als ältere Tiere im Gewicht von 35 g (Stokinger, 1957). Adrenalin wirkt in der Regel nur bei Nagetieren, vor allem bei Kaninchen ödemauslösend (Luisada, 1950) (aber auch beim Menschen), Hunde und Katzen verenden unter anderen Symptomen (Drenckhahn, 1958). Für centrogenes Lungenödem sind Sprague-Dawley-Ratten wesentlich anfälliger als Wistarratten (Maire u. Patton, 1954).

Die Versuchstiere sollen gesund, vor allem frei von Lungenkrankheiten sein. Diese Vorbedingung kann häufig nicht ohne weiteres erfüllt werden. Elmes u. Bell (1962) haben gezeigt, daß ein großer Prozentsatz der handelsüblichen Laboratoriumsratten mit chronischen Lungenkrankheiten behaftet ist. Latente oder subklinische Infektionen der Atemwege können die Toxicität ödemerzeugender Noxen steigern. Für Tiere mit derartigen Erkrankungen sind Ozonkonzentrationen, die von gesunden Tieren überlebt werden, tödlich (Stokinger, 1957).

Umweltfaktoren, wie Tierhaltung und -ernährung, können die Ausbildung des Ödems modifizieren. Ihr Einfluß muß durch standardisierte Klima- und Fütterungsbedingungen ausgeschaltet werden (s. z. B. Hemingway, 1952; Henschler u. Laux, 1960). Steigerung der Umgebungstemperatur (Luisada u. Sarnoff, 1956) oder Erwärmung der Atemluft fördert die Ödementwicklung (Haddy *et al.*, 1949). Befeuchtung der Atemluft hat keine deutliche Wirkung (Haddy *et al.*, 1949). Unterkühlung schützt vor dem Ammoniumchloridödem (Koenig u. Koenig, 1949) und O_2-Ödem (Campbell, 1937a; Grossmann u. Penrod, 1949a). Stoffwechselsenkung bedingt im allgemeinen eine Verminderung, Steigerung des Grundumsatzes eine Zunahme der Ödembereitschaft (Campbell, 1937b; Grossmann u. Penrod, 1949b; Gerschman *et al.*, 1954; Gottsegen *et al.*, 1958). Nach Trockendiät wird die Phosgenvergiftung besser toleriert als nach Normalkost (Cameron u. Courtice, 1946). Bei hungernden Tieren war die Sterblichkeit an O_2-Vergiftung geringer als bei normal ernährten Tieren (Campbell, 1937).

Saisonbedingte Einflüsse sind, soweit sie das Lungengewicht betreffen, auf S. 180 besprochen worden. Auch die Reaktivität gegenüber ödemauslösenden Reizen wird von der Jahreszeit beeinflußt (Gottsegen *et al.*, 1958).

Die Folgen der Narkoseschädigung, der künstlichen Atmung, des Operationstraumas für die Ödembereitschaft sind in Abschnitt A 11 S. 174f. abgehandelt. Körperliche Aktivität kann die Ödementwicklung fördern. So erhöht z. B. die durch eine Lauftrommel erzwungene Motilität die Empfindlichkeit von Ratten gegen Ozon (Stokinger, 1957). Radioaktive Strahlen können prädisponierend wirken (Cassen u. Kistler, 1954a). Andererseits kann die wiederholte Einwirkung subletaler Konzentrationen mancher Ödemnoxen, insbesondere von Reizgasen, Toleranz gegen die gleiche und andere Noxen erzeugen (s. z. B. Box u. Cullumbine,

1947; Henschler, 1960; Henschler u. Laux, 1960; Matzen, 1957; Mendenhall u. Stokinger, 1959).

Entsprechend der Heterogenität der Ödemnoxen sind an der Pathogenese der einzelnen Ödemformen unterschiedliche Faktoren beteiligt. Symptomatik und Morphologie des Lungenödems sind dagegen im großen und ganzen verhältnismäßig uniform; in Einzelheiten können die verschiedenen Ödemformen jedoch von einander abweichen. So kann z.B. die Latenzzeit zwischen der Applikation der Noxe und der vollen Ausbildung des Ödems zwischen wenigen Minuten und Stunden differieren. Auch in der Zusammensetzung der Ödemflüssigkeit hinsichtlich der begleitenden Hyperämie oder der Hämorrhagien findet man individuelle Abweichungen.

B. Beschreibung der Methoden

I. Hämodynamische Veränderungen

Als erster hat wahrscheinlich Welch (1878) das hämodynamische Lungenödem an Kaninchen und Hunden eingehender studiert. Nach Unterbindung der Aorta ascendens oder der Aorta descendens und eines Teils der vom Arcus aortae entspringenden Hauptarterien entwickelte sich bei Kaninchen regelmäßig innerhalb weniger Minuten ein starkes Lungenödem. Ähnliche Resultate werden nach Quetschung des linken Ventrikels erzielt (Alexandrow, 1893; Welch, 1878). Beim Hund ist es nicht so leicht möglich, auf diese Weise Lungenödem hervorzurufen. Sahli (1885) und Grossmann (1889) erzeugten Lungenödem durch Kompression des linken Vorhofs, Lichtheim (1879) beobachtete es nach Unterbindung der Lungenvenen, Rosenbach (1878) bei artefizieller Aorten- und Mitralinsuffizienz. Bei diesen älteren Versuchen wurde das „Lungenödem“ aus dem makroskopischen Befund diagnostiziert, ein Vorgehen, bei dem nur schwerere Formen erkennbar sind (Sahli, 1885). Zusammenstellung der älteren Literatur bei Visscher u. Mitarb. (1956).

In den letzten Jahren sind Eingriffe an Herz und Gefäßen weniger häufig zur Erzeugung von Lungenödem ausgeführt worden. Sie haben für Routineuntersuchungen mancherlei Nachteile: Der Operationsaufwand erschwert Serienversuche; die operativen Veränderungen lassen sich nicht genau dosieren; Narkose und Operation wirken zusätzlich schädigend und dies von Tier zu Tier in unterschiedlichem Ausmaß. Zudem ist es schwierig, allein durch hämodynamische Veränderungen Lungenödem hervorzurufen. Die Tiere müssen entweder so schwer geschädigt werden, daß nicht nur die hämodynamischen Behandlungsfolgen, sondern auch sonstige, z.B. Dyspnoe und Anoxie ödemprovozierend mitwirken (Cameron, 1948) oder zusätzliche Schädigungen müssen artefiziell herbeigeführt werden, z.B. Sauerstoffmangel (Warren u. Drinker, 1942; Drinker, 1950). Andererseits können klinische Lungenödemfälle, die auf hämodynamische Störungen zurückgehen, durch derartige Modellversuche recht gut nachgeahmt und hinsichtlich ihrer pathophysiologischen Mechanismen untersucht werden. Man muß nur berücksichtigen, daß derartige Lungenödemformen beim Menschen häufig am Ende langdauernder Herz- oder Kreislauferkrankungen auftreten, die vorausgehend morphologische Veränderungen des Lungengewebes hervorgerufen haben (Meessen, 1956).

Die Technik der experimentellen Herzchirurgie ist kürzlich von Markowitz *et al.* (1959) dargestellt worden. Die Beschreibung der operativen Maßnahmen wird daher knapp gehalten. Geeignete Versuchstiere sind Hund, Katze, Kaninchen; auch Ratten sind gelegentlich verwendet worden.

1. Eingriffe an der Aortenklappe

a) Aortenklappeninsuffizienz nach Paine u. Mitarb. (1952)

Hunden in Nembutalnarkose, heparinisiert und über eine Trachealkanüle beatmet, wird der Thorax durch Längsspaltung des Sternums geöffnet. Blutdruckkontrolle mit Hg- bzw. Wassermanometern in der rechten oberen Lungenlappenarterie, im linken Vorhofohr und in einer Femoralarterie. Die rechte Arteria carotis communis wird isoliert und unterbunden; eine lange Biopsiezange (für urologische Zwecke) mit abgerundeten stumpfen Branchen wird durch die Arteria carotis und die Aorta ascendens bis in die Höhe der Aortenklappen vorgeschoben und in die gewünschte Stellung gebracht. Man faßt einen Klappenzipfel und reißt ihn ab. Nur selten ist es möglich, mehr als einen Klappenzipfel zu zerstören, ohne sofortiges Herzversagen auszulösen. Folge der Valvulotomie ist eine Vergrößerung des linken Ventrikels und in einem Teil der Fälle Abfall des arteriellen Blutdrucks; die Druckwerte in Pulmonalarterie und -vene bleiben im Normbereich. Ein Lungenödem wird noch nicht erzeugt, aber es wird eine Prädisposition geschaffen, denn nach Adrenalingaben (0,25 mg in den linken Vorhof) oder nach Erzeugung einer Hirnembolie (5% $BaSO_4$-Lösung; s. S. 211) tritt es auf, während diese Maßnamen bei Tieren ohne vorausgehende Herzschädigung in der Regel kein Ödem provozieren.

b) Verfahren nach Hawthorne *et al.* (1956a)

Bastardhunde in Na-Pentobarbitalnarkose (30 mg/kg) und mit 0,5 mg Digoxin i.m. 15—30 min vor der Operation behandelt, werden unter künstlicher Beatmung mit einem Narkoseapparat im 3. oder 4. Zwischenrippenraum links thorakotomiert. Die Oberfläche des linken Ventrikels wird durch Auftropfen von 2—4 ml 2% Butacainsulfat anaesthesiert. Dann wird ein spezielles Valvulotom mit einem Außendurchmesser von 5mm nach der Technik von Smithy *et al.*(1948) durch die Muskulatur des linken Ventrikels hindurch zur Aortenklappe vorgeschoben. Seine Lage wird an extrakardialen Orientierungspunkten (Verlauf der Hauptcoronararterie, Aortenwurzel) kontrolliert. Aus jedem der 3 Zipfel der Aortenklappe kann ein halbmondförmiger Sektor, dessen Größe u.a. von den Maßen des Valvulotoms abhängt, ausgeschnitten werden. Die Tiere überleben derartige Operationen monatelang. Die Aortenklappendefekte reichen nicht aus, um Lungenödem hervorzurufen. Paine u. Mitarb. schädigen die voroperierten Tiere daher zusätzlich, indem sie sie einseitig nephrektomieren und die Nierenarterie der Gegenseite mit einer modifizierten Goldblattklemme soweit einengen, daß zwischen den Pulsationen vor und hinter der Klemme keine Differenzen fühlbar sind. Nach dieser zusätzlichen Schädigung sterben die Tiere innerhalb von 2 Tagen an Lungenödem, während Kontrolltiere ohne Klappeninsuffizienz, aber mit gleicher Nierenschädigung im Verlauf von 4 Tagen bis zu mehreren Wochen an maligner Hypertonie eingehen. Die Ödembildung wird als Folge von Linksversagen bei Drucksteigerung im linken Vorhof, in den Lungenvenen und -capillaren aufgefaßt. Wird außer dem Aortenklappendefekt noch ein Vorhofseptumdefekt gesetzt, der dem regurgitierenden Blut einen anderen Abflußweg eröffnet, so bleibt das Lungenödem aus (Hawthorne *et al.*, 1956b).

2. Eingriffe an der Mitralklappe

a) Mitralinsuffizienz nach Rusznyák *et al.* (1957)

Der Thorax wird im 4. Intercostalraum geöffnet und das Herz freigelegt. In die Vorderwand des linken Ventrikels werden 2 Haltefäden eingezogen. Mit einer feinen Schere dringt man zwischen den Fäden in die Kammer ein und schädigt die Klappe. Eine ausführlichere Darstellung der operativen Technik geben Markowitz *et al.* (1959).

b) Mitralstenose (Rusznyák *et al.*, 1957)

Das linke Herzohr wird in das Mitralostium hineingezogen und dort durch Nähte fixiert. Als Folge der Operation erweitern sich die Hauptlymphwege (Ductus thoracicus, Truncus lymphaceus dexter) stark. Doch erst wenn diese in einer weiteren Operation unterbunden werden, bildet sich Lungenödem aus. Haddy *et al.* (1953) engen den Mitralring durch Seidennähte ein.

3. Eingriffe an der Aorta

Verschluß der Aorta nach Paine u. Mitarb. (1950)

Hunden in Pentobarbitalnatrium-Narkose wird unter Überdruckbeatmung der Brustkorb durch einen Längsschnitt geöffnet. Blutdruckmessung mit Wasser- bzw. Hg-Manometern im rechten und linken Vorhof, in der Arteria carotis oder femoralis und der rechten Lungenoberlappenarterie. Mit einer gewöhnlichen Schraubklemme, vor dem Abgang der Kopf- und Armarterien um die Aorta ascendens gelegt, wird das Gefäß graduell komprimiert. Es kommt zur Dilatation des linken Ventrikels und zur Drucksteigerung in den Lungengefäßen. Lungenödem tritt erst bei hochgradiger Kompression der Aorta auf. Ödembildung wird anhand der Lymphflußrate und des histologischen Bildes beurteilt.

4. Eingriffe an den Lungengefäßen

a) Lungenvenenverschluß nach Cheng (1950)

Männliche Ratten, mit Nembutal und Äther narkotisiert und über einen Trachealkatheter unter Überdruck (z.B. mit dem Gerät nach Porter u. Small, 1947) beatmet, werden auf der linken Seite im 4. oder 5. Intercostalraum durch einen etwa 2 cm langen Schnitt thorakotomiert. Die untere Hälfte der linken Lunge wird nach außen verlagert; um die Vena pulmonalis wird eine lockere Ligatur gelegt, deren Enden in Höhe des Hilus durch die vordere und hintere Brustwand nach außen geführt werden. Nach Reposition der Lunge wird die Operationswunde unter lokaler Antibiotica-Applikation schichtweise geschlossen und die Thoraxhöhle durch eine in die Wunde eingenähte Injektionskanüle vor Ausführung der Hautnaht mit einer Saugpumpe evakuiert; Kanüle und Trachealkatheter werden entfernt, die Enden der Venenligatur an der Haut fixiert. Bis zum Abklingen der Narkose verbleibt das Tier in einer Sauerstoffkammer. Röntgenologische Kontrolle während der folgenden Tage zeigt in der Regel eine normale Belüftung der Lunge. 3—4 Tage nach der Operation wird die um die Pulmonalvene gelegte Ligatur durch kräftigen Zug an ihren nach außen geführten Enden geschlossen. Innerhalb der anschließenden Stunde entwickeln sich ein massives intraalveoläres Ödem und Hämorrhagien. In den folgenden Stunden treten mehr und mehr entzündliche und nekrotische Vorgänge in den Vordergrund.

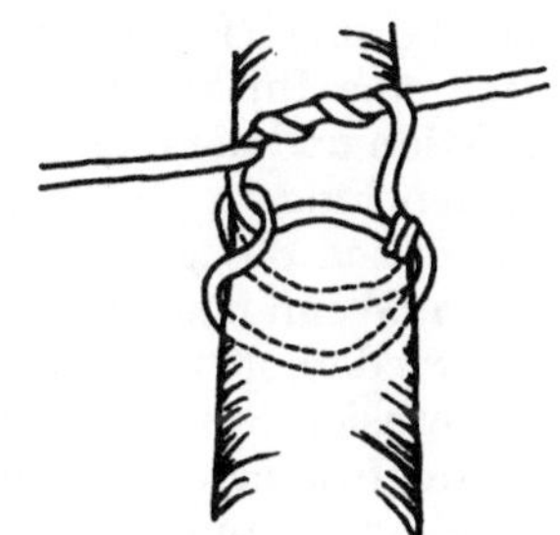

Abb. 7. Knoten zur partiellen Unterbindung der Vena pulmonalis. (Aus: Cheng, 1950)

Eine Verengung der Vene durch partielle Unterbindung kann mit Hilfe des in Abb. 7 wiedergegebenen Knotens erzielt werden. Sie hat ähnliche Folgen; Ödembildung und Entzündung verlaufen allerdings langsamer und weniger regelmäßig.

b) Lungenödem durch pulmonale Hypertonie nach Ferguson u. Berkas (1957)

Hunde im Gewicht von 10—15 kg werden mit Pentobarbital narkotisiert und über einen Trachealtubus mit maximal 15 mm Hg Überdruck beatmet. Nach Eröffnung des Thorax, Unterbindung und Durchtrennung der linken Arteria brachialis und pulmonalis werden proximales Ende der Brachial- und distales Ende der Pulmonalarterie miteinander verbunden. Druckmessung in einem Gefäß des oberen Segments des linken Lungenoberlappens; die beiden restlichen Segmente des Lappens stehen zur Beobachtung der Ödementwicklung zur Verfügung. Der Blutdruck in der Oberlappenarterie wird durch ein an der Unterlappenarterie angelegtes Tourniquet reguliert. Wird er über ein bestimmtes Niveau erhöht, so bildet sich in den beiden durchbluteten Segmenten des Oberlappens ein Ödem aus. Wenn die Lungensegmente vorausgehend denerviert werden, tritt das Ödem schon bei wesentlich niedrigeren Druckwerten auf. Zur Denervierung wird die Blutzufuhr durch die Arteria brachialis für etwa 5 min abgeklemmt und die Segmentarterien, -venen und -bronchien werden in dieser Zeit von allem adventitiellen Gewebe einschließlich der Nerven, Lymphgefäße und Bronchialgefäße freipräpariert.

5. Eingriffe an den Coronargefäßen

Verschluß der Coronararterien

Bei einem erheblichen Prozentsatz spontaner Ödemtodesfälle entsteht das Lungenödem auf dem Boden schwerer Coronarinsuffizienz (Cameron, 1948; Hegglin, 1956). Bei Bemühungen um ein tierexperimentelles Krankheitsmodell hat man versucht, durch Unterbindung der Coronararterien Ödem hervorzurufen. Die Operationstechnik ist von Markowitz *et al.* (1959) beschrieben worden. Unterbindung der Coronararterien verursacht jedoch gewöhnlich Blutdruckabfall in der Arteria femoralis (und tödlichen Zusammenbruch des Kreislaufs) oder Kammerflimmern (Roos u. Smith, 1948; Rössler, 1930; Markowitz *et al.*, 1959), bevor sich ein Lungenödem entwickelt. Roos und Smith (1948) modifizierten daher die Technik: Man beatmet narkotisierte (Pentobarbital-Natrium) Hunde im Gewicht von 5—15 kg über eine Trachealkanüle, spaltet das Sternum und eröffnet das Perikard durch feine Einschnitte über dem linken Ventrikel und dem rechten Herzohr. Nach der Blutstillung erhalten die Tiere 30—50 mg Heparin i.v. Dann werden 1—4 ml einer 3,3%igen Kartoffelstärkesuspension in physiologischer NaCl-Lösung (Partikeldurchmesser 12—72 μ; ca. 1000000 Partikel pro mm^3) durch eine Injektionskanüle in die linke Ventrikelhöhle gespritzt. Während der Injektion und der folgenden 2—3 sec muß die Aorta unmittelbar über dem Herzen mit den Fingern abgeklemmt werden. Die Autoren nehmen an, daß unter diesen Umständen der größte Teil, wenn nicht alle Partikel in die Coronargefäße gelangen. Wenn nötig kann die Injektion in Intervallen von einigen Minuten mehrmals wiederholt werden. Wird zusätzlich das zirkulierende Blutvolumen durch die i.v. Infusion von 250—300 ml Blut erhöht, so reicht eine geringere Zahl von Stärkeinfusionen aus, um den Druck im rechten Vorhof zu erhöhen, eine Herzdilatation, Stauung in der Lunge und Leber und Lungenödem hervorzurufen. Der arterielle Blutdruck bleibt verhältnismäßig lange im Normbereich. Der Tod der Tiere tritt in der Regel innerhalb kurzer Zeit ein, so daß die anatomischen Veränderungen des Myokards noch nicht sehr auffallend sind.

6. Hypervolämie, Hyposmie

In der Pathogenese des Lungenödems können Veränderungen des zirkulierenden Flüssigkeitsvolumens oder des kolloidosmotischen Plasmadruckes eine Rolle spielen. Dieser Mechanismus hat wegen der breiten Anwendung i.v. Infusionen in der Klinik praktische Bedeutung. Altschule u. Mitarb. (1942) haben bei gesunden Versuchspersonen zwar vergeblich versucht, durch rasche Infusion (185 ml/min) von 1800 ml NaCl-Lösung Lungenödem hervorzurufen, glauben aber, daß der Versuch bei Patienten mit chronischen Herz-, Lungen- oder Nierenkrankheiten geglückt wäre. In der Tat ist über derartige Infusionszwischenfälle berichtet worden (Gibbon u. Gibbon, 1942). Akute Blutverluste, die der Infusion vorausgehen, verstärken beim Hund die Ödemneigung (Eaton, 1950). Der Verlust größerer Teile des Lungengewebes (Lobektomie) begünstigt die Ödembereitschaft ebenfalls (Gibbon *et al.*, 1942; Gibbon u. Gibbon, 1942). Hypoxie, vorausgehende Adrenalingaben, Thoraxverletzungen, Atemwiderstandserhöhung und Vagotomie haben dieselben Folgen. Beim gesunden Versuchstier kann man nur durch Infusion sehr großer Flüssigkeitsmengen Lungenödem erzeugen. Neben der Flüssigkeitsmenge ist ihre Zusammensetzung, die Infusionsgeschwindigkeit und der Ort der Infusion bedeutungsvoll. Infusion in die Arteria carotis ruft leichter Ödem hervor als Infusion in die Femoralarterie oder in eine Vene (Luisada u. Sarnoff, 1946a—c).

Nach Courtice u. Korner (1952) sowie Korner (1953) infundiert man Kaninchen im Gewicht von 1,2—3,0 kg angewärmte (32—34° C) Ringer-Locke-Lösung durch eine Injektionskanüle in die Ohrvene oder durch einen Polyäthylenschlauch in die rechte Vena jugularis externa. Der Eingriff an der Jugularvene wird in leichter Narkose (20 mg/kg Nembutal) unter Lokalanaesthesie (Infiltration des Operationsgebietes mit 5—8 ml 1%iger Cocain·HCl-Lösung) ausgeführt. Wenn der Blutdruck während des Versuches kontrolliert werden soll, muß ein weiterer Polyäthylenschlauch in die Arteria carotis eingebunden und die Operationswunde anschließend vernäht werden. Ist die Narkose 1—2 Std nach der Operation abgeklungen, wird mit der Infusion begonnen. Hierzu werden die Tiere auf einem weichen Ledertuch, das in einen Metallrahmen gehängt ist, so gelagert, daß die Atemexkursionen des Thorax nicht behindert werden. Das Körpergewicht wird weitgehend von den Extremitäten — durch Öffnungen der Unterlage gesteckt und am Metallrahmen fixiert — aufgefangen. Bei günstiger Lagerung verhalten sich die Tiere während der Infusionsperiode von 5 Std ruhig, so daß auf Narkose verzichtet werden kann. Wenn mit einem Bluttransfusionsapparat während dieses Zeitraumes etwa 330 ml Infusionslösung/kg in kontinuierlichem Strom zugeführt werden, bildet sich in der Regel ein mittelschweres Lungenödem aus. Die Ödembildung in der Lunge beginnt, wenn die übrigen Körperteile etwa 140 ml Flüssigkeit/kg Gewebe aufgenommen haben. Bis zum Ende der Infusion wird das Plasmavolumen des Blutes (bestimmt aus dem Hämoglobingehalt oder dem Hämatokrit) um durchschnittlich 25% vermehrt; der Venendruck (gemessen in der Ohrvene bzw. in der Jugularvene) steigt im Mittel auf 11,4 cm/H_2O; der kolloidosmotische Plasmadruck fällt um durchschnittlich 30%. Läßt man außerdem O_2-arme Luft atmen (Gasgemisch mit 11% O_2, s. S. 206) so genügt die Hälfte des Infusionsvolumens, um die gleiche Wirkung zu erzielen; die Ödembildung beginnt nach einer Akkumulation von 50 ml zusätzlicher Flüssigkeit/kg Gewebe. Noradrenalin, in der Menge von 0,3 µg/kg/min mit der Infusionsflüssigkeit zugeführt, begünstigt die Ödembildung, vermehrt aber auch die Blutfüllung der Lungengefäße. Hohe Dosen von Noradrenalin (10—20 µg/kg/min) verhindern dagegen die Entstehung von Lungenödem, verursachen aber große Ergüsse in die Pleura- und Peritonealhöhle. (Tötung der Tiere durch i.v. Injektion von 80 mg Nembutal/kg. Bewertung des Ödems nach makroskopischen und mikroskopischen Obduktionsbefunden und dem relativen Lungengewicht).

Courtice u. Mitarb. (1954) übertrugen dieses Verfahren auf Ratten. Man führt Wistarratten im Gewicht von 180—340 g in Äthernarkose einen feinen Polyäthylenschlauch in eine der äußeren Jugularvenen ein. Nach dem Abklingen der

Narkose werden die Tiere in Spezialkäfige (nach Bollman, 1948) gesetzt. In den Käfigen ist die Bewegungsfreiheit der Ratten soweit begrenzt, daß die Infusion, mit der 2 Std nach der Operation begonnen werden kann, ohne zusätzliche Restriktion möglich ist. Die Infusionsflüssigkeit wird aus einer Bürette mit Infusionsraten von 1,5—12 ml/h 5 Std lang infundiert. Man kann sterile Ringer-Locke-Lösung, frisch gewonnenes artgleiches Blut oder Plasma oder mit Plasma verdünntes Blut verwenden. Infusionsblut bzw. -plasma und Empfängerblut müssen vor Beginn der Infusion der Kreuzprobe unterworfen werden. Nach Beendigung der Infusion tötet man die Tiere durch Injektion von Nembutal und obduziert sie sofort. Bewertung des Ödems nach dem makroskopischen Befund, dem histologischen Bild und dem relativen Lungengewicht. Werden Ringer-Locke-Lösung bzw. Plasma als Infusionsflüssigkeit verwendet, so kann man die durch die Infusion bedingten Veränderungen des Blutvolumens aus der Differenz des Hämoglobingehaltes vor und nach der Infusion abschätzen. Plasma oder Blut rufen schwerere Ödeme hervor als Ringer-Locke-Lösung. Bei einem mittleren Infusionsvolumen von 137 ml Ringer-Locke-Lösung/kg stieg das relative Lungengewicht von 4,9 (Kontrollen) auf 6,3 g/kg; 70 ml Plasma bzw. 73 ml Blut/kg Körpergewicht bewirkten Zunahmen auf 8,9 bzw. 9,4 g/kg. Auch das Blutvolumen stieg stärker an. Bei Blut- und Plasmainfusion scheint die Flüssigkeitsanreicherung des Gewebes auf die Lunge beschränkt zu sein, bei Ringer-Locke-Infusion erstreckt sie sich über den gesamten Organismus. Die stärker Lungenödem induzierende Wirksamkeit von Plasma und Blut scheint hämodynamische Ursachen zu haben. Eine Erhöhung des Blutvolumens um mehr als 40—50% steigert offensichtlich den Lungencapillardruck so stark, daß Lungenödem entsteht.

Die Ratte besitzt offensichtlich eine größere Ödembereitschaft als das Kaninchen; die Ödembildung in der Lunge beginnt bei einer wesentlich geringeren Flüssigkeitsanreicherung des Organismus (Courtice *et al.*, 1954). Der Hund scheint dagegen resistenter als das Kaninchen zu sein (Luisada u. Sarnoff, 1944); es müssen größere Volumina pro Gewichtseinheit zugeführt oder zusätzliche Schädigungen gesetzt werden.

Daniel u. Cate (1948) und Haddy *et al.* (1950) verabreichten narkotisierten (Pentobarbital-Natrium 30 mg/kg) Hunden isotonische NaCl-Lösung. Daniel u. Cate infundieren die Lösung durch eine Glaskanüle in die linke Femoralvene, variieren das Infusionsvolumen zwischen 100 und 560 ml/kg und die Infusionsraten zwischen 5 und 12 ml/kg/min. Lungenödem tritt unter diesen Bedingungen nur in Einzelfällen auf; es wird regelmäßiger bei gleichzeitiger O_2-Mangelatmung (13% O_2) gefunden, auch dann, wenn die infundierte Flüssigkeitsmenge, für sich allein verabreicht, unwirksam ist.

Jordan u. DeLaney (1951) versuchten die ödemprovozierenden Maßnahmen physiologischer zu gestalten. Es gelang ihnen aber weder bei Hunden durch schnelle Injektion von 30 ml Blut/kg Gewicht, noch durch O_2-Mangelatmung (10—17% O_2) und gleichzeitige Infusion von 200 ml Kochsalzlösung/15 min/kg Gewicht regelmäßig Lungenödem zu erzeugen. Auch die Kombination von Infusion und Erhöhung des Atemwiderstandes befriedigte nicht. Erst wenn Hypoxie, Erhöhung des Atemwiderstandes und Infusion zusammen angewandt wurden, trat mit ziemlicher Regelmäßigkeit Lungenödem auf, wobei unklar blieb, welcher der entscheidende Faktor ist. Narkotisierte Hunde (18—25 mg/kg Pentobarbital-Natrium i.v.) werden mit einem möglichst großen Intratrachealkatheter intubiert. Der Katheter wird im Pharynxbereich gegen die Umgebung abgedichtet. Wenn Herz- und Atemfrequenz wieder ein stabiles Niveau erreicht haben, wird der Katheter über eine Wasserflasche an einen mit einem Sauerstoff-Stickstoff-Gemisch (O_2-Konzentration 10%) gefüllten Douglasschen Atemsack angeschlossen.

In den Katheter ist ein (widerstandsfreies ?) Ausatmungsventil eingeschaltet. Die Einatmung erfolgt gegen einen Widerstand von 16 cm Wasser, der mit Hilfe einer Waschflasche eingestellt wird. 20 min nach Beginn der O_2-Mangelatmung werden pro kg Körpergewicht 200 ml isotonische Kochsalzlösung innerhalb von 15 min in die Vena jugularis infundiert. Werden die Tiere stark cyanotisch, kann man anstelle des O_2N_2-Gemisches vorübergehend atmosphärische Luft atmen lassen. Jordan und DeLaney erzielten mit diesem Verfahren bei 93% ihrer Versuchstiere schweres Lungenödem. (Bewertung nach dem makroskopischen Obduktionsbefund und Wassergehalt des Lungengewebes).

Harrison und Liebow (1954) analysierten die Faktoren, die an der Ausbildung infusionsbedingten Lungenödems beteiligt sind. Sie fixierten bei Bastardhunden im Gewicht von 8—21 kg in einer Voroperation Nadelführer in der Pulmonalarterie und im linken Vorhof (Methode s. S. 212f.). 8 Tage später wurden die Tiere mit Chloralose (25 mg/kg) und evtl. zusätzlich mit kleinen Dosen Pentobarbital narkotisiert. Dann wurden Polyäthylenkatheter in die Femoralarterie und in die Brustaorta eingeführt. Gerinnungshemmung durch Heparin. Durch die Nadelführer wurden Injektionsnadeln in die Pulmonalarterie und den linken Vorhof geschoben und zur Infusion von Tyrode- und physiologischer NaCl-Lösung verwendet. Infusion nach vorausgehender Berechnung der Zuflußrate, die 5 Std lang aufrecht erhalten werden sollte. Halbstündliche photokymographische Registrierung der Druckwerte in Aorta, Femoralvene, Pulmonalarterie und linkem Vorhof mit einer Batterie von Manometern; Katheterisierung der Harnblase, wobei die ausgeschiedene Urinmenge und das spezifische Gewicht des Urins halbstündlich gemessen wurden. Die Änderungen des Blutvolumens wurden anhand von Hämatokritbestimmungen verfolgt. Ödembewertung nach dem relativen Lungengewicht (s. S. 177ff.). Die Entwicklung des Lungenödems war im großen und ganzen von der pro Zeit- und Gewichtseinheit zugeführten bzw. retinierten Flüssigkeitsmenge und der Zunahme des Blutvolumens abhängig. Aus Tabelle 6 sind diese Zusammenhänge aus den Mittelwerten der registrierten Parameter ersichtlich.

Tabelle 6. *Faktoren der Ödementstehung nach Harrison u. Liebow (1954). Einzelheiten im Text*

Schweregrad des Lungenödems	Relatives Lungengewicht in %	Infundierte Flüssigkeit in ml/kg/h	Ausgeschiedene Flüssigkeit in ml/kg/h	Retinierte Flüssigkeit in ml/kg/h	Anstieg des Blutvolumens in %
Kein Ödem	1,20	64,2	29,8	34,4	19
Fragliches Ödem	1,21—1,40	68,0	23,8	44,2	23
Mäßiges bis schweres Ödem	1,60	85,8	21,2	64,6	39

Bei den Tieren mit dem stärksten Lungenödem (relatives Lungengewicht über 1,60%) wurde ein besonders starker Anstieg des Druckes im linken Vorhof auf über 20 cm H_2O beobachtet. Bei den Tieren der beiden anderen Gruppen blieben die Werte unter 10 cm H_2O. Voraussetzung für die Entstehung infusionsbedingten Lungenödems ist demnach Druckanstieg im linken Vorhof in Verbindung mit der Herabsetzung des kolloidosmotischen Druckes infolge Blutverdünnung[1].

Auch im Herz-Lungen-Präparat kann durch Vermehrung der dem rechten Herzen angebotenen Flüssigkeitsmenge Lungenödem erzeugt werden (Paine *et al.*, 1949a). Die Herstellung des Präparates und die Registriervorgänge werden auf

[1] Genaue Angaben mit NaCl-Lösungen verschiedener Konzentration s. Senga.

S. 169f. beschrieben. Bewertung des Ödems anhand der Lymphflußrate und des histologischen Bildes (wiederholte Probeexcisionen während des Versuches). Bei Steigerung des venösen Zuflusses von 200—300 ml/min auf 600—700 ml/min entstand Lungenödem, das von einer starken Blutfüllung der Lungencapillaren begleitet war. In der abfließenden Lymphe wurden bis zu 600000 Erythrocyten im Kubikmillimeter gezählt.

Paine *et al.* (1949a) beschreiben ferner eine Methode zur Erzeugung von Lungenödem im Herz-Lungen-Präparat durch Herabsetzung des kolloidosmotischen Druckes des Blutes. Hunde werden in Nembutalnarkose zur Lymphstrommessung vorbereitet (s. S. 169f.). Dann wird unter Überdruckatmung der Thorax geöffnet und das Perikard incidiert. Nach Blutstillung und Heparininjektion werden Kanülen zur Blutdruckregistrierung in die linke Arteria subclavia, in die rechte obere Lungenlappenarterie und in das linke Herzrohr eingebunden. Anschließend wird ein gewöhnliches Herz-Lungen-Präparat hergestellt. Eine dem Kreislaufvolumen entsprechende Blutmenge wird zentrifugiert, das überstehende Plasma abgesaugt und durch angewärmte Locke-Lösung ersetzt. Man füllt nach einer Kontrollperiode 200—300 ml der Erythrocytenaufschwemmung anstelle des normalen Blutes in das venöse Vorratsgefäß ein und ersetzt dabei schätzungsweise die Hälfte des Kreislaufvolumens. Unter diesen Bedingungen entsteht Lungenödem, ohne daß die Blutdruckwerte wesentliche Veränderungen erfahren. Die Ödementstehung kann an der Lymphflußrate, am makroskopischen und mikroskopischen (wiederholte Excisionen) Organbefund verfolgt werden. Aber beim Herz-Lungen-Präparat ist es schwieriger, ein Lungenödem zu vermeiden als zu erzeugen.

7. Lymphgefäßunterbindung

Nach der Methode von Rusznyák u. Mitarb. (1957) wird der Thorax narkotisierter Hunde (Überdruck-Äther-O_2-Narkose) im 3. Intercostalraum geöffnet. Der Truncus lymphaceus dexter, der Ductus thoracicus und evtl. auch größere Lymphknoten im hinteren Mediastinum werden unterbunden, die Brusthöhle anschliessend unter gleichzeitiger Evakuation geschlossen. Ausführlichere Darlegungen operativer Maßnahmen an den Lymphgefäßen in der Thoraxhöhle finden sich bei Markowitz *et al.* (1959) und Hansen (1958). Rusznyák *et al.* töteten die Tiere 24 Std oder auch erst mehrere Tage nach der Operation durch Luftembolie oder Barbituratinjektion. In der Mehrzahl der Fälle hatte sich leichtes oder mittelschweres Lungenödem entwickelt; einzelne Tiere waren ödemfrei geblieben. Die Versager werden mit der außerordentlichen Variabilität der anatomischen Verhältnisse der Thoraxlymphgefäße erklärt. Es gelingt nicht immer, außer den großen Lymphgefäßen auch eine ausreichende Anzahl von Lymphknoten abzubinden. Werden zusätzlich zur Lymphgefäßunterbindung Herzklappenfehler erzeugt, dann entsteht in der Regel Lungenödem schwereren Grades (s. S. 196f.).

Die Kenntnis der Pathogenese des Lungenödems ist durch die Einführung dieser Methode erweitert worden. Für Routineuntersuchungen eignet sie sich wegen des Operationsaufwandes und der Unregelmäßigkeit der Ergebnisse weniger gut.

8. Schock und Blutverlust

Blutverluste und Schockzustände begünstigen die Ausbildung von Lungenödem (Eaton, 1950; Moon u. Kennedy, 1932; Moon u. Morgan, 1936a, b). Von dieser Erkenntnis ausgehend, versuchten Moon u. Morgan (1936a, b) bei Hunden durch protrahierte Schockzustände Lungenödem zu erzeugen. Hunden in leichter Äthernarkose wurden 1,5—3,5 g/kg zerkleinerte Muskelsubstanz durch einen

Trichter in die Peritonealhöhle eingeführt. Die Muskelsubstanz wurde unter aseptischen Kautelen aus dem Glutäalmuskel eines frisch getöteten Hundes gewonnen, im Homogenisator steril zerkleinert und im Verhältnis 1:4 in physiologischer Kochsalzlösung suspendiert. 1,5—2,5 g/kg Muskelsubstanz riefen akute Krankheitserscheinungen hervor, wurden in der Regel aber überlebt, 3—3,5 g/kg führten innerhalb von 2—4 Tagen zum Tod der Tiere. Bei der Sektion wurden ausgeprägtes Lungenödem, Hyperämie der Capillaren und Venolen sowie Hämorrhagien in der Lunge, der Leber, den Nieren und im Darmbereich gefunden. Hämoglobingehalt und Erythrocytenzahl waren als Ausdruck einer zunehmenden Bluteindickung bis zum Ende des Versuches um etwa 30% angestiegen.

Prinzipiell ähnliche Ergebnisse wurden bei Hunden erzielt, wenn

1. die Tiere mit etwa einem Drittel ihrer Körperoberfläche für einige Sekunden in heißes Wasser (knapp unter 100° C) getaucht wurden;
2. eine etwa 25 cm lange Schlinge des Jejunums mit einem Leinenband abgebunden wurde;
3. 0,4 g Natriumglykocholat/kg in 10%iger Lösung 6mal i.v. an aufeinanderfolgenden Tagen injiziert wurde oder wenn 1 g Natriumglykocholat/kg auf einmal i.v. verabfolgt wurde;
4. 100—200 ml verdünnte, sterile Hundegalle (insgesamt ca. 200 ml unverdünnter Galle) an mehreren aufeinanderfolgenden Tagen i.v. oder i.p. injiziert wurden;
5. 300 mg Phenobarbital-Natrium/kg 2mal täglich 3 Tage lang gefüttert wurden oder 300 mg Phenobarbital-Natrium/kg auf einmal injiziert wurden;
6. Histamin wiederholt injiziert wurde (s. S. 242f.).

Ursache des im Verlauf von Schockzuständen auftretenden Lungenödems dürfte in erster Linie eine Zunahme der Capillarpermeabilität sein. Bei verzögertem Verlauf können sekundäre Erkrankungen, z.B. Bronchopneumonie, hinzukommen.

Die Bedeutung von Blutverlusten für die Ödementstehung wurde von Eaton (1950) untersucht. Er ließ gesunde Hunde in Nembutalnarkose aus der Femoralarterie bluten, bis sie 25% ihres Blutes verloren hatten und opferte die Tiere in verschiedenen Abständen nach dieser Prozedur durch intraventriculäre Injektion von 10 ml Chloroform. Der Blutverlust ließ den Wassergehalt der Lunge vorübergehend leicht ansteigen. Nach 2—4 Std war er wieder zur Norm zurückgekehrt. Parallel gingen eine temporäre Zunahme der Hämatokritwerte und eine Abnahme des Plasmaproteingehaltes. Im histologischen Bild der Lunge waren allerdings noch mehrere Tage später ödematöse Herde nachweisbar. Verglichen mit den mit anderen Methoden erzielten Resultaten erscheint das Ausmaß des durch Blutverlust erzeugten Lungenödems geringgradig. Der durchschnittliche Wassergehalt der Lungen war 75 min nach der Blutentnahme von 79,34% auf maximal 80,98% angestiegen. Für Routineuntersuchungen dürfte sich diese Methode daher — wie auch andere Autoren (Visscher *et al.*, 1956) ausführen — wenig eignen.

Eine stärkere Anreicherung der Lunge mit Flüssigkeit trat in der Regel auch dann nicht ein, wenn unmittelbar nach Beendigung der Blutentnahme Blut, Plasma oder NaCl-Lösung im Überschuß (etwa das $2^1/_2$fache des verlorenen Quantums) infundiert wurden.

II. Eingriffe am Respirationssystem

1. Steigerung des inspiratorischen oder exspiratorischen Atemwiderstandes

Verfahren nach Reichsman (1946). Ratten (150—250 g) in Urethannarkose wird eine Y-förmige Metallkanüle in die Trachea eingebunden. Beide Schenkel der

Kanüle werden durch Gummischläuche in der in Abb. 8 dargestellten Anordnung an Mariottesche Flaschen angeschlossen. Durch Verschiebung des freien Glasrohres in der Flasche A kann der Inspirationswiderstand variiert werden. In gleicher Weise kann der Exspirationswiderstand mit Hilfe des entsprechenden Glasrohres in der Flasche B verändert werden.

Nach einer Vorperiode von 15—45 min mit freiem Luftaustausch wird der Inspirationswiderstand auf eine Höhe (zwischen 4 und 8,5 cm H_2O) eingestellt, die das Tier gerade noch überwinden kann, was am Durchtritt von Luftblasen durch das Wasser in Flasche A kontrolliert werden kann. Tritt während des Versuchs

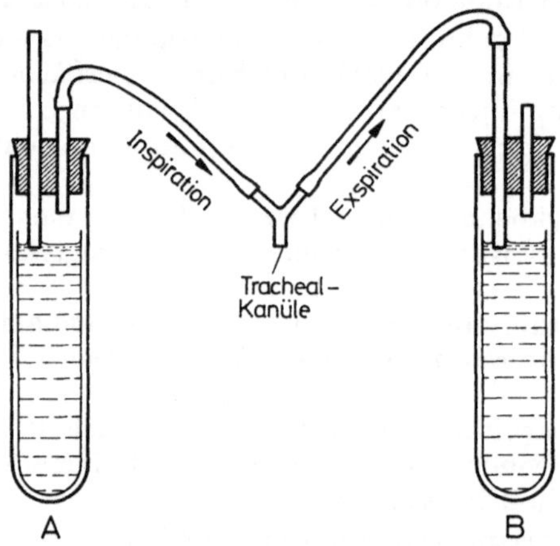

Abb. 8. Versuchsanordnung nach Reichsman (1946) zur Steigerung des inspiratorischen und exspiratorischen Atemwiderstandes

Asphyxie auf, so wird der Inspirationswiderstand vorübergehend vermindert. Unter diesen Bedingungen beträgt die durchschnittliche Überlebenszeit 4 Std.

Atemfrequenz und Atemtiefe werden durch die Erhöhung des Inspirationswiderstandes nur unwesentlich verändert. Erst in der Endphase wird die Atmung langsam und oberflächlich, der Inspirationswiderstand kann nicht mehr kontinuierlich überwunden werden und die Tiere sterben innerhalb weniger Minuten, wenn der Widerstand nicht herabgesetzt wird. Tiere, die in dieser Weise behandelt werden, haben hyperämische und ödematöse Lungen. Die Veränderungen sind aber nicht hochgradig. Zwischen Ödemgrad und Überlebenszeit läßt sich keine Beziehung herstellen. Bei härteren Versuchsbedingungen, die schon nach 2—3 Std den Tod herbeiführten, wurde häufig kein Lungenödem, sondern nur Hyperämie der Lunge gefunden. Zusätzliche Erhöhung des Exspirationswiderstandes verändert dic Überlebenszeit nicht, aber nur bei einem Teil der Tiere wird ein Lungenödem gefunden. Zusätzliche Flüssigkeitsinfusion verkürzt den Zeitraum bis zum Auftreten des Ödems, bleibt aber ohne Einfluß auf den Ödemgrad. Als Infusionsrate werden 1,5—2,0 ml/min vorgeschlagen. Es wird physiologische NaCl-Lösung unter konstantem Druck in die Vena jugularis externa infundiert. Der Tod tritt nach 25—40 min, wenn 45—60 ml Flüssigkeit eingelaufen sind, ein.

Verfahren nach Zinnberg *et al.* (1948). Narkotisierte Hunde (30 mg/kg Nembutal i.p.) werden tracheotomiert. Die größte Glaskanüle (Durchmesser 1—1,6 cm), die eingeführt werden kann, wird in der Trachea fixiert. Sie wird über ein 8 mm starkes, 15—17 cm langes Glasrohr und ein T-Stück mit einem Einwegventil und einer Wasserflasche verbunden (s. Abb. 9). Das Ventil dient je nach Anordnung der widerstandsfreien Ein- oder Ausatmung. Über die Wasserflasche kann sowohl der In- als auch der Exspiration ein Widerstand bis zu 20 cm Wasser entgegengesetzt werden. Bei den angegebenen Abmessungen des Systems ist sein Totluftraum kleiner als der von Kehlkopf, Rachen und Nase oder Mund. Die Tiere atmen Raumluft gegen einen inspiratorischen oder exspiratorischen Widerstand von 20 cm Wasser. Werden die Tiere diesen Bedingungen für mehrere Stunden unterworfen, so tritt in der Mehrzahl der Fälle Lungenödem auf. Einzelne Tiere überlebten unter diesen Verhältnissen 2—3 Tage.

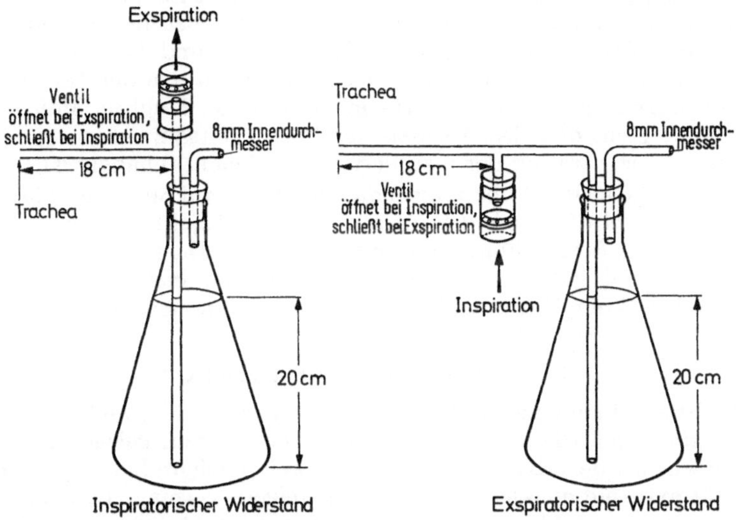

Abb. 9. Versuchsanordnung nach Zinnberg *et al.* (1948) zur Erhöhung des Inspirations- bzw. Exspirationswiderstandes. Einzelheiten im Text

Der Mechanismus der Ödembildung steht in der Diskussion. Eine Verminderung des intrathorakalen bzw. intrapulmonalen Druckes und Vergrößerung des Druckgradienten zwischen capillärem und extravasculärem Raum wäre nur bei erhöhtem Inspirationswiderstand zu erwarten, doch wird nach Untersuchungen von Haddy *et al.* (1950) sowie Haddy u. Campbell (1953) bei gleichzeitiger Erhöhung des in- und exspiratorischen Atemwiderstandes auch der Pulmonalvenendruck angehoben. In ihren Versuchen war das Ausmaß des Lungenödems von der Erhöhung des Pulmonalvenendruckes abhängig (Technik der Atemwiderstandserhöhung nach Zinnberg *et al.*, 1948; arterielle und venöse Blutdruckmessung mit Kathetern nach Haddy *et al.*, 1949).

2. Injektion von Flüssigkeit in die Trachea (Laqueur, 1920; Laqueur und de Vries Reilingh 1920a, b)

Leicht narkotisierte Katzen und Kaninchen werden mit erhöhtem Oberkörper gelagert. Alle 2 min wird mit einer Injektionsspritze isotonische NaCl-Lösung oder Aqua dest. in 5 ml-Portionen bis zu einem Gesamtvolumen von 25 ml in die freigelegte Trachea injiziert (Injektionsdauer jeweils 15 sec). Soll streng quantitativ verfahren werden, muß der Oesophagus unter Schonung des Nervus recurrens durchtrennt werden. Das untere Ende wird abgebunden und der obere Stumpf in die Halswunde eingenäht, so daß ein Zurücklaufen von Flüssigkeit aus der Trachea ins Maul und die Speiseröhre kontrolliert werden kann. Werden nur kleinere Volumina verabreicht, erübrigt sich diese Maßnahme. Die Resorption der instillierten Flüssigkeit geht schnell vonstatten; innerhalb von 30 min verschwindet mehr als die Hälfte aus der Lunge. Hypertonische Lösungen (z.B. 10—15%ige Glucoselösungen) rufen eine beträchtliche, länger anhaltende Flüssigkeitsanreicherung hervor. Werden hochkonzentrierte Lösungen (z.B. 50—60%ige Glucoselösungen) verwendet, so rufen kleinere Mengen (1—1,5 ml) innerhalb von 1—$1^1/_2$ Std ein „osmotisches Lungenödem" durch Flüssigkeitsaustritt aus den Capillaren hervor, das mehrere Stunden lang nachweisbar ist.

Länger als hypertonische Kochsalzlösung wird eiweißhaltige Flüssigkeit in der Lunge zurückgehalten. Courtice und Simmonds (1949a) instillierten in die Trachea von Kaninchen Wasser, physiologische NaCl-Lösung und Serum. Wasser und NaCl-Lösung verschwanden innerhalb weniger Stunden aus der Lunge; die Resorption des injizierten Serums dauerte mehrere Tage. Hughes, May u. Widdicombe (1958) zeigten, daß das Ausmaß der Flüssigkeitsanreicherung der Lunge von der Eiweißkonzentration der instillierten Flüssigkeit abhängig ist.

Harford und Hara (1950) übertrugen das Verfahren auf Mäuse und fanden, daß die Alveolen noch 24 Std nach der intrabronchialen Injektion von 0,1—0,15 ml sterilem artgleichem Serum Flüssigkeit enthielten. Die Flüssigkeitsverteilung läßt sich im Röntgenbild gut sichtbar machen, wenn der instillierten Lösung ein Kontrastmittel (z.B. ein Wismutsalz) zugesetzt wird (Laqueur u. Magnus, 1921a).

3. Sauerstoffmangel der Atemluft

Hypoxie ist als Ödemursache in Betracht gezogen worden, weil bei der Sektion von Flugzeuginsassen, die an O_2-Mangel gestorben waren, gelegentlich Lungenödem gefunden wurde (Kritzler, 1944) und weil hochgradige Hypoxämie die Permeabilität extrapulmonaler Capillaren zu steigern vermag (Landis, 1928). Im Tierversuch gelang es nicht, durch Zuführung O_2-armer Atmungsluft Lungenödem hervorzurufen, aber die Ödembereitschaft wird offensichtlich gefördert, denn Sauerstoffmangel läßt die ödemerzeugende Wirkung anderer Maßnahmen überschwellig werden.

Courtice u. Korner (1952) ließen nicht narkotisierte Kaninchen im Gewicht von 1,2—3,0 kg 5 Std lang ein Gasgemisch mit 11% O_2 durch eine luftdicht schließende Maske oder Trachealkanüle einatmen. Das Gasgemisch wurde aus einer Gasflasche über einen Atmungsbeutel der Maske zugeführt. Diese war mit widerstandsarmen Gummiventilen ausgestattet und hatte einen geringen Totraum (3—4 ml). Ein O_2-Mangelödem entstand bei keinem Tier. Die ödemfördernde Wirkung der Hypoxie wurde erst erkennbar, wenn bei den Tieren gleichzeitig Hypervolämie erzeugt wurde. Dabei genügten wesentlich kleinere Infusionsvolumina als bei Tieren mit Normalatmung (s. S. 199). Über gleiche Erfahrungen bei anderen Tierarten berichten Daniel u. Cate (1948), Hemingway (1952) sowie Poulsen (1954b) (s. Tabelle 7).

Die Gasgemische werden durch Mischung von Luft oder Flaschensauerstoff mit Stickstoff hergestellt. Daniel u. Cate (1948) benutzen hierfür ein Spirometersystem, ersetzen den verbrauchten Sauerstoff und entfernen das CO_2 kontinuierlich, Poulsen (1954b) verwendet den auf S. 234 beschriebenen Apparat nach Poulsen u. Secher (1949). Über eine Atemmaske oder in einer Gaskammer wird das Gasgemisch dem Tier zugeführt.

Nach Untersuchungen von Courtice und Korner (1952) wirkt Hypoxie nicht permeabilitätssteigernd (Drinker, 1950; Jordan u. De Laney, 1951). Hypoxie ruft Herzinsuffizienz hervor, die zu einer Vermehrung des Lungenblutvolumens führt (s. auch Cournand, 1950; Hemingway, 1952). Infolgedessen hebt schon eine ge-

Tabelle 7. *Ödemfördernde Wirkung O_2-armer Atmungsluft*

Tierart	O_2-Konzentration der Atemluft (%)	Einwirkungsdauer	Zusätzliche Schädigung	Lungenödem	Literatur
Hund	12	bis zum Eintritt	—	nein	Daniel u. Cate
	7	des Todes	—	nein	(1948)
	12		Infusion	ja	
	7		Infusion	ja	
Kaninchen	11	5 Std	—	nein	Courtice u.
	11	5 Std	Infusion	ja	Korner (1952)
Meerschweinchen		getötet vor dem Auftreten hypoxischen Herzversagens	—	nein	Hemingway (1952)
Maus	12	15 min	—	nein	Poulsen (1954b)
	8	15 min	—	nein	
	5	bis zum Eintritt des Todes (3—8 min)	—	angedeutet	

ringere Menge infundierter Flüssigkeit den Capillardruck über das Niveau des kolloidosmotischen Drucks. Für hämodynamische Ursachen der Ödembereitschaft sprechen Drucksteigerungen, die bei O_2-Mangel im großen und kleinen Kreislauf beobachtet wurden (z.B. Lewis u. Gorlin, 1952; Stroud u. Rahn, 1953; Aviado, 1961). Drinker (1950) sowie Jordan u. DeLaney (1951) vertreten die Ansicht, daß die Inhalation von O_2-armer Luft die Permeabilität der Lungencapillaren steigert.

4. Lungenödem als Folge von Thoraxverletzungen

Nach Thoraxoperationen oder -verletzungen werden nicht selten Flüssigkeitsansammlungen in der Lunge gefunden, die aus Blut, Transsudat, Exsudat und Schleim bestehen können (Daniel u. Cate, 1948). Derartige Flüssigkeitsansammlungen im Wundbereich rechtfertigen nicht immer die Bezeichnung „Lungenödem"; ödematöse Veränderungen breiten sich aber von den verletzten Partien in das intakte Gewebe aus (Luisada u. Cardi, 1956).

Daniel und Cate (1948) verletzten narkotisierte Bastardhunde im Bereich der rechten Thoraxhälfte durch ein fallendes Gewicht oder einen tangential treffenden Pistolenschuß. Die Verletzungsfolgen wurden anhand der makroskopisch gefundenen intrapulmonalen Flüssigkeitsansammlung in 4 Schweregrade eingestuft. Sie stimmten mit dem Ausmaß der Verletzung überein. Mikroskopisch wurden neben ödematösen Veränderungen, die sich auch auf unverletzte Lungenpartien erstreckten, Alveolarrupturen mit Blutaustritten in die Lufträume beobachtet. Zusätzliche i.v. Infusion (Technik s. S. 198ff.) verstärkte das Lungenödem. Blutungen in die Bauchhöhle, z.B. als Folge von Leberruptur verminderten die Flüssigkeitsansammlung in der Lunge. Cate u. Daniel (1948) nehmen an, daß traumatisch ausgelöstes Lungenödem zum Teil reflektorisch bedingt ist, da Sympathektomie seine Entstehung in den unverletzten, nicht jedoch in den verletzten Lungenteilen hemmt.

5. Lungenödem durch Dampfinhalation

Die Einwirkung hoher Temperaturen auf den Atemtrakt narkotisierter Hunde wurde von Moritz *et al.* (1945) untersucht. Einatmung erhitzter Luft (etwa 300°C beim Eintritt in die Trachea) oder Wärmezufuhr mit der Flamme eines Gebläsebrenners (500° C an der Austrittsöffnung der Kanüle) schädigte die Schleimhaut des oberen Teils der Trachea, der unmittelbar an die isolierte Inhalationskanüle anschloß, hatte aber gewöhnlich keine nachteiligen Folgen für die tieferen Teile der Atemwege oder das Lungenparenchym, weil die Temperatur trockenheißer Luft in der Trachea sehr rasch reduziert wird. Dagegen bewirkte die Inhalation von Dampf, der beim Austritt aus der caudal des Kehlkopfes endenden Kanüle eine Temperatur von etwa 100° C hatte, häufig Ödem, Hyperämie und Hämorrhagien der Lunge. Das Verfahren der Dampfinhalation wurde von Aviado und Schmidt (1952) ausgebaut. Hunde in Morphin-Chloralose-Narkose (2 bzw. 50—100 mg/kg) wurden mittels einer Trachealkanüle an die in Abb. 10 dargestellte Versuchsanordnung angeschlossen. Bei Betätigung der entsprechenden Ventile

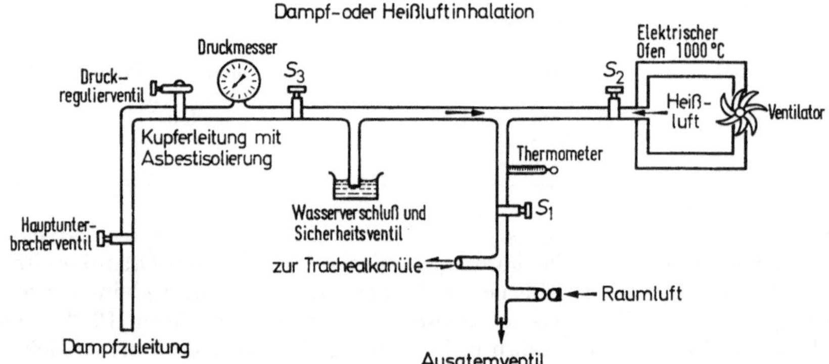

Abb. 10. Versuchsanordnung nach Aviado und Schmidt (1952) zur Dampf- bzw. Heißluftinhalation. Beschreibung im Text

atmeten die Tiere Raumluft (S_1 gesperrt), erhitzte Luft (S_3 und Raumluftverbindung gesperrt) oder Dampf (S_2 und Raumluftverbindung gesperrt) ein. Das Leitungssystem bestand aus asbestisolierten Kupferrohren. Die Heißluft gelangte aus einem elektrischen Ofen mittels Druckventilator, der Dampf aus dem Heizungskessel des Gebäudes in das System. Der Dampfdruck wurde durch Reduzierventile auf Atmosphärendruck gemindert; ein nachgeschaltetes Sicherheitsventil glich etwa noch überhöhte Druckwerte aus. Die Exspirationsluft entwich durch ein Ausatemventil aus hitzebeständigem Material.

Die Dauer der Dampfinhalationen, die wirkungsvoller als trockene Hitze waren, wurde zwischen 15 und 120 sec variiert. Einzelne Tiere starben innerhalb weniger Minuten an Atem- oder Kreislaufversagen, die Mehrzahl im Verlauf von 1—2 Std. Eine Korrelation zwischen Inhalations- und Überlebensdauer bestand nicht. Zu Beginn der Dampfinhalation reagierten die Tiere zunächst mit reflektorischer Apnoe, Bradykardie, Drucksteigerung in den Körperarterien und anschließend mit Polypnoe und Tachykardie. Der Kontakt des Blutes mit dem Dampf verursachte eine beträchtliche Hämolyse; die Bluttemperatur (gemessen in der Aorta) stieg während der Inhalation erheblich an. Etwa 30 min nach Beendigung der Inhalation wurde in der Trachea Schaum sichtbar. Hämatokrit, Hämoglobingehalt des Blutes und spezifisches Gewicht des Plasmas erhöhten sich zunehmend, während die O_2-Sättigung des Blutes fortschreitend abfiel. In den Lungen aller Tiere wurden außer ödematösen Veränderungen hyperämische Erscheinungen und Hämorrhagien gefunden. Das thermische Lungenödem kommt nach Meinung der Autoren als Folge einer Hyperämie der Lungencapillaren und einer Steigerung der Capillarpermeabilität zustande. Da der Pulmonalarteriendruck erhöht, der Druck im linken Vorhof unverändert, das Lungenblutvolumen vergrößert und die Durchströmung der Lunge vermindert war, wurde auf eine Constriction der Lungenvenen geschlossen.

Fineberg *et al.* (1954) modifizierten das Verfahren, weil sie bei willkürlicher Dampfinhalation beträchtliche Schwankungen der Atemfrequenz beobachteten. Um die Dampfaufnahme genauer dosieren zu können, versuchten sie zunächst die Atmung durch Stimulation der Nervi phrenici zu steuern; das Verfahren hatte einige Nachteile. Besser bewährte sich künstliche Beatmung. Ein narkostisierter Hund wurde nach Einbindung einer Trachealkanüle in der Atemkammer der in Abb. 11 dargestellten Versuchsanordnung gelagert, so daß er nur über die

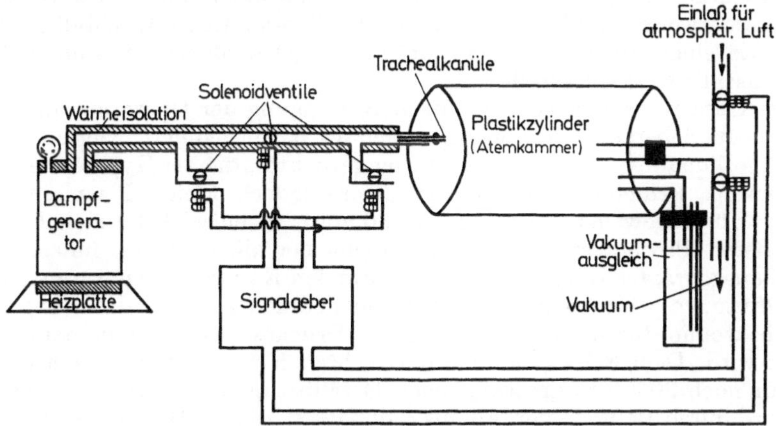

Abb. 11. Schematische Darstellung der Versuchsanordnung nach Fineberg *et al.* (1954) zur Dampfinhalation. Erklärung im Text

Trachealkanüle mit der Umgebung in Verbindung stand. Zwei Solenoidventile, die von einem Signalgeber gesteuert wurden, verbanden die Atemkammer alternierend mit einem Vakuum, das den Druck in der Kammer um 29 cm Wasser reduzierte, und mit atmosphärischer Luft. Die Beatmung war so bemessen, daß das Tier innerhalb von 2 min alle willkürlichen Atemanstrengungen einstellte. Bei vorübergehender Unterbrechung der Beatmung trat eine kurzdauernde Apnoe auf. Dieser Augenblick wurde benutzt, um den Dampfgenerator, einen transportablen Autoklaven, über ein isoliertes Rohr mit der Trachealkanüle zu verbinden. Anschließend wurde die Beatmung wieder in Gang gesetzt und das die Dampfzufuhr freigebende Solenoidventil mit dem Inspirations-(Vakuum-)ventil synchronisiert. Zur Exspiration wurden diese beiden Ventile geschlossen und die drei anderen Ventile des Systems geöffnet, die Druckdifferenz zwischen Atemkammer bzw. Dampfgenerator und atmosphärischer Luft wurde dadurch ausgeglichen, die Ausatmung ermöglicht.

In der Regel wurde der Dampf für 6 Inspirationen von je 2,2 sec Dauer zugeführt; die korrespondierenden Exspirationen währten 3,8 sec. Einige Minuten nach der Dampfapplikation waren Rasselgeräusche über den Lungen hörbar; nach 30 min floß schaumige Flüssigkeit aus der Trachealkanüle ab. Die Überlebenszeit betrug 4—5 Std. Das relative Lungengewicht war auf etwa das 2—2,5-fache der Norm erhöht. Bei einem Teil der Tiere hatte sich ein Pleuraexsudat entwickelt.

6. Verlust von Lungengewebe

Nach der Resektion größerer Lungenpartien besteht in den verbliebenen Teilen des Organs eine gesteigerte Ödembereitschaft (Gibbon *et al.*, 1942; Gibbon u. Gibbon, 1942), die sich besonders dann auswirkt, wenn zusätzliche Maßnahmen, wie z. B. Infusionen, diese Tendenz unterstützen.

Gibbon u. Gibbon (1942) öffneten bei Katzen in Natrium-amytal-Narkose (50 mg/kg) unter künstlicher Beatmung durch eine Trachealkanüle beide Pleurahöhlen im Bereich des 6. Intercostalraumes. Die Lungenwurzelorgane der zu resezierenden Lappen wurden am Hilus mit kräftigen Seidenfäden abgebunden. Der rechte Mittel- und beide Unterlappen, insgesamt etwa 70% des Lungenparenchyms, wurden entfernt. Im 8. Intercostalraum wurde ein dünner Katheter in jede Pleurahöhle eingeführt. Die Operationswunden im 6. Intercostalraum wurden schichtweise geschlossen, der Druck im Thorax durch Anschluß der beiden Katheter an einen konstanten Sog von 7 cm H_2O reguliert, die künstliche Beatmung anschließend eingestellt.

Einige Katzen starben 1—2 Std nach Beendigung der Operation an Lungenödem. Die überlebenden Tiere wurden nach 4—6 Std geopfert, zeigten aber nur eine mäßige Zunahme des relativen Lungengewichtes, die als Hyperämiefolge gedeutet wurde. Erhielten lobektomierte Tiere jedoch kleine Plasmainfusionen (15 ml/kg Körpergewicht innerhalb von 30 min), so entwickelte sich bei einem weit größeren Prozentsatz, wenn auch nicht bei allen Tieren, innerhalb von 1—2 Std ausgeprägtes Lungenödem. Bei normalen Kontrolltieren waren derartige Plasmainfusionen wirkungslos. Die Autoren nehmen an, daß das Lungenödem nach Lobektomie durch eine Erhöhung des Druckes in den Pulmonalcapillaren ausgelöst wird. Dem Schlagvolumen des rechten Herzens stehen nach der Operation nur noch 30% des ursprünglichen Gefäßbettes zur Verfügung. Diese Annahme wird durch Befunde von Adams *et al.* (1953), die bei Hunden nach Lungenresektionen Gefäßdrucksteigerungen erheblichen Ausmaßes beobachteten, gestützt.

7. Einwirkung explosionsähnlicher Luftdruckschwankungen

Explosionsbedingte Druckschwankungen können pathologische Veränderungen an verschiedenen Organen auslösen. In der Lunge bewirken sie die Entstehung von Emphysem, Hämorrhagien und Ödemherden. Eine ausführliche Darstellung der Problematik einschließlich methodischer Angaben stammt von Clemedson (1949). Bei der von ihm gewählten Versuchsanordnung trat das Ödem jedoch hinter anderen Erscheinungen an der Lunge zurück oder fehlte ganz. Deshalb soll auf sein Verfahren nicht näher eingegangen werden.

Ähnliche Erfahrungen machten zunächst auch Cassen u. Mitarb. (1952a, b). Sie fanden bei Mäusen, die in einer Druckkammer frei beweglich Druckwellen verschiedener Intensität ausgesetzt worden waren, in erster Linie Lungenhämorrhagien. Lungenödem trat dagegen bei einem größeren Prozentsatz der Tiere auf, wenn diese während der Explosion auf ihrer Unterlage fixiert waren (Cassen *et al.*, 1952c). Zu diesem Zweck wurden die Extremitäten mit Klebestreifen auf einer massiven Platte befestigt. In Freiluftexperimenten wurden die tierbesetzten Platten an einem Gestell über einer Explosionsladung aufgehängt. Die Stärke der Ladung und ihr Abstand von den Tieren (5—8 m) wurden so gewählt, daß diese für etwa 3 msec einer positiven Druckeinwirkung von 0,4—1,4 atm ausgesetzt waren. Unter diesen Bedingungen starb ein großer Teil der Tiere 10—15 min nach erfolgter Explosion unter Zeichen von Dyspnoe. Druckwerte von 1 atm oder mehr wirkten fast immer tödlich. Das durchschnittliche Lungengewicht der Tiere war auf das 2—3fache der Norm erhöht. Hämoglobinbestimmungen des Lungenparenchyms zeigten, daß die Zunahme des Lungengewichts auch bei dieser Arbeitsweise zu einem großen Teil auf Hämorrhagien zurückgeführt werden muß. Vergleichbare Ergebnisse konnten im Laboratorium in einer röhrenförmigen Druckkammer erzielt werden, wenn die das Tier tragende Platte senkrecht montiert wurde, so daß die Druckwelle das Tier dorsal traf. Es ist fraglich, ob die beschriebenen Lungenveränderungen Folge einer direkten Druckwirkung sind oder, wie weitere Versuche der gleichen Autoren vermuten lassen, in erster Linie über das Zentralnervensystem ausgelöst werden. Das Ausmaß der Lungenveränderungen konnte nämlich reduziert werden, wenn der Kopf des Tieres durch eine Schutzplatte abgeschirmt wurde. Eine entsprechende Abdeckung des Thorakalbereichs war dagegen erfolglos.

III. Eingriffe am zentralen und peripheren Nervensystem

Die Auslösung von Lungenödem durch zentralnervöse Faktoren ist häufig diskutiert und als möglich erachtet worden (Literatur zum Thema u.a. bei Cameron, 1948; Schwab u. Denninger, 1956; Sturm, 1948). Von einigen Autoren wird eine Schädigung des Zentralnervensystems als alleinige Ursache eines Lungenödems in Frage gestellt. Paine u. Mitarb. (1952b) fanden z.B., daß das bei cerebralen Störungen auftretende Lungenödem häufig von Herz- und Kreislaufkrankheiten begleitet war. Beim statistischen Vergleich cerebral und extracerebral bedingter Todesfälle zeigte sich sogar, daß Erkrankungen des Zentralnervensystems weniger häufig mit Lungenödem einhergingen als Krankheiten anderer Organe.

Im Experiment ist neurogenes Lungenödem im Gefolge artefizieller Hirnverletzungen wahrscheinlich erstmalig von Brown-Séquard (1871) beobachtet worden. Einige der seitdem entwickelten Techniken fördern nur die Ödembereitschaft und erfordern unterstützende Maßnahmen. In diesem Abschnitt sollen nur solche Methoden besprochen werden, die durch direkte Eingriffe am Zentralnervensystem Lungenödem hervorrufen. Der Ödem erzeugende Effekt einiger extracerebral angewandter Pharmaka kommt wahrscheinlich ebenfalls ganz oder teilweise über einen Angriff am Zentralnervensystem zustande. Derartige Verfahren werden in Abschnitt IV behandelt.

Die Ursache des neurogenen Lungenödems wird in der Regel in hämodynamischen Veränderungen zu suchen sein. Dagegen wurde nie nachgewiesen, daß es neurogenes Lungenödem als Folge direkt zentralnervös gesteuerter Veränderungen der Capillarpermeabilität gibt (s. z.B. Cameron, 1948; Halmágyi, 1957). Sarnoff u. Sarnoff (1952) schlagen daher vor, den Begriff „neurogenes Lungenödem" durch den Ausdruck „neurohämodynamisches Lungenödem" zu ersetzen.

1. Multiple Hirnembolie

(Paine *et al.*, 1952a.) Vorbereitung der Tiere und Registriertechnik entsprachen dem auf S. 196 beschriebenen Vorgehen der Autoren bei der experimentellen Valvulotomie. Die rechte Arteria carotis communis wurde unterbunden; oberhalb der Ligatur wurde eine Injektionskanüle eingestochen und fixiert. Sodann wurden 0,5 ml einer 5%igen Aufschwemmung von Bariumsulfat in NaCl-Lösung injiziert und mit 5—8 ml Blut in den Hirnkreislauf gespült. Die Tiere reagierten mit tonischen Krämpfen und nachfolgender Erschlaffung. Der Blutdruck im großen Kreislauf (gemessen in der Femoralarterie) stieg in allen Fällen an; Lungenarterien- und Lungenvenendruck blieben in der Mehrzahl der Fälle unverändert. Lungenödem, beurteilt nach dem makroskopischen und mikroskopischen Obduktionsbefund, trat nur ausnahmsweise auf. Erst wenn die Bariumsulfatinjektionen bei Tieren vorgenommen wurden, bei denen zuvor Aorteninsuffizienzen (s. S. 196) erzeugt worden waren, entstand Lungenödem.

2. Erhöhung des intrakraniellen Druckes

Verfahren nach Campbell u. Mitarb. (1949). Der Schädel mit Pentobarbital-Na narkotisierter und in einem Teil der Versuche künstlich beatmeter Bastardhunde wurde neben der Scheitellinie trepaniert. Durch die Trepanationsöffnung (Durchmesser 1 cm) wurde ein kleiner Latexballon extradural unter die Schädelkapsel geschoben. Ein durchbohrtes Metallplättchen (Durchmesser 1,5 cm), das einen Schlauch zum Ballon führte und diesen nach der Füllung am vorbestimmten Ort hielt, wurde mit kleinen Schrauben über der Öffnung befestigt. Die durch den Schlauch erfolgende Flüssigkeitsfüllung des Ballons wurde so bemessen, daß Bradykardie und Pulmonalvenendrucksteigerung, aber keine Apnoe auftraten (Arterien- bzw. Venendruckmessung mit Hilfe von Kanülen oder Herzkathetern). Die Hirndrucksteigerung bewirkte außer Bradykardie eine verminderte Förderleistung des Herzens und eine — von der künstlichen Atmung unabhängige — Drucksteigerung in Pulmonalvenen und -arterien. Bei der Autopsie wurde gewöhnlich dann Lungenödem gefunden, wenn der Pulmonalvenendruck während des Versuches mehr als 20 mm Hg betragen hatte.

Ein ähnliches Verfahren wandten Campbell u. Visscher (1949) bei Meerschweinchen an. Durch eine Trepanationsöffnung von 1,5 mm Durchmesser wurde ein mit einem Plastikschlauch verbundener Ballon unter die Schädelkapsel geschoben und mit 1,5 ml Luft aufgeblasen. Bei der Hälfte der 5 min später getöteten Tiere wurden Ödem, Hyperämie und Hämorrhagien der Lungen gefunden.

Harrison u. Liebow (1952) modifizierten das Verfahren, weil ihre Versuche mit auffüllbaren Polyäthylensäcken, die sub- oder epidural in die Schädelhöhle eingefügt wurden, nicht sehr erfolgreich verliefen. Sie narkotisierten Hunde im Gewicht von 7—20 kg mit Chloralose (50 mg/kg) und unmittelbar vor dem Eingriff zusätzlich mit Pentothal. Nach wirksamer Erhöhung des intrakraniellen Drucks war eine Fortsetzung der Narkose in der Regel nicht mehr erforderlich. Um die Aspiration von Speichel und anderen Sekreten zu verhindern und den Effekt eines evtl. auftretenden Laryngospasmus aufzuheben, kann ein Trachealtubus eingelegt werden. Kompression des Gehirns wurde durch subdurale oder intrazisternale Einspritzung von Tyrodelösung unter Druck erzielt. Die Kompression der Flüssigkeit hat allerdings den Nachteil, daß die Füllungen unter Umständen wiederholt werden müssen. Bei intrazisternaler Injektion können außerdem leicht Hirnverletzungen vorkommen. Um diese Störfaktoren zu umgehen, verfahren die Autoren folgendermaßen: Das linke Scheitelbein wird trepaniert, die Dura geöffnet und ein Metallröhrchen in den Knochen festschließend eingeschraubt. Durch das Röhrchen wurde unter konstantem Druck Tyrodelösung (pH 7,4) gepreßt. Der mit einem Manometer registrierte Druck in der Vorratsflasche wurde durch Preßluft, die über ein Quecksilberventil entweichen konnte, konstant gehalten. Der intrakranielle Druck wurde gewöhnlich auf Werte von 100—150 mm Hg erhöht. Nach Beendigung der Flüssigkeitsfüllung wurde eine Kanüle in die Cisterna magna eingestochen, um zu kontrollieren, ob freie Verbindung besteht und die Druckwerte übereinstimmen. Druckmessungen in der Schädelkapsel, der Pulmonalarterie, im linken Vorhof, in der Femoralarterie und der Femoralvene wurden optisch mit Hamilton-Manometern vorgenommen. Vorhof- und Pulmonalarteriendruckmessung erfolgten bei geschlossenem Thorax über lange Spinalkanülen, die mit Hilfe von „Nadelführern" in die gewünschte Position gebracht wurden. Die Nadelführer bestehen aus endständig verschlossenen Polyäthylenschläuchen, die in einer Voroperation einerseits in die Wand von Pulmonalarterie oder Vorhof, andererseits in die Subcutis eingenäht worden waren (Harrison u. Liebow, 1949).

Die Hirndrucksteigerung bewirkte Bradykardie, Blutdrucksteigerung und sekundär Erhöhung des Druckes im linken Vorhof. Die Bewertung des Lungenödems wurde nach dem Tod der Tiere anhand des relativen Lungengewichtes und des mikroskopischen Bildes durchgeführt. Unter den beschriebenen Bedingungen entstand nur in einem geringen Prozentsatz der Fälle Lungenödem. Positiv verliefen die Versuche in der Regel dann, wenn der Druck im linken Vorhof während einer Periode von mehr als 15 min auf über 20 cm Wasser erhöht war. Um die Ödembereitschaft zu steigern, müßten daher zusätzliche Eingriffe (z. B. Flüssigkeitsinfusion), die für sich allein nicht ödemauslösend wirken, vorgenommen werden.

Andere Untersucher (Surtshin u. Mitarb., 1948) ziehen Hirndrucksteigerung als ödemauslösenden Faktor in Zweifel, weil es ihnen nicht gelang mit diesbezüglichen Maßnahmen Lungenödem hervorzurufen, sondern nur starke Salivation mit Speichelaspiration, wodurch ein ödemähnliches Bild vorgetäuscht wurde.

3. Intrazisternale Fibrininjektionen

Nach einem erstmalig von Cameron und De (1949) beschriebenen Verfahren kann Lungenödem bei mehreren Tierarten durch intrazisternale Fibrininjektionen provoziert werden. Ratten (in leichter Äthernarkose) oder Kaninchen (Nembutal-Äthernarkose) werden im Nacken- und Hinterhauptsbereich geschoren. Das Foramen atlanto-occipitale wird aufgesucht und durch eine kurz abgeschliffene Kanüle werden 0,2 ml (Ratten) bzw. 3 ml (Kaninchen) Fibrinlösung langsam in die basale Zisterne injiziert. Bei zu schneller Zufuhr sterben die Tiere an Atemversagen. Die Fibrinlösung wird unmittelbar vor Gebrauch aus 4 Teilen Fibrinogen (1:10 in sterilem destilliertem Wasser) und einem Teil Thrombin (1:5 in steriler Kochsalzlösung) hergestellt. Während der Injektion der Fibrinlösung traten tonische Kontraktionen der Skeletmuskulatur, Piloarrektion, Pupillenerweiterung und Exophthalmus auf, 1—5 min danach Relaxation sowie Schaumaustritt aus Mund und Nase. Bei fehlendem Schaumaustritt konnte Lungenödem in der Regel post mortem nachgewiesen werden. Die Obduktion ergab neben schwerem Ödem Hyperämie und Blutextravasate in der Lunge sowie eine Dilatation der rechten Herzhälfte. Das Lungen-Herzgewichtsverhältnis war auf 3:1 bis 5,2:1 (normal 2,4:1) angestiegen. Das histologische Bild der Lunge zeigte mit eiweißreichem Exsudat und stellenweise mit Erythrocyten gefüllte Lufträume, stark hyperämische Gefäße, aber keine Gefäßrupturen, beträchtlich erweiterte Lymphgefäße und unveränderte Bronchien. Der Proteingehalt der zellfreien Ödemflüssigkeit lag zwischen 4 und 7%. Intrazisternale Kontrollinjektionen mit Vollblut oder Tusche (partikelhaltig) führten zu ähnlichen, wenn auch nicht so konstanten Resultaten. Dagegen erzeugten Injektionen von Plasma, Serum, heparinisiertem Blut, Kochsalz-, Thrombin- oder Fibrinogenlösung kein Lungenödem. I.p. Verabreichung entsprechender oder größerer Mengen Fibrinogen, Thrombin oder Fibrin waren wirkungslos, so daß resorptive Einflüsse ausgeschlossen werden konnten.

Sarnoff u. Sarnoff (1952a, b) sowie Sarnoff u. Berglund (1952) wandten die Technik in etwas abgewandelter Form bei Kaninchen und Hunden an. Kaninchen im Gewicht von 1,6—2,9 kg wurden mit 4 ml/kg einer 25%igen Urethanlösung i.v. narkotisiert. Durch die Membrana atlanto-occipitalis wurden 0,2—0,5 ml Thrombin und unmittelbar anschließend durch dieselbe Kanüle 1—2 ml Fibrinogen injiziert. Herstellung der Lösungen: 0,12 g Thrombin (500 E) wurden in

5 ml, 0,4 g Fibrinogen in 15 ml isotonischer Kochsalzlösung gelöst. Die Tiere reagiertem mit generalisiertem Rigor, Opisthotonus, Defäkation, Urinabgang und Veränderungen des Atemmodus. Nach Eintritt des Todes (2—35 min nach der Injektion) konnte in der Regel mäßiges bis schweres Lungenödem nachgewiesen werden.

Hunde im Gewicht von 10—20 kg erhielten 4 mg/kg Morphinsulfat i.m. und 30 min später 48 mg/kg Chloralose und 480 mg/kg Urethan i.v. Die Membrana atlanto-occipitalis wurde in einer Länge von 1,5 cm gespalten. Durch einen Katheter wurden dann 3 ml Thrombin und 10—13 ml Fibrinogen (Lösungen wie vorstehend) über die dorsale Fläche der Medulla in Richtung auf das Tentorium gespritzt. Durch diese Modifikation der Methode wurde einer intrazisternalen Drucksteigerung vorgebeugt. Vor der Fibrinapplikation erhielten die Tiere außerdem 1—3 i.v. Infusionen von 10 ml/kg isotonischer NaCl-Lösung zur Steigerung der Ödembereitschaft.

Um die Pathogenese dieser Ödemform zu klären, nahmen Cameron u. De (1949) an Kaninchen und Sarnoff u. Berglund (1952) an Hunden Kreislaufuntersuchungen vor. Der Druck im rechten Vorhof heparinisierter (1 mg) Kaninchen wurde über einen Plastikschlauch (innerer Durchmesser 1 mm, äußerer Durchmesser 1,8 mm), der in die rechte untere Vena jugularis externa eingeführt, ca. 6 cm in Richtung Herz vorgeschoben und in situ mit einem kräftigen Faden fixiert worden war, mit einem mit NaCl-Lösung gefüllten Manometer gemessen; Druckregistrierung in der Arteria carotis mittels Hg-Manometer. Der Carotisdruck stieg nach der Fibrininjektion um 20—50 mm Hg und fiel später unter die Norm, während der Druck im rechten Vorhof ebenfalls erheblich anstieg, aber bis Ende des Versuches erhöht blieb. Ähnliche Befunde wurden bei künstlich beatmeten Hunden, an denen Druckmessungen in verschiedenen Teilen des Kreislaufsystems z.T. bei geöffnetem, z.T. bei geschlossenem (Druckmessung mit Kathetern) Thorax vorgenommen wurden, erhoben. Die intrazisternale Fibrininjektion stimulierte offensichtlich die kardiovasculären Zentren: Arterieller und venöser Druck im großen und kleinen Kreislauf waren erhöht, die Blutvolumina in Lungenvenen und linkem Vorhof vergrößert.

Nach vorheriger Vagusdurchtrennung und nach i.p. Injektion von Atropinsulfat (1,25 mg/kg) konnte durch den Eingriff kein Lungenödem erzeugt werden; auch Cocain-HCl (200 mg/kg i.p.) hatte eine Schutzwirkung. Eine im Gefolge der Fibrininjektion auftretende Liquordrucksteigerung hat wahrscheinlich keine kausale Bedeutung, weil sie auch nach NaCl-Injektionen beobachtet wurde, ohne Ödementstehung nach sich zu ziehen. Da das injizierte Fibrin sich vor allem am Boden des 4. Ventrikels im Bereich der Vaguskerne anlagerte, vermuteten Cameron u. De (1949) eine Vagusreizung, zumal Vagusdurchtrennung das Lungenödem verhinderte. Doch kommt eine Einengung der Atemwege als Ödemursache wohl nicht in Frage, denn durch zunehmende Einschnürung der freipräparierten Trachea konnte innerhalb einer vergleichbaren Zeitspanne kein Lungenödem provoziert werden. Auch Stimulation der peripheren Vagusenden verursachte kein Lungenödem. Cameron u. De (1949) nehmen deshalb an, daß die Fibrininjektionen zentrale Impulse auslösen, die direkt auf die Capillaren einwirken und das Gleichgewicht zwischen hydrostatischem und osmotischem Plasma- bzw. Gewebedruck stören, so daß Plasma oder Vollblut in die Alveolen dringt und infolge akuter Asphyxie der Tod eintritt.

4. Suboccipitale Veratrininjektion

Nach der Technik von Jarisch *et al.* (1939) sowie Richter u. Thoma (1939) legt man bei Katzen in Chloralosenarkose die Membrana occipitalis frei, spaltet sie in

Querrichtung, schiebt eine stumpfe Kanüle in den 4. Ventrikel vor und injiziert 40—50 μg Veratrin in einem Volumen von 0,1—0,2 ml Ringerlösung. Ein Teil der Flüssigkeit läuft dabei wieder ab, so daß ein Aufsteigen zum Diencephalon vermieden wird. Innerhalb weniger Minuten sterben die Tiere an Lungenödem. Auch bei Hunden, Kaninchen, Meerschweinchen und Ratten läßt sich auf diese Weise Lungenödem erzeugen.

Riechert (1951) fixierte Meerschweinchen im Gewicht von etwa 300 g in Bauchlage, so daß der Kopf nach vorn gebeugt werden konnte. Ohne vorherige operative Maßnahmen tastete er sich mit einer Injektionskanüle nach Durchstechung der Haut im Bereich des Hinterhauptsbeines caudalwärts gegen das Foramen occipitale vor, drang in den Duralsack ein und verabreichte 50 μg Veratrin in 0,02 ml NaCl-Lösung. Die Tiere starben innerhalb von 4 min; das relative Lungengewicht hatte sich gegenüber der Norm verdoppelt. Bei Kaninchen im Gewicht von 2000—3000 g (Chloralosenarkose: 0,5 g/kg i.v.) entwickelte sich unmittelbar nach suboccipitaler Injektion von 50 μg Veratrin schweres Lungenödem, dem innerhalb von 4—7 min der Tod folgte (Ödembeurteilung post mortem nach dem mikroskopischen und makroskopischen Bild und dem Lungengewicht) (Horst *et al.*, 1950). Aravanis *et al.* (1957) sowie Testelli *et al.* (1960) verabfolgten künstlich beatmeten Hunden in Chloralosenarkose (0,1 g/kg i.v.) 40—100 μg/kg Veratrin intrazisternal. Die Tiere reagierten mit schwerem Lungenödem; das relative Lungengewicht war auf das 3fache der Norm erhöht. Das Verhalten der Tiere während bzw. nach der Veratrinapplikation kann durch die Narkose in unterschiedlicher Weise beeinflußt werden. Bei nicht narkotisierten Tieren gehen dem Tod motorische Reizerscheinungen (Muskelzuckungen, Krämpfe) voraus (Riechert, 1950). Aber auch hinsichtlich der Ödementwicklung bestehen species- und narkoticumabhängige Differenzen (Jarisch *et al.*, 1939; s. S. 174).

Die Ursache des Veratrinlungenödems sehen Jarisch *et al.* (1939) in einer zentralen Sympathicuserregung, durch die vasopressorische Blutverschiebungen aus dem großen in den kleinen Kreislauf und Überdehnungen der kleinen Lungengefäße infolge Tonusverlust bewirkt werden. Horst u. Mitarb. (1950) schließen sich aufgrund ihrer Versuchsergebnisse (Hemmung des Veratrinlungenödems durch Vorbehandlung der Tiere mit Hydergin) dieser Deutung an und auch Aravanis *et al.* (1957) sowie Testelli *et al.* (1960) folgern aus Druckmessungen im linken Herzventrikel, im linken Vorhof und im rechten Ventrikel, daß Blutverschiebungen aus dem großen in den kleinen Kreislauf ursächlich an der Entstehung des Veratrinlungenödems beteiligt sein müssen. Offenbar handelt es sich bei dieser Art der Ödemprovokation nicht um einen spezifischen Veratrineffekt. Suboccipitale Gaben von Strophanthin und Aconitin waren in gleicher Weise wirksam, Kontrollinjektionen eines entsprechenden Volumens physiologischer Kochsalzlösung hatten dagegen keinen nennenswerten Einfluß (Jarisch *et al.*, 1939; Riechert, 1951).

5. Infusionen in den Hirnkreislauf

Rasche Infusion größerer Flüssigkeitsmengen in die Arteria carotis communis in Richtung Gehirn verursacht bei Hunden innerhalb weniger Minuten die Entstehung von akutem Lungenödem (Luisada u. Sarnoff, 1944, 1946a; Luisada, 1950a). Hunde im Gewicht von 5—20 kg (narkotisiert mit 3 mg/kg Morphin s.c. und 1 g/kg Urethan p.o.) erhalten in Abständen von 10 bzw. 5 min drei Infusionen durch in beide Arteriae carotis communes eingebundene Glaskanülen. Der Infusionsdruck, der 280—300 mm Hg betragen muß, wird durch eine mit der Luftkammer des Flüssigkeitsreservoirs verbundene Pumpe aufrechterhalten und durch ein Manometer kontrolliert. Als Infusionsmengen werden 85, 80 bzw. 65% des mit 10% des Körpergewichtes veranschlagten Blutvolumens, als Infusionsflüssigkeiten temperierte (37° C) physiologische NaCl-Lösung, Tyrodelösung, 5%ige Rinderalbumin-NaCl-Lösung oder O_2-angereichertes Hundeblut empfohlen. Die Tiere sterben in der Regel innerhalb weniger Minuten, überlebende werden 7 min nach Beendigung der letzten Infusion getötet. Unter diesen Bedingungen wurden Zunahmen des mittleren relativen Lungengewichtes von 0,8% (Kontrolltiere) auf 5,6% beobachtet. Infusion von Blut oder Albuminlösung verursacht das schwerere Ödem, Zufuhr isotonischer Salzlösungen dagegen die stärkere Begleitdyspnoe. Die Tiere können (z.B. zwecks Inhalation von ödemhemmenden Pharmaka) ohne erkennbaren Einfluß auf die Ödementstehung tracheotomiert werden (Luisada, 1950a). Künstliche Atmung unter erhöhtem Druck (8 cm H_2O) hemmte, unter vermindertem Druck (Sog) förderte die Ödembildung jedoch (Luisada u. Sarnoff, 1946b). Cheng (1948) hat die gleiche Technik zur Ödemerzeugung mit Erfolg bei Kaninchen angewandt.

Der Entstehungsmechanismus des auf diese Weise hervorgerufenen Lungenödems ist ungeklärt. Gleiche Flüssigkeitsmengen haben bei Infusion in Femoralarterie oder -vene einen wesentlich gringeren Effekt. Der arterielle und venöse Druck im großen Kreislauf steigt nur vorübergehend an. Luisada u. Sarnoff (1946a, b) vermuten, daß neben der rein mechanischen Dehnung der Lungengefäße kardiovasculären Reflexen, die durch die plötzliche Druck- und Volumensteigerung ausgelöst werden und die Pulmonalgefäße beeinflussen, eine kausale Bedeutung zukommt. Denervation des Carotissinus sowie Morphin- und Phenobarbital-Medikation hemmten die Ödementstehung, während Vagotomie wirkungslos war.

6. Massive Hirnverletzungen

Lungenödem ist eine häufige Begleiterscheinung schwerer Kopfverletzungen (MacKay, 1950; dort weitere Lit.). MacKay (1950) versuchte auf dieser Grundlage bei Ratten Lungenödem zu erzeugen. Der Kopf des Tieres wurde zwischen einem fixierten und einem verschiebbaren Holzblock gelagert und durch einen plötzlich ausgeübten Druck auf den beweglichen Block so schwer geschädigt, daß augenblicklich Bewußtlosigkeit und innerhalb einiger Sekunden oder Minuten unter klonischen Krämpfen der Tod eintrat. Der makroskopische Obduktionsbefund und das relative Lungengewicht ließen in der Regel Lungenödem mittleren Grades erkennen. Durch Vorbehandlung der Tiere mit Pentobarbital, Äther oder Chloralhydrat in narkotischen Dosen wird die Entstehung des Lungenödems gehemmt (vgl. S. 174).

7. Umschriebene Hirnläsionen

Gamble u. Patton (1953) sowie Maire u. Patton (1954, 1956a) entdeckten im Hypothalamusbereich von Ratten mehrere umschriebene Bezirke, deren Zerstörung Lungenödem nach sich zog. Männliche Sprague-Dawley-Ratten im Gewicht von 200—450 g wurden durch Evipal (120 mg/kg i.p.) narkotisiert. Mit Hilfe des Stereotaxiegerätes nach Horsley-Clarke wurden in den Hypothalami beidseitig auf elektrolytischem Weg (unipolare Elektrode; Stromstärke 4 mA; Einwirkungszeit 21 sec) umschriebene Läsionen gesetzt. Etwa 60% der Tiere starben 30 min bis 24 Std nach dem Eingriff an Lungenödem. Bei der Obduktion bzw. der mikroskopischen Untersuchung konnten alveoläres Ödem, Schaum in Trachea und Bronchien, erweiterte, flüssigkeits- bzw. zellgefüllte perivasculäre Räume, aber auch massive Hämorrhagien, Atelektasen und Emphysem, bei einigen Tieren auch Pleuraexsudate nachgewiesen werden. Die Lungengewichte waren auf mehr als das Doppelte erhöht. Das Resultat des Eingriffes ist von der genauen Lokalisation und der Größe der Läsionen abhängig. Bei den Ödemtieren fanden sie sich — wie aus Serienschnitten des Gehirns hervorging — im basalen Teil der Regio praeoptica, etwas dorsal vom rostralen Drittel des Chiasma opticum, 1 mm seitlich der Mittellinie. Von diesem Bereich abweichende oder einseitige Läsionen hatten keinen ödemauslösenden Effekt. Die bläschenförmigen Defekte ließen eine Zone totaler Zerstörung mit einem Durchmesser von 0,6—1 mm und einer Tiefe von 2 mm, die von einem 0,5—1 mm breiten Hof mit deutlicher Gewebsschädigung umgeben war, erkennen. Ein zweites Zentrum, dessen Zerstörung die regelmäßige Ausbildung von Lungenödem bewirkte, wurde in der Regio periventricularis (dorsal, medial und caudal vom vorstehend definierten Ort) entdeckt (Maire u. Patton, 1956a).

Weiterhin konnte gezeigt werden, daß im Hypothalamus unmittelbar caudal vom Chiasma ein sog. „Ödemzentrum" liegen muß, das normalerweise von einem Hemmzentrum in der Regio praeoptica unter Kontrolle gehalten wird. Nach Zerstörung des Hemmzentrums oder der Bahnen zwischen Hemm- und Ödemzentrum entwickelt sich typisches Lungenödem. Die Zerstörung des Ödemzentrums oder der absteigenden Bahnen hemmt dagegen dieses, einer Schädigung der Regio praeoptica folgende Ödem. Der periphere Mechanismus dieser Ödemform ist ungeklärt. Offensichtlich spielen efferente Impulse, die entweder infolge Stimulation nervöser Strukturen in der Umgebung der Läsionen oder nach Zerstörung hemmender Neuren entstehen, eine entscheidende Rolle. Nach Durchtrennung des Cervicalmarkes blieb das Lungenödem ebenso aus wie nach Splanchnektomie. Daher vermuten Maire u. Patton (1956b), daß es, bedingt durch Splanchnicusimpulse, zu einer Entleerung visceraler Venenreservoire mit gleichzeitiger Überladung des Lungenkreislaufs kommt. Wie weit die an Ratten gesammelten Erfahrungen auf andere Tierspecies übertragbar sind, ist nicht abzuschätzen, da die Reaktionsweise der Tiere sogar von Rassenunterschieden abhängig ist. So waren Wistarratten mit gleichartigen Hirnläsionen sehr viel resistenter gegen die Ödementwicklung als Sprague-Dawley-Ratten.

8. Vagotomie

Schädigung der Lungenäste des Nervus vagus kann neben anderen Veränderungen der Lunge auch Ödem hervorrufen, hat für die Pathogenese des Lungenödems beim Menschen aber nur ausnahmsweise Bedeutung. Über einen derartigen Fall, bei dem beide Nervi vagi beim Bougieren des durch Carcinomgewebe eingeengten Oesophagus geschädigt wurden, hat Grögler (1935) berichtet. Im Tierexperiment führte Vagotomie in Abhängigkeit von der Species und den Versuchsbedingungen zu recht unterschiedlichen Ergebnissen. Die ältere Literatur zu diesem Thema wurde von Reichsman (1946) und Short (1944) diskutiert.

Bei Kaninchen (im Gewicht von 800—2500 g) durchtrennte Farber (1937a) in Lokalanaesthesie (Infiltration der Haut mit 1%iger Procainlösung) beide Nervi vagi so weit thorakalwärts im Halsbereich wie möglich. Innerhalb von 8—24 Std, in Einzelfällen bis zu 62 Std nach der Operation, starben die Tiere unter Symptomen von Dyspnoe, wobei der Austritt schaumiger Flüssigkeit aus Mund und Nase auffiel. Bei der Obduktion bzw. mikroskopischen Lungenuntersuchung wurden ausgeprägtes Ödem und erhebliche Hyperämie der Lunge, aber auch bronchopneumonische Herde unterschiedlicher Ausdehnung sowie aspirierte Nahrungsbestandteile und Sekrete in den Luftwegen gefunden. Prinzipiell gleiche Ergebnisse wurden von anderen Autoren (Brunn, 1933; Lorber, 1939a, b; Short, 1944) bei leichter Abwandlung des Verfahrens (z.B. Nembutalnarkose; Vagotomieort 1—1,5 cm unterhalb des Larynx; zusätzliche Flüssigkeitsverabreichung) erzielt.

Mit derselben Technik ließ sich bei Meerschweinchen (im Gewicht von 250—700 g) Lungenödem erzeugen (Farber, 1937b). Die Tiere starben $2^1/_2$—4 Std nach der Operation (Lungenbefund wie oben geschildert). Ein ähnliches Resultat wurde erzielt, wenn die Nerven im Bereich der Lungenwurzeln durch Lokalanaesthesie ausgeschaltet wurden. Dazu wurde der Thorax narkotisierter (Urethan) und künstlich beatmeter Meerschweinchen geöffnet; um die Lungenwurzeln wurden mit 1%iger Procainlösung getränkte Wattestreifen gelegt, die halbstündlich erneuert wurden (Farber, 1937b). Ähnlich verfuhren Plester u. Rummel (1951). Sie durchtrennten bei Meerschweinchen in Äthernarkose beide Nervi vagi dicht oberhalb des Ansatzes des Musc. sternocleidomastoideus an das Brustbein oder legten eine Procain-Kollidonplombe um die Nerven. Das spezifische Gewicht der Lungen der $1^1/_2$ Std nach der Operation getöteten Tiere hatte sich von 0,52 (Kontrolltiere) auf 0,73 erhöht. Bickel u. Dieckhoff (1954) beobachteten innerhalb 1 Std eine Zunahme von 0,59 (Kontrollen) auf 0,71. Schmitt u. Meyers (1957), die Meerschweinchen in Äthernarkose tracheotomierten, proximal und distal intubierten und anschließend bilateral vagotomierten, registrierten bei einer durchschnittlichen Überlebenszeit von 4 Std einen Anstieg des mittleren relativen Lungengewichtes auf das 2,5fache der Norm. Im histologischen Bild dominierte die pulmonale Hyperämie über das alveoläre Ödem. Weiser (1933) wandte die Methode bei Ratten an. 3—6 Std nach Durchtrennung beider Nervi vagi starben die Tiere unter Anzeichen von Dyspnoe. Die Sektion ergab Ödem, Hyperämie und Hämorrhagien der Lunge. Zusätzliche Hypervolämie nach i.v. Flüssigkeitsinfusion (Technik s. S. 198ff.) beschleunigte die Entstehung des Lungenödems und den Eintritt des Todes bei vagotomierten Ratten (Reichsman, 1946). Auch bei Mäusen verursacht Vagotomie Lungenveränderungen. Cassen u. Kistler (1954b) legten die Halseingeweide von Mäusen in Pentobarbital-Na-Narkose vom oberen Thoraxrand bis zum Unterkiefer frei, lagerten die Speicheldrüsen zur Seite, suchten die Art. carotis auf, präparierten den Vagus frei und excidierten ein Stück des Nerven. Die Tiere starben 30 min bis 4 Std nach der Operation; die Lungengewichte waren mäßig erhöht.

Bei Hunden und Katzen verliefen Versuche, durch Vagotomie Lungenödem auszulösen, weniger erfolgreich (Schafer, 1920), vermutlich deshalb, weil die größeren Luftwege dieser Tiere funktionell nicht so leicht eingeengt werden können wie die von Ratten oder Meerschweinchen (Lorber, 1939a, b; Reichsman, 1946). So konnten Cate und Daniel (1948) bei bilateral vagotomierten Hunden selbst durch zusätzliche i.v. Infusion von 100—330 ml physiologischer NaCl-Lösung pro kg Körpergewicht nur bei einem Teil der Tiere Lungenödem erzeugen und auch Luisada u. Sarnoff (1946) konnten infusionsbedingtes Lungenödem beim Hund durch Vagotomie nicht verstärken.

Der Entstehungsmechanismus des Vagotomielungenödems konnte bisher nicht endgültig geklärt werden. Bilaterale Vagotomie kann theoretisch verschiedene Funktionen bzw. Organe innerhalb des Respirations- und Zirkulationssystems beeinflussen, die bei der Entstehung von Lungenödem eine Rolle spielen können (Reichsman, 1946). Besonders eingehend wurden die Vorgänge an den Atemwegen untersucht. Farber (1937a, b) folgert aus seinen Resultaten, daß die nach Vagusausschaltung auftretende Kehlkopflähmung und Einengung der Atemwege keine wesentliche Bedeutung besitzt, weil durch den Einsatz einer Trachealkanüle die Überlebenszeit zwar um durchschnittlich 20% verlängert und der Aspiration und Bronchopneumonie vorgebeugt wurde, die Entwicklung von Ödem und Hyperämie jedoch unverändert ablief. Im Gegensatz dazu stehen die Befunde anderer, auch älterer Untersucher (Drenckhahn, 1958; Esser, 1903; Frey, 1877; Short, 1944), die bei vagotomierten Tieren kein Lungenödem beobachteten, wenn die

Aspiration von Schleim und Nahrungsbestandteilen bzw. eine Einengung der Atemwege verhindert wurden. So erzielte Lorber (1939a, b) bei Ratten, Meerschweinchen und Kaninchen ähnliche Ergebnisse wie Farber (1937a). Wenn er jedoch die Luftwege der vagotomierten Tiere mittels Tracheotomie (ohne Verwendung einer Kanüle) und mechanischer Trachealreinigung freihielt, trat entweder gar kein oder nur geringgradiges Lungenödem auf. Short (1944) konnte diese Befunde bestätigen und darüber hinaus zeigen, daß an der Einengung der Luftwege offensichtlich nicht nur der Laryngospasmus, sondern auch eine Ansammlung viscösen Sekretes in der Luftröhre beteiligt ist. Isolierte Durchtrennung der Nervi recurrentes, die eine Verengung der Stimmritze bewirkt, hatte kein Lungenödem zur Folge, spätere Vagotomie verursachte bei solchen Tieren jedoch innerhalb weniger Stunden den Tod an Lungenödem. Für einen derartigen Pathomechanismus spricht weiterhin, daß Tracheotomie bei langdauernden Versuchen von sich aus zu Lungenödem führen kann (Short, 1944). In solchen Fällen wurden in der Trachea unterhalb der Kanüle mit Zellfragmenten untermischte Schleimpfröpfe gefunden, die nicht weiterbefördert werden konnten und die Luftpassage erschwerten. Die Ursache der Sekretansammlung wird in der Ausschaltung des Kehlkopfes bzw. der normalen Transportmechanismen gesehen[2]. Speciesbedingte Differenzen der Reaktionsweise erklären sich teilweise sicherlich durch strukturelle Unterschiede der Bronchialschleimhaut, die z.B. beim Kaninchen im Vergleich zu anderen Tierarten (Ratte, Katze) nur spärlich Schleimzellen und fast keine Schleimdrüsen enthält (Short, 1944). Zur weiteren Klärung des pathogenetischen Einflusses der Vagotomie trug Reichsman (1946) bei. Er fand nur bei einem Teil seiner in Äther- oder Urethannarkose vagotomierten Ratten Lungenödem und konnte laryngoskopisch nachweisen, daß die Intensität des durch den Eingriff bedingten Laryngospasmus variieren kann und offensichtlich in Korrelation zum resultierenden Lungenödem steht. In Urethannarkose, die den Laryngospasmus hemmt, war der Prozentsatz ödemfreier Tiere größer. Zusätzliche Sympathektomie veränderte das Ergebnis nicht. Lungenödem entstand auch, wenn der Nervus vagus auf einer Seite im Hals-, auf der Gegenseite im Brustbereich unterhalb des Abganges des Nervus recurrens durchtrennt wurde, die Stimmritze also nicht eingeengt war. Auch unter diesen Bedingungen soll eine Erhöhung des Inspirationswiderstandes die ursächliche Rolle spielen. Ansammlung zähen Sekretes in den Luftwegen, das bei der Einatmung ventilartig aus größeren in kleinere Bronchien verlagert wird, erschwert die Gaspassage während dieser Phase; bei der Exspiration würde sich der Sekretpfropf in der entgegengesetzten Richtung bewegen und den Durchlaß freigeben. Der Einfluß künstlicher Beatmung auf das Vagotomielungenödem wird unterschiedlich beurteilt. Während Farber (1937b) die Ödementstehung auf diese Weise nicht verhindern konnte, kamen Susman *et al.* (1948) zu gegensätzlichen Resultaten. Sie konnten weder bei vagotomierten Meerschweinchen in Nembutalnarkose (nach der Methode von Farber) noch bei Kontrolltieren Lungenödem nachweisen, wenn sie mit geringem Druck (6 mm Hg) beatmeten, selbst nicht bei Ausdehnung der Versuchsdauer auf 25 Std. Lungenödem entwickelte sich dagegen unterschiedslos bei Vagotomie- und Kontrolltieren, wenn der Beatmungsdruck 20 mm Hg betrug.

Eine vagotomiebedingte Permeabilitätssteigerung der Lungencapillaren wurde von Plester u. Rummel (1951) sowie Weiser (1933) als ödemauslösender Faktor diskutiert. Histamin dürfte an diesem Mechanismus nicht beteiligt sein, da sich weder eine Erhöhung des Histamingehaltes der Lunge noch ein ödemhemmender

[2] Dabei ist die Austrocknung der Atemwege durch zu trockene Einatmungsluft nach der Tracheotomie maßgeblich. Führt man tracheotomierten Tiere eine gut mit Wasserdampf gesättigte Luft zu, dann bleiben sie am Leben (Höbel u. Eichler).

Effekt von Antihistaminica feststellen ließ. Eine Beobachtung von Drenckhahn (1958) weist auf die Mitwirkung einer Capillardrucksteigerung an der Ödemgenese hin. Er sah bei einem vagotomierten Meerschweinchen wechselnde Erhöhungen des Pulmonalvenendruckes, die offenbar von der jeweiligen Intensität der Atemstörung abhängig waren.

Eine weitere Ursache für speciesbedingte Unterschiede der Reaktionsweise dürfte in Modifikationen der nervösen Atmungssteuerung zu suchen sein. Während Hunde, Katzen und Kaninchen auch nach Vagusausschaltung rhythmisch atmen, ist das bei Meerschweinchen nicht der Fall (Oberholzer u. Schlegel, 1956). Bei ihnen treten minutenlange Phasen exspiratorischen Atemstillstandes auf, die nur von gelegentlicher Schnappatmung unterbrochen werden und schließlich unter Asphyxie zum Tod führen. Das Phänomen wird mit dem Ausfall afferenter Vagusfasern, die bei dieser Tierart für die einwandfreie Funktion des inspiratorischen Atemzentrums erforderlich sind, erklärt. Auch die prohibitive Wirkung der künstlichen Beatmung (s.o.) würde dadurch verständlich. Schmitt u. Meyers (1957) sind ebenfalls der Meinung, daß die Lungenveränderungen nach Vagotomie Folge einer afferenten Denervation sind, messen jedoch Kreislaufeffekten größere Bedeutung bei. Die Durchtrennung sensorischer Vagusfasern führt zu einem Verlust sympathischer Aktivität, die für die Aufrechterhaltung des normalen Tonus der glatten Bronchiolen- bzw. Gefäßmuskulatur notwendig ist.

9. Denervation der Lunge

Eine Ausschaltung der gesamten nervösen Versorgung eines Lungenlappens ist im Zusammenhang mit anderen ödemprovozierenden Maßnahmen vorgenommen worden (s. S. 198).

IV. Einwirkung toxischer Konzentrationen chemischer Elemente oder Verbindungen

Lungenödem ist eine häufige Begleiterscheinung zahlreicher Vergiftungen. Es kann ganz im Vordergrund der Symptomatik stehen (wie z.B. bei der Phosgenvergiftung) oder hinter anderen Intoxikationsfolgen zurücktreten. Im vorliegenden Kapitel werden die experimentellen Methoden besprochen, bei denen ein Gifteffekt als solcher zur Ödemauslösung führt, unabhängig davon, ob der primäre Angriffspunkt in der Lunge, an den Zirkulationsorganen oder im Zentralnervensystem liegt. Es kann nur auf solche Noxen eingegangen werden, die systematisch zur Erzeugung von experimentellem Lungenödem verwendet worden sind. Verbindungen, die nur in Gemeinsamkeit mit anderen Maßnahmen (z.B. Anwendung spezieller Applikationstechniken) Ödem hervorrufen, sind in den vorstehenden Kapiteln angeführt. Auf zahlreiche weitere ödemprovozierende Verbindungen ist in der Literatur hingewiesen worden; eine ältere — sicher auch für die damaligen Kenntnisse unvollständige — Übersicht stammt von Petri (1930), weitere Angaben sind in den Arbeiten von Cameron (1948), Sylla (1952), Visscher *et al.* (1956) und in der toxikologischen Literatur (s. z.B. Lehmann u. Flury, 1938; Moeschlin, 1964) enthalten.

1. Inhalation von Giftstoffen

Zur experimentellen Erzeugung von Lungenödem geeignete inhalierbare Gifte finden sich einerseits unter den normalen Atmosphärengasen (Sauerstoff, Kohlendioxyd), andererseits unter den sog. Reizgasen (Musterbeispiel: Phosgen). Während die atmosphärischen Gase aufgrund überhöhter Konzentrationen wirken, entfalten die Reizgase ihre toxischen Effekte bereits in einem relativ niedrigen

Konzentrationsbereich. Diese Eigenschaft der Reizgase macht gewisse Sicherheitsvorkehrungen (Installation der Versuchsanordnung unter einem Abzug usw.) erforderlich. Giftige Konzentrationen irritierender Gase können Reizwirkungen an der Haut, den tangierten oder passierten Schleimhäuten (Conjunctiven und Schleimhäute der Atemwege), Veränderungen am Lungengewebe und — nach Resorption — Allgemeinwirkungen verursachen (Laqueur u. Magnus, 1921a). Der Angriffsort eines Gases innerhalb des Respirationssystems wird vor allem von seiner Löslichkeit bestimmt. Gute Wasserlöslichkeit bedingt bei Kontakt mit den Schleimhäuten u.U. eine so weitgehende Elimination des Gases aus der Atemluft, daß keine wirksamen Gasmengen in die Alveolen gelangen.

Zur rechnerischen Bewertung der Wirkung eines Gases auf den Organismus dient häufig die $c \cdot t$-Formel; sie stellt die Wirkungsintensität in Beziehung zur Gaskonzentration c (in mg/m^3) und zur Einwirkungsdauer t (in min) (s. z. B. Flury, 1921a; Laqueur und Magnus, 1921a, b). Die ct-Formel gilt jedoch nur für einen bestimmten Konzentrationsbereich (Wirth, 1936). Sie wird ferner bei Gasen mit vorwiegend resorptiver Wirkung, die im Organismus entgiftet werden, versagen. Gaskonzentrationen werden angegeben in: ppm (parts pro million bei 25° C und 760 mm Hg) = ml Gas pro m^3 Luft; $^0/_{00}$ (%); mg/m^3 oder mg/l.

Die tatsächliche Reizgaskonzentration im Expositionsraum muß durch wiederholte Gasanalysen ermittelt werden. Dazu werden in der Regel mittels geeichter, evakuierter Gaspipetten von etwa 0,5—2 Liter Inhalt Gasproben entnommen und mit einem abgemessenen Volumen Reaktionslösung versetzt. Nach der erforderlichen Reaktionszeit wird die Gaskonzentration titrimetrisch, colorimetrisch, potentiometrisch usw. bestimmt (Grundlagen der gasanalytischen Technik bei Gage, 1961).

Die Einwirkung der Giftgase kann grundsätzlich nach dem statischen oder dynamischen Prinzip erfolgen. Beim statischen Versuch werden die Tiere dem zu Beginn eingestellten Gasgemisch in dicht schließenden Atemkammern ausgesetzt. Die Methode, die einen verhältnismäßig geringen technischen Aufwand erfordert, eignet sich vorwiegend für kurzdauernde Experimente, weil die anfängliche Konzentration mit der Zeit infolge Aufnahme und Abbau des Gases durch die Tiere, Adsorption an Kammerwände, abgesetzte Exkremente, Körperoberfläche der Tiere usw. mehr und mehr reduziert wird. Gleichzeitig verarmt das Kammerinnere fortschreitend an Sauerstoff und reichert sich mit Kohlendioxyd und Wasserdampf an. Um derartige Störfaktoren so weit wie möglich zu mindern, empfahlen Laqueur und Magnus (1921a) die Verwendung großer Kammern. Ein großes Kammervolumen gestattet außerdem wiederholte Probenentnahmen für die Analyse ohne wesentliche Beeinträchtigung der Gaskonzentration. Die von Laqueur und Magnus für die Exposition von Katzen benutzte Kammer hatte ein Fassungsvermögen von 8 m^3, andere in der Literatur beschriebene Kammern variieren zwischen einem solchen von wenigen Litern und mehreren m^3. Sie sind in der Regel aus Glaswänden aufgebaut, mit einem Ventilator zur Durchmischung der Kammerluft mit dem Reizgas, einer Absaugvorrichtung, Bohrungen zur Analysenentnahme und einer Schleuse (z.B. Fallschleuse) zum Einbringen der Versuchstiere ausgerüstet. Für Tiere wie Ratten und Meerschweinchen ist Hineinschieben der Tiere mit einer Art großer Spritze besser geeignet, weil der Schock durch das Herabfallen vermieden wird.

Das dynamische Prinzip basiert auf der Anwendung strömender Gasgemische und erfordert eine Versuchsanordnung, die eine kontinuierliche Dosierung der Gase zuläßt und das Gemisch durch den Versuchsraum treibt. Das Verfahren ermöglicht lange Expositionszeiten und ist von den vorgenannten Fehlerquellen der statischen Methode weitgehend frei, benötigt aber erheblich größere Gasmengen als diese.

Ältere Techniken, bei denen gewöhnlich Raumluft nebst beigemischtem Giftgas mittels einer Pumpe durch die Expositionskammer gesaugt wurde (Laqueur u. Magnus, 1921b; Lehmann u. Hasegawa, 1912) sind von Gross und Hebestreit (1932) ausführlich besprochen worden. Heute werden gewöhnlich Apparate angewandt, die das Gasgemisch mit Hilfe von Preßluft durch die Kammer treiben. Derartige Einrichtungen sind z. B. von Henschler *et al.* (1960b), Klimmer (1956), Neumann und Klimmer (1939), Wirth (1930) beschrieben oder diskutiert worden. Komprimierte Gase, die handelsüblichen Stahlflaschen entnommen werden, können mit Hilfe von Reduzierventilen und Rotametern dosiert und in Mischkugeln mit Luft oder anderen Gasen vereint werden, wie es z. B. die in Abb. 12 wiedergegebene schematische Darstellung nach Klimmer (1943) zeigt.

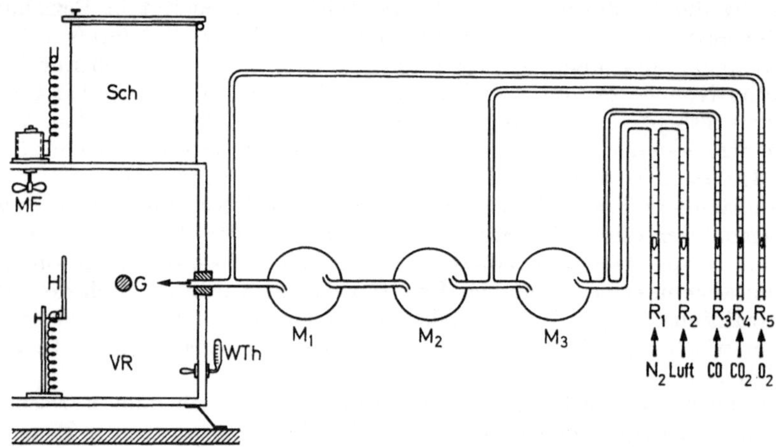

Abb. 12. Schematische Darstellung der Strömungsapparatur nach Klimmer (1943). R_1—R_5 Rotameter; M_1—M_3 Mischkugeln; *VR* Versuchsraum; *Sch* Schleuse

Ein Gas, das nur unter Atmosphärendruck zur Verfügung steht, läßt man gewöhnlich durch eine kontinuierlich arbeitende Vorrichtung (Kolben, Sperrflüssigkeit) aus einem Meßzylinder in eine Mischkugel hineindrücken, wo es von der durchfließenden Luft aufgenommen wird (z.B. Klimmer, 1956; Neumann und Klimmer, 1939; Wirth, 1930). Am Beispiel der von Henschler *et al.* (1960b) sowie von Klimmer (1956) angegebenen Strömungsapparaturen werden die Möglichkeiten zur Gasdosierung genauer dargestellt. Weitere Apparate werden im Rahmen ihrer experimentellen Anwendung beschrieben (s. S. 229, 234).

Verfahren nach Henschler *et al.* (1960b). Die Apparatur (s. Abb. 13), die aus einem System von Rotametern und Mischkugeln besteht, wird zweckmäßigerweise in toto unter einem Abzug aufgebaut. Durch das Rotameter R_1 gelangt ein dosierter Reizgasstrom, durch Rotameter R_2 Frischluft in eine Mischkugel (M_1). Dieses primäre Gasgemisch wird in den Mischkugeln M_2 und M_3 durch Zufuhr weiterer Frischluft (R_4 und R_6) verdünnt. Jeweils vor dem Eintritt in diese Mischkugeln M_2 und M_3 wird ein gemessener Teil des Gasgemisches über die Rotameter R_3 bzw. R_5 in den Abzug geleitet. Die Menge der abgeleiteten Gase kann mittels der Glashähne H_1 und H_2 kontrolliert werden. Aus der Mischkugel M_3 strömt das Gemisch über ein etwa 4 m langes Glasrohr in die Mischtrommel MT, wo es mit einem größeren Luftvolumen zum endgültigen Gas-Luftgemisch vereinigt wird. Die Frischluft zur Vorverdünnung, die z. B. einer druckkonstanten Hausleitung entnommen werden kann, wird mit Hilfe der Reduzierventile RV_{1-3} reguliert;

sie soll öl- und geruchfrei sein und eine relative Feuchte von 40—45% haben. Die Luft zur endgültigen Verdünnung des Gemisches in der Trommel *MT* wird von einem Ventilator *V* geliefert und kann durch den Schieber *S* vor dem Saugstutzen in Verbindung mit dem Nebenstrommesser *RN* genau dosiert werden. Die Mischtrommel war aus Zinkblech, alle anderen Teile der Apparatur waren aus Glas gefertigt; zur Verbindung der Rohrleitungen eignen sich Polyvinylchloridschläuche. Durch Veränderung der Frischluftzufuhr und der abgeleiteten Anteile der Gasgemische läßt sich jede gewünschte Gaskonzentration herstellen und bei Kenntnis der Einstellwerte jederzeit reproduzieren. Die Strömungsgeschwindigkeit ist von der Größe des Versuchsraumes und der Häufigkeit des Luftwechsels

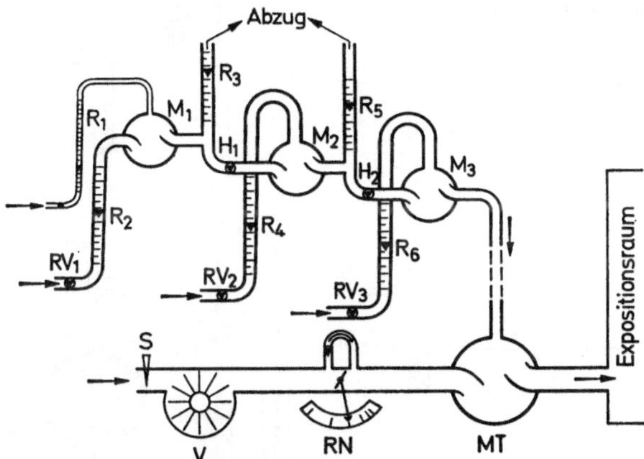

Abb. 13. Schema der Apparatur zur Herstellung hochverdünnter Gas-Luftgemische nach Henschler *et al.* (1960b). Erläuterungen im Text

(14—22mal pro Stunde) abhängig. Sie beträgt z.B. bei einem Versuchsraum von 8 m³ Inhalt und 22fachem Luftwechsel 176 m³/Std.

Die in Abb. 14 dargestellte Apparatur nach Klimmer (1956) eignet sich zur kontinuierlichen Dosierung von Gasen, die unter Normaldruck zur Verfügung stehen. Die aus einer Steuerungs- und Dosierungseinrichtung und einer Expositionskammer bestehende Apparatur soll aus Sicherheitsgründen unter einem Abzug installiert werden. Das Reizgas wird aus einem Meßzylinder (*MZ*) von 1—3 Liter Inhalt durch eine kontinuierlich zulaufende Druckflüssigkeit verdrängt. Nach Passage eines als Ventil wirkenden Blasenzählers (*BZ*) vereinigt es sich mit einem rotametrisch (*R*) kontrollierten Luftstrom (500—5000 l/h) in der Mischkugel (*MK*), von wo es in den Versuchsraum (*VR*) und weiter in den Abzug gelangt. Der Druck im Gasreservoir (*MZ*) wird mit Hilfe des kontinuierlich angehobenen Niveaugefäßes (*NG*) konstant gehalten (Kontrolle des Gasdruckes durch das Gasmanometer *WM*); der Querschnitt beider Gefäße ist gleich groß. Das Aufsteigen des Niveaugefäßes wird durch einen Sperr- und Steuermechanismus geregelt. Dieser besteht aus einer mit Arretierungszapfen (*AZ*) bewehrten Sperrscheibe (*SP*), auf deren Achse die Nylonbremsschnur (*Sch*) aufgewickelt ist, und einer Vorrichtung zur alternierenden Freigabe bzw. Arretierung der Zapfen. Die sich abspulende Bremsspur reguliert in Abhängigkeit vom Durchmesser der Sperrscheibenachse, von der Winkelgeschwindigkeit der Sperrscheibe, der Anzahl der Arretierungszapfen (36—90) und der pro Zeiteinheit freigegebenen Arretierungen das Ansteigen des Niveaugefäßes. Zur Sperrung bzw. Freigabe der Zapfen dient die mit dem Weicheisenanker (*W*) und dem Kipphebel (*A*) verbundene

Messingachse (*MA*), die mit Hilfe des Elektromagneten (*M*) verschoben werden kann. Bei Stromschluß gibt die Achse den jeweils blockierten Zapfen frei, während die Stahlfeder (*St*) des Kipphebels (*A*) gleichzeitig einen der folgenden Zapfen vorübergehend abfängt, bis die Achse (*MA*) von der Feder (*F*) wieder in die Ruhelage befördert wird. Die Steuerung bzw. Speisung des Elektromagneten (*M*) erfolgt über den käuflichen Zeitgeber (*Z*) (Fa. Braun, Melsungen; 220/6 V, Impulse 0,5—60 sec) und das Relais (*Re*).

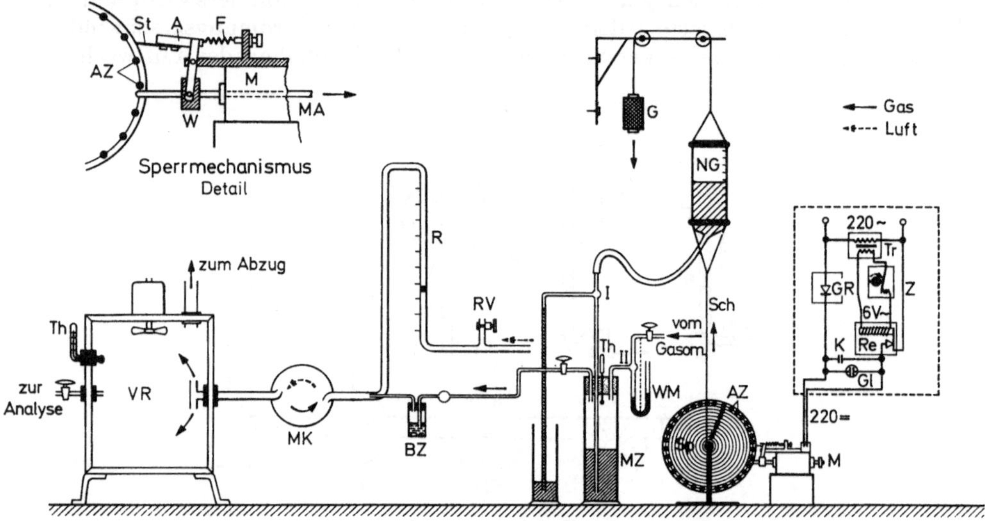

Abb. 14. Schema der Strömungsapparatur nach Klimmer (1956). Erklärungen im Text

a) Phosgen und Diphosgen

Phosgen ($COCl_2$), eine farblose Flüssigkeit mit einem Siedepunkt von 8° C und einem spezifischen Gewicht von 1,4, ist bei Zimmertemperatur ein farbloses, schlecht wasserlösliches Gas. Aus der großen Zahl der bekannten Reizgase (ältere Übersicht s. Flury, 1921a) ragt Phosgen insofern heraus, als seine Einwirkung primär fast ausschließlich Schädigungen des Lungengewebes verursacht. Krankheitserscheinungen an anderen Organen sind sekundäre Folgen der Lungenschäden.

Phosgenvergiftung nach dem statischen Prinzip. Laqueur u. Magnus (1921a) benutzten für die Phosgenexposition eine Gaskammer von 8 m³ Inhalt. Durch eine Schleuse konnten gleichzeitig mehrere Tiere eingebracht werden. Phosgengas aus Gaspipetten (in der Regel 200 ml = 800 mg) wurde mit Preßluft in die Kammer eingeblasen und mit Hilfe eines Ventilators in der Kammer verteilt. Bei Katzen entwickelte sich nach einer Einwirkungsdauer von 15—20 min in der Regel eine ausgeprägte, häufig tödliche Vergiftung, deren Schweregrad nach der *ct*-Formel vorausberechnet werden konnte. Wenn das $c \cdot t$-Produkt den Wert 450 überschritt, konnte in der Regel schweres Lungenödem erwartet werden; die Streubreiten waren jedoch erheblich, große Versuchsreihen daher erforderlich. Zwischen verschiedenen Tierarten — untersucht wurden Mäuse, Ratten, Meerschweinchen, Kaninchen, Katzen, Hunde, Pferde und Affen — bestehen nur geringe Empfindlichkeitsunterschiede. Auch in neuerer Zeit gelangten Autoren, die nach demselben Prinzip vorgingen, zu ähnlichen Resultaten. Rothlin (1941), der Ratten paarweise in einer Gaskammer von 30 Liter Inhalt für 20 min der Einwirkung verschiedener Phosgenkonzentrationen aussetzte, fand z. B., daß 30 mg/m³ ($c \cdot t = 600$) in der Regel von allen und 100 mg/m³ von 50% der Tiere überlebt wurden, während 150 mg/m³ für alle Tiere tödlich waren. Bei Kaninchen (Kammer von 400 Liter Inhalt, Expositionszeit 30 min) betrug die Mortalität unter der Einwirkung einer Phosgenanfangskonzentration von 270 mg/m³ 80—100% (Boyd u. Perry, 1960), bzw. unter einer solchen von 400—550 mg/m³ 70% (Halpern *et al.*, 1950). Kaninchen reagieren auf Phosgen nicht mit solcher Regelmäßigkeit wie andere Versuchstiere, weil der die Nasenschleimhaut treffende Reiz eine reflektorische Atmungsverlangsamung bzw. vorübergehenden Atemstillstand verursacht. Die während der Expositionszeit in die Lunge eindringende Phosgenmenge unterliegt daher von Tier zu Tier großen Schwankungen. Der Ablauf des Reflexes kann jedoch unterbrochen werden, wenn man die Nasenschleimhaut vor der Vergiftung anaesthesiert. Laqueur u. Magnus (1921b) bliesen Osmosilpulver (feinzerstäubte kolloidale Kieselsäure) mit 10% Cocain in die Nase und erzielten bei der nachfolgenden Vergiftung einheitlichere Resultate.

Phosgenvergiftung nach dem dynamischen Prinzip. Wenn möglich wird man dem Durchströmungsversuch den Vorzug vor dem statischen Versuch geben, weil die experimentellen Bedingungen dabei besser kontrollierbar sind. Auf das Prinzip der älteren Methoden sei nur kurz anhand des Vorgehens von Laqueur und Magnus (1921b) hingewiesen. Eine mit zwei verschließbaren Ausgängen versehene Glasflasche von 84 Liter Inhalt wurde evakuiert, mit 50 ml Phosgen aus einer Gaspipette beschickt und anschließend über einen Dreiwegehahn, eine mit konzentrierter Schwefelsäure gefüllte Waschflasche und ein Strömungsmanometer mit dem unteren Zugang einer 50 Liter fassenden Glasglocke verbunden. Die als Expositionsraum dienende Glasglocke war auf eine (nach Einfetten) luftdicht schließende Glasplatte aufgeschliffen und stand über eine zweite (obere) Öffnung mit einer Saugpumpe, der ein weiteres Strömungsmanometer vorgeschaltet war, in Verbindung. Mit Hilfe der Pumpe wurde das Gasgemisch (1,5 l/min; 20 min lang) aus der Vorratsflasche durch die Glasglocke gesaugt. Exponierte Kaninchen starben unter diesen Bedingungen regelmäßig an schwerem Lungenödem; ihre relativen Lungengewichte waren auf das 3—7fache der Norm angestiegen.

Heute wird man sich nach Möglichkeit einer der modernen Durchströmungsapparaturen bedienen, z. B. der auf S. 222f. ausführlich beschriebenen Apparatur nach Henschler *et al.* (1960b). Mit ihrer Hilfe stellten Henschler u. Laux (1960) strömende Phosgen-Luftgemische mit einer Phosgenkonzentration von 10—20 ppm her und ließen sie 30 min lang auf Wistarratten im Gewicht von 120—150 g in einer Gaskammer von 200 Liter Inhalt (Gaswechsel 12—15mal pro Stunde) einwirken. Gasanalysen wurden nach dem unten geschilderten Verfahren (Wirth, 1936) in 10 min-Intervallen ausgeführt. Konzentrationen von 10—15 ppm waren für etwa 75%, Konzentrationen von 20 ppm Phosgen für alle Tiere tödlich. Die durchschnittliche Überlebenszeit betrug 5—6 Std, bei den niedrigeren Konzentrationen bis zu 30 Std. Das relative Lungengewicht war z. T. auf mehr als 40 g/kg erhöht.

Die lungenschädigende Phosgenminimalkonzentration versuchte Wirth (1936) an Katzen zu bestimmen. Er dosierte das Phosgen nach dem später von Henschler *et al.* (1960b) weiterentwickelten Prinzip (s. S. 222f.). Ein gemessener trockener Phosgenstrom aus einer Stahlflasche wurde mit einem dosierten Luftstrom gemischt und ein kleiner Teil dieses Gemisches weiter mit Luft verdünnt. Das Endgemisch wurde in Gaskammern von 200 Liter oder 1 m³ Inhalt, die in der üblichen Weise ausgestattet waren, eingeleitet. Die Strömungsgeschwindigkeit des Phosgens war zwischen 0,1 und 1 l/Std, die der Frischluft zwischen 500 und 5000 l/Std variierbar. Phosgenkonzentrationen von 0,5—2 mg/m³ riefen auch bei vielstündiger Einwirkung nur ausnahmsweise intraalveoläres Ödem hervor; fast immer wurde interstitielles Ödem mit Verbreiterung der Alveolarsepten gefunden. Bei Konzentrationen von 5—7 mg/m³ und Einwirkungszeiten von 3—8 Std wurde regelmäßiger intraalveoläres Ödem beobachtet. Aus den Ergebnissen ist zu folgern, daß das tödlich wirkende *ct*-Produkt bei Einwirkung schwacher Konzentrationen höhere Werte erreicht.

Phosgenzufuhr durch eine Trachealkanüle. Schwierigkeiten bei der Phosgeninhalation können auftreten, wenn — wie es bei Therapieversuchen gelegentlich erforderlich ist — dem Versuchstier eine genau dosierte, hoch konzentrierte Gasmenge innerhalb kurzer Zeit zugeführt werden soll. Unter der Einwirkung des konzentrierten, stark reizenden Gases kann die Atemgröße und abhängig davon die in der Zeiteinheit eingeatmete Gasmenge besonders während der ersten Minuten der Expositionszeit beträchtlich variieren. Eine einfache Methode, die es gestattet, die verabreichte Gasmenge zu messen, hat Gildemeister (1921) angegeben. Man fixiert in der Trachea narkotisierter Versuchstiere (Urethan 0,5 g/kg) eine T-förmige Kanüle; ein Schenkel der Kanüle wird über ein Einatmungsventil (Müllersche Flasche mit Quecksilberfüllung) mit dem Vorratsgefäß für die Gasmischung, der andere mit einem Spirometer zur Messung des Exspirationsluftvolumens verbunden. Als Spirometer benutzte der Autor einen wassergefüllten, mit seiner Öffnung umgekehrt in eine pneumatische Wanne eintauchenden Glaszylinder, in den der entsprechende Kanülenschenkel einmündete. An die als Vorratsgefäß dienende, 6 Liter fassende Glasflasche wird ein Atembeutel von 2 Liter Inhalt angeschlossen, der das Eindringen atmosphärischer Luft in das Vorratsgefäß verhindern soll. Das Vorratssystem von insgesamt 8 Liter Inhalt wird mit Phosgen (10 ml) beschickt. Die Tiere atmen im Verlauf von $^1/_2$—1 min die vorbestimmte, mit Hilfe des Spirometers registrierte Gasmenge ein. 67—240 ml des Gasgemisches/kg Gewicht riefen in fast allen Fällen Lungenödem hervor.

Phosgenanalyse nach Wirth (1936) (in Anlehnung an das Verfahren von Kölliker). Das phosgenhaltige Gasgemisch wird nacheinander durch ein Trockenröhrchen mit gekörntem $CaCl_2$, durch eine Gaswaschflasche mit Silbersulfat in konzentrierter H_2SO_4 (3 g Silbersulfat auf 100 ml Schwefelsäure 1,84), durch zwei Gasfilter mit Glaswolle und durch zwei Gaswaschflaschen mit je 150 ml n/10 Natriumäthylatlösung in absolutem Alkohol geleitet. Anschließend wird die Natriumäthylatlösung quantitativ mit destilliertem Wasser in ein Becherglas (600 ml) gespült und mit 20 ml verdünnter HNO_3 angesäuert (Gesamtflüssigkeitsmenge 350—400 ml). Potentiometrische Titration der Cl-Ionen mit n/10 Silbernitrat an Platin- bzw. Kalomelelektroden. 1 ml n/10 Silbernitrat entspricht 4,95 mg Phosgen.

Die mit der Phosgenvergiftung verbundenen pathologisch-anatomischen und funktionellen Veränderungen im Organismus sind eingehend untersucht worden (Heitzmann, 1921; Laqueur u. Magnus, 1921a). Neuere Arbeiten (Lit. s. Cameron, 1948) haben die alten Auffassungen über den Pathomechanismus des Phosgenödems bestätigt. Einwirkung schwacher Konzentrationen führt nach einer gewissen Latenzzeit zur Ausbildung von Lungenödem. Es kommt zunächst zum Aus- bzw. Übertritt von zellfreiem Exsudat, dann auch von Leukocyten und Fibrin aus den Capillaren in die Alveolen; Erythrocyten sind im Exsudat in der Regel nicht enthalten. Der Angriffsort des Phosgens liegt offensichtlich in der alveolocapillären Membran. Nach Short (zit. nach Cameron, 1948) treten an den Mitochondrien des Capillarendothels Schädigungen auf, bevor der Flüssigkeitsaustritt aus den Capillaren beginnt. Direkte Einflüsse des Phosgens auf den Kreislauf oder auf nervöse Receptoren der Lunge konnten nicht nachgewiesen werden (Patt *et al.*, 1946; Whitteridge, 1948). Bei der Inhalation von Phosgen sind Giftwirkungen an lungenfernen Organen schon deshalb nicht zu erwarten, weil das Gas bei der Passage der Alveolar-Capillarwand rasch hydrolysiert und mithin unwirksam wird, toxische Konzentrationen also nicht in andere Organe gelangen. Das gesamte Krankheitsbild ist eine Folge der Lungenschädigung, Störungen anderer Organe sind sekundär bedingt. Der Verlauf der experimentellen Phosgenvergiftung ist von der angewandten Gaskonzentration abhängig. Nur wenn diese nicht zu hoch (über 300 mg/m³) gewählt wird, bleiben komplizierende Reizwirkungen auf die Bronchialschleimhaut und -muskulatur aus. In dieser Hinsicht bestehen jedoch erhebliche Speciesdifferenzen. So reagieren Meerschweinchen z. B. schon auf sehr viel geringere Phosgenkonzentrationen mit Bronchialmuskelkrämpfen als die meisten anderen Versuchstiere. Unter dem Einfluß hoher Phosgenkonzentrationen schließlich kann der Tod sehr schnell eintreten, ohne daß es zur Ausbildung von Lungenödem kommt.

Diphosgen ($Cl—COOCCl_3$[3]). Die Symptomatik der Phosgen- und Diphosgenvergiftung ähneln einander bis in Einzelheiten hinein. Auch die ödemauslösenden Konzentrationen beider Gase liegen in der gleichen Größenordnung. Bei Einwirkungszeiten von 10 min waren Diphosgenkonzentrationen zwischen 330 und 490 mg/m³ für 30—100% der exponierten Mäuse, 520 mg/m³ für 80% der Ratten und 520—690 mg/m³ für Hunde (Exposition 30 min) tödlich (Postel *et al.*, 1946). Um Lungenödem zu provozieren, darf die angewandte Diphosgenkonzentration einen bestimmten Bereich nicht überschreiten. Überhöhte Konzentrationen bewirken den Tod durch Unterbrechung der Lungenzirkulation infolge intravasaler Hämolyse und Agglutination. Diphosgen wirkt offensichtlich — ebenso wie es für Phosgen angenommen wird — rein lokal, greift bei Inhalation also am Lungenparenchym an; pathologische Veränderungen an anderen Organen sind sekundär bedingt. Nach i.p. Injektion entstanden Nekrosen in der Bauchhöhle, Lungenveränderungen wurden nicht beobachtet (Tobias *et al.*, 1949).

b) Chlorpikrin

Chlorpikrin (CCl_3NO_2), eine farblose Flüssigkeit mit einem Siedepunkt von 113° und einem spezifischen Gewicht von 1,69, ist schwer wasserlöslich, jedoch gut mit Äther mischbar. In mittelhohen Dosen angewandt, ruft Chlorpikrin beim Versuchstier Lungenödem hervor, das in ähnlicher Form abläuft wie das Phosgenödem. Jedoch zeigt es eine Reizwirkung auf die Atemwege (Husten). Die Chlorpikrinvergiftung kann in einer Atemkammer der oben (S. 221) beschriebenen Art erfolgen. Das Gift wird dann in Form einer ätherischen Lösung in der Kammer zerstäubt (Gildemeister u. Heubner, 1921). Bei Katzen, die nach dieser Technik für 30 min einer Chlorpikrin-Konzentration zwischen 200 und 500 mg/m³ ausgesetzt wurden ($c \cdot t = 6000—15000$), entwickelte sich regelmäßig Lungenödem; die individuelle Ansprechbarkeit ist jedoch ähnlich wie bei der Phosgenvergiftung recht unterschiedlich. Die Empfindlichkeit von Mäusen gleicht derjenigen von Katzen, während Hunde bei gleicher Einwirkungszeit etwas höhere Konzentrationen vertragen. Die Ausbildung des Lungenödems scheint etwas schneller vor sich zu gehen als bei der Phosgenvergiftung. Von dieser unterscheidet sich die Chlorpikrinvergiftung ferner durch eine Neigung zu Lungenblutungen, durch das Fehlen von Fibrin im Exsudat und durch resorptive Giftwirkungen, die sich an anderen Organen manifestieren.

Halmágyi *et al.* (1956) modifizierten das Verfahren der Chlorpikrinverteilung im Versuchsraum. Sie bedienten sich einer Gaskammer von 30 Liter Inhalt, die in der üblichen Weise mit einem elektrischen Windflügel, einer Absaugvorrichtung und einer Fallschleuse ausgestattet war; in der Kammer befand sich weiterhin eine

---

[3] Der Siedepunkt von 127,5° verlangt eine besondere Vorrichtung zur Herstellung der Gasmischungen, die leichter im statischen Prinzip zu erreichen ist.

von einem Drahtkäfig umschlossene elektrische Heizplatte, auf der ein Becherglas Platz fand, das mittels einer Pipette mit 0,1—0,3 ml einer gesättigten wäßrigen Lösung von Chlorpikrin beschickt wurde. Bei vorübergehendem Aufheizen der Platte verdampfte die Chlorpikrinlösung; der Ventilator sorgte für eine gleichmäßige Verteilung der Dämpfe in der Kammer. Nach einer Vorperiode von 4 min wurden die in der Fallschleuse befindlichen Tiere in die Kammer befördert und bei Raumtemperatur für 5 min der Gaseinwirkung ausgesetzt. Bei männlichen oder weiblichen Ratten (150—350 g) wurde unter diesen Bedingungen eine durchschnittliche Überlebenszeit von etwa 20 min beobachtet, das relative Lungengewicht der Tiere hatte sich auf das 2—2,5fache der Norm erhöht.

c) Chlor

Chlor, (Cl_2, Siedepunkt —34° C, Dichte 2,5) kann in geeigneter Konzentration Lungenödem auslösen. Es verursacht daneben Reizerscheinungen an den Schleimhäuten, Bronchospasmen, Lungenhämorrhagien und Pleuraexsudate. Da das Gas verhältnismäßig gut wasserlöslich ist, wird es in niedrigen Konzentrationen durch die Schleimhäute der Atemwege so weitgehend aus der Atemluft eliminiert, daß keine wirksamen Mengen in die Alveolen gelangen. Diese Eigenschaft des Chlors bedingt beim statischen Versuch außerdem eine allmähliche Abnahme seiner anfänglichen Konzentration im Versuchsraum (vgl. S. 221) und erklärt, daß diese Arbeitsweise (z.B. Nickerson u. Curry, 1955; Testelli *et al.*, 1960b) scheinbar höhere Konzentrationen erfordert als das dynamische Verfahren. Nickerson u. Curry setzten Ratten im Gewicht von 200—400 g paarweise in einer Gaskammer von 8 Liter Inhalt für 15 min Cl_2-Konzentrationen von 500—2000 ppm aus. Die abgemessenen Gasvolumina wurden mit einer Spritze in die Gaskammer eingeblasen und mittels eines Ventilators verteilt. Konzentrationen von mehr als 1000 ppm waren unter diesen Bedingungen fast immer tödlich, bei 500 ppm betrug die Mortalität 17%. Unter der Einwirkung der höheren Konzentrationen stieg das relative Lungengewicht der Tiere auf mehr als 20 g/kg. Testelli *et al.* (1960b) beließen Ratten bis zu 1 Std in einer Gaskammer mit einer Cl_2-Anfangskonzentration von 0,005%. Die mittlere Überlebenszeit betrug unter diesen Bedingungen 40—60 min; der Lungengewichtsindex der Tiere war auf etwa das Doppelte der Norm erhöht (von 0,5 auf über 1,0%). Bei Anwendung der Durchströmungstechnik erzielten Henschler *et al.* (1960a) bei Ratten durch Cl_2-Konzentrationen zwischen 570 und 880 ppm (Einwirkung 15 min) schweres Lungenödem und eine hohe Mortalitätsrate. Die mittlere Überlebenszeit betrug etwa 4 Std, das durchschnittliche relative Lungengewicht erreichte Werte von etwa 25 g/kg. Das aus handelsüblichen Stahlflaschen entnommene Chlor wurde mit Hilfe der auf S. 223 geschilderten Apparatur dosiert (Gaskammer von 200 Liter Inhalt, Gaswechsel 12—15mal pro Stunde).

Chloranalyse. Entnahme der Gasproben aus dem Versuchsraum mit hochevakuierten, geeichten Rundkolben von 0,5 oder 1 Liter Inhalt. Mittels geeichter Spritze wird n/10 Kaliumjodidlösung zugesetzt; nach wiederholtem Umschütteln wird das freigesetzte Jod mit n/100 Natriumthiosulfatlösung titriert.

d) Nitrose Gase

Nitrose Gase setzen sich gewöhnlich aus mehreren Komponenten zusammen. Neben Stickstoffmonoxyd (NO), Stickstoffdioxyd (NO_2), Stickstofftetroxyd (N_2O_4) können sie Salpetersäure und salpetrige Säure in Gas- oder Nebelform enthalten (Flury, 1930). In Abhängigkeit vom prozentualen Anteil der einzelnen Komponenten wird das unter der Einwirkung nitroser Gase entstehende Vergiftungsbild variieren. Lungenödem wird durch die oxydierten Formen, hauptsächlich das Stickstoffdioxyd hervorgerufen; Stickstoffmonoxyd verursacht dagegen innerhalb kurzer Zeit den Tod an Erstickung mit Methämoglobinbildung ohne ödematöse Veränderungen der Lunge herbeizuführen. Da Stickstoffmonoxyd gewöhnlich als Ausgangsprodukt für die Herstellung der anderen nitrosen Gase dient und seine Oxydation verhältnismäßig langsam verläuft, muß die Versuchsanordnung so gestaltet werden, daß sein Anteil am endgültigen Gasgemisch nicht ins Gewicht fällt. Stickstoffmonoxyd wird im Laboratorium in der Regel aus Natriumnitrit, das mit der doppelten Menge Wasser überschichtet wird, durch Eintropfen von konzentrierter Schwefelsäure gewonnen (Noyes, 1925), durch Passage von 2 Waschflaschen mit konzentrierter Schwefelsäure gereinigt und im Gasometer über gesättigter Kochsalzlösung aufbewahrt (s. z.B. Henschler *et al.*,

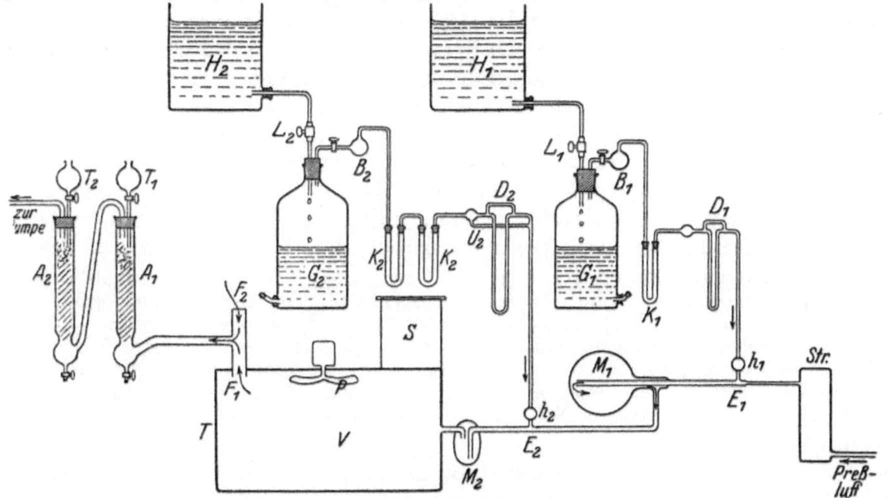

Abb. 15. Schematische Darstellung der Strömungsapparatur nach Wirth (1930). Erklärungen im Text

1960b; Wirth, 1930). Über frischer Kochsalzlösung ist Stickstoffmonoxyd nur wenige Tage haltbar; seine Zersetzung wird hinausgezögert, wenn stets dieselbe Kochsalzlösung im Gasometer verbleibt (Wirth, 1930).

Die Gasdosierung kann z.B. mit Hilfe der auf S. 223f. beschriebenen Apparatur nach Klimmer (1956) erfolgen. Wirth (1930) verwandte die in Abb. 15 schematisch wiedergegebene Versuchsanordnung, die auf einem ähnlichen Prinzip basiert. Ein öl-, staub- und wasserfreier Preßluftstrom wird nach Passage eines Strömungsmessers (*Str*) bei E_1 mit einem konstanten Strom des Reizgases vereint. Das im Gasometer G_1 aufbewahrte Stickstoffmonoxyd wurde durch aus dem Reservoir H_1 zutropfende Kochsalzlösung (regulierbar mittels Schraubhahn L_1) über das Differentialmanometer D_1 (zur Messung der Strömungsgeschwindigkeit) in den Preßluftstrom gedrückt und mit diesem der Mischkugel M_1 und von dort dem Versuchsraum V zugeleitet. Auf diesem Weg — vor allem in der Mischkugel — erfolgt die Oxydation des Stickstoffmonoxyds zu Stickstoffdioxyd. (Bei E_2 kann bedarfsweise ein weiteres Gas beigefügt werden.) Der in der üblichen Weise ausgestattete Versuchsraum hatte ein Fassungsvermögen von 100 Liter. Zur Vernichtung der nitrosen Gase wurde das Gemisch aus dem Versuchsraum mittels einer Pumpe durch den Stutzen F_1 über die mit Bimsstein gefüllten Absorptionstürme A_1 und A_2 gesaugt; jeweils vor Versuchsbeginn wurde der Bimsstein mit Natronlauge bzw. konzentrierter Schwefelsäure berieselt. Die Pumpleistung übertraf den Gaszustrom zum Versuchsraum geringfügig, der Mehrbedarf wurde durch Raumluft über F_2 gedeckt.

Um eine quantitative Umwandlung von Stickstoffmonoxyd in Stickstoffdioxyd zu erreichen, leiteten Henschler *et al.* (1960b) entsprechend dem Vorgehen von Beyer (1943) rotametrisch dosierte Ströme von NO (0,5 l/h) und O_2 (20 l/h) nach Trocknung an Schwefelsäure gemeinsam durch ein 1 m langes, 5 cm weites mit Raschig-Ringen gefülltes Reaktionsrohr. Das Stickstoffdioxyd wurde mit Hilfe der auf S. 223 beschriebenen Apparatur, die sich zur Herstellung dosierter Gasgemische jeder gewünschten Konzentration eignet, weiter verdünnt und anschließend dem Versuchsraum zugeführt.

Gasanalyse. Wirth (1930) oxydierte die mit evakuierten Gaspipetten aus dem Versuchsraum entnommenen nitrosen Gase durch Wasserstoffsuperoxyd zu Salpetersäure, setzte Kaliumjodid und n/10 Ammoniummolybdat zu und titrierte das abgeschiedene Jod mit n/100 Natriumthiosulfat. Das durch entsprechende Mengen Wasserstoffsuperoxyd und Ammoniummolybdat in Abwesenheit nitroser Gase freigesetzte Jod wurde in der gleichen Weise bestimmt und als Leerwert vom Analysenwert subtrahiert. — Von einigen Autoren (z.B. Henschler *et al.*, 1960a) wurde das colorimetrische Verfahren nach Rimarski u. Konschak (1940) bzw. nach Beyer (1943) angewandt. — Zur Ermittlung der NO_2-Konzentration stark verdünnter Gasgemische eignet sich das empfindlichere Verfahren nach Saltzman (1954), das Henschler *et al.* (1960b) in nachstehender Modifikation anwandten.

Die Gasproben wurden mit hochevakuierten Gaspipetten (0,5—2,0 Liter Inhalt) aus dem Versuchsraum entnommen und mittels geeichter Spritze mit 20 ml Absorptionslösung (0,5% Sulfanilsäure und 0,002% N-(1-Naphthyl)-äthylendiamin in 14%iger Essigsäure) versetzt. Nach 15 min (wiederholt umschütteln) wurde spektrophotometrisch bei einer Wellenlänge von 550 mμ und einer Schichtdicke von 1 cm die Extinktion gemessen. Die Berechnung der Analysenwerte wurde an Hand einer Eichkurve für Standard-$NaNO_2$-Lösung vorgenommen, wobei ein Molverhältnis Nitrit zu NO_2-Gas von 0,72 zugrunde gelegt wurde.

Henschler *et al.* (1958, 1960a, b) setzten Albinoratten im Gewicht von 120—160 g 30 min lang Stickstoffdioxydkonzentrationen zwischen 119 ppm (220 mg/m³) und 344 ppm (560 mg/m³) aus. (Gaswechsel 12—15mal pro Stunde.) Die Konzentration von 119 ppm wurde von allen Tieren überlebt; im Bereich von 135—203 ppm betrug die Mortalität 40%, im Bereich von 240—344 ppm bis zu 100% bei einer mittleren Überlebenszeit von 2,1 Std. Das relative Lungengewicht war auf mehr als das dreifache der Norm erhöht.

Wirth (1930) verwandte Katzen als Versuchstiere. Er ließ den Versuchsraum vor dem Einschleusen der Tiere 1 Std lang mit dem gewünschten Gasgemisch (Stickstoffdioxydkonzentration 400—4000 mg/m³) durchströmen. NO_2-Konzentrationen bis zu 500 mg/m³ waren bei einer Expositionszeit von 90 min nicht tödlich; Konzentrationen von 600—900 mg/m³ führten nach einer Latenzzeit von mehreren Stunden, Konzentrationen von mehr als 1300 mg/m³ schon während der Expositionszeit zum Tod der Tiere infolge Lungenödem. Letzteres dokumentierte sich in einem Anstieg des relativen Lungengewichtes auf das 2—3,5fache der Norm.

Das Phänomen der Entstehung von Toleranz gegen ödemauslösende Noxen, auf das oben (S. 194) bereits hingewiesen wurde, ist am Beispiel von Stickstoffdioxyd eingehender studiert worden. Henschler *et al.* (1964a) haben weibliche Mäuse (Durchschnittsgewicht: 20 g) einmalig 6 Std lang mit Stickstoffdioxyd in Konzentrationen zwischen etwa 2,4 und 62,0 ppm vorbehandelt. Wurden die so vorbehandelten Tiere nach einem Intervall von 4 Tagen 30 min lang der Einwirkung einer hohen (100%ig letalen) Stickstoffdioxydkonzentration (ca. 650 ppm) ausgesetzt, so war ihre Überlebenszeit im Vergleich zu Kontrolltieren erheblich (auf das 1,6—4,7fache) verlängert, und zwar in deutlicher Abhängigkeit von der im Vorversuch angewendeten Stickstoffdioxydkonzentration. Wenn vorbehandelte Tiere unter im übrigen gleichen Bedingungen einer ödemprovozierenden, jedoch nicht letalen Stickstoffdioxydkonzentration (ca. 180 ppm) ausgesetzt wurden, so war bei ihnen eine deutliche Reduktion der Ödementwicklung (beurteilt aufgrund des Wassergehaltes der Lunge) nachweisbar; auch bei dieser Versuchsanordnung bestand eine deutliche Korrelation zwischen Vorbehandlungskonzentration und Ödemminderung: nach Vorbehandlung mit 2,4 ppm NO_2 war die Ödementwicklung um etwa 10%, nach Vorbehandlung mit ca. 60 ppm um 80% gehemmt.

Die Schutzwirkung ist nicht nur nach einer relativ langen Vorexponierung nachweisbar, sondern kann auch bei kurzdauernder (10 min) Einwirkung höherer Reizgaskonzentrationen (400 ppm NO_2) erzielt werden. Demnach ist nicht die Vorbehandlungsdauer, sondern die Vorbehandlungsdosis der maßgebliche Faktor. Die gleichen Autoren haben weiterhin festgestellt, daß die Toleranz 6 Std nach der Vorbehandlung noch nicht eindeutig nachweisbar ist, sondern sich erst im Verlauf von etwa 24 Std entwickelt, zwischen dem 2. und 5. Tag ein Maximum erreicht, um sich anschließend innerhalb von ungefähr 4 Wochen wieder zurückzubilden.

Die Toleranzsteigerung dürfte im wesentlichen auf einer Verlängerung der Diffusionsstrecke (des Luft-Blut-Weges) beruhen, die ihrerseits aufgrund einer ödematös entzündlichen Reaktion, die nach dem ersten Kontakt mit dem Reizgas im Alveolarseptum abläuft, entsteht (Henschler *et al.*, 1964b). Es kommt auf diese Weise zur Ausbildung eines Schutzwalles, der bei nachfolgender Exponierung die Diffusion des Reizgases aus den Alveolen zu den Capillaren hemmt. In Übereinstimmung mit dieser durch morphologische und funktionelle Befunde gestützten Annahme steht die Tatsache, daß die Toleranz nicht auf das induzierende Reizgas beschränkt ist, sondern sich auch auf andere Ödemnoxen, die vom Alveolarraum aus wirksam werden, erstreckt. Umgekehrt hat diese Form der Toleranz keinen Einfluß auf die durch hämatogen verbreitete Noxen oder hämodynamisch ausgelösten Ödemformen.

e) Ozon

Sauerstoff ist in seiner dreiatomigen Form, dem Ozon, ein stechend riechendes, schlecht wasserlösliches Gas mit stark irritierenden Eigenschaften. Sein Einfluß auf den menschlichen bzw. tierischen Organismus hat in den letzten Jahren vor allem aus arbeits- und flugmedizinischen Gründen Interesse gefunden, ist aber auch im Rahmen der allgemeinen Lufthygiene von Bedeutung, weil in der Atmosphäre von Großstädten gelegentlich kritische Ozonkonzentrationen nachgewiesen wurden (s. z.B. Mittler *et al.*, 1956; Stokinger, 1954; Stokinger *et al.*, 1957; Svirbely u. Saltzman, 1957). Lange Zeit war es allerdings umstritten, ob die toxischen Effekte ozonhaltiger Gasgemische dem Ozon selbst oder einer Verunreinigung mit anderne Komponenten, insbesondere mit nitrosen Gasen, zuzuschreiben sei. Eine Übersicht über diesbezügliche ältere Literatur hat Stokinger (1954) gegeben. In den folgenden Jahren konnte jedoch gezeigt werden, daß auch hochgereinigtes Ozon in einem verhältnismäßig niedrigen Konzentrationsbereich den Tod von Versuchstieren herbeiführen kann, und zwar vor allem infolge von Lungenödem und -hämorrhagien (Svirbely u. Saltzman, 1957). Neben diesen Veränderungen wurden Reiz- und Entzündungserscheinungen an den Luftwegen beobachtet, Schädigungen, die auch bei chronischer Einwirkung subletaler Dosen (etwa 1 ppm) auftreten (Stokinger *et al.*, 1957). Symptomatik und Verlauf der Vergiftung ähneln dem durch andere Reizgase verursachten Krankheitsbild. Der Mechanismus der Ödementstehung konnte bisher nicht geklärt werden. Skillen *et al.* (1961a, b) diskutierten eine Mitwirkung von endogenem 5-Hydroxytryptamin (vgl. S. 242).

Die Herstellung von Ozon im Laboratorium erfolgt gewöhnlich mit Hilfe käuflicher Ozonisatoren (z.B. Modell O_Z3, Fa. Siemens) aus gereinigter, getrockneter Luft oder getrocknetem Sauerstoff; letzterer ist vorzuziehen, weil die Gefahr der Entstehung verunreinigender Komponenten geringer ist. Doch spielt bei den heute üblichen Methoden die Kontamination des Ozons mit anderen Gasen auch bei Verwendung von Luft als Ausgangsmaterial offensichtlich keine Rolle mehr (Stokinger, 1957). Vor Eintritt in den Ozonisator muß Preßluft gesäubert werden, indem sie durch eine Lösung von Kaliumbichromat oder Kaliumpermanganat in konzentrierter Schwefelsäure und anschließend durch eine Lage Glaswolle und eine Silikagelsäule (Matzen, 1957a, b; Svirbely u. Saltzman, 1957) oder durch ein Spezialfiltersystem (Mittler *et al.*, 1956, 1957) geschickt wird. Flaschensauerstoff wird gewöhnlich an konzentrierter Schwefelsäure getrocknet (Henschler *et al.*, 1960a). Aus dem Ozonisator entnommene, gemessene Gasvolumina werden mit gefilterter Luft gemischt, auf die gewünschte Konzentration eingestellt (z.B. mit Hilfe der auf S. 223 beschriebenen Versuchsanordnungen nach Henschler *et al.*, 1960b) und dem Expositionsraum zugeführt oder mit einem Exhaustor durch ihn hindurchgesaugt (Mittler *et al.*, 1957). Skillen *et al.* (1961) leiteten das Ozonluftgemisch von der Kammerdecke (Kammergröße 76·76·79 cm) her ein und pumpten es von den 4 Bodenecken aus ab (Gaswechsel 15—60mal/Std).

Die Toxicität des Ozons befolgt im Konzentrationsbereich zwischen 2,5 und 50 ppm die *ct*-Formel verhältnismäßig genau; das Ergebnis wird jedoch von verschiedenen Faktoren, wie vom Alter und vom Gesundheitszustand (Erkrankungen der Respirationsorgane; vorangegangene Exposition: Toleranz) der Versuchstiere mit bestimmt. Die in der Literatur angegebenen mittleren Letalkonzentrationen (LC_{50}) für Tiere der gleichen Species differieren beträchtlich. So ermittelte Stokinger (1954) bei 4stündiger Exposition für Mäuse im Gewicht von 22 g einen Wert von 3,8 ppm, für Ratten (250 g) einen solchen von 4,8 ppm und für Hamster (75 g) von 10,5 ppm; ähnliche Resultate erzielten Svirbely und Saltzman (1957). Matzen (1957a) errechnete dagegen bei gleicher Einwirkungszeit für Mäuse eine LC_{50} von 8,0—8,5 ppm. Mittler *et al.* (1956) benötigten noch höhere Konzentrationen, und zwar bei 3stündiger Exposition für Mäuse 21,0 ppm und für Ratten 21,8 ppm; der entsprechende Wert für Meerschweinchen betrug 51,7 ppm, für Kaninchen 36,0 ppm und für Katzen 34,5 ppm. Bei kürzerer Versuchsdauer (30 min) mußten Henschler *et al.* (1960a) bei Mäusen ebenfalls relativ hohe Konzentrationen anwenden: 100—200 ppm Ozon verursachten bei einer mittleren Überlebenszeit von 7—8 Std eine Mortalität zwischen 65 und 90%. Die Diskrepanzen zwischen den Ergebnissen der einzelnen Untersucher wurden von Mittler *et al.* (1957) auf unterschiedliche Analysenmethoden (s. u.) zurückgeführt. Bei kontinuierlicher Einwirkung niedriger Konzentrationen während mehrerer Tage verliert die *ct*-Formel ihre Gültigkeit. Ozonkonzentrationen von 2,4 ppm wurden von über 90% der exponierten Mäuse 98 Std lang ertragen (Mittler *et al.*, 1957).

Nach 4stündiger Einwirkung von 5—10 ppm Ozon war der Wassergehalt der Mäuselungen von 78,4% (mittlerer Normalwert) auf 85—88% gestiegen (Matzen, 1957a). Bei Ratten (Körpergewicht 325—375 g) erhöhte sich das relative Lungengewicht unter annähernd gleichen Bedingungen auf das 3fache der Norm (Skillen *et al.*, 1961). Eine ähnliche Zunahme des relativen Lungengewichtes sahen Henschler und Jacob (1958) und Henschler und Laux (1960) bei Ratten im Gewicht von 120—160 g, die einer Ozonkonzentration von 100 ppm für nur 30 min ausgesetzt worden waren (maximale Überlebenszeit 3,5 Std); 25 ppm bewirkten bei gleicher Versuchsdauer einen Anstieg auf das Doppelte.

Ozonanalyse. Kritische Bemerkungen zu verschiedenen Methoden der Ozonanalyse finden sich in den Arbeiten von Mittler *et al.* (1957), Stokinger (1954), Svirbely u. Saltzman (1957).

Gegenwärtig wird häufig das Verfahren nach Byers u. Saltzman (1958) angewandt. Den mit evakuierten Gaspipetten aus der Kammer entnommenen Proben wird 1%ige neutral gepufferte (Phosphatpuffer nach Sörensen) Kaliumjodidlösung zugesetzt. Nach wiederholtem Schütteln wird mit n/100 Natriumthiosulfatlösung titriert (z.B. Henschler *et al.*, 1960a) oder das freigesetzte Jod photometrisch bei einer Wellenlänge von 352 mμ gemessen (z.B. Skillen *et al.*, 1961).

f) Verschiedene Gase und Dämpfe

Durch Inhalation von Dichloräthylsulfid in niedrigen Konzentrationen kann bei Versuchstieren Lungenödem hervorgerufen werden (Flury und Wieland, 1921). Bei Katzen bewirkten Konzentrationen von 10—100 mg/m³ bei Expositionszeiten zwischen 100 und 5 min schwere Krankheitserscheinungen, die sich im Verlauf von 18—24 Std entwickelten. Im Vordergrund des Vergiftungsbildes steht jedoch nicht immer ein Lungenödem, sondern häufig andere Krankheitszustände der Lunge (Emphysem, diphtherische Veränderungen der Bronchien, Bronchopneumonie) oder weiterer Organe. Dichloräthylsulfid scheint sich daher zur Erzeugung von experimentellem Lungenödem weniger zu eignen als andere Reizgase.

Die toxikologischen Eigenschaften einer größeren Zahl organischer Arsenverbindungen hat Flury (1921b) beschrieben. Ihr Wirkungscharakter entspricht teils dem des Phosgens, teils dem des Dichloräthylsulfids. Sie verursachen neben akutem Lungenödem Capillarschädigungen sowie Irritation der Haut, Schleimhäute und sensiblen Nerven; daneben werden resorptive Giftwirkungen beobachtet. Lungenödem provozierende Eigenschaften scheinen vor allem bei folgenden Arsenverbindungen im Vordergrund zu stehen: Arsentrichlorid in Konzentrationen von 50—100 mm³/m³, Exposition 20—60 min; Kakodylchlorid ($(CH_3)_2AsCl$) 100—1000 mm³/m³, Exposition 20—60 min; Kakodylcyanid ($(CH_3)_2AsCN$) 100—1000 mm³/m³, Exposition 3—20 min; Kakodylrhodanid ($(CH_3)_2AsSCN$) 100 mm³/m³, Exposition 5—15 min; Diphenylarsinchlorid ($(C_6H_5)_2AsCl$) 50 bis 100 mm³/m³, Exposition 30 min. Die aufgeführten Werte wurden in allen Fällen an Katzen ermittelt.

Keten (CH_2CO) besitzt, wie Cameron und Neuberger (1937) gezeigt haben, ödemprovozierende Eigenschaften. Inhalation des Gases in einer Konzentration von 100 ppm führte bei Expositionszeiten von 5—20 min innerhalb von 2—4 Std den Tod der Versuchstiere (Mäuse und Ratten) herbei. Es wurden ähnliche Lungenveränderungen beobachtet wie nach Phosgenapplikation.

Cadmiumoxydrauch kann, wie aus der Gewerbetoxikologie bekannt ist, Lungenödem auslösen (s. z.B. Kleinfeld *et al.*, 1958). Ein Verfahren zur experimentellen Ödemerzeugung durch Cadmiumoxyd haben Henschler *et al.* (1964b) angegeben. Der durch Verbrennung von feinen Cadmiumfeilspänen im Kohlenlichtbogen hergestellte Cadmiumoxydrauch wird mit strömender Luft gemischt und dem Expositionsraum zugeleitet. Für Mäuse waren 16 mg Cd/m³ in Form von Cadmiumoxydrauch bei einer Einwirkung von 30 min in 100% der Fälle letal, wobei der Tod nach durchschnittlich 72 Std eintrat. Das durch Cadmiumoxydrauch verursachte Lungenödem ähnelt dem Phosgenödem. Die Cadmiumoxydkonzentration kann mit Hilfe der Dithizonmethode nach Church (1947) bestimmt werden.

In Form von Aerosolen zugeführt, konnte mit $CoCl_2$ bei Ratten und Meerschweinchen Lungenödem erzeugt werden (Eichler *et al.*, 1967a, b). Zur Vernebelung diente eine Vorrichtung von Palmer u. Kingsbury (1952), die Aerosole mit einem Partikeldurchmesser von 1—2 μ lieferte. Im Liter zugeführte Luft befand sich 0,2 mg Co, das verschieden lange angeboten wurde. Nach Einwirkung von $^1/_2$ Std waren kaum histologische Veränderungen zu sehen, obwohl sich eine Änderung der Atmung bereits ankündigte. Nach $1^1/_2$ Std Exposition entwickelte sich das Ödem erst in Stunden. Wenn die Tiere nach 3 Std der Einatmung getötet wurden, war auch noch kein Ödem bemerkbar, das sich erst später voll entwickelt. Die in den ersten 3 Tagen sterbenden Tiere zeigten bei der Sektion und histologisch das klassische Bild des Lungenödems. Später kommen mehr und mehr bronchopneumonische Bilder zum Vorschein. Das Sekret wurde fibrinhaltig und schließlich sah man ein introvertiertes Ödem mit Fibroblasten und Schaumzellen. Wurde das Kobalt komplex mit Äthylendiamintetraessigsäure (ÄDTE), dann nahm die Toxicität ab. Bei einem Co auf 1 ÄDTE waren kaum Lungenveränderungen merkbar. Auch die Verteilung änderte sich (Eichler *et al.*, 1967).

g) Kohlendioxyd

Überhöhte Kohlendioxydkonzentrationen der Atemluft können bei Versuchstieren (bisher beobachtet bei Mäusen, Ratten, Meerschweinchen, Kaninchen, Katzen und Hunden) Lungenödem hervorrufen. Dieser schon länger bekannte Effekt des Kohlendioxyds ist in neuerer Zeit von Poulsen (1952a, 1954b) (hier auch Hinweise auf ältere Lit.) eingehend studiert und methodisch verwertet worden.

Zur Herstellung des aus O_2 und CO_2 zusammengesetzten Gasgemisches benutzte Poulsen (1954b) eine von Poulsen u. Secher (1949) aus einer älteren Apparatur (Kochmann, 1912) entwickelte Versuchsanordnung. Die in Abb. 16 schematisch wiedergegebene Einrichtung eignet

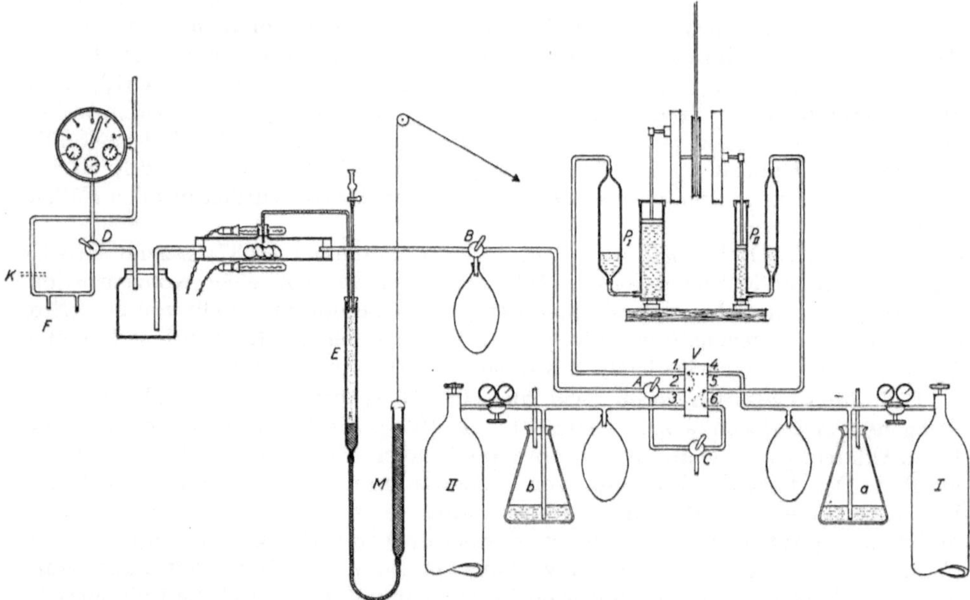

Abb. 16. Schematische Darstellung der Versuchsanordnung nach Poulsen und Secher (1949) zur Gasdosierung und Durchströmung. Erläuterungen im Text

sich zur getrennten Dosierung und Mischung von 2 Gasen und einem flüssigen Bestandteil (in flüchtiger Form); ihre Förderleistung ist so abgestimmt, daß größere Versuchstiere über eine Trachealkanüle direkt an das Rohrleitungssystem (Durchmesser der Rohre etwa 20 mm) angeschlossen, kleinere Tiere in Atemkammern exponiert werden können. Die Gase gelangen aus den Stahlflaschen I und II über Reduzierventile und die Waschflaschen a und b, mit deren Hilfe der Gasdruck auf 1 cm H_2O eingestellt wird, in 2 Gummisäcke. Die miteinander synchronisierten Pumpsysteme P I und P II (Metallpumpen mit angeschlossenen Glaszylindern; Füllflüssigkeit: Wasser) saugen das Gas aus den beiden Gummisäcken über das Ventil an und drücken es in die am Dreiwegehahn A beginnende Hauptleitung, und zwar System P I über

Einlaßventil 4—1 und Auslaßventil 1—2, System P II über Einlaßventil 3—5 und Auslaßventil 5—6. Durch den Dreiwegehahn C kann das Gas aus der Flasche II bedarfsweise ins Freie geführt werden; wenn gleichzeitig die Rohrverbindung bei 4 unterbrochen wird, fördert das System Raumluft. Die Pumpen werden durch einen Elektromotor betrieben, der gleichzeitig das mit den Pumpenhuben synchronisierte Gleitventil V betätigt. Die Hubhöhe (und damit das Hubvolumen) kann durch Verschiebung des Drehpunktes der Kolbenstange am Schwungrad verändert werden. Die Hubfrequenz der Pumpe wird mit Hilfe eines Rheostaten reguliert und durch ein Zählwerk kontrolliert. Je nach dem gewünschten Mischungsverhältnis der Gase können beide Pumpsysteme außerdem unterschiedlich groß gewählt werden. Durch die Rohrverbindung zwischen A und B gelangt das Gasgemisch in einen weiteren Gummisack bei B, der die Pumpenhube bzw. die Druckschwankungen ausgleicht, und weiter in eine Mischkammer. (Hier kann den Gasen bei Bedarf eine flüchtige Flüssigkeit beigefügt werden. Zu diesem Zweck wird das Quecksilberreservoir M mit Hilfe des Pumpmotors kontinuierlich angehoben, so daß die Flüssigkeit aus dem Glasbehälter E verdrängt wird und in die Mischkammer tropft. Zwei Heizlampen fördern das Verdampfen der zutropfenden Flüssigkeit.) Eine 5 Liter-Flasche dient als weiteres Misch- und Druckausgleichgefäß. Über den Dreiwegehahn D kann das Gasgemisch der Atemkammer bzw. dem Tier (Ausgang F) oder einer Gasuhr (zur Bestimmung des Minutenvolumens der Apparatur) zugeleitet werden.

Poulsen (1954b) benutzte für die Exposition von Mäusen, die er vor dem Versuch mindestens 48 Std unter konstanten Bedingungen bei einer Temperatur von 25° C gehalten hatte, Glasgefäße mit einem Fassungsvermögen von 375 ml; das CO_2-angereicherte Gasgemisch strömte vom Boden des Behälters her ein und durch eine Öffnung im Oberteil aus. Unmittelbar nach Beendigung der CO_2-Einwirkung wurden die Tiere durch i.p. Injektion einer 25%igen KCN-Lösung getötet. Auswertung aufgrund des Verhältnisses von relativem Gewicht zu Wassergehalt der Lunge (s. S. 182ff.). Der CO_2-Gehalt des Gasgemisches wurde zwischen 10 und 40% variiert. Das resultierende Vergiftungsbild war innerhalb eines bestimmten Bereiches konzentrationsabhängig: Durch Inhalation von 10—15% CO_2 wurde kein oder nur geringgradiges, durch 20% CO_2 Lungenödem aller Schweregrade ausgelöst. Bei einem Anteil von 25% CO_2 war die maximale Wirkung erreicht. Höhere Konzentrationen (30—40%) verursachten zwar eine weitere Zunahme des relativen Lungengewichtes, aber keinen zusätzlichen Anstieg des Wassergehaltes der Lunge; in diesem Konzentrationsbereich bewirkt CO_2 außerdem tiefe Narkose mit Aufhebung der Reflexe (s. auch Poulsen, 1952a). Das Ödem entwickelte sich innerhalb von 5—15 min bis zu seiner endgültigen Stärke. Ausdehnung der Expositionszeit auf 60 min änderte das Ergebnis nicht. Die niedrigste der geprüften Konzentrationen (10%) rief auch bei einer Verlängerung der Versuchsdauer auf 4 Std kein Ödem hervor. In der Anfangsphase ist der Lungengewichtsanstieg mehr durch Hyperämie der Lungen, späterhin vor allem durch zunehmende extravasale Flüssigkeitsakkumulation bedingt.

Der Pathomechanismus der Ödementstehung ist ungeklärt. Die Verschiebung des pH-Wertes des Blutes, die mit der CO_2-Zufuhr einhergeht (Poulsen, 1952a), dürfte keine kausale Bedeutung besitzen, denn nach i.v. Injektion von Salzsäure wurde kein Lungenödem beobachtet (Poulsen, 1952b; s. auch Koenig und Koenig, 1949). Veränderungen der Capillarpermeabilität und des kolloidosmotischen Plasmadruckes spielen wohl ebenfalls keine Rolle. Poulsen (1954b) vermutet als Ödemursache eine Erhöhung des Pulmonalcapillardruckes und eine Verminderung des intrapleuralen Druckes. Die Beteiligung hämodynamischer Faktoren wird durch Befunde von Aviado (1961) wahrscheinlich gemacht, der bei Beatmung von Versuchstieren mit CO_2-reicher (10%) Luft Drucksteigerungen im kleinen und großen Kreislauf registrierte. Die als weitere Ödemursache postulierte Verminderung des intrapleuralen Druckes erklärt Poulsen mit einer vor allem inspiratorisch auftretenden Bronchoconstriction bei gleichzeitig forcierten Atemanstrengungen. Bronchoconstriction und Atmungsstimulation wurden als direkte CO_2-Effekte auf die Bronchialmuskulatur bzw. das Respirationszentrum angesehen. Die Literaturangaben zur Frage des CO_2-Einflusses auf die Bronchialweite sind allerdings widersprüchlich; es wird sowohl über eine bronchoconstrictorische (Lit. bei Poulsen, 1954b) als auch eine bronchodilatatorische Aktivität des Kohlendioxyds (s. z.B. Wick, 1952a) berichtet. Nach Allgood *et al.* (1968) wirkt CO_2 lokal erschlaffend auf die Bronchialmuskeln. Wieweit die durch CO_2 bewirkte Verminderung der Oberflächenspannung der Alveolen und die Zunahme der Alveolarweite (Wick, 1952b, c) als ödemgenetische Faktoren in Frage kommen, ist nicht bekannt.

h) Sauerstoff

Die Atmung eines Gasgemisches, dessen Sauerstoffgehalt den der Luft wesentlich übersteigt, kann pathologische Veränderungen verschiedener Organe zur Folge haben. Dieses seit langem bekannte (s. z.B. Smith, 1899) und häufig diskutierte Phänomen (s. Ohlsson, 1947) ist in neuerer Zeit u.a. von Clamann und Becker-Freyseng (1940), Liebegott (1941), Pichotka (1941), Pichotka und Kühn (1947) eingehend studiert worden. Symptomatik und Pathomorphologie der O_2-Vergiftung sind vom Sauerstoffpartialdruck, vom Gesamtdruck im Versuchsraum und von der Einwirkungszeit abhängig. Lungenödem entwickelt sich nur unter bestimmten Versuchsbedingungen bevorzugt vor sonstigen Schäden der Respirations- oder anderer Körperorgane (Cameron, 1948; Pichotka und Kühn, 1947). Unter dem Einfluß höheren Druckes (3,5—6 atm) entstehen in erster Linie Störungen des Nervensystems, die sich in Form von Reiz- und Lähmungserscheinungen äußern, während pathologische Befunde an anderen Organen (einschließlich der Lunge) zurücktreten. Bean u. Johnson (1955) fanden z.B. bloß bei 21% der Ratten, die sie einem O_2-Druck von 5,6 atm aussetzten, ein Lungenödem. Längere Expositionszeiten, die bei Anwendung normalen oder nur wenig erhöhten Druckes notwendig sind, fördern dagegen das Auftreten komplizierender Sekundärerkrankungen (s. z.B. Gottsegen *et al.*, 1956, 1958). Für die Erzeugung von Lungenödem wird sich daher vor allem ein möglichst hoher O_2-Partialdruck bei mäßig erhöhtem Gesamtdruck (bis 3,5 atm) und kurzer Versuchsdauer eignen.

Die Versuchseinrichtung kann verhältnismäßig einfach gestaltet sein, wenn die Sauerstoffeinwirkung unter Normaldruck erfolgen soll. Pichotka u. Kühn (1947) benutzten für die Exposition von Meerschweinchen und Kaninchen Glaskammern von 60 bzw. 150 Liter Inhalt; Sauerstoff aus Stahlflaschen strömte kontinuierlich durch einen Stutzen am Kammerboden ein und durch eine Öffnung in der Kammerdecke ab. Die O_2-Konzentration in der Kammer lag zwischen 85 und 95%. Einer ähnlichen Versuchsanordnung bedienten sich Hemingway u. Williams (1952). Sie wandten zur Vergiftung von Meerschweinchen jedoch etwas höhere O_2-Konzentrationen (95—99%; Barometerdruck 730—750 mm Hg) an. Zur Beseitigung freiwerdenden Kohlendioxyds kann ein Absorptionsmittel in die Kammer eingebracht werden. Die tatsächliche Zusammensetzung des Gasgemisches muß durch O_2- und CO_2-Analysen ermittelt werden. Unter ihren Bedingungen konnten Hemingway u. Williams (1952) Lungenödem in der Regel erst nach mehr als 60stündiger Exposition nachweisen. Todesfälle traten erstmalig am 5. Versuchstag auf. Der Ödemgrad war von der Versuchsdauer abhängig. Am 6. Tag erreichte das relative Lungengewicht das 2,5fache der Normwerte. Da der Hämoglobingehalt der Lunge keine signifikanten Veränderungen aufwies und auch mikroskopisch Hyperämie oder Hämorrhagien nur vereinzelt gefunden wurden, führen die Autoren den Anstieg des Lungengewichtes auf das Ödem zurück. Kühn u. Pichotka versuchten die Beziehungen zwischen der Dauer der O_2-Einwirkung und den resultierenden morphologischen Veränderungen zu klären. Die Organe von Tieren, die während der Exposition (Versuchsbedingungen s.o.: Pichotka u. Kühn, 1947) spontan eingegangen oder in bestimmten Intervallen zwischen 60 und 120 Std getötet worden waren, wurden histologisch aufgearbeitet. Bei allen Tieren wurde mehr oder weniger stark ausgeprägtes alveoläres Ödem, das z. T. durch eine Beimischung fibrinöser und cellulärer Elemente charakterisiert war, festgestellt, daneben Schädigungen der Bronchialschleimhaut und hyaline Veränderungen der Wände der Alveolen, Alveolargänge und Bronchiolen. Bei den frühzeitig (innerhalb von 60 Std) gestorbenen oder geopferten Tieren wurde in erster Linie Lungenödem beobachtet; die übrigen Veränderungen traten vor allem in späteren Phasen hinzu.

Um komplizierende Sekundär- und Begleiterkrankungen der O_2-Vergiftung hintanzuhalten, arbeiten einige Autoren mit erhöhten O_2-Druckwerten. Bei diesem Vorgehen kann die Expositionszeit beträchtlich verkürzt werden. Gottsegen *et al.* (1956, 1958) setzten Ratten (im Gewicht von 175—275 g) 2,5—3 Std in einer Druckkammer von 60 Liter Inhalt einem O_2-Druck von 3,5 atm aus. Die Kammer wurde vor Beginn des Versuches zunächst mit Sauerstoff durchströmt; anschließend wurde der Kammerdruck mehrmals alternierend auf 3,5 atm erhöht und langsam auf etwas über 1 atm vermindert. Der N_2-Partialdruck konnte auf diese Weise unter 70 mm Hg abgesenkt, der O_2-Druck auf über 2600 mm Hg erhöht werden. Während des Versuches stand die Gasflasche ständig mit der Kammer in Verbindung, um aussickerndes Gas kontinuierlich zu ersetzen. Die Tiere — von einzelnen Ausnahmen abgesehen — starben entweder während des Aufenthaltes in der Kammer oder innerhalb der folgenden 60 min. Dekompressionsschäden wurden nicht beobachtet. Auch unter diesen Bedingungen waren im mikroskopischen Bild der Lunge neben Ödemherden Hyperämie, perivasculäre Infiltrationen, degenerative Veränderungen des Alveolarepithels und der Bronchiolen sowie Dilatation der Lymphgefäße nachweisbar.

Bean u. Johnson (1952, 1955) sowie Johnson u. Bean (1957) ließen auf Ratten (200—300 g) Sauerstoff unter einem Druck von 5,6 atm bei Temperaturen von 24—29° C einwirken, bis Krämpfe auftraten; unter stufenweiser Druckminderung (8 min Dauer) wurden die Tiere ausgeschleust. Das mittlere relative Lungengewicht war auf 1,39 ($\pm$0,41) gestiegen (Kontrollen 0,63).

Der Pathomechanismus des Sauerstoffödems ist nicht geklärt. Die Hauptursache dürfte in einer bronchopulmonalen Gewebsschädigung (s. z. B. Gottsegen *et al.*, 1956, 1959), speziell wohl in einer Capillarschädigung (Kühn und Pichotka, 1948) zu suchen sein; möglicherweise spielt die Entstehung von Atelektasen dabei eine Rolle (Penrod, 1956). Eine Constriction der Lungengefäße wurde von Cameron (1948) in Betracht gezogen; andere Autoren messen jedoch hämodynamischen Faktoren ebenso wie einer Lymphstauung keinen entscheidenden sondern höchstens akzessorischen Einfluß bei (Gottsegen *et al.*, 1956). Die kausale Bedeutung hormonaler (Hypophyse, Nebennieren, Schilddrüse; Bean und Bauer, 1952; Bean und Johnson, 1952, 1955; Bean und Smith, 1953), enzymatischer (Hemmung SH-haltiger Enzyme; Gerschman *et al.*, 1954) und neurogener Mechanismen (Bean, 1956; Gottsegen *et al.*, 1959) sowie der CO_2-Stauung im Gewebe (Seelkopf und Werz, 1948) wurde diskutiert. Auch bei der O_2-Vergiftung wird der Tod — wie das Auftreten hypoxämisch bedingter Zellschäden in Leber und Herzmuskel vermuten läßt — wahrscheinlich durch O_2-Mangel im Gewebe verursacht (Pichotka und Kühn, 1947).

2. Extrapulmonale Giftapplikation

a) Phenylalkylamine

aa) Adrenalin. Adrenalin in hohen (toxischen bzw. letalen) Dosen kann bei Laboratoriumstieren verschiedener Species Lungenödem hervorrufen. Diese Eigenschaft des Adrenalins wurde schon bald nach seiner Reindarstellung für experimentelle Zwecke ausgenutzt (s. z.B. Heinz, 1906; Trendelenburg, 1924) und z.Z. dürfte der Wirkstoff die am häufigsten angewandte Ödemnoxe sein. Auch beim Menschen kann die Verbindung Lungenödem verursachen. So wurde über tödlich verlaufende Lungenödemfälle nach Injektion toxischer oder therapeutischer Dosen von Adrenalin oder Adrenalin-verwandten Substanzen berichtet (Hess, 1956; Wichels u. Lauber, 1934) und bei Phäochromocytomkranken wurde Lungenödem infolge paroxysmaler Adrenalin- bzw. Nor-Adrenalinausschüttung beobachtet (z.B. Harrison u. Seward, 1954; Schwab u. Denninger, 1952a, b, 1956; Schwiegk, 1959).

Versuchstieren wird gewöhnlich das synthetische l-Adrenalin in Form des Hydrochlorids in einer Konzentration von 1:1000 in physiologischer Kochsalzlösung intravenös, gelegentlich auch intraperitoneal, intramuskulär (Drenckhahn, 1958) oder intrakardial (MacKay u. Pecka, 1949) verabreicht. Subcutane Injektionen sind ebenfalls wirksam; es müssen jedoch wesentlich höhere Dosen verabfolgt werden und die Ergebnisse variieren infolge von Resorptionsunterschieden stärker (Drenckhahn, 1958). Die optimal ödemprovozierende Adrenalindosis ist nicht nur nach unten, sondern auch nach oben begrenzt; überhöhte Dosen wirken so schnell tödlich, daß für die Ödementwicklung nicht genügend Zeit bleibt (MacKay u. Pecka, 1949). In der Reaktionsweise bestehen erhebliche Speciesdifferenzen. Bei Kaninchen, Meerschweinchen, Ratten und Mäusen entwickelt sich nach Adrenalinzufuhr Lungenödem beträchtlichen Grades, während Hunde und Katzen gewöhnlich an Herzversagen oder Erstickung sterben (Drenckhahn, 1958; Trendelenburg, 1924). Bei den beiden letztgenannten Species kann gewöhnlich nur durch modifizierte Applikation oder bei gleichzeitiger Anwendung zusätzlicher Maßnahmen Lungenödem ausgelöst werden (Paine *et al.*, 1952). So injizierten Cassen u. Kistler (1954a) z.B. den Wirkstoff bei Katzen in den Hypothalamus. Die initiale Apnoe kann durch langsame intravenöse Infusion des Adrenalins umgangen werden (Eichler u. Barfuss, 1940); allerdings wurde nach 1—3stündiger Zufuhr von 10—28 μg/kg/min Adrenalin auch nur bei einem Teil der so behandelten Katzen Lungenödem gefunden. Bei den restlichen Tieren waren Herzbeutelergüsse entstanden, die durch Herztamponade den Tod herbeiführten und die Ausbildung von Lungenödem erschwerten.

Für *Kaninchen* liegt die ödemauslösende Adrenalindosis bei i.v. Applikation zwischen 0,2 und 2 mg/kg. Die Höhe der erforderlichen Dosis ist wahrscheinlich z.T. von der Injektionsdauer, die in der Regel 15—60 sec beträgt, abhängig. Luisada (1928) beobachtete bei Tieren im Gewicht von 1000—2000 g nach langsamer (1 min) i.v. Injektion von 0,35—0,55 mg Adrenalin eine Moralität von 90%. Zu ähnlichen Ergebnissen kamen Nickerson u. Curry (1955): 0,1—0,15 mg/kg i.v. waren unwirksam; 0,25—0,5 mg/kg verursachten eine Letalität von 88%, und 1—2 mg/kg eine solche von 100%. Glass (1928) benötigte bei 700—1000 g schweren Kaninchen 2 mg i.v., um alle Tiere mit Sicherheit zu töten. Unter den geschilderten Bedingungen sterben einige Tiere innerhalb von 2—10 min, die Mehrzahl nach 30—60 min, einzelne erst nach mehreren Stunden. Autoptisch ist in der Regel ausgeprägtes Lungenödem nachweisbar. Einige Autoren warten nicht den Spontaneintritt des Todes ab, sondern opfern überlebende Tiere nach einer bestimmten Einwirkungszeit, z.B. 15 min (Stone u. Loew, 1949). Innerhalb dieser Zeitspanne war das Lungengewicht von Kaninchen (im Gewicht von 2—3 kg), die 0,375 mg/kg Adrenalin (bezogen auf Base) in 0,1%iger Lösung i.v. (Injektionsdauer 15 sec) erhalten hatten, auf das Doppelte der Norm angestiegen.

Bei *Meerschweinchen* liegt der wirksame Dosenbereich des Adrenalins zwischen 0,2 und 0,6 mg/kg i.v. bzw. 1 und 2 mg/kg i.m. (Winter, 1949; MacKay u. Pecka, 1949; Drenckhahn, 1958). Winter (1949) injizierte Meerschweinchen im Gewicht von 300—500 g 0,6 mg/kg Adrenalin-HCl i.v.; die mittlere Überlebenszeit seiner Tiere betrug 7 min, ihr relatives Lungengewicht 19,7 g/kg (Normalwert: 6,8 g/kg). MacKay u. Pecka (1949) erzielten mit einer Dosis von 0,0015 mM/kg (etwa 0,3 mg/kg) einen maximalen Effekt; das relative Lungengewicht stieg auf das dreifache der Norm. Bei weiterer Dosissteigerung auf 0,0020 mM/kg trat der Tod so rasch ein, daß dieser Wert nicht mehr ganz erreicht wurde.

Ratten reagieren auf i.v. Adrenalingaben von 0,3—2 mg/kg (z.B. Cassen u. Kistler, 1954a; Eichholtz u. Hoppe, 1933; Halmágyi *et al.*, 1956; Henschler u. Reich, 1959) oder i.m. Injektion von 4—5 mg/kg (Riechert, 1951; Drenckhahn, (1958) mit schwerem Lungenödem, das bereits 15 min nach i.v. Applikation voll ausgebildet ist. Die rasche Entwicklung des Adrenalinlungenödems demonstrierten Cassen u. Kistler (1954a). Sie injizierten Ratten in Minutenabständen nach i.v. Adrenalingabe (0,6 mg/kg) Evans-Blau. Nur der innerhalb der ersten 3 min verabfolgte Farbstoff war in der Ödemflüssigkeit nachweisbar. Nach der 4. min trat kein Farbstoff mehr aus dem Blut in die Ödemflüssigkeit über, weil der Krankheitszustand bis dahin offenbar seine volle Stärke erreicht hatte.

Kovanov (1966) gab Ratten 4 mg/kg Adrenalin i.p. Zuerst kam es zu motorischer Erregung, dann zu allmählicher Zunahme der Atemfrequenz bis zu Atemnot. Die Agonie war stets von Krämpfen begleitet. Der Tod erfolgte 21—50 min nach der Adrenalingabe. Die Lungen waren histologisch blutgefüllt, die Atemwege voll weißlich schaumiger Flüssigkeit. Die Entwicklung des Ödems ließ sich durch Phenothiazine (Chlorpromazin, Perphenazin, Trifluorperazin) auch 15 min nach Adrenalin verhüten, ebenso durch Dihydroergotoxin. Ganglienblocker (Pentamin und Pyrilen) wirkten nicht.

Mäuse müssen etwas höhere Adrenalindosen erhalten: 5 mg/kg i.v. verursachen schweres Lungenödem mit einem Anstieg des mittleren Lungengewichtes von 160 auf 370 mg (Cassen u. Kistler, 1954b). Poulsen (1954b) injizierte den Wirkstoff i.p. und tötete überlebende Tiere 5 oder 15 min nach der Injektion. Dosen bis zu 1,0 mg/kg waren wirkungslos. Nach der Injektion von 10 mg/kg entwickelte sich schweres Lungenödem, das in der Mehrzahl der Fälle schon 5 min später nachweisbar war und während der folgenden 10 min an Stärke zunahm. Eine Analyse der Befunde nach den auf S. 183f. geschilderten Verfahren desselben Autors zeigte, daß die Gewichtszunahme der Lunge bei dieser Ödemform zu einem erheblichen Teil eine Hyperämiefolge ist.

Die ödemprovozierende Adrenalindosis kann bei gleichzeitiger Verabreichung verschiedener anderer Verbindungen, die für sich allein in dieser Hinsicht unwirksam sind, erheblich reduziert werden. So konnten Eichholtz u. Hoppe (1933) bei Ratten (80—90 g) bereits mit einer Adrenalindosis von 0,05 mg/kg schweres Lungenödem auslösen, wenn sie gleichzeitig Cocain in krampferzeugender Dosis injizierten. Der Ödemgrad erreichte dieselbe Stärke (Anstieg des relativen Lungengewichtes auf das 2,5fache der Norm) wie nach alleiniger Zufuhr von 1,6 mg Adrenalin/kg. Andere Lokalanaesthetica zeigten den Effekt in geringerem Maß. Riechert u. Schmieder (1941) konnten diesen Befund bestätigen und auf adrenalinverwandte Substanzen mit ödemprovozierender Eigenschaft ausdehnen. — In ähnlicher Weise fördern Bradykinin (25—50 µg/kg i.v.) die Ödembereitschaft, so daß (normalerweise unwirksame) Adrenalindosen von 0,05—0,10 mg/kg i.v. bei Kaninchen Ödem erzeugen (Di Mattei, 1962).

Der Entstehungsmechanismus des Adrenalin-Lungenödems wird wahrscheinlich durch mehrere Faktoren bestimmt. Häufig ist ein zentralnervöser Angriffspunkt angenommen worden, da artifizielle Läsionen bestimmter Teile des Zentralnervensystems (Glass, 1928) oder Durchtrennung des Rückenmarks (Cassen *et al.*, 1956; Luisada, 1928; Odake, 1960) sowie Vorbehandlung mit zentraldämpfenden

Pharmaka (Barbiturate) (z.B. Luisada, 1928) die Ödementstehung hemmten. Der letztgenannte Befund konnte von anderen Untersuchern allerdings nicht bestätigt werden (Stone u. Loew, 1949; Cassen *et al.*, 1956). Eine Schutzwirkung übten aber auch Operationen in anderen Körperbereichen aus, wie Splenektomie, Nephrektomie oder Scheinoperationen, bei denen die Abdominalorgane lediglich durch Manipulationen gereizt wurden (Polli u. Luisada, 1957); die Autoren erklären den Effekt als Folge einer unspezifischen Stressreaktion. Direkte Beweise für die Beteiligung eines „Permeabilitätszentrums" (z.B. Luisada, 1928) konnten bisher nicht erbracht werden. Cassen u. Kistler (1954a) sowie Cassen *et al.* (1956) vermuten eine Einwirkung des Adrenalins auf die zentralnervöse Steuerung des präcapillaren Sphinctersystems. Denkbar wäre auch eine direkte oder indirekte Beeinflussung des Lymphabflusses aus der Lunge (Altschule, 1956; Drenckhahn, 1958; Rusznyák *et al.*, 1957; Smith, 1949) oder eine peripher ausgelöste Steigerung der Capillarpermeabilität. Ob der Freisetzung von Histamin im Organismus durch Adrenalin (Eichler u. Barfuss, 1940; Staub, 1946) dabei eine Rolle zukommt, ist ungeklärt. Vorbehandlung von Versuchstieren mit Antihistaminica, einschließlich Phenothiazinen, die in der Hand einiger Autoren das Adrenalinödem hemmte (z.B. Corelli, 1951; Halpern *et al.*, 1950; Kovanov, 1966; Poulsen, 1954e; Schmitterlöw u. Wessman, 1951), erwies sich in anderen Untersuchungen als wirkungslos (Stone u. Loew, 1949; Winter, 1949). An der isolierten perfundierten Lunge konnte weder durch Adrenalin noch durch Histamin Lungenödem provoziert werden (Born, 1954). Die Mitwirkung von Kininen an der Ödementstehung wurde von Di Mattei (1962) diskutiert; er konnte nach Verabreichung ödemauslösender Adrenalindosen (Kaninchen) eine beträchtliche Bradykininanreicherung in Lunge, Leber und Trachealflüssigkeit nachweisen; durch Unterbindung der Lebervenen wurde die Entstehung des adrenalinbedingten Lungenödems verhindert und eine Herabsetzung des Bradykiningehaltes des Plasmas und der Lunge verursacht.

Entscheidend für die Ödemgenese dürften hämodynamische Faktoren sein (Drenckhahn, 1958; Gilbert *et al.*, 1958; Paine *et al.*, 1952). So konnte Drenckhahn (1958) zeigen, daß eine direkte Beziehung zwischen dem Einfluß ödemprovozierender Adrenalindosen auf den Pulmonalvenendruck und dem resultierenden Lungenödem besteht. Er registrierte bei Kaninchen und Meerschweinchen den Gefäßdruck unter weitgehender Schonung der Tiere. In oberflächlicher Narkose (Pernocton bzw. Chloralose) wurde bei geschlossenem Thorax und Spontanatmung von der geöffneten Trachea aus eine Spezialkanüle rechts neben der Bifurcatio tracheae durch die mediale Wand des rechten Bronchus in die großen Pulmonalvenen oder in den linken Vorhof eingeführt. Die richtige Position der Kanüle wurde durch eine Verdickung des Kanülenrohres, die ein zu weites Vordringen verhinderte, gewährleistet. Der Pulmonalvenendruck von Meerschweinchen (250 bis 750 g) stieg nach Adrenalingabe (1—2 mg/kg s.c.) innerhalb weniger Minuten von einem mittleren Ausgangswert von $3{,}8 \pm 2$ mm Hg bis auf maximal 52 mm Hg an. Lungenödem wurde immer dann beobachtet, wenn der Pulmonalvenendruck 30 mm Hg überschritt und damit den kolloidosmotischen Plasmadruck, der bei dieser Tierspecies etwa 23—27 mm Hg beträgt, übertraf. Zwischen der Höhe des Pulmonalvenendruckes und dem post mortem festgestellten relativen Lungengewicht bestand eine positive Korrelation. Bei Kaninchen (3 mg/kg Adrenalin i.m.) wurden ähnliche Ergebnisse erzielt. Der Steigerung des Pulmonalvenendruckes ging eine Erhöhung des arteriellen Druckes im großen Kreislauf voraus (Zeitintervall 10—60 sec), deren Ausmaß das der pulmonalen Kreislaufveränderungen bestimmte. Der Venendruck im Körperkreislauf war nur um wenige mm Hg erhöht. Eine derartige Druckzunahme genügt jedoch, um das venöse Angebot an die rechte Herzhälfte beträchtlich zu vergrößern und eine Verschiebung von Blut aus dem großen in den kleinen Kreislauf zu bewirken. Eine zusätzliche Beanspruchung des Lungenkreislaufes kommt retrograd als Folge der Überlastung des linken Ventrikels zustande.

In Übereinstimmung mit der hämodynamischen Hypothese steht der Befund, daß das Adrenalin-Lungenödem durch Ganglienblocker und Sympatholytica besser bekämpft werden kann als durch andere Pharmaka (z. B. Cassen u. Kistler, 1954; Correlli, 1951; MacKay u. Pecka, 1949; Paine *et al.*, 1952, Riechert, 1951; Stone u. Loew, 1949; Testoni u. Lomeo, 1953). Das wirksame Prinzip dieser Substanzen ist die Hemmung der adrenalinbedingten arteriellen Drucksteigerung (Paine *et al.*, 1952) (s. auch die Versuche von Kovanov: S. 239).

Endogenes Adrenalin spielt als Mediator der Ödemauslösung wahrscheinlich auch bei anderen Formen des experimentellen Lungenödems eine Rolle. So war z. B. der Katecholamingehalt im Blut von Kaninchen nach Erzeugung von ödemprovozierenden Läsionen im Bereich der Area praeoptica des Gehirns beträchtlich erhöht (Ueba, 1962).

bb) Noradrenalin. L-Noradrenalin wirkt in ähnlicher Weise ödemprovozierend wie Adrenalin; es muß jedoch — wie MacKay und Pecka (1949) in vergleichenden Untersuchungen an Meerschweinchen gezeigt haben — höher dosiert werden als dieses. Bei intrakardialer (weibliche Tiere) oder intravenöser (männliche Tiere) Applikation verursachten 0,004 mM/kg Noradrenalin annähernd den gleichen Effekt wie 0,001 mM/kg Adrenalin, nämlich eine Zunahme des relativen Lungengewichtes um etwa 130% (Tötung der Tiere 1 Std nach der Injektion durch Ätherinhalation). Gelegentlich wurde Noradrenalin in Form von Dauerinfusionen als ödemförderndes Agens eingesetzt. Korner (1953) provozierte bei Kaninchen Lungenödem durch 5stündige Infusion von Ringer-Locke-Lösung mit einem Zusatz von 0,3 μg/kg/min Noradrenalin (Infusionstechnik s. S. 199). Gleiche Flüssigkeitsvolumina ohne Noradrenalin waren bei Kontrolltieren nahezu wirkungslos. Hochdosierte Noradrenalininfusionen (10—20 μg/kg/min) verhinderten dagegen die Entstehung hypervolämischen Lungenödems. Es entwickelten sich statt dessen große Ergüsse in der Pleura- und Peritonealhöhle (s. auch Eichler u. Barfuss, 1940).

Dem Noradrenalinödem dürfte derselbe Pathomechanismus zugrunde liegen wie dem Adrenalinödem. Es wurden Drucksteigerungen im arteriellen und venösen Teil des großen Kreislaufes sowie eine Blutvolumenzunahme im Lungenkreislauf beobachtet (Korner, 1953). Wie beim Adrenalinödem geht auch bei dieser Ödemform ein Teil der Lungengewichtszunahme auf das Konto der Hyperämie.

cc) Verschiedene Verbindungen. Offenbar wirken nur wenige adrenalinverwandte Verbindungen ödemprovozierend. Riechert und Schmieder (1941), die mehrere Phenyl- bzw. Oxyphenylalkylamine vergleichend an Ratten prüften, sahen nur nach i.v. Applikation letaler Dosen von Adrenalin (2 mg/kg), Dioxynorephedrin (Corbasil; 12 mg/kg) und (in geringem Maß) Synephrin (Sympatol; 1500 mg/kg) die Entstehung von Lungenödem, während p-Oxyephedrin (Suprifen), Pholedrin (Veritol), Ephedrin, Amphetamin (Benzedrin) und Methamphetamin (Pervitin) in dieser Hinsicht wirkungslos waren. Ähnliche Resultate erzielten Heim und Bänder (1950) bei der Verwendung von Mäusen als Versuchstiere. Lungenödem entwickelte sich nur nach s.c. Injektion der LD_{50} von Adrenalin und Synephrin. Dagegen verursachten die entsprechenden Dosen von Pholedrin, Ephedrin und Methamphetamin zwar Verquellung der Alveolarsepten und Veränderungen an den elastischen Fasern, gelegentlich auch Erythrocytendiapedese in den Alveolen, nicht jedoch alveoläres Ödem.

Soweit Phenylalkylaminderivate ödemerzeugende Eigenschaften besitzen, scheinen diese auf die (—)-Isomeren beschränkt zu sein. Luduena (1962), der die

Aktivität von Isoproterenol (Aludrin) unter diesem Gesichtspunkt untersuchte, beobachtete bei Ratten nur nach Verabreichung letaler Dosen der linksisomeren Form Lungenödem. Applikation der rechtsisomeren oder racemischen Form führte zum Tod an Atemversagen.

b) 5-Hydroxytryptamin

Die Bedeutung von 5-Hydroxytryptamin (5-HT) als Mediator bei der Entstehung von Lungenödem verschiedener Genese ist wiederholt diskutiert worden. Einige Untersucher erhoben auch Befunde, die für einen derartigen Effekt von endogenem 5-Hydroxytryptamin sprechen. So beobachteten Skillen *et al.* (1961a, b), daß ozonbedingtes Lungenödem bei Ratten mit einer 5-HT-Anreicherung der Lunge und einer Verminderung des 5-HT-Gehaltes des Gehirns einhergeht. Bei anaphylaktischem Lungenödem von Mäusen (ausgelöst durch Injektion von Kaninchenantiserum gegen Ehrlich-Ascitestumorzellen der Maus) konnte ebenfalls eine beträchtliche Erhöhung des 5-HT-Gehaltes der ödematösen Lunge nachgewiesen werden (Kind *et al.*, 1961). Definitive Schlußfolgerungen aus diesen Befunden konnten bisher nicht gezogen werden. Kabins *et al.* (1959) haben jedoch gezeigt, daß durch Injektion von 0,5—6,5 mg 5-Hydroxytryptamin in die Arteria pulmonalis narkotisierter, künstlich beatmeter Hunde Lungenödem hervorgerufen werden kann. Aus Kreislaufuntersuchungen wurde geschlossen, daß der Wirkstoff eine Constriction der Lungenarterien und -venen bewirkt (Gilbert *et al.*, 1958; Kabins *et al.*, 1959); diesem Effekt liegt möglicherweise ein sympathischer Reflex zugrunde. Als weiterer ödemgenetischer Faktor wurde eine direkt durch 5-Hydroxytryptamin oder durch sekundäre Histaminausschüttung bedingte Änderung der Capillarpermeabilität in Betracht gezogen (Kabins *et al.*, 1959). Zumindest beim anaphylaktischen Lungenödem (s.o.) scheint Histamin jedoch keine Rolle zu spielen; denn bei dieser Ödemform war zwar der 5-HT- nicht jedoch der Histamingehalt der Lungen erhöht (Kind *et al.*, 1961).

c) Histamin

Histamin ist aufgrund seiner pharmakologischen Eigenschaften häufig als ödemauslösendes Agens in Betracht gezogen worden und bei Versuchstieren wurde nach Histaminverabreichung gelegentlich auch die Entstehung von Lungenödem beobachtet. Doch scheint es nicht möglich zu sein, durch einmalige Injektion einer höheren Histamindosis mit Regelmäßigkeit Lungenödem hervorzurufen (s. Eichler und Speda, 1940). So sah Rühl (1930) bei narkotisierten, künstlich beatmeten Katzen mit geöffnetem Thorax nach i.v. Injektionen von 0,5—1,5 mg/kg Histamin nur präödematöse Veränderungen oder Lungenödem leichteren Grades, das in der Regel nur im histologischen Präparat, nicht an einer Zunahme des Lungengewichtes erkennbar war. Bei modifizierter Applikation läßt sich durch Histamin offensichtlich auch Lungenödem schweren Grades auslösen. Eichler (1937), Eichler und Barfuss (1940) sowie Eichler und Speda (1940) verabfolgten Katzen Histamin durch i.v. Infusion (Infusionsrate: 1—4 μg/kg/min). Gleichzeitige Infusionen von Histamin und Adrenalin oder adrenalinverwandten Substanzen wirkten hinsichtlich der Ödementstehung synergistisch. Moon und Morgan (1936a, b) injizierten Hunden 5—8 Tage lang 1- oder 2mal täglich 7,5—15 mg/kg Histaminphosphat s.c. und töteten die Tiere nach der letzten Injektion. Neben ausgeprägtem Lungenödem und erheblicher Hyperämie der Lungencapillaren und -venolen hatten sich allerdings auch pathologische Veränderungen an Leber, Nieren und Därmen entwickelt. Hämoglobingehalt und Erythrocytenzahl waren als Ausdruck einer zunehmenden Bluteindickung bis zum Ende des Versuches um etwa 30% angestiegen. Bei Meerschweinchen wurden ähnliche Ergebnisse erzielt, wenn den Tieren 2mal täglich 0,5 mg Histamin pro kg Körpergewicht verabreicht wurden.

Der Pathomechanismus des Histaminlungenödems hängt wahrscheinlich nicht nur mit einem direkten Einfluß dieser Verbindung auf die Gefäßwände, sondern auch mit einer Beeinträchtigung der Herzfunktion zusammen (s. Rühl, 1929, 1930). Die Beteiligung körpereigenen Histamins an der Entstehung von Lungenödem, das primär unter der Einwirkung anderer Noxen zustande kommt, ist wiederholt diskutiert worden. Einige Autoren interpretieren die Schutzwirkung, die Antihistaminica bei manchen Formen des Lungenödems auszuüben scheinen, in diesem Sinn (s. S. 240). Weiterhin werden verschiedene ödemprovozierende Maßnahmen, z.B. Adrenalin- (Eichler und Barfuss, 1940; Staub, 1946) oder Ammoniumchloridverabreichung (Jaques, 1952), von einer Erhöhung des Bluthistamingehaltes begleitet. Jaques (1954) konnte darüber hinaus nachweisen, daß das Ausmaß der durch Ammoniumchlorid bewirkten Ödemreaktion bei Ratten dem Histamingehalt ihrer Lungen korreliert war. Bei jungen Tieren, deren Lungen nur wenig Histamin enthielten, war auf diesem Weg kein Lungenödem auslösbar.

d) Insulin (Hypoglykämie)

Schwere Hypoglykämie kann, wie MacKay und Pecka (1950) gezeigt haben, bei Versuchstieren zu einem Lungenödem führen. Die Autoren injizierten Ratten beiderlei Geschlechts nach 24stündigem Nahrungsentzug je 2 E Altinsulin und Protamininsulin pro 100 g Körpergewicht. Die im hypoglykämischen Schock gestorbenen Tiere wiesen schweres Lungenödem auf; das relative Lungengewicht war von 0,60% (Kontrollen) auf 1,29% angestiegen. An der Ödemauslösung ist wahrscheinlich eine durch die Hypoglykämie bedingte Adrenalinausschüttung beteiligt; denn durch Adrenalektomie oder Demedullierung der Nebenniere (einen Tag bzw. eine Woche vor der Insulinbehandlung vorgenommen) konnte die Entstehung des Lungenödems eingeschränkt, durch Vorbehandlung mit einem Antiadrenergicum völlig verhindert werden. Der primäre ödemgenetische Faktor wird jedoch in einer Stimulierung autonomer Zentren des Hirnstammes infolge Glucosemangel gesehen.

e) Ammoniumsalze

Die ödemprovozierende Wirkung von Ammoniumsalzen ist seit längerer Zeit bekannt. So beobachtete Modrakowski (1914) die Entwicklung von Lungenödem am Herzlungenpräparat, wenn das Perfusionsblut Ammoniumchlorid enthielt. Auch beim Menschen kann auf dieser Basis, z.B. im Gefolge von Ammoniakvergiftungen (v. Fazekas, 1934) Lungenödem entstehen.

Zur Erzeugung von Lungenödem bei Versuchstieren wird gewöhnlich Ammoniumchlorid in 6—25%iger wäßriger Lösung und Dosen von 0,4—1,2 g/kg Körpergewicht angewandt. Andere Ammoniumsalze wirken ähnlich, wenn die Konzentration des Ammoniumions in der gleichen Größenordnung liegt (Koenig und Koenig, 1949a, b). Cameron u. Sheikh (1951) konnten z.B. bei Ratten mit einem mittleren Gewicht von etwa 150 g durch i.p. oder p.o. Gabe 6%iger Lösungen (8—10 ml/kg=0,5—0,6 g/kg) von Ammoniumchlorid, -carbonat, -sulfat, -phosphat [$(NH_4)_2HPO_4$], -nitrat, -acetat, -citrat und -bromid Lungenödem provozieren. Der Effekt tritt nach p.o., s.c., i.m., i.p. und i.v. Applikation auf. Die wirksame Dosis liegt innerhalb enger Grenzen und wird wesentlich von der Resorptionsgeschwindigkeit bestimmt. Zu hohe Dosen oder zu schnelle Resorption führen zum Tod, bevor Lungenödem entstehen kann. Bei zu niedriger Dosierung oder verzögerter Resorption bleiben Lungenveränderungen (oder andere Vergiftungserscheinungen) ganz aus. Der Ausbildung des Lungenödems bzw. dem Tod können Reizerscheinungen von seiten des Zentralnervensystems (Muskelschwäche, gesteigerte Erregbarkeit auf akustische, taktile und Schmerzreize, Muskelzuckungen, tonische Krämpfe und Koma) sowie Atemstörungen (Dyspnoe, Stridor, Atemversagen) voraus- oder nebenhergehen (Bersaques u. Leusen, 1954; Cameron u. Sheikh, 1951; Sarnoff u. Kaufman, 1951). Diese Vergiftungsfolgen können unabhängig von der Ödementwicklung den Tod herbeiführen. In der Reaktionsweise der Versuchstiere bestehen offensichtlich erhebliche Art-, Rassen- und Altersdifferenzen. Jaques (1954) konnte zeigen, daß die Ansprechbarkeit von Ratten auf die Ödemnoxe dem Histamingehalt ihrer Lungen parallel ging. Bei jungen Tieren mit histaminarmen Lungen ließ sich durch Ammoniumchlorid kein Ödem provozieren.

Bei *Katzen* ist es prinzipiell möglich, Lungenödem durch Ammoniumsalze hervorzurufen (Koenig u. Koenig, 1949a, b). Die Tiere reagieren jedoch häufig sowohl bei oraler als auch bei intraperitonealer Verabreichung mit Erbrechen oder starkem Speichelfluß, wodurch Dosierung und Ödembewertung erschwert werden.

Kaninchen scheinen als Versuchstiere ebenfalls wenig geeignet zu sein. Den meisten Untersuchern gelang es selbst mit letalen Dosen nicht, bei dieser Species Lungenödem auszulösen (z.B. Koenig u. Koenig, 1949a, b). Die Reaktionsweise wird jedoch offensichtlich weitgehend von Rassenunterschieden bestimmt; denn MacKay *et al.* (1949) konnten mit Dosen von 1,25 g/kg Ammoniumchlorid (in 25%iger Lösung p.o.) auch bei dieser Tierart Ödem provozieren.

Meerschweinchen beantworten dagegen die orale (Magensonde: 0,9—1,2 g/kg) oder i.p. Zufuhr von 0,5—0,7 g Ammoniumchlorid/kg Körpergewicht regelmäßig mit der Ausbildung von Lungenödem (s. z.B. Koenig u. Koenig, 1949a, b; MacKay *et al.*, 1949).

Auch bei *Ratten* kann nach i.p. Injektion von 0,4—0,6 g/kg Ammoniumchlorid die Entwicklung von Lungenödem erwartet werden (z.B. Koenig u. Koenig, 1949a, b; Cameron u. Sheikh, 1951). Auf Ausnahmen (altersbedingte Empfindlichkeitsunterschiede) ist oben hingewiesen worden.

Die Vergiftungserscheinungen einschließlich des Lungenödems laufen bei Ratten und Meerschweinchen innerhalb von 15—60 min nach der Ammoniumchloridzufuhr ab; der Tod tritt im Durchschnitt nach etwa 30 min ein (Cameron u. Sheikh, 1951; Gottsegen *et al.*, 1958, desgl. Kovanov, 1966). Katzen überleben etwas länger. Das entstandene Lungenödem kam in einem Anstieg des relativen Lungengewichtes auf durchschnittlich das doppelte der Norm zum Ausdruck (s. z.B. Gottsegen *et al.*, 1958; Halmágyi *et al.*, 1956; Jaques, 1952; MacKay *et al.*, 1949). Im histologischen Bild der Lungen waren neben massivem Ödem, Emphysem, vasculären Schädigungen und Hämorrhagien unterschiedlichen Ausmaßes Erweiterungen der perivasculären und peribronchialen Lymphgefäße nachweisbar (Cameron u. Sheikh, 1951; Koenig u. Koenig, 1949a, b; Luisada, 1950). Die Ödemflüssigkeit hat von Anfang an einen hohen Eiweißgehalt (Cameron u. Sheikh, 1951); das Blut erfährt eine erhebliche Eindickung (Jaques, 1952).

Das Lungenödem kann — wahrscheinlich infolge verlängerter Überlebenszeit — schwerere Grade erreichen, wenn die zentralnervösen Erscheinungen durch Vorbehandlung der Tiere mit Barbituraten hintangehalten werden. Bei Ratten bewirkte i.p. Injektion von 0,4 g/kg Ammoniumchlorid z.B. einen Anstieg des relativen Lungengewichts von 0,85 (Kontrollen) auf 1,51%, nach Vorbehandlung mit Phenyläthylbarbitursäure (10 mg/kg s.c.) dagegen auf 2,26% (Halmágyi *et al.*, 1956).

Die Ammoniumchloridkonzentration des Blutes muß eine bestimmte Höhe erreichen und diese für einige Zeit (mindestens 15 min) beibehalten, damit Lungenödem entstehen kann. Wahrscheinlich ist — wie die gleichartige Wirksamkeit der verschiedenen Ammoniumsalze vermuten läßt — das Ammonium und nicht eine etwaige Acidose (pH des Blutes 6,8—7,2) oder Alkalose (Bersaques u. Leusen, 1954; Winterstein u. Gökhahn, 1953) der für die Vergiftungserscheinungen verantwortliche Faktor, denn die Verabreichung größerer Mengen von Säuren oder Alkalien verursachte kein Lungenödem (Koenig u. Koenig, 1949b; Cameron u. Sheikh, 1951). Nach Untersuchungen von Sarnoff u. Kaufman (1952) ist ein Versagen des linken Ventrikels ursächlich an der Entstehung des Ammoniumchloridlungenödems beteiligt. Auch Gottsegen *et al.* (1957) ziehen Kreislaufstörungen als Ödemursache in Betracht; sie beobachteten bei Ratten nach Ammoniumchloridverabreichung Bradykardie und Veränderungen des Elektrokardiogramms. Cameron u. Sheikh (1951) vermuten, daß das Ammonium die Capillarpermeabilität erhöht. Jaques (1952, 1954) folgert aus seinen Untersuchungen, daß körpereigenes Histamin und Adrenalin bei der Ödementstehung mitwirken. Da unter dem Einfluß von Antiadrenergica und Sympatholytica sowie andauernder Chloralose- oder Äthernarkose die Ödementstehung (nicht jedoch der Tod der Tiere) verhindert werden konnte, nehmen einige Untersucher an, daß das sympathische Nervensystem bzw. adrenergische System am Pathomechanismus beteiligt sind (Cameron u. Sheikh, 1951; Koenig u. Koenig, 1949b; MacKay *et al.*, 1949). In den Versuchen von Kovanov (1966) mit i.p. Gabe von 0,24 g/kg NH_4Cl konnte das Ödem durch Phenothiazine, aber auch durch Ganglienblocker gehemmt werden, nicht aber durch Dihydroergotamin.

f) Natriumcarbonat, Natriumbicarbonat

Die Verabreichung von Natriumcarbonat und Natriumbicarbonat kann unter bestimmten Voraussetzungen Lungenödem zur Folge haben. Koenig *et al.* (1952) infundierten narkotisierten (35 mg/kg Pentobarbital-Na) und teilweise künstlich beatmeten Katzen 5%ige Na_2CO_3- oder 8%ige $NaHCO_3$-Lösungen in die Vena femoralis. Tiere, die innerhalb von 20—100 min 50—100 ml der 8%igen $NaHCO_3$-Lösung erhalten hatten, reagierten mit tetanischen Krämpfen; der pH-Wert des Blutes stieg von 7,45 (Normalwert) auf 7,85—7,95; post mortem wurde bei allen Tieren Lungenödem nachgewiesen. Nach Zufuhr kleinerer Mengen der Lösung (40—45 ml innerhalb von 2 Std) blieb der Blut-pH-Wert unter 7,75; Lungenödem trat unter diesen Bedingungen nicht auf. 35—100 ml der 5%igen Na_2CO_3-Lösung innerhalb von 120 min verabfolgt, bewirkten eine Verschiebung des pH-Wertes auf 7,80—7,90 und in der Mehrzahl der Fälle ebenfalls Lungenödem. Künstliche Beatmung modifizierte das Versuchsergebnis nicht. Der Eiweißgehalt der aus der Trachea gewonnenen Ödemflüssigkeit betrug 0,8—1,4%. Die Autoren nehmen an, daß die Alkalose an der Ödementstehung ursächlich beteiligt ist. Die alkalotische Tetanie scheint dagegen nur eine unabhängige Begleiterscheinung zu sein; andere Tetanieformen (z.B. nach Injektion von Natriumcitrat) gingen ohne Lungenödem einher.

g) Thioharnstoff und Thioharnstoffderivate

Thioharnstoff und einige seiner Derivate können bei Versuchstieren Lungenödem hervorrufen. Am deutlichsten scheint diese Eigenschaft beim α-Naphthylthioharnstoff ausgeprägt zu sein (Richter, 1952), aber auch Thioharnstoff, β-Naphthylthioharnstoff, $\alpha\alpha$- und $\beta\beta$-Dinaphthylthioharnstoff (Cameron, 1948; Dieke, 1949) sowie Thiosemicarbazid (Dieke, 1949; Tennekoon, 1954) sind in ähnlicher Weise wirksam.

α-Naphthylthioharnstoff ist schlecht wasserlöslich. Für die gewöhnlich geübte i.p. oder i.v. Injektion wird die Substanz in Olivenöl suspendiert (Richter, 1952) oder mit Hilfe von Propylenglykol in Lösung gebracht (Drinker und Hardenbergh, 1949; Halmágyi *et al.*, 1956; Williams, 1953). Nicht alle Tierarten reagieren auf die Verabreichung von α-Naphthylthioharnstoff in gleicher Weise mit Lungenödem; als Versuchstiere eignen sich in erster Linie Ratten bestimmter Rassen, ferner Hunde, Katzen und Mäuse. Auf Art-, Rassen- und Altersunterschiede in der Ansprechbarkeit ist oben (S. 193f.) hingewiesen worden; sie kommen insbesondere in der Höhe der Letaldosis zum Ausdruck. Allgemeingültige Angaben über die erforderlichen Dosen können daher nicht gemacht werden. Dieke und Richter (1946) ermittelten an ihrem Tiermaterial bei i.p. Verabreichung von α-Naphthylthioharnstoff z.B. die folgenden mittleren Letaldosen (LD_{50}): für norwegische Ratten verschiedener Stämme 2,5—6,25 mg/kg; für eine andere Rattenrasse (R. rattus subsp.) 250 mg/kg; für Hunde weniger als 16 mg/kg; für Mäuse 56 mg/kg. Nicht nur tödliche Gaben wirken ödemprovozierend; mäßige Grade von Lungenödem treten bereits unter dem Einfluß subletaler Dosen auf.

Für Hunde liegen die ödemauslösenden Dosen von α-Naphthylthioharnstoff (als 2%ige Lösung in Propylenglykol) zwischen 7 und 20 mg/kg i.v. (Drinker und Hardenbergh, 1949; Halmágyi *et al.*, 1956; Williams, 1953).

Bei Ratten umspannen die in der Literatur angegebenen Werte einen größeren Bereich. Starzecki und Halmágyi (1961) verabfolgten als Standarddosis von α-Naphthylthioharnstoff z.B. 100 mg/kg i.p., Dieke und Richter (1946) Dosen zwischen 2,5 und 250 mg/kg i.p. (s.o.). Richter (1952) versuchte die Beziehungen zwischen Dosis, Zeit und Wirkung genauer abzugrenzen. Er verabreichte Ratten im Gewicht von 200—300 g, die er durch 4tägige Unterbringung in Einzelkäfigen in einem ruhigen gleichmäßig temperierten Raum konditioniert hatte, α-Naphthylthioharnstoff in Dosen von 1—50 mg/kg i.p. (als Suspension in Olivenöl; Dosis in 1 ml/100 g Körpergewicht), tötete die Tiere durch Entbluten in stündlichen Intervallen und verfolgte die Entwicklung des Lungenödems anhand der Veränderungen des relativen Lungengewichtes. Während Dosen von 1 mg/kg keine Wirkung hatten, war das relative Lungengewicht 1 Std nach Injektion von 3—50 mg/kg deutlich gesteigert. Das Ödem erreichte 2—4 Std nach der Injektion maximale Intensität und begann sich anschließend wieder zurückzubilden, sofern die Tiere überlebten.

Mäuse reagierten auf i.p. Injektion von 0,5—4,5 mg α-Naphthylthioharnstoff pro Tier mit der Ausbildung von Lungenödem (Harford und Hara, 1950).

Die wirksamen Dosen von Thioharnstoff lassen sich ebenfalls nicht genau festlegen. Koch (1956) verabreichte Ratten im Gewicht von 115—220 g 75 mg/kg i.p. Innerhalb von 48 Std starben 75% der Tiere; das relative Lungengewicht war signifikant auf 1,89% (Normalwert 0,86%) gestiegen. Henschler und Reich (1959) benötigten bei Tieren der gleichen Gewichtsklasse bei gleicher Applikationsart 500 mg/kg, nahmen die Auswertung allerdings schon nach etwa 1 Std vor. Luisada (1950) beurteilt die Thioharnstoffmethode negativ, weil die Resultate, die er bei Ratten durch i.p. Injektion von 200 mg/kg Thioharnstoff erzielte, quantitativ und chronologisch so stark variierten, daß eine einwandfreie Bewertung therapeutischer Maßnahmen schwierig war.

Der Pathomechanismus des durch Thioharnstoff und seine Derivate hervorgerufenen Lungenödems ist nicht vollständig geklärt. Es wird angenommen, daß die Verbindungen einen reversiblen Anstieg der Permeabilität der Lungencapillaren bewirken, ohne Dauerschäden an den Gefäßen zu hinterlassen. Für diese Annahme spricht u.a. der hohe Eiweißgehalt (4—4,5%) der aus der Trachea gewonnenen Ödemflüssigkeit (Williams, 1953). Als Ursache der Capillarschädigung vermuten Gruhzit *et al.* (1951) eine Hemmung der Sulfhydrylenzyme. Die Capillaren anderer Organe werden offensichtlich nicht beeinträchtigt (Drinker, 1950). Ödem bzw. Exsudat bilden sich nur in der Lunge und der Thoraxhöhle aus. Neben diesen Veränderungen beobachtete Koch (1956) entzündliche Infiltration des interstitiellen Lungengewebes, Peribronchitis und Bronchitis. Der Druck in den Pulmonalgefäßen wird durch die Verbindungen wahrscheinlich nicht nennenswert beeinflußt (Dawes *et al.*, 1951; Gruhzit *et al.*, 1951; Halmágyi *et al.*, 1955).

h) Thiosemicarbazid

Thiosemicarbazid ($H_2NNH \cdot CSNH_2$) besitzt ödemerzeugende Eigenschaften, entfaltet diese jedoch — soweit bisher bekannt — nur bei Ratten; alle anderen überprüften Tierarten (Affen, Hunde, Katzen, Meerschweinchen) reagierten unter dem Einfluß der Verbindung nicht mit Lungenödem. Auch in anderer Hinsicht unterscheidet sich Thiosemicarbazid von den vorangehend besprochenen Thioharnstoffderivaten (Dieke, 1949): Die mittlere Letaldosis läßt sich besser abgrenzen (LD_{50} i.p. bzw. p.o. 10—25 mg/kg) und der Mechanismus der Ödementstehung ist wahrscheinlich grundsätzlich different (s. u.). Die Thiosemicarbazidvergiftung geht außerdem mit zentralnervösen Reiz- bzw. Lähmungserscheinungen einher. Einige Thiosemicarbazone (p-Acetylaminobenzaldehydthiosemicarbazon [Conteben] und p-Acetylsulfonylbenzaldehydthiosemicarbazon) wirken in ähnlicher Weise ödemprovozierend wie Thiosemicarbazid (Francis und Spinks, 1950).

Tennekoon (1954) untersuchte die Bedingungen, unter denen sich das Thiosemicarbazidödem entwickelt und arbeitete ein offensichtlich zuverlässiges Verfahren zur Ödemprovokation bei Ratten aus. Er injizierte ausgewachsenen Wistar-Ratten i.p. 30 mg Thiosemicarbazid pro kg Körpergewicht als 1%ige Suspension in 10%iger Gummi arabicum-Lösung. Innerhalb von 50—100 min starben die Tiere an Lungenödem. Das Lungen-Herzgewichtsverhältnis bewahrte während einer Latenzperiode von 30—45 min seinen normalen Wert von etwa 1,5 und stieg anschließend rasch an. Während dieser Phase befindet sich das Tier zunächst in einem Zustand gesteigerter Erregbarkeit und Krampfbereitschaft, der von Dyspnoe, Bewußtseinsverlust und Atemversagen abgelöst wird. Das Tier stirbt an Erstickung, wenn die Ödemflüssigkeit sich in die Bronchien ergießt. Pleuraexsudate und Schädigungen anderer Organe wurden nicht beobachtet. Am Herz-Lungen-Präparat von Ratten und Kaninchen in der Anordnung nach Born (1954) (s. S. 188f.) konnte durch 15—60 min dauernde Perfusion mit 10^{-3} mol Thiosemicarbazid kein Lungenödem erzeugt werden. Eine direkte Einwirkung auf die Lungencapillaren ist daher unwahrscheinlich. Da zentraldämpfende Maßnahmen sowie Sympatholytica und Ganglienblocker die Ödementwicklung hemmten, sieht Tennekoon das Thiosesemicarbazidlungenödem als hydrostatisch bedingt an (Blutverschiebung aus dem großen in den kleinen Kreislauf).

i) Chloroform

Die i.v. Zufuhr von Chloroform in geeigneter Dosis kann, wie Testelli und Musiker (1960) sowie Testelli *et al.* (1960) gezeigt haben, bei Hunden und Kaninchen Lungenödem hervorrufen. Die Autoren injizierten 0,1 ml Chloroform pro kg Körpergewicht in die Ohrrandvene (Kaninchen) bzw. die Vena saphena (Hunde); die Injektionsdauer betrug 60—120 sec. Die Mehrzahl der Tiere verendete innerhalb 1 Std. Auch bei den überlebenden Tieren, die 60 min nach der Injektion geopfert wurden, war Lungenödem nachweisbar. Das mittlere relative Lungengewicht war auf etwa das doppelte der Norm erhöht. Wirksame Dosis und Injektionsgeschwindigkeit liegen innerhalb eines engen Bereiches. Zu hohe Dosen oder zu schnelle Injektion führen so rasch zum Tod, daß kein Lungenödem entstehen kann.

Chloroform soll eine direkte depressorische Wirkung auf das Myokard ausüben, und zwar auf den linken Ventrikel in stärkerem Maß als auf den rechten. Als Folge dieser unterschiedlichen Beeinflussung beider Herzhälften kommt es zu einer Drucksteigerung in den Pulmonalcapillaren mit Flüssigkeitstranssudation in die Alveolen. Für einen derartigen Pathomechanismus sprechen auch die Resultate intrakardialer Druckmessungen: Der systolische Druck war vermindert, und zwar vor allem in der linken Kammer, während der Druck im linken Vorhof erhöht war.

j) Chlorpikrin

Chlorpikrin wirkt nicht nur bei Inhalation (vgl. S. 227f.), sondern auch bei i.v. Injektion ödemprovozierend. Bei beiden Applikationsarten sind die klinischen und morphologischen Befunde der Chlorpikrinvergiftung identisch. Auch nach Injektion greift Chlorpikrin wahrscheinlich direkt am Lungengewebe an (Gildemeister u. Heubner, 1921). Die Verbindung wird gewöhnlich in Form einer 1%igen Lösung in 50%igem Äthanol verabfolgt. Kaninchen, die 15 mg/kg Chlorpikrin i.v. erhalten hatten, starben innerhalb von 15—240 min an Lungenödem (Halpern *et al.*, 1950). Bei Meerschweinchen entwickelte sich nach i.v. Zufuhr von 4,2 mg/kg (LD_{50}) schweres Lungenödem, charakterisiert durch Schaumaustritt aus Nase und Mund und einen Anstieg des mittleren relativen Lungengewichtes auf mehr als das 3fache der Norm (Prasad, 1958). Ratten (im Gewicht von 120 bis 160 g) reagierten auf Dosen von 15 mg/kg i.v. mit Lungenödem; das relative Lungengewicht erhöhte sich innerhalb von 20 min auf das doppelte der Norm (Henschler u. Reich, 1959).

k) Pentetrazol und andere Analeptica

Pentetrazol (Pentamethylentetrazol, Cardiazol) in letalen sowie subletalen, aber schon krampferzeugenden Dosen verursacht bei Versuchstieren Atemstörungen und Lungenödem. Jarisch u. Thoma (1940) verabreichten Kaninchen Dosen von 20—30 mg/kg i.v.; tödlich verlaufendes Lungenödem entwickelte sich allerdings nur bei einzelnen Tieren. Bei Meerschweinchen (150 mg/kg) und Ratten (200 mg/kg i.v.) wirkt Pentetrazol offensichtlich regelmäßiger ödemerzeugend. Die Ausbildung des Ödems verläuft rasch; bei Kaninchen drang schon 4 min nach der i.v. Gabe Schaum aus der Nase. Das histologische Bild der Lungen zeigt Ödem, Hyperämie, Hämorrhagien sowie stark eingeengte Bronchien. Riechert (1941) untersuchte die Beziehungen zwischen krampf- und ödemprovozierenden Eigenschaften von Pentetrazol. Die untere i.v. Krampfdosis für Ratten betrug bei einer Injektionsdauer von 1 min 40 mg/kg; Lungenödem oder -hyperämie waren unter diesen Bedingungen nicht nachweisbar. 60 mg/kg verursachten mittelschweres Ödem (Anstieg des relativen Lungengewichtes auf etwa das doppelte der Norm). Kurz nach Ablauf der Krampfphase war das Ödem am stärksten ausgeprägt, klang dann aber bald wieder ab; 7—8 Std nach der Pentetrazolzufuhr war das Lungengewicht wieder normal. Bei narkotisierten Tieren (Tribromäthanol) lösten die gleichen Pentetrazoldosen weder Krämpfe noch Lungenödem aus. Auch wiederholte i.p. Gaben unterschwelliger Pentetrazoldosen (2—6 Einzeldosen von 20—40 mg/kg in Intervallen von 30—90 min) wirkten krampf- und ödemprovozierend.

Andere Verbindungen aus der Gruppe der zentralen Analeptica besitzen ebenfalls ödemerzeugende Eigenschaften, wenn auch in nicht sehr ausgeprägter Form. Hahn (1947, 1948) konnte bei Kaninchen mit krampfwirksamen Nikethamiddosen

(Coramin) nur in Einzelfällen Lungenödem auslösen; bei Ratten gelang es selbst mit tödlichen Dosen nicht (Riechert, 1951). Letale Dosen von Homocamfin (Hexeton) verursachten nur bei einem Teil der behandelten Ratten Lungenödem. Pikrotoxin (4—5 mg/kg i. v.) bewirkte bei der gleichen Species regelmäßiger allerdings nur geringgradiges Lungenödem (Riechert, 1951).

Dem Pentetrazollungenödem liegt nach Ansicht von Jarisch u. Thoma (1940) eine Blutüberfüllung und Drucksteigerung im kleinen Kreislauf sowie ein lokaler vasomotorischer Mechanismus zugrunde. Nach Riechert (1951) ist an diesen Vorgängen eine zentrale Sympathicuserregung maßgeblich beteiligt; die Schutzfunktion, die das sympatholytisch wirkende Ergotamintartrat (Gynergen) bei der Pentetrazolvergiftung besitzt, wird in diesem Sinn verstanden. Bronchoconstriction und Hypersekretion üben einen zusätzlich schädigenden bzw. komplizierenden Einfluß aus. Bei narkotisierten Tieren (besonders in Chloralosenarkose) kann durch Nicethamid- und in geringem Maß auch durch Pentetrazolgaben die Speichelsekretion so gesteigert sein, daß bedingt durch die Aspiration größerer Sekretmengen Lungenödem vorgetäuscht wird (Hahn, 1948).

l) Verschiedene chemische Verbindungen

Weitere chemische Verbindungen, die ödemprovozierende Eigenschaften besitzen, sind bisher nur vereinzelt als experimentelle Ödemnoxe verwendet worden; über andere liegen lediglich Zufallsbeobachtungen vor, die kein Urteil über ihren Wert für Versuchszwecke zulassen. Auf einige dieser Verbindungen wird anhand von Literaturzitaten hingewiesen.

Alloxan verursacht, in Dosen von 50—100 mg/kg i.v. verabreicht, bei Hunden Lungenödem (Gruhzit *et al.*, 1951; Aviado, 1953; Aviado und Schmidt, 1957). Unmittelbar nach der Injektion reagierten die narkotisierten Tiere mit einer passageren Apnoe, nach 10—30 min mit progressiv zunehmender Polypnoe; innerhalb der folgenden 30 min wurde Schaum in der Trachealkanüle sichtbar. Als Ödemursache wird eine Capillarschädigung (Gruhzit *et al.*, 1951) sowie eine lokale Constriction der Lungenvenen (Aviado, 1953; Aviado und Schmidt, 1957) in Erwägung gezogen.

Verschiedene *Barbiturate* sind als Ödemnoxe verwendet worden. Moon und Morgan (1936a, b) verabreichten Hunden 2mal tgl. 3 Tage lang 300 mg Phenobarbital-Natrium pro kg Körpergewicht p.o.; der Tod trat nach 5 Tagen ein. Bei Kaninchen entwickelte sich nach i.v. Injektion von 200—600 mg/kg Aprobarbital (Somnifen) oder 500—800 mg/kg Phenobarbital (Luminal, Gardenal) akutes Lungenödem (Bariéty und Kohler, 1951).

Parasympathicomimetica. Acetylcholinchlorid, in letalen Dosen (40—420 mg/kg) i.m. injiziert, bewirkte bei mehr als der Hälfte der so behandelten Ratten und Meerschweinchen (in einem geringeren Prozentsatz auch bei Kaninchen) Ödem, Hyperämie und Hämorrhagien der Lunge (Altschul und Laskin, 1946). Mit tödlichen *Neostigminmethylsulfatdosen* (0,2—3 ml einer Lösung 1:2000) wurden ähnliche Resultate erzielt (Altschul und Laskin, 1946). Andere Cholinesterasehemmer wie Physostigmin, Parathion und weitere anticholinesteratische Insecticide sowie Pilocarpin verursachen ebenfalls lungenödemähnliche Bilder (Aviado und Schmidt, 1959). Auch *Muscarin* besitzt nach Grossmann (1887, 1889) ödemprovozierende Eigenschaften. Der Autor injizierte Hunden 0,25—0,5%ige Lösungen (genauere Dosierung nicht ersichtlich) und stellte die Diagnose aufgrund des Obduktionsbefundes. Als Ödemursache wird eine Drucksteigerung im Pulmonalkreislauf angenommen. Muscarin bewirkt ähnlich wie Acetylcholin Bradykardie, die für die Drucksteigerung in den Pulmonalvenen verantwortlich sein könnte (Campbell *et al.*, 1951). Wieweit die durch Muscarin (s. Waser, 1961) bzw. Pilocarpin und

Cholinesterasehemmer (s. Aviado und Schmidt, 1959) ausgelöste Hypersekretion der cholinergisch innervierten Bronchial- und Speicheldrüsen zur Flüssigkeitsansammlung in den Luftwegen beiträgt bzw. das Krankheitsbild komplizierend beeinflußt, ist nicht geklärt.,

Jod und einige *Jodverbindungen* können Lungenödem auslösen. Zeissl (1895) beobachtete es bei Hunden nach i.v. Zufuhr von 1 ml einer Lösung von 2,1 g Jod und 2,2 g Natriumjodid in 100 ml Aqu. dest. Bei Ratten — allerdings nur oberhalb einer gewissen Altersgrenze — traten Lungenödem und Pleuraexsudate nach i.p. Gabe von 1,5 g/kg Natriumjodid auf (Trotter, 1952). Auch bei Katzen und Kaninchen läßt sich durch parenterale Zufuhr von Natriumjodid Lungenödem provozieren (Dessnitzkaja, 1960). *Jodacetamid* (2—4 mg/kg i.v.) wurde von Gruhzit *et al.* (1951) zur Ödemerzeugung bei Hunden verwendet.

Silbernitrat ($AgNO_3$) wirkt bei verschiedenen Applikationsweisen ödemerzeugend. Das ursprünglich von Coelho und Rocheta (1933) angegebene Verfahren ein- oder mehrfacher Injektionen einer 10%igen Silbernitratlösung (1mal 0,5 ml/kg bzw. 10—15 Injektionen von je 0,1—0,2 ml innerhalb von 5—10 min) in die Wand des linken Herzventrikels narkotisierter Hunde, wie es von Luis und Duarte (1960) bzw. von Testelli *et al.* (1960) geübt wurde, scheint nur eine geringe Erfolgsquote zu besitzen; häufiger sterben die Tiere an Herzflimmern. Besser wirksam ist offensichtlich die Injektion in die Arteria pulmonalis (Luis und Duarte, 1960) oder auch in eine Vene (0,8 ml/kg einer 0,4%igen $AgNO_3$-Lösung) (Serebrovskaya, 1960). Romanov (1967) injizierte in 20—30 sec in die Vena femoralis 0,15 ml/kg einer 0,1 n $AgNO_3$-Lösung. Die Überlebensdauer betrug im Durchschnitt 24 min; Tod unter typischem Lungenödem. Wenn 2—3 min nach der Silbernitratgabe Unitiol (2,3-Dimercaptopropan-1-Sulfonsäure) in der Menge von 100 mg/kg i.v. gegeben wurde, konnte das Ödem verhindert werden. Als Ödemursache werden hämodynamische Veränderungen im Pulmonalkreislauf angenommen.

Die Entstehung von Lungenödem bei Versuchstieren wurde ferner beobachtet nach Verabreichung von Neosalvarsan i.v., besonders in gealtertem Zustand (Krayer, 1930), verschiedenen Eisenpräparaten i.v. (Nissim, 1954), Galle und Gallensalzen i.v. oder i.p. (Moon u. Morgan, 1936a, b), Monomethylthioacetamid i.p. (Femmer, 1958), Methylsalicylat (Kotowschtschikow, 1913; Lomeo *et al.*, 1960), Phosgenoxim i.v. (Mikhailow, 1957; Mitsov, 1957), Methylenblau und Methylenviolett (Lagrange und Promel, 1949), verschiedenen basischen Farbstoffen (Visscher *et al.*, 1962; Goetzman, 1962). Weitere Daten finden sich bei Petri (1930) sowie Visscher *et al.* (1956).

V. Sonstige Ödemursachen

1. Allergie und Anaphylaxie

Anaphylaxie und anaphylaktischer Schock gehen bei Versuchstieren in der Regel nicht mit Lungenödem einher (Kind *et al.*, 1961; Treadwell *et al.*, 1960). Unter besonderen Voraussetzungen kann die Injektion heterologer Sera jedoch Lungenödem auslösen. Kind *et al.* (1961, 1964) benutzten zur Ödemprovokation bei Mäusen Kaninchen-Antiserum gegen Zellen in vitro gezüchteter experimenteller Mäusetumoren. Zur Gewinnung des Antiserums erhielten Kaninchen zunächst in 4tägigen Intervallen 4 i.v. Injektionen einer Aufschwemmung von je 10^4 in vitro kultivierter Ehrlich-Ascitestumorzellen, anschließend 2mal wöchentlich ein Gemisch von Ehrlich-Zellen (10^7) und Freundschem Adjuvans subcutan. Nach frühestens 8wöchiger Behandlung wurde den Kaninchen Blut entnommen, von dem das Serum abgetrennt wurde. Mäuse im Gewicht von etwa 20 g wurden zunächst durch i.p. Inoculation von Pertussiserregern (Bordetella pert., etwa

$5 \cdot 10^9$ pro Tier) in einen Zustand erhöhter Empfindlichkeit versetzt. 5—8 Tage nach dieser Vorbehandlung erhielten die Mäuse je 0,5 ml des Kaninchenantiserums gegen Ehrlich-Zellen i.v. Wenige Minuten (5—20) nach der Injektion starben die Tiere unter Austritt schaumig-blutiger Flüssigkeit aus der Nase. Das mittlere Lungengewicht war auf 350 mg angestiegen (Kontrollen 186 mg). Die Injektion von normalem Kaninchenserum und Kaninchenantiserum gegen Mäuseglobulin hatte kein Lungenödem zur Folge.

Das Antiserum gegen Globulin führte jedoch ebenfalls innerhalb von 5—15 min den Tod der Tiere herbei. Die Vorbehandlung mit Pertussiserregern steigert die Empfindlichkeit der Tiere für Histamin, 5-Hydroxytryptamin und anaphylaktische Prozesse (Kind, 1958), ist jedoch keine unabdingbare Voraussetzung für die Ausbildung des Lungenödems (Kind *et al.*, 1964). Bei der experimentellen Prüfung von Kaninchenantiseren gegen verschiedene andere Mäusegewebe erwiesen sich weiterhin nur Antiseren gegen Zellen des Mastocytoms P-815 (ein experimenteller Mastzellentumor der Maus) und gegen in vitro gezüchtete Zellen des permanenten Fibroblastenstammes L der Maus als ödemprovozierend (Kind *et al.*, 1964).

Möglicherweise ist endogenes 5-Hydroxytryptamin (5-HT) an der Auslösung dieser Form des Lungenödems beteiligt. Der 5-HT-Gehalt der Lungen von Mäusen, die Antiserum gegen Ehrlich-Zellen erhalten hatten, war jedenfalls im Vergleich zu unbehandelten Kontrollen beträchtlich erhöht. Veränderungen des Histamingehaltes der Lungen waren dagegen nicht nachweisbar.

2. Urämie

Urämisches Lungenödem gilt als eine häufig vorkommende Komplikation schwerer Nierenerkrankungen (Lit. s. Lindquist, 1964). Bei Versuchstieren läßt sich Lungenödem auf dem Boden einer experimentellen Urämie dagegen nur in Einzelfällen auslösen. Urämie kann aber eine prädisponierende Rolle bei der Entstehung von experimentellem Lungenödem verschiedener Genese spielen, während sie in anderen Fällen die Ödementwicklung sogar zu hemmen scheint.

Lindquist (1964) hat die Bedeutung der experimentellen Urämie für die Ausbildung von Lungenödem eingehend studiert und insbesondere Wechselbeziehungen zwischen Urämie und einer Reihe von Ödemursachen herauszuarbeiten versucht. Die Untersuchungen wurden an Kaninchen beiderlei Geschlechts im Gewicht von 2,2—2,5 kg durchgeführt; die Tiere wurden vor Versuchsbeginn unter Standardbedingungen in Einzelställen gehalten und hinsichtlich ihres Wohlbefindens kontrolliert (Körpergewicht, klinischer Befund). Urämie wurde durch bilaterale Ureterunterbindung herbeigeführt. Der Eingriff wurde oberhalb der Schambeine unter Lidocain-(Xylocain-)Anaesthesie der Blase vorgenommen. Die Tiere wurden am Operationstag sowie 1, 2, 3 oder 4 Tage nach der Operation durch Entblutung getötet, soweit sie nicht bereits spontan an Urämie gestorben waren. Zur Ödembewertung diente ein breites Spektrum diagnostischer Verfahren. Zur Diagnose in vivo: Erscheinung und Verhalten des Tieres, Atemfrequenz, Herzfrequenz, Elektrokardiogramm, Thorax-Röntgenbefund. Zur postmortalen Beurteilung: Makroskopischer Autopsiebefund der Lunge, Ausdehnung und Menge der Ödemflüssigkeit in der Lunge, Lungengewicht, Wassergehalt der Lunge, Lungenvolumen, mikroskopischer Lungenbefund. Der Urämiegrad wurde aufgrund des Serumkaliumgehaltes und des Nichteiweißstickstoffgehaltes des Blutes bewertet.

Nach der beidseitigen Ureterunterbindung kam es bei allen Tieren als Ausdruck der Urämie zu einem graduell bis zum 4. Tag zunehmenden Anstieg der Reststickstoff- und Serumkaliumwerte. Röntgenologische Lungenveränderungen waren dagegen nur bei maximal 3% der Tiere (am 3. Tag) nachweisbar. Auch andere Ödemsymptome wurden in vivo nicht beobachtet. Ebenso konnte post mortem bei der großen Mehrzahl der Versuchstiere mit verschiedenen diagnostischen Verfahren (s.o.) kein Lungenödem festgestellt werden. Als Beispiel werden die Werte für das Lungengewicht und den Wassergehalt der Lunge von Kontroll- und Urämietieren angeführt.

	Lungengewicht in g/kg Körpergewicht	Wassergehalt der Lunge in %
Kontrolltiere	4,17 ± 0,53	81,0 ± 0,9
Urämietiere	4,25 ± 0,45	80,0 ± 1,3

Im Gegensatz zu diesem negativen Lungenbefund zeigten die urämischen Tiere eine beträchtliche, mit der Urämiedauer zunehmende Ansammlung von Ascitesflüssigkeit (am 3. bzw. 4. Tag post operationem durchschnittlich 108 ml Ascitesflüssigkeit je Tier). Pleuraexsudate waren nur bei einem Teil der Tiere (45%) und nur in geringem Ausmaß (durchschnittlich 3 ml) nachweisbar.

Aus diesen Resultaten ist zu folgern, daß durch bilaterale Ureterunterbindung verursachte Urämie für sich allein nicht ausreicht, um bei Kaninchen ein Lungenödem herbeizuführen.

Bilaterale Ureterunterbindung steigerte jedoch die Neigung zur Entwicklung von Lungenödem, das durch Flüssigkeitsüberladung mittels Dextraninfusion (6% Dextran in 0,9% NaCl-Lösung mit Zusatz von 0,24 g $CaCl_2$ und 0,42 g KCl; Infusionsvolumen: 12% des Körpergewichts; Infusionsrate: 1,3 ml/min/kg) provoziert wurde. Auch bei dem durch Narkotalnarkose (Isopropyl-β-bromallyl-N-malonylcarbamid-Na 0,055 g, Phenazon 0,08 g, Glycerin 0,05 g, Aqu. steril. ad 1 ml; 1,7 ml/kg Körpergewicht) induzierten Lungenödem förderte Urämie die Ödemausbildung. In beiden Fällen bestand eine Parallelität zwischen der Neigung zur Ödementstehung und dem Urämiegrad. Die Urämie hatte dagegen keinen Einfluß auf das durch Bivagotomie und durch Adrenalininjektion verursachte Lungenödem. Auch bei der Kombination von Flüssigkeitsüberladung und Adrenalininjektion steigerte Urämie die Ödementwicklung nicht. Aus diesen Befunden folgert Lindquist, daß bilaterale Ureterunterbindung nur unter bestimmten Bedingungen die Ödembereitschaft erhöht, unter anderen Bedingungen dieselbe jedoch reduzieren kann. So führt Urämie in Verbindung mit Flüssigkeitsüberladung offenbar nur dann zu erhöhter Ödembereitschaft, wenn damit eine Zunahme des Blutvolumens einhergeht.

VI. Ödem der perfundierten Lunge

Isolierte perfundierte Lungen, perfundierte Lungen in situ oder Herz-Lungenpräparate sind in der Vergangenheit häufig zur Analyse der bei der Lungenödementstehung wirksamen lokalen Faktoren verwendet worden. Einige technische Hinweise für die Herstellung derartiger Präparate sind auf S. 188—191 und 201f. gegeben worden. Weitere Angaben finden sich in der Literatur z.B. bei Flury (1925), der die älteren Arbeiten einschließlich methodischer Vorschriften gesammelt und besprochen hat. Man kann die ödemerzeugende Noxe auf die isolierten Thoraxorgane eines vorher gesunden Tieres einwirken lassen oder die Lunge lebender Tiere schädigen und die weiteren Untersuchungen am isolierten Organ vornehmen. Zur Ödemprovokation am isolierten Organ eignen sich vor allem hämodynamische Maßnahmen sowie direkt am Lungenparenchym angreifende chemische Noxen.

Verfahren zur Ödemauslösung am Herz-Lungen-Präparat durch Hypervolämie und Hyposmie (Paine *et al.*, 1949a) sind auf S. 201f. im Zusammenhang mit der Erzeugung derartiger Zustände beim intakten Tier beschrieben worden.

Die Grundlagen für die Ödementwicklung in der perfundierten Lunge in Abhängigkeit vom Perfusionsdruck haben Hughes, May u. Widdicombe (1958a) eingehend studiert. Zur Gewinnung der Präparate wurden Kaninchen im Gewicht von 2—2,4 kg narkotisiert (35 mg/kg Pentobarbital-Na), heparinisiert (10 mg/kg) und nach Einbindung einer Trachealkanüle unter Überdruckbeatmung in der Medianlinie thorakotomiert. In der Pulmonalarterie und im linken Herzohr wurde je ein Polyäthylenschlauch fixiert und um den Sulcus atrioventricularis eine fest schließende Ligatur gelegt. Unmittelbar darauf begann die Perfusion, so daß der

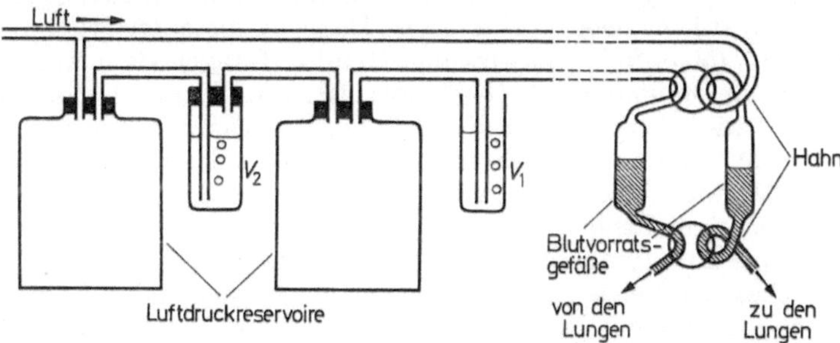

Abb. 17. Schematische Darstellung des Perfusionsapparates nach Hughes *et al.* (1958a). Erläuterungen im Text

Lungenkreislauf nicht länger als 1—2 min unterbrochen war. Der Perfusionsapparat erzeugte einen pulsationsfreien Blutstrom. Die Druckdifferenz zwischen Arterien und Venen betrug 2—4 mm Hg. Auf diese Weise konnte der mittlere Capillardruck, angenommen als Mittelwert zwischen arteriellem und venösem Druck verhältnismäßig genau abgeschätzt werden. In Abb. 17 ist der Perfusionsapparat schematisch wiedergegeben. Der mittlere Perfusionsdruck wurde durch Ventil V_1, die Druckdifferenz zwischen Arterie und Vene durch Ventil V_2 reguliert. Ein zweifacher Vierwegehahn zur gleichzeitigen Umschaltung von Luftdruck und Blutstrom erlaubte jedes der beiden Blutreservoire alternierend als Zu- bzw. Rückflußgefäß zu verwenden. Die Umschaltung erfolgte, wenn der Flüssigkeitsspiegel zwischen beiden Gefäßen um 1—2 cm differierte. Mit Hilfe einer Meßskala konnte das jeweils im Apparat befindliche Flüssigkeitsvolumen sowie die Flußrate geschätzt werden. Der Perfusionsdruck wurde mit einem Hg-Manometer in unmittelbarer Nachbarschaft der Lungen gemessen. Die Vorratsgefäße, die das heparinisierte Blut eines Spenderkaninchens enthielten, wurden in einem Wasserbad temperiert, so daß das Blut beim Eintritt in die Lunge eine Temperatur von 37—38° C hatte. Die Beatmung erfolgte mit einer Frequenz von 20/min und einem Druck von 12 cm H_2O; der Exspirationsdruck betrug 2 cm H_2O, so daß kein vollständiger Kollaps der Lunge eintreten konnte. Der mittlere Perfusionsdruck betrug während einer anfänglichen Kontrollperiode 10 mm Hg und wurde dann erhöht. Die Geschwindigkeit der Ödementstehung ist von der Höhe des Perfusionsdruckes und von der Zusammensetzung der Perfusionsflüssigkeit abhängig. Bei Druckwerten zwischen 20 und 30 mm Hg verdoppelte sich das Lungengewicht innerhalb von 20 min, bei Werten zwischen 30 und 40 mm Hg erfolgte die Ödementwicklung noch schneller. Ebenso bewirkte die Verwendung von Ringer-Locke-Lösung anstelle von Blut zur Perfusion eine erhebliche Beschleunigung des Prozesses. Die Ödembewertung kann am Ende des Versuches z.B. aufgrund des

Lungen-/Herzgewichtsindexes oder auch während des Versuches nach dem Verfahren von Born (1954) vorgenommen werden (s. S. 188f.). Zwischen vermehrter Gefäßfüllung und Ödem der Lunge versuchten die Autoren aufgrund von Eisenanalysen des Organs zu differenzieren (vgl. S. 189).

Einige der chemischen Verbindungen, die eine weite Verbreitung als Ödemnoxe für intakte Tiere gefunden haben, sind am perfundierten Organ unwirksam. Born (1954) hat mit Hilfe des auf S. 188f. beschriebenen Verfahrens den Einfluß einiger dieser Wirkstoffe auf isolierte Kaninchenlungen vergleichend untersucht. Die ödemerzeugenden Stoffe können den Vorratsflaschen für die Perfusionslösung zugesetzt oder in den Perfusionsschlauch eingespritzt werden. Zusatz von Adrenalin (10^{-4} mol; Einwirkung 3 min) zur Perfusionsflüssigkeit oder Injektion der Verbindung (0,1—1,0 mg) verursachte kein Lungenödem. Auch Histamin (geprüft bis zu Dosen von 0,1 mg) war wirkungslos. Dagegen löste der Histaminliberator Compound 48/80 (50 µg/ml; Einwirkung 10 min) Lungenödem aus. Denselben Effekt hatte Ammoniumchlorid (10^{-3} mol; 10 min). Beide Verbindungen bewirkten einen Anstieg des Perfusionsdruckes. Auch unter dem Einfluß von Chlorpikrin (5×10^{-4} M) wurde ein vorübergehender Anstieg des Perfusionsdruckes und nach wenigen Minuten eine fortschreitende Zunahme des Lungengewichtes beobachtet, die von einer Erhöhung des Atemwiderstandes begleitet war. Perfusion mit 2,4-Dinitrophenol (10^{-3} mol) führte dagegen zu einem graduellen Abfall des Perfusionsdruckes bei gleichzeitigem Anstieg der Perfusionsrate und nach einer Latenzzeit von durchschnittlich 19 min ebenfalls zur Ausbildung von Lungenödem. Niedrigere Konzentrationen (bis zu 10^{-4} mol) hatten keinen Effekt. Lungenödem entwickelte sich ferner innerhalb einiger Minuten, wenn der Perfusionsflüssigkeit Quecksilberverbindungen ($HgCl_2$, Mersalyl) in Konzentrationen von 10^{-4}—10^{-3} mol zugesetzt wurden. Durch Thiosemicarbazid (10^{-3} mol; Einwirkung bis zu 60 min) konnte an perfundierten Ratten- und Kaninchenlungen kein Ödem erzeugt werden (Tennekoon, 1954). Alloxan (Zusatz von 100 mg zum Perfusionsblut) rief dagegen nicht nur in der Lunge des intakten Hundes, sondern auch am perfundierten Organ Ödem hervor (Aviado u. Schmidt, 1957). Verschiedene basische Farbstoffe (wie Methylenblau) sowie einige polybasische makromolekulare Verbindungen (z. B. Protamin) sind ebenfalls am perfundierten Organ wirksam, allerdings nur, wenn die Perfusionsflüssigkeit Erythrocyten enthält (Visscher *et al.*, 1962; Goetzman, 1962).

Ödemprovokation mit inhalierbaren Giftstoffen ist auch am isolierten Organ versucht worden. Ein Verfahren, das die Applikation von Reizgasen unter diesen Bedingungen ermöglicht, ist von Daly *et al.* (1946) angegeben worden. Unter der Einwirkung von Phosgen wurden während der 7—8stündigen Versuchsdauer zwar Schäden an der Bronchialschleimhaut und Bronchoconstriction hervorgerufen; die Ödementstehung war im Vergleich zu Kontrollorganen jedoch nicht beschleunigt.

Die perfundierte Lunge neigt in Abhängigkeit von den Versuchsbedingungen früher oder später spontan zur Ausbildung von Ödem. Mehrere Faktoren können ursächlich daran beteiligt sein: die Zusammensetzung der Perfusionsflüssigkeit und abhängig davon der kolloidosmotische Druck, der pH-Wert des Perfusates, toxische Komponenten der Flüssigkeit, der Perfusionsdruck, die Abbindung der Vena cava und die damit verbundene Abflußbehinderung der Lymphflüssigkeit, mechanische und chemische Umstände der künstlichen Beatmung (insbesondere der CO_2-Gehalt der Atemluft) (Barry, 1923; Courtice u. Phipps, 1946; Daly *et al.*, 1946; Hughes *et al.*, 1958a; Newton, 1932; Piiper, 1960; Rusznyák *et al.*, 1957; Wood u. Moe, 1942). Andererseits lassen mehrere der typischen, am intakten Tier wirksamen Ödemnoxen einen Einfluß auf das isolierte Organ vermissen. Auch dort, wo zwischen der Einwirkung lokal angreifender Gifte und der Ödemmanifestation eine bestimmte Latenzzeit liegt, wie z.B. bei der Phosgenschädigung (8—10 Std), wird die Methode versagen, weil es schon vorher zur spontanen Ödementwicklung kommt (Daly *et al.*, 1946). Die Bedeutung dieser Technik für das Studium von Ödemproblemen ist demnach recht begrenzt; zur Klärung spezieller und geeigneter Fragen wird sie nützlich sein.

Literatur

Adams, W. E., J. F. Perkins, A. Flores, P. Chao, and M. Castellanos: The significance of pulmonary hypertension as a cause of death following pulmonary resection. J. thorac. Surg. **26**, 407—418 (1953).

Alexandrow, T.: Über die Entstehungsweise des Stauungsödems in den Lungen. Zbl. allg. Path. path. Anat. **4**, 691—693 (1893).

Allgood, R. J., W. G. Wolfe, P. A. Ebert, and D. C. Sabiston Jr.: Effects of CO_2 on bronchoconstriction after pulmonary artery occlusion. Amer. J. Physiol. **214**, 772 (1968).

Altschul, R., and M. M. Laskin: Microscopic lesions in acetylcholine shock. Arch. Path. **41**, 11—16 (1946).

Altschule, M. D.: Acute pulmonary edema. New York: Grune & Stratton 1954.

— Neuere Ergebnisse über die Pathogenese des Lungenödems. Klin. Wschr. **34**, 169—174 (1956).

— D. R. Gilligan, and N. Zamcheck: The effects on the cardiovascular system of fluids administered intravenously in man. IV. The lung volume and pulmonary dynamics. J. clin. Invest. **21**, 365—368 (1942).

Aravanis, C., A. Libretti, E. Jona, J. F. Polli, C. K. Liu, and A. A. Luisada: Pulmonary reflexes in pulmonary edema? Amer. J. Physiol. **189**, 132—136 (1957).

Assmann, A.: Krankheiten der Atmungsorgane. In: H. Schwiegk u. A. Jores: Lehrbuch der inneren Medizin, 7. Aufl. Berlin-Göttingen-Heidelberg: Springer 1949.

Aviado, D. M.: Pathogenesis of alloxan pulmonary edema investigated by phosphorus^{32} and iodine^{131}. Fed. Proc. **12**, 299 (1953).

— The pharmacology pf the pulmonary circulation. Pharmacol. Rev. **12**, 159—239 (1960).

— Nervous influences on the pulmonary circulation. Naunyn-Schmiedebergs Arch. exp. Path. Pharmak. **240**, 446—452 (1961).

—, and C. F. Schmidt: Respiratory burns with special reference to pulmonary edema and congestion. Circulation **6**, 666—680 (1952).

— — Pathogenesis of pulmonary edema by alloxan. Circulat. Res. **5**, 180—186 (1957).

— — Physiologic basis for the treatment of pulmonary edema. J. chron. Dis. **9**, 495—509 (1959).

Bariéty, M., et D. Kohler: Action des barbituriques dans l'oedème pulmonaire aigu expérimental du lapin. C.R. Soc. Biol. (Paris) **145**, 182—183 (1951).

Barry, D. T.: Pulmonary oedema and congestion in the heart-lung preparation. J. Physiol. (Lond.) **57**, 368—378 (1923).

Bartels, H., u. G. Rodewald: Die alveolär-arterielle Sauerstoffdruckdifferenz und das Problem des Gasaustausches in der menschlichen Lunge. Pflügers Arch. ges. Physiol. **258**, 163—176 (1953).

Bean, J. W.: Reserpine, chlorpromazine and the hypothalamus in reactions to oxygen at high pressure. Amer. J. Physiol. **187**, 389—394 (1956).

—, and R. Bauer: Thyroid in pulmonary injury induced by oxygen in high concentration at atmospheric pressure. Proc. Soc. exp. Biol. (N.Y.) **81**, 693—694 (1952).

—, and P. C. Johnson: Influence of hypophysis on pulmonary injury induced by exposure to oxygen at high pressure and by pneumococcus. Amer. J. Physiol. **171**, 451—458 (1952).

— — Epinephrine and neurogenic factors in the pulmonary edema and CNS-reactions induced by oxygen at high pressure. Amer. J. Physiol. **180**, 438—444 (1955).

—, and C. W. Smith: Hypophyseal and adrenocortical factors in pulmonary damage induced by oxygen at atmospheric pressure. Amer. J. Physiol. **172**, 169—174 (1953).

Beecher, H. K., M. F. Warren, and A. Murphy: Comparison of cyclopropane and ether anesthesia on lymph production. Amer. J. Physiol. **154**, 475—479 (1948).

Bennhold, H., u. H. Ott: Der Sauerstofftransport. In: Handbuch der allgemeinen Pathologie, Bd. V/1. Berlin-Göttingen-Heidelberg: Springer 1961.

Bersaques, J. de, and I. R. Leusen: The direct influence of ammonium chloride on the respiratory centre. Arch. int. Pharmacodyn. **97**, 13—16 (1954).

Beyer, K.: Zur Bestimmung von „nitrosen Gasen". Z. anorg. allg. Chem. **250**, 321—330 (1943).

Bickel, E., u. J. Dieckhoff: Kollidon und Gefäßabdichtung — zugleich ein Beitrag zur Behandlung des experimentellen Lungenödems. Dtsch. med. J. **5**, 463—465 (1954).

Bollman, J. L.: A cage which limits the activity of rats. J. Lab. clin. Med. **33**, 1348 (1948).
Bondurant, S., J. B. Hickam, and J. K. Isley: Pulmonary and circulatory effects of acute pulmonary vascular engagement in normal subjects. J. clin. Invest. **36**, 59—66 (1957).
Born, G. V. R.: Acute oedema in the isolated, perfused lungs of rabbits. J. Physiol. (Lond.) **124**, 502—514 (1954).
Borst, H. G., E. Berglund, J. L. Whittenberger, I. Mead, M. McGregor, and C. Collier: The effect of pulmonary vascular pressures on the mechanical properties of the lungs of anesthetized dogs. J. clin. Invest. **36**, 1708—1714 (1957).
Bostroem, B., u. J. Piiper: Über arteriovenöse Anastomosen und Kurzschlußdurchblutung der Lunge. Pflügers Arch. ges. Physiol. **261**, 165—171 (1955).
Box, G. E. P., and H. Cullumbine: The effect of exposure to sub-lethal doses of phosgene on the subsequent L(Ct) 50 for rats and mice. Brit. J. Pharmacol. **2**, 38—55 (1947).
Boyd, E. M.: Expectorants and respiratory tract fluid. Pharmacol. Rev. **6**, 521—542 (1954).
—, and M. S. Lapp: On the expectorant action of parasympathomimetic drugs. J. Pharmacol. exp. Ther. **87**, 24—32 (1946).
—, and W. F. Perry: Urethane administration and potassium content of bronchial secretions in the cat. Proc. Soc. exp. Biol. (N.Y.) **57**, 334—335 (1944).
— — Respiratory tract fluid and inhalation of phosgene. J. Pharm. Pharmacol. **12**, 726—732 (1960).
— —, and M. E. T. Stevens: The effect of damage to the tracheal mucosa upon the drainage of respiratory tract fluid. Amer. J. Physiol. **140**, 467—473 (1944).
Brown-Séquard, E.: On the production of haemorrhage, anaemia, oedema and emphysema in the lungs by injuries to the base of the brain. Lancet **1871 I**, 6.
Brunn, F.: Experimentelles zum Lungenödem. Wien. klin. Wschr. **46**, 262—265 (1933).
— Untersuchungen über den elastischen Lungenwiderstand. Helv. physiol. pharmacol. Acta **15**, 315—327 (1957).
Bucher, K.: Pharmakodynamische Alteration des elastischen Lungenwiderstandes. Erhöhung durch Histamin und durch Adrenalin. Helv. physiol. pharmacol. Acta **18**, 1—9 (1960).
Büchner, F.: Spezielle Pathologie, S. 155ff. München u. Berlin: Urban & Schwarzenberg 1955.
Byers, D. H., and B. E. Saltzman: Determination of ozone in air by neutral and alkaline iodide procedures. Amer. ind. Hyg. Ass. J. **19**, 251—257 (1958).
Cameron, G. R.: Pulmonary oedema. Brit. med. J. **1948 I**, 965—972.
—, and F. C. Courtice: The production and removal of oedema fluid in the lung after exposure to carbonyl chloride (phosgene). J. Physiol. (Lond.) **105**, 175—185 (1946).
—, and S. N. De: Experimental pulmonary oedema of nervous origin. J. Path. Bact. **61**, 375—387 (1949).
—, and H. Neuberger: Ketene as a noxious gas. J. Path. Bact. **45**, 653—660 (1937).
—, and A. H. Sheikh: The experimental production of pulmonary oedema with ammonium salts, together with a classification of lung oedemas. J. Path. Bact. **63**, 609—617 (1951).
Campbell, G. S., F. J. Haddy, W. L. Adams, and M. B. Visscher: Circulatory changes and pulmonary lesions in dogs following increased intracranial pressure and the effect of atropine upon such changes. Amer. J. Physiol. **158**, 96—102 (1949).
— —, and M. B. Visscher: Effect of acute bradycardia on pulmonary vascular pressures in anesthetized dogs. Proc. Soc. exp. Biol. (N.Y.) **71**, 52—54 (1951).
—, and M. B. Visscher: Pulmonary lesions in guinea pigs with increased intracranial pressure and the effect of bilateral cervical vagotomy. Amer. J. Physiol. **157**, 130—134 (1949).
Campbell, J. A.: Body temperature and oxygen poisoning. J. Physiol. (Lond.) **89**, 17P—18P (1937a).
— Oxygen poisoning and the thyroid gland. J. Physiol. (Lond.) **90**, 91P—92P (1937b).
Cassen, B., W. Gutfreund, and M. Moody: Demonstration of central nervous mediation of acute pulmonary edema produced by intravenously administered epinephrine. Proc. Soc. exp. Biol. (N.Y.) **93**, 251—253 (1956).
— P. Kalian, and H. Gass: High speed photography of the motion of mice subjected to laboratory produced air blast. J. Aviat. Med. **23**, 104—114 (1952a).
—, and K. Kistler: Development of acute pulmonary edema in mice and rats and an interpretation. Amer. J. Physiol. **178**, 49—52 (1954a).
— — Effects of preadministering various drugs on the acute pulmonary edema produced by blast injury and by the intravenous injection of epinephrine. Amer. J. Physiol. **178**, 53—57 (1954b).
— —, and W. Mankiewiez: Lung hemorrhage produced in heparinized mice by air blast. J. Aviat. Med. **23**, 115—119 (1952b).
— — — Some effects of air blast on mechanically constrained mice. J. Aviat. Med. **23**, 120—129 (1952c).

Cate, W. R., and R. A. Daniel: "Wet Lung" — an experimental study. II. Neurogenic factor. Ann. Surg. **127**, 847—857 (1948).

Ceelen, W.: Lungenödem. In: Handbuch der speziellen pathologischen Anatomie und Histologie, Bd. III/3, S. 132—145. Berlin-Göttingen-Heidelberg: Springer 1931.

Cheng, K. K.: Protein content of oedema fluid from lungs. In: G. R. Cameron, Brit. med. J. **1948 I**, 965—972.

— The effects of obstructing the blood-flow through the pulmonary vessels: an experimental study in rats. Quart. J. exp. Physiol. **36**, 101—117 (1950).

Church, F. W.: A mixed color method for the determination of cadmium in air and biological samples by the use of dithizone. J. industr. Hyg. **29**, 34 (1947).

Clamann, H. G., u. H. Becker-Freyseng: Einwirkung des Sauerstoffes auf den Organismus bei höherem als normalem Partialdruck unter besonderer Berücksichtigung des Menschen. Luftfahrtmedizin **4**, 1—10 (1940).

Clemedson, C. J.: An experimental study on air blast injuries. Acta physiol. scand. **18**, Suppl. **61**, 1—200 (1949).

Clemens, H. J.: Vorkommen, Lokalisation und Bedeutung von sauren Mucopolysacchariden in der Lunge. Acta histochem. (Jena) **2**, 170—195 (1956).

Coelho, E., et J. Rocheta: Études expérimentales sur la pathogenie de l'oedème aigu du poumon. Ann. Méd. **34**, 91—98 (1933).

Corelli, D.: Wirkung des Dihydroergotamin (DHE 45) auf das durch Adrenalin ausgelöste akute Lungenödem, Vergleich zwischen DHE 45 und 3277 RP. Schweiz. med. Wschr. **81**, 881—882 (1951).

Cournand, A.: Some aspects of the pulmonary circulation in normal man and in chronic cardiopulmonary diseases. Circulation **2**, 641—657 (1950).

Courtice, F. C., J. Harding, and P. J. Korner: The experimental production of pulmonary oedema in unanaesthetized rats by means of intravenous infusions of Ringer-Locke solution, plasma and blood. Aust. J. exp. Biol. med. Sci. **32**, 563—570 (1954).

—, and P. I. Korner: The effects of anoxia on pulmonary oedema produced by massive intravenous infusions. Aust. J. exp. Biol. med. Sci. **30**, 511—526 (1952).

—, and B. Morris: The effect of diaphragmatic movement on the absorption of protein and of red cells from the pleural cavity. Aust. J. exp. Biol. med. Sci. **31**, 227—238 (1953).

—, and P. J. Phipps: The absorption of fluid from the lungs. J. Physiol. (Lond.) **105**, 186—190 (1946).

—, and W. J. Simmonds: Absorption from the lungs. J. Physiol. (Lond.) **109**, 103—116 (1949a).

— — Absorption of fluids from the pleural cavities of rabbits and cats. J. Physiol. (Lond.) **109**, 117—130 (1949b).

Dalhamn, T.: Mucous flow and ciliary activity in the trachea of healthy rats and rats exposed to respiratory irritant gases. Acta physiol. scand. **36**, Suppl. 123, 148—152 (1956).

Daly, I. de Burgh: The nervous control of the pulmonary circulation. Naunyn-Schmiedebergs Arch. exp. Path. Pharmak. **240**, 331—445 (1960).

— P. Eggleton, S. R. Elsden, and C. O. Hebb: A biochemical study of isolated perfused lungs with special reference to the effects of phosgene. Quart. J. exp. Physiol. **33**, 215—240 (1946).

Daniel, R. A., and W. R. Cate: "Wet lung" — an experimental study. I. The effects of trauma and hypoxia. Ann. Surg. **127**, 836—847 (1948).

Dawes, G. S., J. C. Mott, and J. G. Widdicombe: Respiratory and cardiovascular reflexes from the heart and lungs. J. Physiol. (Lond.) **115**, 258—291 (1951).

Dessnitzkaja, M. M.: Einfluß von Cholinolytica auf die Entwicklung von toxischem Lungenödem und Pleuritis. Pharmakol. u. Toxikol. **23**, 328—331 (1960). Zit. nach Chem. Zbl. **133**, 1700 (1962).

Dieke, S. H.: Thiosemicarbazide: A new toxic derivative of thiourea. Proc. Soc. exp. Biol. (N.Y.) **70**, 688—693 (1949).

—, and C. P. Richter: Age and species variation in the acute toxicity of α-naphthylthiourea. Proc. Soc. exp. Biol. (N.Y.) **62**, 22—25 (1946).

Dongen, K. van, and H. Leusink: The action of opium alkaloids and expectorants on the ciliary movements in the air passages. Arch. int. Pharmacodyn. **93**, 261—276 (1953).

Drenckhahn, F. O.: Die Ödementstehung beim experimentellen Adrenalinlungenödem. Pflügers Arch. ges. Physiol. **266**, 231—248 (1958).

Driesen, W., u. W. Rummel: Der Einfluß vegetativ-nervös bedingter Permeabilitätsänderungen auf die Sulfonamidverteilung. Dtsch. med. Wschr. **74**, 965—967 (1949).

Drinker, C. K.: Pulmonary oedema and inflammation. Cambridge (Mass.): Harvard University Press 1950.

—, and E. Hardenbergh: Acute effects upon the lungs of dogs of large intravenous doses of α-Naphthylthiourea (ANTU). Amer. J. Physiol. **156**, 35—43 (1949).

Durlacher, S. H., W. G. Bangfield, Jr., and A. D. Bergner: Postmortem pulmonary edema. Yale J. Biol. Med. **22**, 565—572 (1950).

Eaton, R. M.: Pulmonary edema. Experimental observations on dogs following acute peripheral blood loss. Dis. Chest **17**, 95 (1950).

Ehrich, W. E.: Die Entzündung. In: F. Büchner, E. Letterer, F. Roulet, Handbuch der allgemeinen Pathologie, Bd. VII/1. Berlin-Göttingen-Heidelberg: Springer 1956.

Eichholtz, F., u. G. Hoppe: Die Krampfwirkung der Lokalanästhetika, ihre Beeinflussung durch Mineralsalze und Adrenalin. Naunyn-Schmiedebergs Arch. exp. Path. Pharmak. **173**, 687—696 (1933).

Eichler, O.: Zur Pharmakologie des Veritols und zu seiner Einordnung in die Reihe der Adrenalinkörper. Naunyn-Schmiedebergs Arch. exp. Path. Pharmak. **187**, 429—443 (1937).

—, u. F. Barfuss: Untersuchungen über den Histamingehalt des Blutes bei Infusion von Adrenalin und Histamin. Naunyn-Schmiedebergs Arch. exp. Path. Pharmak. **195**, 245—257 (1940).

— F. Glanzmann u. M. Höbel: Wirkungen von Cobaltkomplexsalzen. Im Druck.

— M. Höbel, D. Maroske, K. Wegener u. H. J. Lauer: Quantitative Bestimmung der Aufnahme von Kobalt nach Verabreichung in Aerosolform. I. Beschreibung der Methode und ihre Anwendbarkeit für Toxicitätsbestimmungen. Z. biol. Aerosolforsch. **13**, 526 (1967).

— D. Maroske, M. Höbel u. K. Wegener: Quantitative Bestimmung der Aufnahme von Kobalt nach Verabreichung in Aerosolform. II. Verteilung in Organen und morphologische Veränderungen der Lungen bei Meerschweinchen und Ratten. Z. biol. Aerosolforsch., im Druck.

—, u. G. Speda: Versuche über die Abhängigkeit des Histamingehaltes im Blutplasma von der Atmung. Naunyn-Schmiedebergs Arch. exp. Path. Pharmak. **195**, 152—163 (1940).

Elmes, P. C., and D. Bell: The effect of chlorine on the lungs of rats free of chronic pulmonary disease. Meeting Brit. Pharmacol. Soc., Oxford, Juli 1962.

Ernst, A. M.: Einfluß einiger Narkotika auf den Effekt der Bewegungen des Flimmerepithels in Trachea und Bronchi. Arch. int. Pharmacodyn. **58**, 208—212 (1938).

Esser, J.: Die Beziehungen des Nervus vagus zu Erkrankungen von Herz und Lungen, speziell bei experimenteller chronischer Nikotinvergiftung. Naunyn-Schmiedebergs Arch. exp. Path. Pharmak. **49**, 190—212 (1903).

Euler, U. S. v.: Physiologie des Lungenkreislaufs. Verh. dtsch. Ges. Kreisl.-Forsch. **17**, 8—16 (1951).

Evelyn, K. A., and H. T. Malloy: Microdetermination of oxyhemoglobin and methemoglobin and sulfhemoglobin in a single sample of blood. J. biol. Chem. **126**, 655 (1938).

Eyster, J. A. E.: Zit. von M. C. Winternitz and R. A. Lambert. J. exp. Med. **29**, 537—545 (1919).

Farber, S.: Studies on pulmonary edema. I. The consequences of bilateral cervical vagotomy in the rabbit. J. exp. Med. **66**, 397—404 (1937a).

— Studies on pulmonary edema. II. The pathogenesis of neuropathic pulmonary edema. J. exp. Med. **66**, 405—411 (1937b).

Fazekas, G. J. von: Histologische Veränderungen bei akuten Ammoniak-(Salmiakgeist-)Vergiftungen, mit besonderer Berücksichtigung des Zentralnervensystems. Dtsch. Z. ges. gerichtl. Med. **23**, 225—234 (1934).

Femmer, K.: Über die Giftwirkung von Monomethyl- und Dimethylthioacetamid. Naunyn-Schmiedebergs Arch. exp. Path. Pharmak. **233**, 376—383 (1958).

Ferguson, D. J., and E. M. Berkas: Effect of lung denervation on pulmonary hypertension and edema. Circulat. Res. **5**. 310—314 (1957).

Fineberg, C., B. J. Miller, and F. F. Allbritten: Thermal burns of the respiratory tract. Surg. Gynec. Obstet. **98**, 318—328 (1954).

Flinker, L. M., and J. D. McCarrell: Effect of ether and pentobarbital anesthesia on cervical lymph flow and protein content in the cat. Amer. J. Physiol. **155**, 50—55 (1949).

Flury, F.: Über Kampfgasvergiftungen. I. Über Reizgase. Z. ges. exp. Med. **13**, 1—15 (1921a).

— Über Kampfgasvergiftungen. IX. Lokalreizende Arsenverbindungen. Z. ges. exp. Med. **13**, 523—578 (1921b).

— Gasvergiftungen. In: Handbuch der normalen und pathologischen Physiologie, Bd. II. Berlin 1925.

— Die Rolle des Stickstoffmonoxyds bei der Vergiftung durch nitrose Gase. Naunyn-Schmiedebergs Arch. exp. Path. Pharmak. **157**, 104—106 (1930).

—, u. H. Wieland: Über Kampfgasvergiftungen. VII. Die pharmakologische Wirkung des Dichloräthylsulfids. Z. ges. exp. Med. **13**, 523—578 (1921).

Francis, J., and A. Spinks: The toxic and antituberculous effects of thiosemicarbazones and streptomycin in dogs, monkeys, and guinea pigs. Brit. J. Pharmacol. **5**, 549—564 (1950).

Frey, O.: Die pathologischen Lungenveränderungen nach Lähmung der Nervi vagi. Leipzig 1877.

Friedberg, K. D.: Quantitative Untersuchungen über die Staubelimination in der Lunge und ihre Beeinflußbarkeit im Tierexperiment. Silikose-Forschungsinstitut, Bochum 1960.

Gage, J. C.: Gases, vapors, mists and dusts. In: C. P. Stewart and A. Stolman, Toxicology, vol. II, p. 17—54. New York and London: Academic Press 1961.

Gamble, J. E., and H. D. Patton: Pulmonary edema and hemorrhage from preoptic lesions in rats. Amer. J. Physiol. **172**, 623—631 (1953).

Gerschman, R., D. L. Gilbert, S. W. Nye, P. W. Nadig, and W. O. Fenn: Role of adrenalectomy and adrenal-cortical hormones in oxygen poisoning. Amer. J. Physiol. **178**, 346—350 (1954).

Gibbon, J. H., and M. H. Gibbon: Experimental pulmonary edema following lobectomy and plasma infusion. Surgery **12**, 694—704 (1942).

— —, and C. W. Kraul: Experimental pulmonary edema following lobectomy and blood transfusion. J. thorac. Surg. **12**, 60 (1942).

Giese, W.: Über die Endstrombahn der Lunge. In: Lungen und kleiner Kreislauf, S. 45—53. Bad Oeynhausener Gespräche I. Berlin-Göttingen-Heidelberg: Springer 1957.

— Die Atemorgane. In: M. Staemmler, Lehrbuch der speziellen pathologischen Anatomie, 2. Aufl., Bd. II. Berlin: W. de Gruyter 1960.

— Die allgemeine Pathologie der äußeren Atmung. In: Handbuch der allgemeinen Pathologie, Bd. V/1. Berlin-Göttingen-Heidelberg: Springer 1961.

Gieseking, R.: Das experimentelle Lungenödem im elektronenoptischen Bild. Verh. dtsch. Ges. Path. **42**, 344—349 (1959).

Gilbert, R. P., L. B. Hinshaw, H. Kuida, and M. B. Visscher: Effects of histamine, 5-hydroxytryptamine, and adrenaline on pulmonary hemodynamics with particular reference to arterial and venous segment resistances. Amer. J. Physiol. **194**, 165—170 (1958).

Gildemeister, M.: Zit. in E. Laqueur u. R. Magnus, Über Kampfgasvergiftungen. V. Experimentelle und theoretische Grundlagen zur Therapie der Phosgenerkrankung. Z. ges exp. Med. **13**, 200—290 (1921).

—, u. W. Heubner: Über Kampfgasvergiftungen. VI. Die Chlorpikrinvergiftung. Z. ges. exp. Med. **13**, 291—366 (1921).

Glass, A.: Die Beeinflussung des Adrenalin-Lungenödems durch experimentelle Verletzungen des Hirnstammes und des Sympathikus. Naunyn-Schmiedebergs Arch. exp. Path. Pharmak. **136**, 88—100 (1928).

Goetzman, B.: Polybasic electrolytes and colloid osmotic pressure of plasma, serum and bovine serum albumine solution. Proc. Soc. exp. Biol. (N.Y.) **111**, 43—44 (1962).

Gordonoff, T.: Physiologie und Pharmakologie des Expektorationsvorganges. Ergebn. Physiol. **40**, 53—100 (1938).

Gottsegen, G., I. Szam u. M. Csornay: Zur Pathologie und Therapie des hyperoxischen Lungenödems. Z. ges. inn. Med. **11**, 551—557 (1956).

— — — Wirkung synthetischer Hibernatoren auf das experimentelle Lungenödem. Naunyn-Schmidebergs Arch. exp. Path. Pharmak. **230**, 435—447 (1957).

— — — Wirkung des Methylenblau auf das experimentelle akute Lungenödem. Naunyn-Schmiedebergs Arch. exp. Path. Pharmak. **234**, 126—132 (1958).

— — u. L. Tardos: Über die Rolle nervöser Faktoren in der Entstehung des hyperoxischen Lungenödems. Verh. dtsch. Ges. Kreisl.-Forsch. **25**, 282—284 (1959).

Greenberg, A., and D. Erickson: A method for the quantitative determination of hemoglobin in tissues. J. biol. Chem. **156**, 679—682 (1944).

Grögler, F.: Zur Frage der Entstehung des Lungenödems und der Vaguspneumonie. Med. Klin. **31**, 274—275 (1935).

Gross, E., u. H. Hebestreit: Methoden des Tierversuches in der Arbeitsmedizin. In: Handbuch der biologischen Arbeitsmethoden, Abt. IV, Teil 16. Berlin u. Wien: Urban & Schwarzenberg 1932.

Gross, P.: The mechanism of dust clearance from the lung. A theory. Amer. J. clin. Path. **23**, 116—120 (1953).

Grosse-Brockhoff, F.: Hämodynamik der Lungenkreislaufstörungen. Verh. dtsch. Ges. Kreisl.-Forsch. **17**, 34—67 (1951).

— Pathophysiologie des Lungenkreislaufs. In: Lungen und kleiner Kreislauf. Bad Oeynhausener Gespräche I. Berlin-Göttingen-Heidelberg: Springer 1957.

Grossmann, M.: Das Muskarin-Lungenödem. Z. klin. Med. **12**, 550—591 (1887).

— Experimentelle Untersuchungen zur Lehre vom akuten allgemeinen Lungenödem. Z. klin. Med. **16**, 161—183, 270—310 (1889).

Grossmann, M. S., and K. E. Penrod: Relationship of hypothermia to high oxygen poisoning. Amer. J. Physiol. **156**, 177—181 (1949a).

— — The thyroid and high oxygen poisoning in rats. Amer. J. Physiol. **156**, 182—184 (1949b).

Gruhzit, C. C., B. Peralta, and G. K. Moe: The pulmonary arterial pressor effect of certain sulfhydryl inhibitors. J. Pharmacol. exp. Ther. **101**, 107—111 (1951).
Haddy, F. J., and G. S. Campbell: Pulmonary vascular resistance in anaesthetized dogs. Amer. J. Physiol. **172**, 747—751 (1953).
— — W. C. Adams, and M. B. Visscher: A study of pulmonary venous and arterial pressures and other variables in the anesthetized dog by flexible catheter techniques. Amer. J. Physiol. **158**, 89—95 (1949).
— —, and M. B. Visscher: Effects of changes in body temperature and inspired air humidity on lung edema and hemorrhage. Amer. J. Physiol. **158**, 429—432 (1949).
— — — Pulmonary vascular pressures in relation to edema production by airway resistance and plethora in dogs. Amer. J. Physiol. **161**, 336—341 (1950).
— A. L. Ferrin, D. W. Hannon, I. F. Alden, W. L. Adams, and I. D. Baronofsky: Cardiac function in experimental mitral stenosis. Circulat. Res. **1**, 219—225 (1953).
Hahn, F.: Zur Frage der durch Cardiazol und Coramin auslösbaren Atemstörungen. Klin. Wschr. **24/25**, 276—278 (1947).
— Untersuchungen über die Angriffspunkte von Cardiazol und Coramin. III. Über die Wirkung auf den zentralen Parasympathikus. Naunyn-Schmiedebergs Arch. exp. Path. Pharmak. **205**, 572—581 (1948).
Halmágyi, D.: Die klinische Physiologie des kleinen Kreislaufs. Jena: Gustav Fischer 1957.
— Role of the autonomous nervous system in the genesis of pulmonary hypertension in heart disease. J. chron. Dis. **9**, 525—535 (1959).
— B. Felkai, J. Jványj, T. Zsótér u. S. Szües: Zur Physiologie des Lungenödems nach Verabreichung von α-Naphthylthiourea (ANTU) beim Hund. Verh. dtsch. Ges. Kreisl.-Forsch. **21**, 398—404 (1955).
— A. Kovács, P. Neumann, and S. Kenêz: Protective effect of lobeline in experimental pulmonary edema. Arch. int. Pharmacodyn. **106**, 17—27 (1956).
Halpern, B. N., S. Cruchaud, G. Vermeil et J.-L. Roux: Étude pathogénique et thérapeutique de l'oedème aigu du poumon expérimental. Arch. int. Pharmacodyn. **82**, 425—476 (1950).
Hamilton, F. W., R. G. Ellison, R. W. Pickering, E. E. Hague, and J. T. Rucker: Hemodynamic and endocrine responses to experimental mitral stenosis. Amer. J. Physiol. **176**, 445—451 (1954).
Hansen, H. G.: Die Physiologie des Lymphozytenwechsels und seine Beeinflußbarkeit durch Hormone des Hypophysen-Adrenalsystems. Stuttgart: Georg Thieme 1958.
Harford, C. G., and M. Hara: Pulmonary edema in influenzal pneumonia of the mouse and the relation of fluid in the lung to the inception of pneumococcal pneumonia. J. exp. Med. **91**, 245—259 (1950).
Harrison, B. L., and E. H. Seward: Pulmonary oedema due to latent phaeochromocytoma. Brit. med. J. **1954 I**, 1077.
Harrison, W., and A. A. Liebow: Polyethylene plastic needle guides for angiotomy. Proc. Soc. exp. Biol. (N.Y.) **70**, 226 (1949).
— — The effects of increased intracranial pressure on the pulmonary circulation in relation to pulmonary edema. Circulation **5**, 824—832 (1952).
— — The effects of massive intravenous infusions with special reference to pulmonary congestion and edema. Yale J. Biol. Med. **26**, 372—384 (1954).
Hawthorne, E. W., C. V. Brownlee, and R. S. Jason: Development of acute pulmonary edema and death in dogs with aortic insufficiency following renal artery constriction. Amer. J. Physiol. **185**, 474—478 (1956a).
— —, and M. W. Spelman: Prophylaxis against acute pulmonary edema and death in dogs with aortic insufficiency following renal artery constriction afforded by prior construction of an atrial septal defect. Amer. J. Physiol. **185**, 479—482 (1956b).
Hayek, H. v.: Reaktionsfähigkeit der Alveolarepithelien und Lungenödem. Klin. Wschr. **22**, 637—638 (1943).
— Über die Veränderlichkeit der Oberflächenspannung in den Alveolen und ihre Bedeutung für die Retraktionskraft der Lunge. Naunyn-Schmiedebergs Arch. exp. Path. Pharmak. **214**, 266—268 (1952).
— Die menschliche Lunge. Berlin-Göttingen-Heidelberg: Springer 1953.
— Anatomische Grundlagen der Lungenfunktion. In: Lungen und kleiner Kreislauf. Bad Oeynhausener Gespräche I. Berlin-Göttingen-Heidelberg: Springer 1957.
Hayward, G. W.: Pulmonary oedema. Brit. med. J. **1955 I**, 1361—1367.
Hegglin, R.: Die Zirkulationsstörungen der Lunge. In: Handbuch der inneren Medizin, Bd. IV, Teil 2. Berlin-Göttingen-Heidelberg: Springer 1956.
Heim, F., u. A. Bänder: Über die Beeinflussung hoher Adrenalindosen durch Sympatol, Ephedrin, Veritol und Pervitin. Naunyn-Schmiedebergs Arch. exp. Path. Pharmak. **211**, 287—291 (1950).

Heim, F., u. H. Meves: Die Wirkung von Histamin und Antistin an der in situ durchströmten Froschlunge. Naunyn-Schmiedebergs Arch. exp. Path. Pharmak. **211**, 462 bis 467 (1950).
Heimburg, P., B. Ochwaldt u. W. Schoedel: Über die Durchblutung broncho-pulmonaler Gefäßverbindungen. Pflügers Arch. ges. Physiol. **273**, 264—271 (1961).
Heinz, R.: Handbuch der experimentellen Pathologie und Pharmakologie, Bd. 2/1. Jena: Gustav Fischer 1906.
Heitzmann, O.: Über Kampfgasvergiftungen. IV. Ergänzende Befunde zur pathologischen Anatomie der Phosgenvergiftung. Z. ges. exp. Med. **13**, 180—199 (1921).
Hemingway, A.: A method of chemical analysis of guinea pig lung for the factors involved in pulmonary edema. J. Lab. clin. Med. **35**, 817—822 (1950).
— Pulmonary edema in guinea pigs during severe hypoxia. J. appl. Physiol. **4**, 868—872 (1952).
—, and G. S. Campbell: An analysis of normal guinea pig lung for factors determining pulmonary edema and congestion. J. Lab. clin. Med. **37**, 143—150 (1951).
—, and W. L. Williams: Pulmonary edema in oxygen poisoning. Proc. Soc. exp. Biol. (N.Y.) **80**, 331—334 (1952).
Henschler, D.: Schutzwirkung einer Vorbehandlung mit geringen Gaskonzentrationen gegen tödliche Reizgas-Lungenödeme. Naunyn-Schmiedebergs Arch. exp. Path. Pharmak. **238**, 66—67 (1958).
— Die Diffusionskapazität der Lunge als Maß der Wirkung geringer Reizgaskonzentrationen. Naunyn-Schmiedebergs Arch. exp. Path. Pharmak. **246**, 84 (1964).
— F. Amend u. A. Jüttner: Die Wirkung von Siliconaerosolen auf Reizgaslungenödeme. Naunyn-Schmiedebergs Arch. exp. Path. Pharmak. **239**, 288—298 (1960a).
— E. Hahn u. W. Assmann: Wirkungsbedingungen einer Toleranzsteigerung bei wiederholter Einatmung von Lungenödem erzeugenden Reizgasen. Naunyn-Schmiedebergs Arch. exp. Path. Pharmak. **249**, 325—342 (1964a).
— — H. Heymann u. H. Wunder: Mechanismus einer Toleranzsteigerung bei wiederholter Einatmung von Lungenödem erzeugenden Gasen. Naunyn-Schmiedebergs Arch. exp. Path. Pharmak. **249**, 343—356 (1964b).
—, u. K. O. Jacob: Prednisolon zur Therapie von Reizgaslungenödem. Klin. Wschr. **36**, 684 (1958).
—, u. W. Laux: Zur Spezifität einer Toleranzsteigerung bei wiederholter Einatmung von Lungenödem erzeugenden Gasen. Naunyn-Schmiedebergs Arch. exp. Path. Pharmak. **239**, 433—441 (1960).
—, u. E. Reich: Zum Mechanismus der ödemhemmenden Wirkung von Prednisolon bei toxischen Lungenödemen. Klin. Wschr. **37**, 716—717 (1959).
— A. Stier, H. Beck u. W. Neumann: Geruchsschwellen einiger wichtiger Reizgase (Schwefeldioxyd, Ozon, Stickstoffdioxyd) und Erscheinungen bei der Einwirkung geringer Konzentrationen auf den Menschen. Arch. Gewerbepath. Gewerbehyg. **17**, 547—570 (1960b).
Hess, H.: Eine Methode zur fortlaufenden Registrierung der Veränderungen des Lungenblutvolumens beim Menschen. Verh. dtsch. Ges. Kreisl.-Forsch. **22**, 297—300 (1956).
Heubner, W.: Durchlässigkeit der Lunge für fremde Stoffe. In: Handbuch der normalen und pathologischen Physiologie, Bd. II. Berlin: Springer 1925.
Hilden, T.: On the pathogenesis of acute pulmonary edema. Acta med. scand., Suppl. **234**, 162—171 (1949).
Höbel, M., u. O. Eichler: Persönl. Mitteilung.
Horst, H. G., H. Legeler u. F. Wegener: Hemmung des Veratrinlungenödems des Kaninchens durch dehydrierte Mutterkornalkaloide (Hydergin). Z. ges. exp. Med. **116**, 179—183 (1950).
Hughes, R., A. J. May, and J. G. Widdicombe: Mechanical factors in the formation of oedema in perfused rabbits' lungs. J. Physiol. (Lond.) **142**, 292—305 (1958a).
— — — The effect of pulmonary congestion and oedema on lung compliance. J. Physiol. (Lond.) **142**, 306—313 (1958b).
Hungerford, G. F., and W. O. Reinhardt: Comparison of effects of sodium-pentobarbital and ether-induced anestesia on rate of flow and cell content of rat thoracic duct lymph. Amer. J. Physiol. **160**, 9—14 (1950).
Illig, L.: Untersuchungen über die sogenannten Metarteriolen und Capillarsphincter. Klin. Wschr. **34**, 822 (1956).
— Capillar„Contractilität", Capillar„Sphincter" und „Zentralkanäle" („A.-V.-Bridges"). Klin. Wschr. **35**, 7—22 (1957).
Jaques, R.: Acute pulmonary oedema and histamine. Brit. J. exp. Path. **33**, 484—490 (1952).
— Lung histamine and susceptibility to pulmonary oedema in the rat. Brit. J. exp. Path. **35**, 209—213 (1954).
Jarisch, A., H. Richter u. H. Thoma: Zentrogenes Lungenödem. Klin. Wschr. 18, 1440—1443 (1939).

Jarisch, A., u. H. Thoma: Lungenveränderungen im Cardiazolkrampf. Klin. Wschr. **19**, 76—78 (1940).
Joffe, M. H.: Method of assessing experimental pulmonary edema. Science **120**, 612—613 (1954).
Johnson, P. C., and J. W. Bean: Effect of sympathetic blocking agents on the toxic action of oxygen at high pressure. Amer. J. Physiol. 188, 593—598 (1957).
Jordan, G. L., and A. Y. DeLaney: Standard method for the production of pulmonary edema in the dog. Arch. Surg. **63**, 191—202 (1951).
Kabins, S. A., C. Molina, and L. N. Katz: Pulmonary vascular effects of serotonine (5-OH-tryptamine) in dogs: its role causing pulmonary edema. Amer. J. Physiol. **197**, 955—958 (1959).
Kimmerle, G., u. W. Diller: Die Früherkennung eines toxischen Lungenödems bei Hunden im Röntgenbild. Naunyn-Schmiedebergs Arch. Pharmak. exp. Path. **264**, 255—256 (1969).
Kind, L. S.: The altered reactivity of mice after inoculation with Bordetella pertussis vaccine. Bact. Rev. **22**, 173—182 (1958).
— A. Burkhalter, and R. Sherins: Increased lung serotonin and pulmonary edema in mice injected with antiserum to Ehrlichs ascites tumor. Proc. Soc. exp. Biol. (N.Y.) **108**, 735—737 (1961).
— A. T. Smith, and P. Ellman: Absence of lipoprotein in pulmonary oedema fluid produced by cytotoxic antibody. Nature (Lond.) **201**, 1237—1238 (1964).
Kisch, B.: Elektronenmikroskopische Untersuchungen bei akutem Lungenödem. Medizinische **1958 II**, 1189, 1194.
Kleinfeld, M., J. Messite, and C. P. Giel: Pulmonary edema of non cardiac origin. Amer. J. med. Sci. **235**, 660—667 (1958).
Klimmer, O. R.: Beitrag zur Kenntnis der Vergiftungen durch Verbrennungsgase. Naunyn-Schmiedebergs Arch. exp. Path. Pharmak. **201**, 69—98 (1943).
— Einfache Apparatur zur Konstanthaltung von Gaskonzentrationen bei toxikologischen Untersuchungen. Naunyn-Schmiedebergs Arch. exp. Path. Pharmak. **227**, 467—469 (1956).
Koch, R.: Zur Genese des durch Thioharnstoff und seine Derivate ausgelösten Lungenödems (Pneumonose). Naunyn-Schmiedebergs Arch. exp. Path. Pharmak. **227**, 239—245 (1956).
Kochmann, M.: Über kombinierte Narkose. I. Mitteilung: Über Narkoseapparate. Arch. int. Pharmacodyn. **22**, 487—505 (1912).
Koenig, H., and R. Koenig: Production of acute pulmonary edema by ammonium salts. Proc. Soc. exp. Biol. (N.Y.) **70**, 375—380 (1949a).
— — Studies on the pathogenesis of ammonium pulmonary edema. Amer. J. Physiol. **158**, 1—15 (1949b).
— D. Schildkraut, H. Stahlecker, and R. S. Koenig: Occurrence of acute pulmonary edema in experimental alkalosis. Proc. Soc. exp. Biol. (N.Y.) **80**, 370—372 (1952).
Konzett, H., u. R. Rössler: Versuchsanordnung zur Untersuchung an der Bronchialmuskulatur. Naunyn-Schmiedebergs Arch. exp. Path. Pharmak. **198**, 71—74 (1940).
Korner, P. J.: The effect of noradrenaline-induced systemic vasoconstriction on the function of pulmonary oedema. Aust. J. exp. Biol. med. Sci. **31**, 405—423 (1953).
Kotowschtschikow, A. M.: Zur Frage nach den Veränderungen der Herztätigkeit und des Blutkreislaufs bei akutem Lungenödem. Z. exp. Path. Ther. **13**, 400—460 (1913).
Kovanov, V. V.: Pharmakologija i Toksikologija. (Moskau) **29**, 287—291 (1966).
Krayer, O.: Die akute Kreislaufwirkung des Neosalvarsans. Naunyn-Schmiedebergs Arch. exp. Path. Pharmak. **153**, 50—66 (1930).
Kreuzer, F.: Modellversuche zum Problem der Sauerstoffdiffusion in den Lungen. Helv. physiol. pharmacol. Acta, Suppl. **9**, 1—99 (1953).
Kritzler, R. A.: War Med. (Chic.) **6**, 369 (1944). Zit. nach A. Hemingway. J. appl. Physiol. **4**, 868—872 (1952).
Kühn, H. A., u. J. Pichotka: Über die Morphogenese der Lungenveränderungen bei der Sauerstoffvergiftung. Naunyn-Schmiedebergs Arch. exp. Path. Pharmak. **205**, 667—683 (1948).
Lagerlöf, H.: Methods of investigating pulmonary circulation. Comptes Rendus du IIe Congr. Int. D'Angeiologie. 1955, Fribourg/Suisse. Editions Universitaires, Fribourg 1956.
Lagrange, E., et R. Promel: Intoxication par le violet de méthyle et protection contre cette intoxication. C.R. Soc. Biol. (Paris) **142**, 1582—1583 (1948).
— — Recherches expérimentales sur l'oedème pulmonaire. Arch. int. Pharmacodyn. **79**, 445—453 (1949).
Lambert, R. K., and H. Gremels: On the factors concerned in the production of pulmonary oedema. J. Physiol. (Lond.) **61**, 98—112 (1926).
Landis, E. M.: Micro-injection studies of capillary permeability. III. The lack of oxygen on the permeability of the capillary wall to fluid and to plasma proteins. Amer. J. Physiol. **83**, 528—542 (1928).

Laqueur, E.: Einfluß der künstlichen Füllung der Lunge mit Flüssigkeit, im besonderen durch „osmotisches Ödem", auf Atmung, Kreislauf und Blut. Künstliches (osmotisches) Lungenödem. II. Mitt. Pflügers Arch. ges. Physiol. **184**, 104—133 (1920).

— u. R. Magnus: Über Kampfgasvergiftungen. III. Experimentelle Pathologie der Phosgenvergiftung. Z. ges. exp. Med. **13**, 31—179 (1921 a).

— — Über Kampfgasvergiftungen. V. Experimentelle und theoretische Grundlagen zur Therapie der Phosgenerkrankung. Z. ges. exp. Med. **13**, 200—290 (1921 b).

—, u. D. de Vries Reilingh: Perkussion und Auskultation am normalen Kaninchen und nach Erzeugung von osmotischem Lungenödem als Hilfsmittel beim propädeutischen Unterricht. Zbl. inn. Med. **41**, 81—85 (1920 a).

— — Die klinischen Erscheinungen bei künstlicher Füllung der Lunge mit Flüssigkeit und bei osmotischem Lungenödem. Dtsch. Arch. klin. Med. **131**, 310—329 (1920 b).

Lauche, A.: Trachea, Bronchien, Lungen und Pleura. In: P. Cohrs, R. Jaffé u. H. Meessen, Pathologie der Laboratoriumstiere, Bd. I. Berlin-Göttingen-Heidelberg: Springer 1958.

Lazarus, M. L., u. I. A. Serebrovskaja: Das Lungenösem. Moskau 1962.

Lehmann, K. B., u. F. Flury: Toxikologie und Hygiene der technischen Lösungsmittel. Berlin 1938.

—, u. Hasegawa: Studien über die Wirkung technisch und hygienisch wichtiger Gase und Dämpfe auf den Menschen. Die nitrosen Gase: Stickoxyd, Stickstoffdioxyd, salpetrige Säure, Salpetersäure. Arch. Hyg. (Berl.) **77**, 323—368 (1912).

Lewis, B. M., and R. Gorlin: Effects of hypoxia on pulmonary circulation of the dog. Amer. J. Physiol. **170**, 574—587 (1952).

Lichtheim: Versuche über Lungenatelektase. Naunyn-Schmiedebergs Arch. exp. Path. Pharmak. **10**, 54—100 (1879).

Liebegott, G.: Über Organveränderungen bei langer Einwirkung von Sauerstoff mit erhöhtem Partialdruck im Tierexperiment. Beitr. path. Anat. **105**, 413—431 (1941).

Lindquist, B.: Experimental uraemic pulmonary oedema. Acta med. scand. **176**, Suppl. 418 (1964).

Lochner, W.: Zur Physiologie des kleinen Kreislaufs. In: Lungen und kleiner Kreislauf. Bad Oeynhausener Gespräche I. Berlin-Göttingen-Heidelberg: Springer 1957.

Lomeo, G., P. de Bonis u. G. Cali: Untersuchungen über akutes experimentelles Methylsalicylat-Ödem der Lunge. Z. Naturforsch. **15b**, 65—66 (1960).

Lorber, V.: Lung edema following bilateral vagotomy. Studies on the rat, guinea pig, and rabbit. J. exp. Med. **70**, 117—130 (1939 a).

— Role of respiratory obstruction in neuropathic pulmonary edema following vagotomy. Proc. Soc. exp. Biol. (N.Y.) **40**, 464—465 (1939 b).

Lottenbach, K., J. Noelpp-Eschenhagen u. B. Noelpp: Mechanische Aspekte der Lungenfunktion. In: Handbuch der inneren Medizin, Bd. IV/2. Berlin-Göttingen-Heidelberg: Springer 1956.

Luduena, F. P.: Smooth muscle contracting effects of levo-N-isopropyl arterenol and adrenolytic action of its dextro-isomer. Arch. int. Pharmacodyn. **137**, 155—165 (1962).

Luis, A. S., and C. S. Duarte: Experimental study on the pathogenesis of acute pulmonary edema. I. Pulmonary edema induced by silver nitrate. Mal. cardiovasc. **1**, 39—49 (1960).

Luisada, A.: Beitrag zur Pathogenese und Therapie des Lungenödems und des Asthma cardiale. Naunyn-Schmiedebergs Arch. exp. Path. Pharmak. **132**, 313—329 (1928).

— Therapy of paroxysmal pulmonary edema by antifoaming agents. Circulation **2**, 872—879 (1950 a).

— Therapy of paroxysmal pulmonary edema by anti-foaming agents. Proc. Soc. exp. Biol. (N.Y.) **74**, 215—217 (1950 b).

—, and L. Cardi: Acute pulmonary edema: Pathology, physiology and clinical management. Circulation **13**, 113—135 (1956).

—, and S. J. Sarnoff: Paroxysmal pulmonary edema: a new experimental method. Proc. Soc. exp. Biol. (N.Y.) **57**, 279—280 (1944).

— — Paroxysmal pulmonary edema consequent to stimulation of cardiovascular receptors. I. Effect of intra-arterial and intravenous infusions. Amer. Heart J. **31**, 270—281 (1946 a).

— — Paroxysmal pulmonary edema consequent to stimulation of cardiovascular reflexes. II. Mechanical and neurogenic elements. Amer. Heart J. **31**, 282—292 (1946 b).

— — Paroxysmal pulmonary edema consequent to stimulation of cardiovascular reflexes. III. Pharmacologic experiments. Amer. Heart J. **31**, 293—307 (1946 c).

Mack, J.: Diskussionsbemerkung. Dis. Chest **22**, 697—698 (1952).

MacKay, E. M.: Experimental pulmonary edema. IV. Pulmonary edema accompanying trauma to the brain. Proc. Soc. exp. Biol. (N.Y.) **74**, 695—697 (1950).

— M. D. Jordan, and L. L. MacKay: Experimental pulmonary edema. II. Pathogenesis of pulmonary edema caused by ammonium ion. Proc. Soc. exp. Biol. (N.Y.) **72**, 421—424 (1949).

MacKay, E. M., and E. F. Pecka Jr.: Studies of experimental pulmonary edema. I. Pulmonary edema from 1-epinephrine and 1-nor-epinephrine (arterenol). Proc. Soc. exp. Biol. (N.Y.) 71, 669—670 (1949).
— — Experimental pulmonary edema. III. Hypoglycemia, a cause of pulmonary edema. Proc. Soc. exp. Biol. (N.Y.) 73, 568—569 (1950).
MacKenzie, J. B., and C. G. MacKenzie: Production of pulmonary edema by thiourea in the rat and its relation to age. Proc. Soc. exp. Biol. (N.Y.) 54, 34—37 (1943).
Macklin, C. C.: The pulmonary alveolar mucoid film and the pneumocytes. Lancet **1954 I**, 1099—1104.
Maire, F. W., and H. D. Patton: Hyperactivity and pulmonary edema from rostral hypothalamic lesions in rats. Amer. J. Physiol. **178**, 315—320 (1954).
— — Neural structures involved in the genesis of preoptic pulmonary edema, gastric erosions and behavior changes. Amer. J. Physiol. **184**, 345—350 (1956a).
— — Role of the splanchnic nerve and the adrenal medulla in the genesis of preoptic pulmonary edema. Amer. J. Physiol. **184**, 351—355 (1956b).
Maréchaux, E. W.: Über die Wirkung von Sauerstoff erhöhten Teildruckes auf lungengeschädigte Tiere. Naunyn-Schmiedebergs Arch. exp. Path. Pharmak. **201**, 213—233 (1943).
Markowitz, J., J. Archibald, and H. G. Downie: Experimental surgery. Baltimore: Williams and Wilkins Co. 1955.
Mattei, P. Di: Occurence of kinines in epinephrine induced pulmonary edema in rabbits. Arch. int. Pharmacodyn. **140**, 368—373 (1962).
Matzen, R. N.: Development of tolerance to ozone in reference to pulmonary edema. Amer. J. Physiol. **190**, 84—88 (1957a).
— Effect of vitamin C and hydrocortisone on the pulmonary edema produced by ozone in mice. J. appl. Physiol. **11**, 105—109 (1957b).
Meessen, H.: Die Lunge bei der Mitralstenose. Dtsch. med. Wschr. 81, 1445—1448 (1956).
—, u. H. Schulz: Elektronenmikroskopische Untersuchungen des experimentellen Lungenödems. In: Lungen und kleiner Kreislauf. Bad Oeynhausener Gespräche I. Berlin-Göttingen-Heidelberg: Springer 1957.
Meier, M.: Pharmakodynamische Alteration der Lungenelastizität. Untersuchungen an der isolierten Kaninchenlunge. Helv. physiol. pharmacol. Acta 18, 112—118 (1960).
Mendenhall, R. M., and H. E. Stockinger: Tolerance and cross-tolerance development to atmospheric pollutants ketene and ozone. J. appl. Physiol. **14**, 923—926 (1959).
Mikhailov, S.: Pathomorphological changes in phosgenoxime intoxication (1957). Ref. Chem. Abstr. **55**, 21350 (1961).
Mitsov, Z.: Experimental data on phosgenoxime intoxication (1957). Ref. Chem. Abstr. **55**, 21350 (1961).
Mittler, S., D. Hedrick, M. King, and A. Gaynor: Toxicity of ozone. I. Acute toxicity. Industr. Med. Surg. **25**, 301—306 (1956).
— M. King and B. Burkhardt: Toxicity of ozone. III. Chronic toxicity. Arch. industr. Hlth. **15**, 191—197 (1957).
Modrakowski, G.: Beobachtungen an der überlebenden Säugetierlunge. 2. Mitteilung. Über die experimentelle Erzeugung von Lungenödem. Pflügers Arch. ges. Physiol. **158**, 527—554 (1914—1917).
Moeschlin, S.: Klinik und Therapie der Vergiftungen. Stuttgart: Georg Thieme 1964.
Moon, V. H., and P. J. Kennedy: Pathology of shock. Arch. Path. **14**, 360—371 (1932).
—, and D. R. Morgan: Experimental pulmonary edema. Proc. Soc. exp. Biol. (N.Y.) **33**, 560—562 (1936a).
— — Experimental pulmonary edema. Arch. Path. **21**, 565—577 (1936b).
Moore, J. C., and M. S. Sexter: Changes in lung compliance during development of ANTU pulmonary edema. Fed. Proc. **15**, 132—133 (1956).
Moritz, A. R., F. C. Henriques, and R. C. McLean: The effects of inhaled heat on the air passages and lungs, an experimental investigation. Amer. J. Path. **21**, 311—331 (1945).
Mürtz, R.: Veno-venöse Kurzschlußdurchblutung in der Lunge. In: Physiologie und Pathologie des Gasaustausches in der Lunge. Bad Oeynhausener Gespräche IV. Berlin-Göttingen-Heidelberg: Springer 1961.
Neumann, W., u. O. Klimmer: Apparaturen zur Dosierung von Flüssigkeiten und Gasen. Naunyn-Schmiedebergs Arch. exp. Path. Pharmak. **191**, 501—504 (1939).
Newton, W. H.: Pulmonary oedema in the cat heart-lung preparation. J. Physiol. (Lond.) **75**, 288—304 (1932).
Nickerson, M., and C. F. Curry: Control of pulmonary edema with silicone aerosols. J. Pharmacol. exp. Ther. **114**, 138—147 (1955).
Nissim, J. A.: The mechanisms of toxicity of some iron preparations. Brit. J. Pharmacol. **9**, 103—105 (1954).

Noyes, W. A.: The preparation of nitric oxide from sodium nitrite. J. Amer. chem. Soc. **47**, 2170 (1925).
Oberholzer, R., u. H. Schlegel: Einfluß der beidseitigen Vagusausschaltung auf die spontane Atmungstätigkeit des Meerschweinchens. Ber. ges. Physiol. **180**, 134 (1956).
Odake, T.: Role of the central nervous system on adrenaline pulmonary edema. I. Influence of blocking of the central nervous system on adrenaline pulmonary edema. Jap. Circulat. J. (Ni.) **24**, 781—789 (1960).
Ohlsson, W. T. L.: A study on oxygen toxicity at atmospheric pressure. Acta med. Scand. **128**, Suppl. **190**, 1—93 (1947).
Paine, R., H. R. Butcher, F. A. Howard, and J. R. Smith: Observations on mechanisms of edema formation in the lungs. J. Lab. clin. Med. **34**, 1544—1553 (1949a).
— — — — A technique for the collection of lymph from the right thoracic duct in dogs. J. Lab. clin. Med. **34**, 1576—1578 (1949b).
— — J. R. Smith, and F. A. Howard: Observations on the role of pulmonary congestion in the production of edema of the lungs. J. Lab. clin. Med. **36**, 288—296 (1950).
— J. R. Smith, H. R. Butcher, and F. A. Howard: Heart failure and pulmonary edema produced by certain neurologic stimuli. Circulation **5**, 759—765 (1952a).
— —, and F. A. Howard: Pulmonary edema in patients dying with disease of the central nervous system. J. Amer. med. Ass. **149**, 643—646 (1952b).
Palmer, F., and St. S. Kingsbury: Particle size in nebulized aerosols. Amer. J. Pharm. **124**, 112—124 (1952).
Patt, H. M., J. M. Tobias, M. N. Swift, S. Postel, and R. W. Gerard: Hemodynamics in pulmonary irritant poisoning. Amer. J. Physiol. **147**, 329—339 (1946).
Penrod, K. E.: Nature of pulmonary damage produced by high oxygen pressure. J. appl. Physiol. **9**, 1—4 (1956).
Perry, W. F., and E. M. Boyd: A method for studying expectorant action in animals by direct measurement of the output of respiratory tract fluids. J. Pharmacol. exp. Ther. **73**, 65—77 (1941).
Petri, E.: Pathologische Anatomie und Histologie der Vergiftungen. In: Handbuch der speziellen pathologischen Anatomie und Histologie, Bd. 10. Berlin: Springer 1930.
Pichotka, J.: Über die histologischen Veränderungen der Lunge nach Atmung von hochkonzentriertem Sauerstoff im Experiment. Beitr. path. Anat. **105**, 381—412 (1941).
— u. H. A. Kühn: Experimentelle und morphologische Untersuchungen zur Sauerstoffvergiftung. Naunyn-Schmiedebergs Arch. exp. Path. Pharmak. **204**, 336—366 (1947).
Piiper, J.: Die funktionellen Abschnitte des Lungengefäßsystems. Silikose-Forschungsinstitut Bochum 1960.
— O_2-Austausch in der funktionell inhomogenen Lunge, S. 20—29. In: Physiologie und Pathologie des Gasaustausches in der Lunge. Bad Oeynhausener Gespräche IV. Berlin-Göttingen-Heidelberg: Springer 1961.
Plester, D., u. W. Rummel: Pharmakologisches zum Problem: Vegetative Innervation und Permeabilität. Arch. int. Pharmacodyn. **85**, 431—437 (1951).
Polli, J. F., and A. A. Luisada: Effect of splenectomy, nephrectomy and other procedures on epinephrine-induced pulmonary edema. Amer. J. Physiol. 188, 599—603 (1957).
Ponder, E.: The relation of red blood cell density and corpuscular haemoglobin concentration. J. biol. Chem. **144**, 333—338 (1942).
Porter, C. B., and J. T. Small: A method for intrathoracic operation in the rat. Proc. Soc. exp. Biol. (N.Y.) **64**, 239—241 (1947).
Postel, S., J. M. Tobias, H. M. Patt, and R. W. Gerard: The effect of exercise on mortality of animals poisoned with diphosgene. Proc. Soc. exp. Biol. (N.Y.) **63**, 432—436 (1946).
Poulsen, T.: Investigations into the anaesthetics properties of carbon dioxide. Acta pharmacol. (Kbh.) 8, 30—46 (1952a).
— Investigations into reflex irritability during intravenous infusion of hydrochloric acid. Acta pharmacol. (Kbh.) 8, 254—262 (1952b).
— Quantitative estimation of pulmonary oedema in mice. Acta pharmacol. (Kbh.) **10**, 117—126 (1954a).
— Investigations into the pulmonary oedema produced in mice by carbon dioxide. Acta pharmacol. (Kbh.) **10**, 204—222 (1954b).
— Experimental investigations into the effects of morphine and aprobarbital on carbon-dioxide provoked pulmonary oedema in mice. Acta pharmacol. (Kbh.) **10**, 246—252 (1954c).
— Experimental investigations into the effect of ether on carbon dioxide provoked pulmonary oedema in mice. Acta pharmacol. (Kbh.) **10**, 253—260 (1954d).
— Investigations into the effects of atropine, sympatholytics, sodium nitrite, and promethazine on pulmonary oedema provoked by carbon dioxide. Acta pharmacol. (Kbh.) **10**, 379—389 (1954e).

Poulsen, T., and O. Secher: Apparatus for experimental anaesthesia. Acta pharmacol. (Kbh.) **5**, 189—195 (1949).
Prasad, B. N.: Role of prednisone in acute pulmonary oedema. Arch. int. Pharmacodyn. **114**, 146—151 (1958).
Qualls, G., H. J. Curtis, and G. R. Meneely: Rate of uptake of fluid from lung measured with radioisotopes; comparison of rapid rate for water with slower rate for saline. Amer. J. Physiol. **172**, 221—225 (1953).
Radford, E. P., and N. M. Lefcoe: Effects of bronchoconstriction on elastic properties of excised lungs and bronchi. Amer. J. Physiol. **180**, 479—484 (1955).
Reichsman, F.: Studies on the pathogenesis of pulmonary edema following bilateral vagotomy. Amer. Heart J. **31**, 590—616 (1946).
Renkin, E. M., u. J. R. Pappenheimer: Wasserdurchlässigkeit und Permeabilität der Capillarwände. Ergebn. Physiol. **49**, 59—126 (1957).
Richter, C. P.: The physiology and cytology of pulmonary edema and pleural effusion produced in rats by alpha-naphthylthiourea (ANTU). J. thorac. Surg. **23**, 66—91 (1952).
Richter, H., u. H. Thoma: Zentrale Wirkungen des Veratrins. Naunyn-Schmiedebergs Arch. exp. Path. Pharmak. **193**, 622—628 (1939).
Riechert, W.: Beitrag zum Cardiazol-Lungenödem. Naunyn-Schmiedebergs Arch. exp. Path. Pharmak. **197**, 620—628 (1941).
— Beitrag zur Genese des toxischen Lungenödems. Naunyn-Schmiedebergs Arch. exp. Path. Pharmak. **212**, 108—110 (1950).
— Genese und Behandlung des toxischen Lungenödems. Naunyn-Schmiedebergs Arch. exp. Path. Pharmak. **212**, 321—330 (1951).
— u. H. Schmieder: Vergleichende pharmakologische Untersuchungen der Adrenalin-Ephedrinkörper. Naunyn-Schmiedebergs Arch. exp. Path. Pharmak. **198**, 121—139 (1941).
Rimarski, W., u. M. Konschak: Auftreten von Stickoxyden und von Kohlenoxyd beim Schweißen, Schneiden und Richten in engen Räumen. Autogene Metallbearbeitung **33**, 29 (1940).
Robin, E. D., and E. D. Thomas: Some relations between pulmonary edema and pulmonary inflammations (pneumonia). Arch. intern. Med. **93**, 713—724 (1954).
Rössler, R.: Über experimentelle Herzschädigung durch Koronargefäßverengung und ihre Beeinflussung durch Pharmaka. Naunyn-Schmiedebergs Arch. exp. Path. Pharmak. **153**, 1—35 (1930).
Romanov, S. S.: Pharmacologija i Toksikologija (Moskau) **30**, 237 (1967).
Roos, A., and J. R. Smith: Production of experimental heart failure in dogs with intact circulation. Amer. J. Physiol. **153**, 558—566 (1948).
Rosenbach, O.: Über artefizielle Herzklappenfehler. Naunyn-Schmiedebergs Arch. exp. Path. Pharmak. **9**, 1—30 (1878).
Rosenbluth, M. B., F. H. Epstein, and D. J. Feldman: Study of antifoaming agents and preliminary evaluation of their use in experimental pulmonary edema. Proc. Soc. exp. Biol. (N.Y.) **80**, 691—693 (1952).
Rossier, P. H., A. Bühlmann u. K. Wiesinger: Physiologie und Pathophysiologie der Atmung, 2. Aufl. Berlin-Göttingen-Heidelberg: Springer 1958.
Rothlin, E.: Experimenteller Beitrag zur Pathologie und Therapie der Spätfolgen des durch Phosgen erzeugten Lungenödems. Schweiz. med. Wschr. **70**, 641—647 (1940).
— Pathogénie et thérapeutique de l'intoxication par le phosgène. Schweiz. med. Wschr. **71**, 1526—1535 (1941).
Rühl, A.: Über Herzinsuffizienz durch Histamin. Naunyn-Schmiedebergs Arch. exp. Path. Pharmak. **145**, 255—276 (1929).
— Über Störungen des Sauerstoffdurchtritts in der Lunge. Naunyn-Schmiedebergs Arch. exp. Path. Pharmak. **158**, 282—303 (1930).
Rusznyák, I., M. Földi u. G. Szabo: Physiologie und Pathologie des Lymphkreislaufs. Jena: Gustav Fischer 1957.
Sahli, H.: Zur Pathologie und Therapie des Lungenödems. Naunyn-Schmiedebergs Arch. exp. Path. Pharmak. **19**, 433—482 (1885).
Saltzman, B. E.: Colorimetric microdetermination of nitrogen dioxide in the atmosphere. Analyt. Chem. **26**, 1949—1955 (1954).
Sarnoff, S. J., and E. Berglund: Pressure volume characteristics and stress relaxation in the pulmonary vascular bed of the dog. Amer. J. Physiol. **171**, 238—244 (1952).
—, and H. E. Kaufman: Elevation of left auricular pressure in relation to ammonium pulmonary edema in the cat. Proc. Soc. exp. Biol. (N.Y.) 78, 829—832 (1951).
—, and L. C. Sarnoff: Neurohemodynamics of pulmonary edema. I. Autonomic influence on pulmonary vascular pressures and the acute pulmonary edema state. Dis. Chest **22**, 685—698 (1952a).

Sarnoff, S. J., and L. C. Sarnoff: Neurohemodynamics of pulmonary edema. II. The role of sympathetic pathways in the elevation of pulmonary and systemic vascular pressures following the intracisternal injections of fibrin. Circulation **6**, 51—62 (1952b).

Scatchard, G., A. C. Batchelder, and A. Brown: Chemical, clinical and immunological studies on the products of human plasma fractionation. VI. The osmotic pressure of plasma and of serum albumin. J. clin. Invest. **23**, 458—464 (1944).

Schafer, E. S.: Experiments on the cervical vagus and sympathetic. Quart. J. exp. Physiol. **12**, 231—301 (1920).

Schlipköter, H. W.: Elektronenoptische Untersuchungen ultradünner Lungenschnitte. Dtsch. med. Wschr. **79**, 1658—1669 (1954).

Schmitt, G. H., and F. H. Meyers: Characterization of the acute pulmonary edema that follows vagal section in the guinea pig. Amer. J. Physiol. **190**, 89—92 (1957).

Schmitterlöw, C. G., and C. G. Wessman: The protective action of phenergan against acute pulmonary edema produced in the guinea-pig by large doses of adrenaline. Acta physiol. scand. **23**, 31—43 (1951).

Schoedel, W.: Nachweismethoden der arterio-venösen Anastomosen. Comptes Rendus du IIe Congr. Int. D'Angéiologie 1955, Fribourg/Suisse. Editions Universitaires, Fribourg 1956.

— G. Baltzer, G. Gade u. J. Piiper: Über die Durchblutung prä- und postcapillärer Verbindungen zwischen Bronchial- und Pulmonalgefäßsystem. Pflügers Arch. ges. Physiol. **273**, 272—280 (1961).

— u. F. Grosse-Brockhoff: Die Orthologie und Pathologie der Kreislauffunktion. In: Handbuch der allgemeinen Pathologie, Bd. V/1. Berlin-Göttingen-Heidelberg: Springer 1961.

Schulz, H.: Die submikroskopische Anatomie und Pathologie der Lunge. Berlin-Göttingen-Heidelberg: Springer 1959.

Schwab, R., u. K. Denninger: Paroxysmale Hypertonie und Nebennierenmark. Z. ges. inn. Med. **7**, 592 (1952a).

— — Über die Behandlung hyper- und hypotonischer Blutdruckkrisen. Dtsch. med. Wschr. **77**, 1472—1475 (1952b).

— — Lungenödem. Z. ges. inn. Med. **11**, 341—350 (1956).

Schwiegk, H.: Die Störungen der hormonalen Regulation des Kreislaufs. Verh. dtsch. Ges. Kreisl.-Forsch. **25**, 202—222 (1959).

Seager, C. D., and C. D. Wood: Aconitine induced pulmonary edema. Proc. Soc. exp. Biol. (N.Y.) **111**, 120—121 (1962).

Seelkopf, K., u. R. von Werz: Über die Rolle der Kohlensäure bei der Sauerstoffvergiftung. Naunyn-Schmiedebergs Arch. exp. Path. Pharmak. **205**, 351—366 (1948).

Senga, H.: Zit. nach O. Eichler, Die Pharmakologie anorganischer Anionen. Handbuch der experimentellen Pharmakologie, Erg.-W. Bd. X, S. 379. Berlin-Göttingen-Heidelberg: Springer 1950.

Serebrovskaya, J. A.: Investigation of the protein metabolism of blood plasma and edema fluid in some types of experimental pulmonary edema. Pat. Fiziol. éksp. Ter. **4**, 60—65 (1960). Ref. Chem. Abstr. **54**, 25206 (1960).

Short, R. H. D.: Pulmonary change in rabbits produced by bilateral vagotomy. J. Path. Bact. **56**, 355—363 (1944).

Sjöstrand, T.: On the principles for the distribution of the blood in the peripheral vascular system. Skand. Arch. Physiol. **71**, Suppl. 5 (1935).

Skillen, R. G., C. H. Thienes, J. Cangelosi, and L. Strain: Lung 5-hydroxytryptamine and ozone induced pulmonary edema in rats. Proc. Soc. exp. Biol. (N.Y.) **107**, 178—180 (1961a).

— — — — Brain 5-hydroxytryptamine in ozone-exposed rats. Proc. Soc. exp. Biol. (N.Y.) **108**, 121—122 (1961b).

Smith, J. L.: The pathological effects due to increase of oxygen tension in the air breathed. J. Physiol. (Lond.) **24**, 19—35 (1899).

Smith, R. O.: Lymphatic contractility, a possible intrinsic mechanism of lymphatic vessels for the transport of the lymph. J. exp. Med. **90**, 497—509 (1949).

Smithy, H. G., H. R. Pratt-Thomas, and H. P. Deyerle: Aortic valvulotomy. Surg. Gynec. Obstet. **86**, 513—523 (1948).

Spector, W. G.: Substances which affect capillary permeability. Pharmacol. Rev. **10**, 475—505 (1958).

Spector, W. S. (Ed.): Handbook of biological data. Philadelphia and London: W. B. Saunders Co. 1956.

Spencer, H.: Pathology of the lung. Oxford-London-New York-Paris: Pergamon Press 1962.

Stary, Z.: Mucosaccharides and glycoproteins. Chemistry and physiopathology. Ergebn. Physiol. **50**, 174—408 (1959).

Starzecki, B., and D. F. J. Halmágyi: Absorption of inhaled water in experimental pulmonary edema and embolism. Amer. J. Physiol. **201**, 762—764 (1961).

Staub, H.: Histaminämie nach Adrenalin. Expereintia (Basel) **2**, 29 (1946).
Stephenson, R. P.: An apparatus for recording the output and coronary flow in the heart-lung preparation. J. Physiol. (Lond.) **108**, 102—103 (1949).
Stokinger, H. E.: Ozone toxicity. Arch. industr. Hyg. **9**, 366—383 (1954).
— Evaluation of the hazards of ozone and oxides of nitrogen. Arch. industr. Hlth. **15**, 181—190 (1957).
— W. D. Wagner, and O. J. Dobrogorski: Ozone toxicity studies. III. Chronic injury to lungs of animals following exposure at low level. Arch. industr. Hlth. **16**, 514—522 (1957).
Stone, C. A., and E. R. Loew: Effect of various drugs on epinephrine-induced pulmonary edema in rabbits. Proc. Soc. exp. Biol. (N.Y.) **71**, 122—126 (1949).
Stroud, R. C., and R. Hahn: Effect of O_2 and CO_2 tensions upon the resistance of pulmonary blood vessels. Amer. J. Physiol. **172**, 211—220 (1953).
Sturm, A.: Die klinische Pathologie der Lunge. Stuttgart: Wissenschaftl. Verlagsges. 1948.
Surtshin, A., L. N. Katz, and S. Rodbard: An attempt to produce pulmonary edema by increased intracranial pressure. Amer. J. Physiol. **152**, 589—590 (1948).
Sussman, A. H., A. Hemingway, and M. B. Visscher: Importance of pressure factors in the genesis of pulmonary edema following vagotomy. Amer. J. Physiol. **152**, 585—588 (1948).
Svirbely, J. L., and B. E. Saltzman: Ozone toxicity and substances associated with its production. Arch. industr. Hlth. **15**, 111—118 (1957).
Sylla, A.: Lungenkrankheiten. München u. Berlin 1952.
Tennekoon, G. E.: Pulmonary oedema due to thiosemicarbazide. J. Path. Bact. **67**, 341—347 (1954).
Testelli, M. R., and S. Musiker: Paroxysmal pulmonary edema by intravenous chroroform. Proc. Soc. exp. Biol. (N.Y.) **104**, 109—110 (1960).
— — and A. A. Luisada: Effect of digitalis glycosides in paroxysmal pulmonary edema. J. appl. Physiol. **15**, 83—86 (1960).
Testoni, F., e G. Lomeo: L-azione di alcuni alcaloidi diidrogenati della segale cornuta nell'edema polmonare acuto sperimentale da adrenalina. Experientia (Basel) **9**, 30—31 (1953).
Thews, G.: Die Sauerstoffdiffusion in den Lungencapillaren. In: Physiologie und Pathologie des Gasaustausches in der Lunge. Bad Oeynhausener Gespräche IV. Berlin-Göttingen-Heidelberg: Springer 1961.
Tobias, J. M., S. Postel, H. M. Pratt, C. C. Lushbaugh, M. N. Swift, and R. W. Gerard: Localization of the site of action of a pulmonary irritant diphosgene. Amer. J. Physiol. **158**, 173—183 (1949).
Treadwell, P. E., R. Wistar, and A. F. Rasmussen: Passive anaphylaxis in mice with homologous antiserum. J. Immunol. **84**, 539—544 (1960).
Trendelenburg, P.: Adrenalin and adrenalinverwandte Substanzen. In: Handbuch der experimentellen Pharmakologie, Bd. II/2, S. 1130—1293. Berlin: Springer 1924.
Trotter, W. R.: A comparison of the acute toxic effects of iodides and thiourea derivatives. Brit. J. exp. Path. **33**, 207—215 (1952).
Ueba, Y.: Pulmonary edema of nervous origin. II. Catechols of blood plasma in preoptic or hypothalamic lesions. Nippon Naika Gakkai Zasshi **49**, 253—258 (1960). Ref. Chem. Abstr. **56**, 867 (1962).
Visscher, M. B., K. Absolon, and H. Ballin: Electrochemical and colloidal phenomena in pulmonary edema. Univ. Minn. med. Bull. **33**, 181—188 (1962).
— F. J. Haddy, and G. Stephens: The physiology and pharmacology of lung edema. Pharmacol. Rev. **8**, 389—434 (1956).
Vitale, A., P. R. Dumke, and J. H. Comroe: Lack of correlation between rates and arterial oxygen saturation in patients with pulmonary congestion and edema. Circulation **10**, 81—83 (1954).
Warren, M. F., and C. K. Drinker: The flow of lymph from the lungs of the dog. Amer. J. Physiol. **136**, 207—221 (1942).
Waser, P. G.: Chemistry and pharmacology of muscarine, muscarone and some related compounds. Pharmacol. Rev. **13**, 465—515 (1961).
Weiser, J.: Zur Frage der sogenannten Vaguspenumonie. Pflügers Arch. ges. Physiol. **231**, 68—76 (1933).
—, u. J. Rienmüller: Über die Innervationswege der Permeabilitätsbeeinflussung der Froschlunge. Pflügers Arch. ges. Physiol. **233**, 386—394 (1933).
Welch, W. H.: Zur Pathologie des Lungenödems. Virchows Arch. path. Anat. **72**, 375—412 (1878).
Whitteridge, D.: The action of phosgene on the stretch receptors of the lung. J. Physiol. (Lond.) **107**, 107—114 (1948).
Wichels, P., u. H. Lauber: Adrenalinvergiftung, tödliche, medizinale. Z. klin. Med. **119**, 42—49 (1932).

Wick, H.: Die Beeinflussung der Tracheobronchial- und Alveolarweite durch lokale Einwirkung des Kohlendioxyds. Arch. int. Pharmacodyn. 88, 461—472 (1952a).
— Über die Änderung der Lungenelastizität durch Kohlensäure. Arch. int. Pharmacodyn. **89**, 21—27 (1952b).
— Die Wirkung der Kohlensäure auf die Weite der Lungenalveolen. Arch. int. Pharmacodyn. **89**, 40—47 (1952c).
Williams, M. H., Jr.: Effect of ANTU-induced pulmonary edema on the alveolar-arterial oxygen pressure gradient in dogs. Amer. J. Physiol. **175**, 84—86 (1953).
Winter, C. A.: Failure of antihistaminic drug "Phenergan" to protect against acute pulmonary edema. Proc. Soc. exp. Biol. (N.Y.) **72**, 122—124 (1949).
Winternitz, M. C., and R. A. Lambert: Edema of the lungs as a cause of death. J. exp. Med. **29**, 537—545 (1919).
Winterstein, H., u. N. Gökhan: Ammoniumchlorid-Acidose und Reaktionstheorie der Atmungsregulation. Arch. int. Pharmacodyn. **93**, 212—232 (1953).
Wirth, W.: Beitrag zur Wirkung von Gasgemischen (nitrose Gase-Kohlenoxyd). Naunyn-Schmiedebergs Arch. exp. Path. Pharmak. **157**, 264—285 (1930).
— Über die Wirkung kleinster Phosgenmengen. Naunyn-Schmiedebergs Arch. exp. Path. Pharmak. **181**, 198—206 (1936).
Wohlzogen, F. X., W. Brandstetter u. E. Kiesewetter: Eine Methode zur quantitativen Beurteilung des Lungenödems. Ber. ges. Physiol. **180**, 136 (1956).
Wood, C. D., L. D. Seager, and G. Ferrell: Influence of autonomic blockade on aconitine induced pulmonary edema. Proc. Soc. exp. Biol. (N.Y.) **116**, 809—811 (1964).
Wood, E. H., and G. K. Moe: The measurement of edema in the heart-lung-preparation. Amer. J. Physiol. **136**, 506—514 (1942).
Zeissl, M. v.: Über Lungenödem infolge von Jodintoxikation. Z. klin. Med. **27**, 363—380 (1895).
Zinberg, S., G. Nudell, W. G. Kubicek, and M. B. Visscher: Observations on the effects on the lungs of respiratory air flow resistance in dogs with special reference to vagotomy. Amer. Heart J. **35**, 774—779 (1948).

Namenverzeichnis

Die *kursiven* Seitenzahlen beziehen sich auf die Literatur.
Die in eckigen Klammern stehenden Ziffern bedeuten die Nummern der entsprechenden Literaturzitate.

Sachverzeichnis

„B" nach den angegebenen Seitenzahlen bedeutet Abbildung bzw. Diagramm, „T" bedeutet Tabelle